Clinical and Translational Medicine

Clinical and Translational Medicine

Editor: Anna Garner

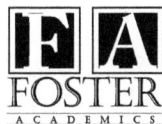

FOSTER
ACADEMICS

www.fosteracademics.com

www.fosteracademics.com

FA
FOSTER
ACADEMICS

Cataloging-in-Publication Data

Clinical and translational medicine / edited by Anna Garner.
    p. cm.
Includes bibliographical references and index.
ISBN 978-1-63242-840-0
1. Clinical medicine. 2. Medicine, Experimental. 3. Medical innovations. 4. Medicine--Research. I. Garner, Anna.
RC66 .C55 2019
616.09--dc23

Foster Academics,
118-35 Queens Blvd., Suite 400,
Forest Hills, NY 11375, USA

ISBN 978-1-63242-840-0 (Hardback)

Contents

Preface

This book has been a concerted effort by a group of academicians, researchers and scientists, who have contributed their research works for the realization of the book. This book has materialized in the wake of emerging advancements and innovations in this field. Therefore, the need of the hour was to compile all the required researches and disseminate the knowledge to a broad spectrum of people comprising of students, researchers and specialists of the field.

Clinical and translational medicine refers to the therapeutic clinical potential and application of translational research that seeks to develop the understanding of mechanisms and treatments of human diseases. The clinical variation between diseases, biomarkers, pathogenesis and therapies are also highlighted through studies of clinical and translational medicine. This is a critical and core component of the full-spectrum of biomedical research. Translational medicine refers to an area of research that seeks to determine the relevance of novel discoveries in the biological science to human disease. It also integrates new knowledge in clinical practice and clinical observations into scientific knowledge. Hence, translational research, facilitates the generation of novel hypotheses and disease characterization based on direct human observation. Translational medicine can work to expedite the incorporation of novel endpoints into clinical testing, thus shortening the duration of clinical trials. This book brings forth some of the most innovative concepts and elucidates the unexplored aspects of clinical and translational medicine. The ever growing need of advanced technology is the reason that has fueled the research in this field in recent times. A number of latest researches have been included to keep the readers up-to-date with the global concepts in this area of study.

At the end of the preface, I would like to thank the authors for their brilliant chapters and the publisher for guiding us all-through the making of the book till its final stage. Also, I would like to thank my family for providing the support and encouragement throughout my academic career and research projects.

Editor

Analysing the role of complexity in explaining the fortunes of technology programmes: empirical application of the NASSS framework

Trisha Greenhalgh[1][*][iD], Joe Wherton[1], Chrysanthi Papoutsi[1], Jenni Lynch[2], Gemma Hughes[1], Christine A'Court[1], Sue Hinder[3], Rob Procter[4] and Sara Shaw[1]

Abstract

Background: Failures and partial successes are common in technology-supported innovation programmes in health and social care. Complexity theory can help explain why. Phenomena may be simple (straightforward, predictable, few components), complicated (multiple interacting components or issues) or complex (dynamic, unpredictable, not easily disaggregated into constituent components). The recently published NASSS framework applies this taxonomy to explain *Non-adoption* or *Abandonment* of technology by individuals and difficulties achieving *Scale-up*, *Spread* and *Sustainability*. This paper reports the first empirical application of the NASSS framework.

Methods: Six technology-supported programmes were studied using ethnography and action research for up to 3 years across 20 health and care organisations and 10 national-level bodies. They comprised video outpatient consultations, GPS tracking technology for cognitive impairment, pendant alarm services, remote biomarker monitoring for heart failure, care organising software and integrated case management via data warehousing. Data were collected at three levels: micro (individual technology users), meso (organisational processes and systems) and macro (national policy and wider context). Data analysis and synthesis were guided by socio-technical theories and organised around the seven NASSS domains: (1) the condition or illness, (2) the technology, (3) the value proposition, (4) the adopter system (professional staff, patients and lay carers), (5) the organisation(s), (6) the wider (institutional and societal) system and (7) interaction and mutual adaptation among all these domains over time.

Results: The study generated more than 400 h of ethnographic observation, 165 semi-structured interviews and 200 documents. The six case studies raised multiple challenges across all seven domains. Complexity was a common feature of all programmes. In particular, individuals' health and care needs were often complex and hence unpredictable and 'off algorithm'. Programmes in which multiple domains were *complicated* proved difficult, slow and expensive to implement. Those in which multiple domains were *complex* did not become mainstreamed (or, if mainstreamed, did not deliver key intended outputs).

Conclusion: The NASSS framework helped explain the successes, failures and changing fortunes of this diverse sample of technology-supported programmes. Since failure is often linked to complexity across multiple NASSS domains, further research should systematically address ways to reduce complexity and/or manage programme implementation to take account of it.

* Correspondence: trish.greenhalgh@phc.ox.ac.uk
[1]Department of Primary Care Health Sciences, University of Oxford, Oxford OX2 6GG, UK
Full list of author information is available at the end of the article

Background

Introduction

Technological innovation is viewed by policymakers as a driver of both health and wealth [1]. Technology is often depicted as 'empowering' for both patients and staff, and has been associated with improved efficiency, quality and safety of care [2–5]. In reality, however, technology start-ups may fail to attract investment [6]; patients may or may not be able or willing to use new technologies [7]; professionals may resist them [8–10]; new technologies may clash with legacy systems and with established routines [11, 12]; a technology may be implemented but fail to deliver the anticipated benefits [13]; and small-scale demonstration projects may fail to scale up locally, spread distantly or be sustained over time [14, 15].

In a recently published systematic review, we synthesised evidence on individual, team, organisational and system influences on the success of technology-supported innovation programmes in health and social care [16]. We drew in particular on published technology implementation frameworks and key theoretical work on diffusion of innovations [17, 18], technological entrepreneurship [6, 19], the patient experience of chronic illness [20], clinician resistance to technologies [21], the social processes of 'normalising' technologies in organisations [22–25], business and financial planning [14], organisational resilience and sustainability [26–28], and theoretical studies on complex adaptive systems [29, 30].

Our synthesis of this diverse literature occurred in parallel with testing of candidate domains and theories from our systematic review on a sample of six empirical case studies. We produced a new multi-level interdisciplinary framework called NASSS (Non-adoption or Abandonment of technology by individuals and difficulties achieving Scale-up, Spread and Sustainability), which incorporates and extends the theoretical frameworks and models listed in the previous paragraph. The NASSS framework is shown diagrammatically in Panel 1 and Fig. 1.

Panel 1: Domains and questions in the NASSS framework
  Domain 1: the condition
    1A. What is the nature of the condition or illness?
    1B. What are the relevant co-morbidities?
    1C. What are the relevant socio-cultural factors?
  Domain 2: the technology
    2A. What are the key features of the technology?
    2B. What kind of knowledge does the technology bring into play?
    2C. What knowledge and/or support is required to use the technology?
    2D. What is the technology supply model?
    2E. Who owns the intellectual property (IP) generated by the technology?
  Domain 3: the value proposition and value chain
    3A. What is the developer's business case for the technology (supply-side value)?
    3B. What is its desirability, efficacy, safety and cost-effectiveness (demand-side value)?
  Domain 4: the adopter system

(Continued)

    4A. What changes in staff roles, practices and identities are implied?
    4B. What is expected of the patient (and/or immediate carer) — and is this achievable by and acceptable to them?
    4C. What is assumed about the extended network of lay carers?
  Domain 5: the organisation(s)
    5A. What is the organisation's capacity to innovate?
    5B. How ready is the organisation for this technology-supported change?
    5C. How easy will the adoption and funding decision be?
    5D. What changes will be needed in team interactions and routines?
    5E. What work is involved in implementation and who will do it?
  Domain 6: the wider system
    6A. What is the political context for programme development, implementation and roll-out?
    6B. What is the regulatory context?
    6C. What is the position of professional bodies?
    6D. What is the socio-cultural context (public perception, interest, expectation)?
    6E. What is the nature and extent of inter-organisational networking?
  Domain 7: Embedding and adaptation over time
    7A. How much scope is there for adapting and co-evolving the technology and the service over time?
    7B. How resilient is the organisation to handling critical events and adapting to unforeseen eventualities?

The original questions guiding our empirical research were the following. (1) How can we improve the process by which health and care technologies are developed and implemented? (2) How can we support the customisation and use of such technologies in the home and/or the health or care setting? (3) How can we ensure that patients' needs and concerns remain central when developing technology-supported service innovations [31, 32]? The study of complexity was not part of our original proposal, but it quickly emerged as the dominant theme in our empirical data (as well as a prominent element in the more recent literature we were identifying for our systematic review [29, 30]).

Our previous publication focused mainly on the secondary research component of the NASSS framework [16]. This paper presents a more detailed account of our empirical findings and illustrates how the framework allowed us to explore complexity in multiple interacting domains.

Complex systems and the NASSS framework

A system is defined as an assembly of agents that interact with each other. In a simple system (few agents and components) or a complicated one (many agents and components), the relationships between agents are well defined and stable, which means the overall behaviour of the system is predictable. In contrast, complex, adaptive systems are composed of agents with ill-defined and unstable boundaries that may act in unexpected ways, whose actions are interconnected so that one agent's actions change the context for other agents [33]. Hence,

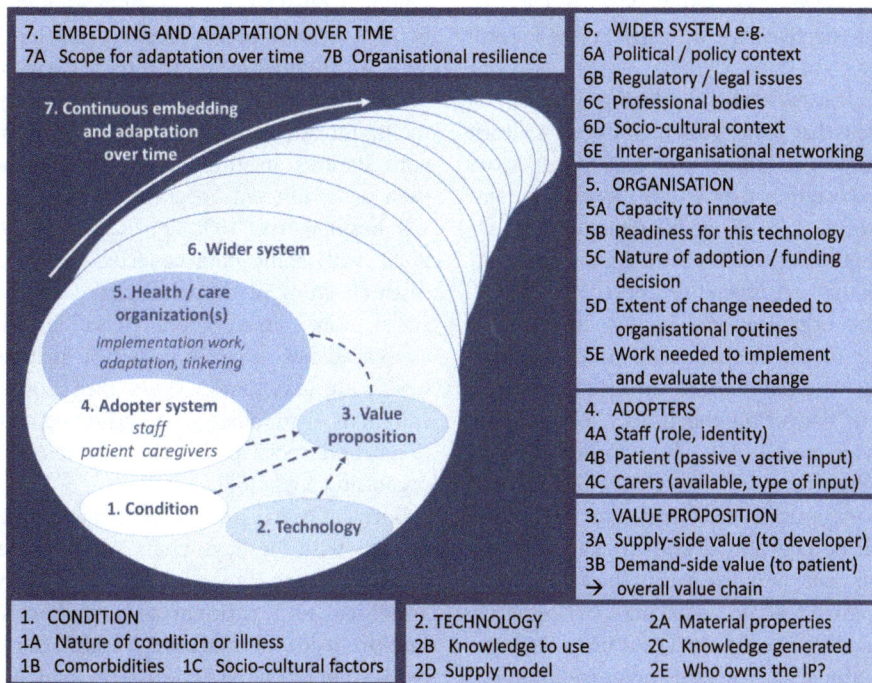

Fig. 1 The NASSS framework for considering influences on the adoption, non-adoption, abandonment, spread, scale-up and sustainability of health and care technologies. Image adapted from J Med Internet Res. 2017; 19: e367

in *complex* systems, agents interact with each other and with other systems in unexpected ways; their component agents (people, cells, technologies) can simultaneously be members of several systems. The complex system works by a fundamentally different logic, since its response to change is—to a greater or lesser extent—unpredictable and non-linear [34].

Against this background, the NASSS framework has been developed to encourage complex thinking (what Tsoukas calls 'conjunctive theorising' [35]) about technological innovations in healthcare. With a view to generating a rich narrative of events unfolding in a real-world setting, aspects of the different domains are first considered in terms of whether they are simple (straightforward, predictable, few components—as in making a sandwich), complicated (remains predictable but there are multiple interacting components or issues—as in building a rocket) or complex (dynamic, unpredictable, not easily disaggregated into constituent components—as in raising a child). Simple and complicated phenomena operate according to linear, Newtonian (predictive, cause-and-effect) logic; they can, for example, be meaningfully analysed in terms of their component parts. Complex phenomena operate according to different (non-linear) logic, in which a given cause may not always have the same effect. They exhibit broad patterns and emerge over time, but they are not predictable.

A simple illness or condition (domain 1 in the NASSS framework) is well characterised, well understood and

predictable (though it may still be *serious*, e.g. deep venous thrombosis); its management is straightforward and is influenced only minimally by co-morbidities or socio-cultural factors. The same goes for a complicated condition (e.g. many cancers), though the logistics may be more challenging. Complex conditions, in contrast, are poorly characterised, poorly understood, unpredictable and/or strongly influenced by co-morbidities and socio-cultural factors (e.g. drug dependency, dementia).

The complexity dimension in domain 2 (technology) may refer to the technology's material (including technical) properties, its ease of use, the kind of data it generates, its supply chain or the intellectual property associated with it. In all these sub-domains, complexity—which is impossible to define in rigid and universal terms—may relate to changeability, unpredictability, contestability (e.g. experts disagree on what the data mean and whether they can be trusted) and interdependence with other changeable, unpredictable or contestable aspects (such as availability of broadband).

The value proposition (domain 3) refers to both supply-side value (whether there is a straightforward and uncontested business case for generating revenue for the developer) and demand-side value (whether there is strong and uncontested evidence that the technology is desirable for patients, effective, safe and cost-effective). Complexity in this domain relates to (for example) multiple and perhaps interdependent assumptions on which the business case is based, a speculative or contested evidence base for effectiveness or cost-effectiveness, or gaps in the overall value chain.

Complexity in relation to intended adopters (domain 4) does not mean merely that some individuals need to learn new skills or procedures or adopt new staff roles. More challenging is the expectation that a staff member, patient or lay carer will need to take on a different identity (e.g. data processer, teacher) alongside their traditional one and/or make judgements that are difficult or unpredictable.

Complexity in the organisational setting (domain 5) relates in particular to the scope, scale, pace, resource requirements, and the logistical uncertainties and interdependencies of delivering the innovation and the associated new service model [36]. The introduction of a 'disruptive' technology (that is, one that enables—and perhaps requires—organisational work to be done differently [37]) will be complex if known preconditions for innovation are not met (e.g. if there is weak leadership, poor managerial relations or severely stretched resources); if the technology is a poor strategic 'fit'; if new work routines and/or inter-organisational co-operation are needed; or if a large amount of work is needed to build a vision, engage staff, implement the programme and develop ways of monitoring its impact.

Complexity in the external context (domain 6) means that there are tricky hurdles to be overcome in relation to political, financial, legal, regulatory or public concerns, or that inter-organisational networking and knowledge sharing are difficult. Again, the key issue is often the interdependency of different influences (which tends to mean that any one problem cannot be addressed without generating other problems elsewhere in the system).

Finally, complexity in domain 7 (adaptation over time) means that further adaptation or co-evolution of the technology is impossible because of lack of material or technical flexibility, and/or because the organisation(s) lack the resilience to adapt to changing external conditions (see Discussion).

Such were the findings of our systematic review that formed the theoretical basis of the NASSS framework [16]. In the remainder of this paper, we describe the empirical testing and refining of the NASSS domains across a maximum-variety sample of technology implementation case studies. The specific research question addressed in this paper was: Given that technology programmes in health and social care are often described as 'complex', what is the nature of this complexity and how might it affect the fortunes of a programme?

Methods
Context, governance and methodology
The research took place in various field sites across the UK. It embraced two research programmes: VOCAL (Virtual

Online Consultations—Advantages and Limitations) and SCALS (Studies in Co-Creating Assisted Living Solutions). VOCAL (funded from 2015 to 2017, with an earlier set-up phase from 2011) was an in-depth study of the development, introduction and local roll-out of remote (video) consultations in three contrasting clinical departments, each on a different geographical site, in a large, multi-site UK hospital trust [38, 39]. SCALS (funded from 2015 to 2020, with some data collected from 2013) is an action research study of the challenges faced by UK health and social care organisations who introduce technology-supported new service models; it includes examples from healthcare (e.g. remote biomarker monitoring, video consultations, technologies for integrating care across organisations) and social care (safety alarms, GPS tracking, care organising apps) [32].

Both VOCAL and SCALS had an external steering group with a lay chair and representation from patients, front-line clinicians, the technology industry and local and national policymakers (including information leads at National Health Service (NHS) England). The VOCAL study also had a separate patient advisory group convened and chaired by a community anthropologist.

Case studies (all of which were drawn from VOCAL and SCALS) were sampled by a combination of responsiveness (health or care organisations sought our input to real-world implementation challenges), convenience (local initiatives caught our interest) and theoretical sampling (later cases were systematically sought to illustrate themes that had come up in our literature review but were not yet represented in our sample). The six prospective case studies reported below have so far been followed for up to 3 years. Additional, theoretically sampled case studies in the SCALS programme (added more recently and not reported here) will be explored in future papers.

Each case study has involved a flexible programme of qualitative interviews and observation (with patients, clinicians, managers, technical designers, commercial partners and—where relevant—investors), analysis of documents (correspondence, business plans, clinical records), ethnography (of technology use by patients/clients and staff, of meetings and events, and of technology design and functionality) and video-recording of both ends of remote consultations [31, 32]. In addition, in order to build up a rich picture of the national context in which technologies evolve, we used a combination of purposive and snowball sampling to identify 45 potential stakeholders from across government (e.g. NHS England), professional organisations (e.g. Royal College of Physicians, Medical Protection Society), patient groups (e.g. National Voices), industry (e.g. Microsoft) and charitable and third sector organisations (e.g. Health Foundation). We invited a maximum variety sample of 39 of these stakeholders to talk informally with the study team, of whom we spoke with 36 (the remaining 3 being uncontactable). We conducted formal semi-structured interviews with a purposive sample of 12 of these stakeholders (ensuring variation of groups and perspectives) and combined this with analysis of approximately 50 key national-level policy and policy-related documents published since 2000.

Data sources for case studies in VOCAL and SCALS used for development and testing of the NASSS framework are summarised in Table 1. The empirical case studies are outlined briefly below and analysed in more detail in the Results section.

Outline of the six case studies

Case A (video outpatient consultations) included four clinical services in the NHS: adult diabetes, antenatal diabetes and cancer surgery, all using Skype™ [38], and a community-based, nurse-led heart failure service, using predominantly FaceTime™. Video consultation was offered to patients for whom it was judged clinically appropriate by the clinician. There was strong support from senior management and many (though not all) clinicians. Almost all patients volunteering for this option experienced it as convenient, technically straightforward and able to meet their clinical needs. But implementation proved logistically difficult, technically challenging, labour-intensive and slow. Video consulting was considered not clinically appropriate for many patients. By the end of the study period, video consultations had been abandoned in the antenatal diabetes service and put 'on hold' in the community heart failure service. In the adult diabetes and cancer surgery services, they continued and were being extended to other clinical services within the trust.

Case B (global positioning system [GPS] tracking for people with cognitive impairment) began when the SCALS team were approached by a local council in a deprived and multi-ethnic inner city borough and asked to help improve the take-up of devices to electronically track people with cognitive impairment who 'wandered' outside the home. We worked with the council and with linked voluntary sector groups to implement and adapt a selection of devices and a linked call centre and monitoring service [40, 41]. Whilst several hundred people in the catchment population had cognitive impairment, only 11 were ever identified as eligible for GPS tracking and 7 assented (of which only 3 continue to use the technology). Successful adoption of the technology was found to require a network of extended family and call centre staff who collectively 'knew' the client and his or her preferred walking route(s).

Case C (pendant alarms): Pendant alarms are worn around the neck (or on the wrist) and connected to a remote call centre. The client should press the alarm if he/she is in difficulty (e.g. fallen and cannot get up); the call

centre will alert either a relative (on a retained contact list) or an emergency service. Pendant alarm services had been in widespread use for some years in two participating organisations in the SCALS study—both urban settings serving a mixed socio-demographic population. Various arrangements were in place for referring clients (including self, GP, social worker and local age charity) and fitting the alarm (typically a commercial supplier). In both sites, alarms were widely supplied and often 'worked' as intended, though they depended on a network of carers and professional staff whose collective knowledge of the client allowed them to interpret remote signals (e.g. judge whether a call was an emergency). In many instances, clients did not activate the alarm when care staff and relatives considered that they should have done so.

Case D (telehealth for heart failure) was the qualitative component of a multi-centre randomised controlled trial of biomarker monitoring (weight, blood pressure, heart rate) in heart failure (SUPPORT-HF). All participants in this trial were supplied with a tablet technology through which they could access their biomarker results, trends and educational material [42]. The intervention arm included active communication of results and recommendations to the patient's general practitioner with the aim of increasing use of recommended medical therapy and improving patients' well-being; in the control arm, data were available for the general practitioner to access if desired. Across participating sites, clinicians engaged variably with the study, occasionally leading to slower than predicted recruitment. Participants' use of the technology also varied widely, influenced by various clinical, technical and logistical issues.

Case E (care organising software) followed the fortunes of two software products, each designed to help relatives and friends organise tasks and visits for someone with health and/or care needs. Product A, a web portal, had been developed in-house by a small software company. The business model was to sell the product (at a cost of several thousand pounds) to care organisations that would then provide it to their clients free of charge. Product B was a smartphone app (with linked web portal) that had been developed via publicly funded R&D using co-design methodology by a national carers' charity; it was made available for individual download (e.g. via the Apple App Store) for £2.99. By the end of the study, very few families were using Product A, but around 7500 were registered to use Product B (a proportion of whom were also receiving a wider package of support from the care charity).

Case F (shared data warehouse for integrated case management of patients at risk of hospital admission) was introduced in 2009 to support a policy of coordinated, multi-disciplinary case management between health and social care services through assessment and care planning. It had been proposed as a solution to the growing

Table 1 Summary of empirical case studies and data sources (adapted from J Med Internet Res. 2017; 19: e367)

Study site(s)	Technology/ies	Participants	Data sources
Case A. Video outpatient consultations			
A1: Acute hospital trust (3 specialties — diabetes, antenatal, cancer — on different sites) A2: Nurse-led heart failure service run from community hospital	Skype™ (acute hospital) and FaceTime™ (community hospital) together with commercially available blood pressure and heart rate monitors, weighing scales and oximeter	A1: 24 staff (9 clinicians, 10 support staff, 5 managers); 27 patients A2: 10 staff (8 nurses, one manager, one administrator); 8 patients Plus 48 national stakeholders and wider informants on remote consulting	35 formal semi-structured interviews plus ~ 100 informal interviews; 150+ hours of ethnographic observation; 40 videotaped remote consultations (12 diabetes, 6 antenatal diabetes, 12 cancer, 10 heart failure); 500+ emails; 30 local documents, e.g. business plans, protocols; 50 national-level documents
Case B. GPS tracking for cognitive impairment			
Social care organisation in deprived borough in inner London	GPS tracking devices supplied by 5 different technology companies, includes GPS tracking with virtual map and 'geo-fence' alert functions	7 index cases; 8 lay carers; 5 formal carers, 3 social care staff; 3 healthcare staff; 3 call centre staff	22 ethnographic visits and 'go-along' interviews with index cases (~ 50 h); 15 ethnographic visits with health and social care staff; 6 staff interviews; 5 team meetings; 3 local protocols
Case C. Pendant alarms			
C1: Healthcare commissioning organisation in deprived borough in outer London C2: Social care organisation in mixed borough in the Midlands	In both sites, pendant alarms and base units were supplied by multiple different technology companies and supported by local councils, each with a different set of arrangements with providers and an 'arms-length management organisation' alarm support service	C1: 8 index cases; 7 lay carers; 12 professional staff C2: 11 index cases; 9 health/social care staff from frontline service delivery to senior board level; 3 representatives from telecare industry	50 semi-structured and narrative interviews; 61 ethnographic visits (~ 80 h of observation) including needs assessments and reviews; 20 h of observation at team meetings
Case D. Remote biomarker monitoring in heart failure			
Acute hospital trusts in six different cities in UK	Tablet computer and Bluetooth-enabled commercially available sensing devices (blood pressure and heart rate monitor, weighing scales)	7 research staff including principal investigator and research coordinator for SUPPORT-HF trial; 7 clinical staff involved in trial; 4 clinical staff not involved in trial; (to date) 18 patient participants and one spouse	1 patient focus group; 8 patient interviews; 24 additional semi-structured interviews; SUPPORT-HF study protocol and ethics paperwork; material properties and functionality of biomarker database
Case E. Care organising software			
E1: Healthcare commissioning organisation in northern England E2: National carer support charity in UK	Product A: Web-based portal developed by small tech company for use by families to help them organise and coordinate the care of (typically) an older relative Product B: Smartphone app co-designed by carer support charity for same purpose	Product A: 2 technology developers and CEO of technology company; 4 social care commissioners; 30 health and social care staff considering using the device; 4 users of the device, one non-user Product B (to date): 2 members of care charity (including CEO); 10 qualitative case studies of users undertaken by another academic team	22 semi-structured and narrative interviews; 16 h ethnographic observations of meetings; auto-ethnographic testing of functionality and usability of devices; secondary analysis of 3rd party evaluation of Product B
Case F. Data warehouse for integrated case management			
1 acute hospital trust, 1 community health trust, 3 local councils, 3 healthcare commissioning organisations	Integrated data warehouse incorporating predictive risk modelling (in theory interoperable with record systems in participating organisations)	14 staff; 20 patient participants	14 semi-structured interviews; 50 ethnographic visits (~ 80 h); 12 h shadowing community staff; 4 h observation of interdisciplinary meetings; 12 local protocols/documents

challenge of emergency hospital admissions in older people with multiple health and care needs, reflecting national policy [43]. The cross-organisation data warehouse incorporating a predictive risk modelling tool was intended to automate the identification and stratification of people at high risk of hospital admission, and enable shared access to care plans, thus facilitating coordinated action and frequent dialogue between primary and secondary care providers and social services. However, the original vision of 'integrated care' achieved *through* the technology was only partially realised because, in practice, high-risk patients were identified and managed through a combination of risk stratification and data entry (using the technology) and clinical judgement and dialogue (bypassing the technology).

Data analysis and testing of the NASSS framework

We sought to analyse our six case studies both individually [44] and also as a theoretically sampled collection of cases representing maximum diversity in each of the NASSS domains [45]. This work both informed, and was informed by, our ongoing systematic review [16]. For example, the addition of domain 1 to the NASSS framework was prompted by a strong theme in our empirical data that non-adoption and abandonment of technologies were often explained by heterogeneity and unpredictability in the patient's illness, co-morbidities and socio-cultural background. The addition of Case F (data warehouse) was prompted by the discovery from our secondary research that technologies intended for sharing data between organisations raised unique logistical, technical and professional challenges.

For each of the six case studies, we analysed qualitative data thematically and produced an initial narrative summary. We wove in quantitative data (e.g. uptake and usage rates) as part of that narrative and used longitudinal methods (e.g. repeat interviews, data trends) to build the narrative over time. We held a series of meetings (approximately monthly) to discuss each of the NASSS domains, singly and in combination, as they pertained to each case study—and tested emerging theory against these domains. Our refinement of the NASSS framework, and in particular the generation of key sub-questions within each domain, owed much to these cross-case meetings.

Results

Below, we apply the different domains of the NASSS framework to our case studies before considering (in the Discussion) the implications of our findings in terms of complexity theory. We have presented Case A (video outpatient consultations) in depth and added additional data from other case studies where they add to the granularity of the analysis.

Domain 1: the condition

Differences in the underlying illness largely explained differences in the fortunes of the video consultation option in the four services studied in Case A. Routine check-ups for adults with diabetes and follow-up consultations after cancer surgery were mostly consistent and predictable (i.e. simple), and most unpredictable eventualities were of low risk. By the end of the study period, approximately 20% of all consultations in these clinics were being conducted by video.

In contrast, diabetes in pregnancy was an example of a complex condition. In pregnancy, diabetes tends to be metabolically volatile and if poorly controlled may lead to foetal abnormalities or death. Many pregnant women had developed diabetes only since becoming pregnant, and so were novices in self-administering insulin. The lead physician felt strongly accountable to the unborn child, and so only offered the video option to patients (3% of the total) judged to be 'low risk' (for example, those with high health literacy, good technological skills and fluency in English).

Heart failure is a serious, unpredictable and often unstable (hence, complex) illness whose effects vary from patient to patient and in the same patient over time [46]. It is mostly a condition of older people and occurs disproportionately in lower socio-economic groups. One of its common side effects is profound tiredness, and it is almost always associated with other co-morbidities (notably kidney disease, diabetes, depression or cognitive impairment). Heart failure nurses in our study made judgements about the stability or otherwise of the illness and about patients' co-morbidities (including cognitive ability and mental health status), health and technological literacy, family support and technical set-up at home and motivation. As a result, the video consultation option was deemed inappropriate for many (at the time of writing, fewer than 20 such consultations had been undertaken across a clinic population of several hundred).

Complexity in the underlying condition was also associated with non-adoption, abandonment or limited usefulness of technologies in Cases B and C (in which dementia or multi-morbidity respectively made the patient unable or unwilling to use the supplied technology) and Case F (in which the predictive risk modelling tool selected multi-morbidity as a risk factor for hospital admission, but few such patients proved to be 'textbook cases' to manage).

Domain 2: the technology

The technologies used for video consultations, Skype™ and FaceTime™, are both mass-market software packages from large multi-national companies, presenting low risk of supplier withdrawal and relatively straightforward substitutability (hence, in these respects they could be classified as simple or complicated). However, there were elements of complexity. For example, they were run from NHS hardware (sometimes many years old) and from patient-held laptops, tablets or smartphones of varying quality and dependability. The software was sometimes logistically difficult to install on NHS computers (e.g. because of limited capacity of the IT support team and maintain 'non-standard' software environments), and even when installed, it was not 100% dependable for both technical (machine 'crashing') and human error (e.g. forgotten password) reasons. Workarounds tended to use low-tech, dependable solutions (e.g. community heart failure nurses defaulted to telephone consultations when video connection failed), thus reducing complexity.

Whilst video transmits speech and visual cues reasonably well (although variations in audio and video quality are quite common), clinical examination sometimes needs other modalities. In heart failure care, for example, the physical examination (e.g. blood pressure, heart rhythm, leg oedema) that the nurses considered essential was not easy in the remote environment—though it was sometimes possible with patient and carer assistance when the nurse knew the patient well. There was no easy or automated way of sharing and recording patient-held data such as home blood pressure readings (patients typically read out numbers but some misinterpreted the digital display or viewed it upside down).

The other case studies illustrated different aspects of complexity in the technology. GPS tracking technology (Case B), pendant alarms (Case C) and care organising software (Case E) all relied on bespoke solutions from small and medium-sized enterprise (SME) companies, and hence were vulnerable to withdrawal; these companies sometimes lacked capacity to meet the bureaucratic requirements for potential spread and scale-up. Case D used software that had been developed as part of an academic research study; importantly, the research nurse and technical team were co-located, allowing minor (but potentially critical) technical issues to be resolved in an ongoing way. Case F featured bespoke software supplied through a longstanding relationship with an SME that was subsequently acquired by a global company. These technologies all required considerable knowledge and skill to use to their full potential. An assumption underpinning the design of patient-held assistive technologies was that a group of relatives and/or friends would exist, live locally, be technology-savvy and be able and willing to collaborate around the care of the index case. In fact, such networks were rarely pre-existing; they often had to be built and nurtured. Cases B, C and D highlighted the role of both lay carers and professional staff in helping to set up and 'service' the technology and keep it in working order, a role that could be particularly onerous if the technology (as in case B) was not dependable.

The data warehouse for integrated case management in Case F was well embedded organisationally (in the sense that it was enshrined in national policy and local subcontracts and data sharing agreements, and staff were employed to work on it). But it was not *technically* well embedded in the sense of seamless interoperability of data between participating organisations; significant workarounds were required to (for example) share care plans. The predictive risk modelling tool generated a different kind of risk estimate than a home visit from a clinician or social worker who knew the individual well and who had the capacity and authority to bear witness to a narrative and make contextual judgements. Our data illustrated that often neither approach alone offered the full picture that was sometimes necessary for making judgements. Thus, the output (risk score) generated by the technology was complex (in the sense that it was incomplete and contested).

Domain 3: the value proposition and overall value chain

The supply-side value proposition for video consulting in Case A currently appears complex. The multi-national companies behind Skype™ and FaceTime™ are also developing multiple other health products, especially directed towards the expanding 'wellness and wearables' market. From a purely financial perspective, such direct-to-consumer products may offer a more lucrative supply-side value proposition than investing in a major business venture to support video consultation products and services in the NHS, because working through technical and information governance challenges is a resource-intensive and time-consuming process with no guarantee of meeting shareholder or executive expectations at the end of it. Our interviews also suggest that companies are aware of the potential for reputational risk associated with seeking to profit from virtual consultations in the NHS.

The demand-side value (to patients) of video consultations is also complex, since the evidence base on which it rests is currently sparse. Whilst around 20 randomised controlled trials in a range of conditions have demonstrated equivalent efficacy and safety between video and face-to-face consultations [38], the samples for these trials are likely to have been carefully selected. Members of our VOCAL patient advisory group raised concerns about the risk of a 'two-tier' service in which demand-side value for a minority of patients will be gained at the expense of service cuts for the majority—a concern which, though speculative, has recently been echoed by professional bodies, clinicians and patients [47, 48].

In Case D, one aspect of the value proposition (which affects both supply- and demand-side value) is the potential of the data collected to inform the development of predictive algorithms based on biomarker changes over time and hence predict and pre-empt decompensation, hence averting hospital admission (rather than just prompting medication changes on the basis of, say, a rise or fall in blood pressure). This option creates new possibilities for 'personalised' medicine, but it also increases complexity. Whilst real-world value is hard to assess in the context of a randomised controlled trial, we note that the promise (or aspiration) of the telehealth package in Case D is highly complex, since it seeks to achieve multiple goals, including: (1) improving heart failure management in the community; (2) reducing demand on services (by allowing nurses to take on higher case loads); (3) preventing unplanned admissions; and (4) developing further predictive capabilities.

Case E illustrates two very different business models (and technology development models) for similar technologies and use cases. In one (Product A), the value proposition was highly speculative and little attempt was made to work with intended end-users to increase the technology's fitness for purpose (and hence its desirability) during development. The implicit assumption was that the technology would be more or less plug-and-play; the business model rested on provider organisations paying for a block contract even though the intended benefits (and/or savings elsewhere in the system) were not clear. Product B included substantial up-front investment (from publicly funded R&D) to under-take co-design work; it was explicitly developed by a charity as a 'public good' in which costs to end-users would be minimal and viewed as a *component* of a wider (and ongoing) charity-supported package. These projects are both ongoing, but at the time of writing we would classify Product A's value proposition as complex and Product B's as complicated.

Domain 4: the adopter system

In the adoption of video consulting (Case A), there was considerable complexity in the adopter system. There was, for example, a striking difference between innovators (who embraced the new technology and way of working with enthusiasm) and other clinicians on the same teams who were reluctant to change, reflecting previous research showing that staff resistance is the single most important reason given for low uptake of remote health care [10, 49]. The hurdle was not merely learning to use a new technology but also accepting changes in identity (e.g. some staff did not view themselves as 'techy') and role (e.g. helping a remote patient troubleshoot technical problems with Skype™ or FaceTime™), dealing with perceptions of overload when running a new virtual service in parallel with a traditional face-to-face one and feeling under pressure to realise efficiency gains before the system had been fully redesigned to maximise such gains. New staff roles were not restricted to clinicians directly using the video technology; receptionists, clerks and technicians all had to accommodate new roles that the technology required in order to 'work'. The same was true of the patient, who could sometimes but not always seek technical help from family members.

The other case studies illustrated additional complexities in the adopter system, such as some staff expressing ethical reservations about 'tagging' clients (Case B) or clinical concerns about the data generated by the technology (Case D—some clinicians were worried about possible legal liability if telehealth data, generated elsewhere and impossible to verify directly, were later found to be flawed). In Case C, clients sometimes rejected a pendant alarm because it symbolised dependence or because they were unwilling to pay a small monthly connection fee or be placed in a dependency relationship with a relative or neighbour.

Domain 5: the organisation(s)

The hospital trust that hosted the VOCAL study had strong leadership and good managerial relations; it met key criteria for technological innovativeness (e.g. it had previously won a national 'Digital Trust of the Year' award), and there was board-level enthusiasm for the introduction of video consultations. Despite these encouraging precondi-tions ('simple' in our taxonomy), other features of the organisation were highly complex. In particular, it had very limited spare staff time and resources (e.g. key posts were unfilled, and many clinic terminals were running outdated versions of software packages)—a problem known as 'lack of organisational slack' [18]. In addition, whilst many senior decision-makers *assumed* that the new service would save money by making services more efficient, the question of whether a video consultation would *actually* cost less to deliver was not easy to answer because of potential knock-ons in the system (e.g. the need for additional IT support and staff training; the fact that rooms still needed to be occupied, records retrieved and appointments booked even when the consultation was virtual; and the theoretical possibility of an increase in appointments as clinicians and patients found it easier to connect).

Another feature of complexity was that whilst video consultations between clinicians and selected patients usually worked well, the linked routines for booking appointments, managing the clinic list (e.g. registering when each patient had 'arrived' and 'left') and organising follow-up did not mesh well with a system that had evolved to process patients using their physical presence (waiting in line at a reception desk), manual transfer of paper records between different plastic 'bins' and sticky notes. Alignment with such routines was initially achieved using workarounds; by the end of the study, new (computer-based) routines had been developed by some but not all participating teams. Whilst Skype functionality increased access (by, for example, allowing patients to send messages to the clinician's Skype account), and whilst this ease of access was sometimes clinically appropriate and encouraged (e.g. "drop me a message to confirm the change of insulin dose was OK"), it generated complexities elsewhere in the system, since the clinician then had to log the message on the medical record.

Similar complexity-related challenges were evident in the community heart failure study. The community trust was a digital innovator and had supplied all nurses with tablet computers to help them with various aspects of their work. Again, whilst video consultations worked well *clinically* for selected patients, at the time of writing they were not well integrated *logistically* with the administra-tive aspects of the service. There was no formal opposition from top management in the community trust to the nurse-led video consultation service. But neither was there strong enthusiasm, and there was limited spare capacity among front-line teams to undertake the work of making sense of the new approach, enrolling and training staff beyond initial enthusiasts, implementing new work routines and evaluating the service.

In our other case studies, enthusiasm at board level was sometimes absent (e.g. because business cases were weak) and/or key opponents were strategically placed and had high wrecking power (specific examples withheld). In Case D, wide variability in clinician engagement among the different study sites could be explained largely in terms of the extent to which the local team shared a vision for how remote biomarker monitoring for heart failure might enhance rather than threaten the existing service, an aspect of implementation work that May calls 'coherence work' [22].

In Case F, establishing integrated case management through shared data and predictive risk modelling technology was extremely complex because multiple organisations needed to be involved; the establishment and development of the programme unfolded over several years and relied on partnership working and contracting arrangements at different levels of multiple organisations. The technology was implemented, but the anticipated reduction in costs from reducing hospital admissions were not realised as real savings because of the complexities of reimbursement mechanisms and because case management was not always successful in avoiding admissions.

Domain 6: the wider system
The most significant system-level challenge to the scale-up and spread of video consultations in Case A was that there was no established national tariff for funding such consultations. In the VOCAL study, the local commissioning organisation proposed reimbursing such consultations at a rate ('pass through tariff' [50]) intermediate between a telephone consultation and a face-to-face one. But even though members of the relevant national policymaking team were on the study steering group and there was no opposition 'in principle' to establishing a national tariff, this had still not been achieved at the time of writing—mainly because data to inform costing calculations were difficult to obtain and contested by some parties. This is a good example of how innovative, technology-supported service models can succeed as demonstration projects through local workarounds but will fail to spread or be sustained unless the regulatory and financial context is supportive [51]. Another contextual factor which added complexity in case study A was a mixed reaction from professional bodies, whose enthusiasm for new, potentially more efficient, models of care was tempered by concerns about workload and threats to equity.

Our national-level stakeholder interviews revealed another aspect of complexity relating to the nature and strength of evidence expected by different stakeholder groups. The technology industry typically moves quickly, with a development model based on rapid iterations of technologies and a pragmatic understanding of what works in practice (the 'fail early, fail often' principle). Policymakers, in contrast, tend to want what they call 'gold standard' evidence (for example, from randomised controlled trials) to 'prove' that a particular technology has the impacts claimed. This mismatch appeared to explain some of the slow progress on national-level policy in relation to video consultations.

The acute trust where our video consultation study was based was one of the first public sector providers in the UK to introduce this service model [39]. In the last year of the VOCAL study, more than 50 organisations contacted the lead clinician seeking advice or asking to visit to see the video consultation service in action. This is an example of the important role of inter-organisational networking in supporting the exchange of both explicit and tacit knowledge [18].

Domain 7: adaptation over time
The video consulting services in Case A illustrated both resistance to adaptation (through material limitations and institutionalised information governance regulations) and adaptiveness (through clinicians' creative and responsive use of the technology). The NHS has a 'locked-down' computer environment in which any new hardware or software must be carefully considered and formally approved before being installed or upgraded (a characteristic that reduces complexity for IT managers but tends to increase complexity for front-line staff). Rapidly evolving software sits awkwardly in such an environment. In the VOCAL study, an automated upgrade to Skype™ made the system non-functional on clinical terminals until re-authorised by someone with administrator-level access rights—a problem that resulted in some remote clinics having to be done by telephone.

The material features of Skype™ enabled the development of 'ad hoc' consulting in the young adult diabetes clinic, for example, when the patient saw that the clinician was online and sent a text (SMS) message asking a question about a recently changed insulin dosage. The clinician could either reply by SMS message (within Skype™) or offer a real-time video consultation (typically very short). This adaptive use of video technology for patient-initiated consultations was viewed by clinicians as a game-changer for 'challenging' patients (characterised by high non-attendance rate at clinic, poor glycaemic control and a history of hospital admission for diabetic emergencies).

Several other cases in our dataset illustrated a similar tension between system rigidity (for contractual or cost reasons) and adaptation (through user creativity). In Case C, for example, potentially remediable problems occurred with some alarms, but adaptation was impossible because of the risk of loss of warranty. A pendant alarm service initially introduced to provide *emergency physical support* (e.g. for falls) was adapted over time to provide *non-emergency emotional support* for certain older people, who were encouraged by call centre staff to press the alarm button to trigger a supportive conversation when feeling lonely.

In Case F, following the introduction of the integrated case management data warehouse technology, clinical and administrative staff across different organisations collectively learnt and redefined what this technology could and could not do. They amended, adapted and worked around it. For example, clinicians and practitioners reviewed the outputs of the data-driven risk stratification model but also supplemented them with other data and used their judgement to target additional patients who had *not* been flagged as 'high risk' by the technological algorithm. Technical developers continually updated the user interface through an ongoing relationship with the procuring body. Notwithstanding these efforts, there was a brittleness about the technology (and the work routines it presupposed) that staff experienced as persistently frustrating. Thus, there was a sense that the technology had been 'successfully' implemented and was for the moment being sustained (because it met policy expectations), but was not truly fit for purpose.

Discussion

Through in-depth, longitudinal ethnography across a maximum-variety sample of local technology-supported innovations, along with an analysis of national context, we have shown that failures, partial successes and unanticipated problems are common. Using the NASSS framework, these outcomes can be explained by complexity across multiple, interacting domains. Technology-supported innovation programmes face particular challenges when:

- *The condition or illness* is complex because it is poorly characterised, poorly understood, unpredictable in its natural history or associated with multiple co-morbidities or socio-cultural concerns (such as poverty, low health literacy or particular beliefs or traditions).
- *The technology* creates additional complexity because it has multiple interacting components, requires close embedding within already-complex technical systems, lacks dependability, provides an unreliable, incomplete or contested picture of the condition, requires advanced knowledge to use it or exists only as a bespoke solution that is vulnerable to supplier withdrawal.

- *The supply-side value proposition* rests on an underdeveloped, implausible or risky business case (hence, is unlikely to attract investment), or the *demand-side value proposition* suggests that (from the patient's perspective) the technology could be undesirable, unsafe, ineffective or unaffordable.
- *The adopter system* is complex because the innovation does not merely require staff to take on new roles but also puts staff under pressure, threatens their professional identity, values or scope of practice, or poses a risk of job loss; because it requires patients to undertake complex tasks such as initiate changes in therapy or make judgements about what is an emergency; or because it presupposes a network of carers who are willing and able to coordinate their input.
- *The organisation(s) is/are complex* as a result of severe resource pressures (e.g. frozen posts), weak leadership and managerial relations and a climate in which creativity and risk-taking are punished; and in situations where, in relation to this particular technology, there is minimal tension for change, poor innovation-system fit and multiple opponents to the programme, some of whom are strategically placed and have wrecking power. Complexity will loom large when new team routines or care pathways predicated on the new technology conflict with established ones, and when significant work is needed to build shared vision, engage staff, enact new practices, monitor impact and support ongoing adaptation. It will be a prominent feature of a programme spanning multiple organisations who have no formal links and/or have conflicting agendas, where funding depends on cost savings across the system, where the costs and benefits to each partner organisation are unclear, and where new infrastructure for the proposed programme conflicts with existing infrastructure and where there are significant budget implications.
- *The wider system* is complex because policy changes that the new service model requires raise tricky political, regulatory, legal, financial or other challenges, because policymakers and industry have different views on what counts as high-quality evidence, because professional bodies and lay stakeholders are currently unsupportive or opposed or because there are barriers to inter-organisational networking and knowledge-sharing.
- *The time dimension* is complex because further adaptation and/or co-evolution of the technology or service is impossible (or only possibly to a limited extent), or because sense-making, collective reflection and adaptive action are discouraged in a rigid, inflexible implementation model.

As the case narratives above illustrate, when there is complexity across *multiple* domains (and this occurs commonly), outcomes become even less predictable, less controllable and (hence) less amenable to conventional planning and implementation logic.

Despite abundant evidence of complexity in multiple domains in all our case studies, our data indicated a tendency of planners, policymakers and technology designers to assume that the issues to be addressed were merely *complicated* (hence, knowable, predictable and controllable) rather than *complex* (that is, inherently not knowable or predictable but dynamic and emergent). What might be called 'complexity work' (adaptation and adjustment to accommodate a host of emergent issues) was absent from policymakers' version of the project but loomed large in the day-to-day experience of front-line staff.

A complicated programme can be managed rationally by careful planning, implementation of agreed procedures and monitoring. Typically, such programmes are divided into discrete work packages (perhaps 'work-as-imagined' packages [52]), each of which can be defined, assigned a leader, undertaken and reported on separately from other work packages. A focus on complicatedness rather than complexity is illustrated, for example, by the digital maturity assessment tools produced by NHS England [53]. The 'de facto standard in UK government' for managing complicated programmes, underpinned by a logic model, is PRINCE2 (PRojects IN Controlled Environments) [54]. PRINCE2 and similar tools focus almost exclusively on an abstracted depiction of process (what needs to be done, by whom and by when).

A *complex* programme, especially one that is designed around clinical or social care of sick or vulnerable people, requires a very different approach. Its management must attend carefully to people, motivations, values and professional norms, and put mechanisms in place to detect deviations from expected outcomes, identify the numerous contributory causes and make timely adjustments by adapting technologies, practices and workflows. This is partly about a different, more flexible, iterative and user-centred approach to programme management (which some have termed 'co-realisation' [55]), partly about a central focus on the *people* involved, including the deeply held professional identities, norms and values that underpin so-called resistance to new technologies [21] and the need for organisational members to *make sense* of technology-supported change in an ongoing, evolving way [23], and partly about the importance of *organisaton and system learning* to ensure that what has been learnt during deployment can be captured and re-used to inform strategies for subsequent scaling up and sustainability [56].

The uncertainty of outcomes in complex programmes means that they are highly likely to witness active experimentation by users as they grapple with the challenges of discovering the capabilities and limitations of a new technology. These experiments might involve reconfiguring the technologies, processes or both. Hence, the phase within a programme that is commonly referred to as 'deployment' needs to be viewed not as its final denouement but as an opportunity for learning, refinement and adaptation. The key to achieving this is the use of a variety of modes of communication, both among programme team members and between the programme team and the users [57].

It is encouraging that some recognition of the need for technology 'deployment' to be iterative, adaptive, people-focused and oriented to social learning is evident in some recent initiatives in healthcare. For example, the NHS Technology Adoption Centre (NTAC), which is part of the UK's National Institute for Health and Care Excellence (NICE), provides innovation process guides that are designed to capture and distill the experiences of early adopters [58]. However, NTAC's primary focus is on tackling organisational issues such as stakeholder recruitment and business case development, rather than, for example, supporting the day-to-day work of monitoring, communicating, evaluating and adapting.

Conclusion

This first empirical application of the NASSS framework has illustrated how complexity characterises multiple dimensions of many technology-supported change programmes. In every case study, the mismatch between work-as-imagined and work-as-done was substantial. Illnesses behaved idiosyncratically, not as depicted in textbooks. Technologies showed promise (including potential value for developers and patients) but also both symbolic and material fickleness. Human agents (staff, patients, technology developers, policymakers) brought their values, motives, capabilities and beliefs to bear on their assessment of local situations, and this affected their resulting action (or inaction), which then had knock-ons across the system. The organisational and wider setting for introducing, implementing and monitoring technologies was characterised by both opportunities and constraints that were multiple and changing. Creative, adaptive solutions and workarounds sometimes but not always helped keep the show on the road.

We conclude that a rationalist approach to implementing technology programmes, based on abstracted principles for managing complicatedness in linear and static deployment models, is unlikely to lead to the large-scale 'disruptive innovation' that policymakers have envisaged, nor will it address the specific challenges of local scale-up, distant spread and long-term sustainability. As Ludwig Wittgenstein commented in 'Philosophical Investigations',

We have got onto slippery ice where there is no friction and so in a certain sense the conditions are ideal, but also, just because of that, we are unable to walk. We want to walk, so we need friction. Back to the rough ground! [59].

Our data suggest that it is towards this 'rough ground' of real-world implementation, collective sensemaking and social learning at the front line that attention should now be turned. Until recently, researchers trod tentatively if at all on such ground, but the shift to complexity thinking in the business and management literature has begun to generate principles, tools and practical approaches that are (at least to some extent) evidence-based.

Whilst we originally developed the NASSS framework to support academic activity (e.g. 'conjunctive theorising' [35] to illuminate and explain our case studies), we have begun to use the framework in more practical ways to try to increase the success of complex programmes in health and social care. Relevant to this practical application (which is currently in its early stages) is the work of Janssen et al. on technology-driven transformation [60]. These authors acknowledge that complexity theory eschews universal solutions and predictive models but maintain that there are nevertheless some core principles of non-linear system change that will increase the chances of programme success.

Adapting these suggestions and taking account of the findings presented here, we propose the following principles for technology adopters, commissioners and policymakers: (1) assess the nature and extent of complexity in the programme and ensure that emergent and adaptive measures are used to address these issues; (2) establish overall leadership (since complex programmes often suffer from outsourcing of control and coordination); (3) craft and sustain a vision (ensure that key players understand and share a sense of why the project is important); (4) create incentives (but leave front-line staff to work out how to deliver); (5) respond adaptively as the programme-in-context evolves (for example, by collecting and reflecting on emerging data and harnessing human creativity); (6) control growth (since projects that evolve organically are vulnerable to over-ambitious extension and scope creep); (7) create slack (to resource adaptive responses); and (8) manage the tension between innovation and implementation, especially when continuing evolution of the technology (e.g. additional functionality) adds to complexity.

Our empirical findings also suggest that it will often be mission-critical to reduce complexity in as many domains and sub-domains as possible. Maylor et al., focusing mainly on commercial projects, recently developed a complexity assessment tool intended to be used prospectively to identify, understand, reduce and/or 'run with' the different aspects of complexity in a technology project or programme [36]. We are currently in the process of using the NASSS framework to adapt this tool to support a systematic approach to complexity reduction in the very different context of health and social care.

Acknowledgements

We are grateful to the participants (patients, carers, stakeholders and staff) in the VOCAL and SCALS studies for their commitment and insights. We are grateful to various colleagues who tested the NASSS framework on their own projects and provided feedback. We drew on a qualitative evaluation of Product B undertaken by researchers at another university and published internally by the carers' charity.

Funding

The VOCAL study was funded through a National Institute for Health Research Health Services and Delivery Research grant to TG (13/59/26). The SCALS program's main funding is from a Senior Investigator Award and Public Engagement Award to TG from the Wellcome Trust in its Society and Ethics Program (WT104830MA). Additional funding for the GPS tracking case study was provided through a Program Development Grant to TG from the National Institute for Health Research (RP-DG-1213-10003). The SCALS study is registered on the Wellcome Trust's Society and Ethics portfolio. TG, SS and JW are part-funded from the National Institute for Health Research Biomedical Research Centre, Oxford, UK (grant NIHR- BRC-1215-20008). The initial draft of this paper was written when TG was on a writing retreat at the Bellagio Center, Italy, funded by the Rockefeller Foundation.

Transparency declaration

TG (lead author and the manuscript's guarantor) affirms that the manuscript is an honest, accurate and transparent account of the study being reported; that no important aspects of the study have been omitted; and that any discrepancies from the study as planned have been explained.

Role of sponsor

The sponsor took no part in data collection, data analysis or writing of the paper.

Authors' contributions

TG was the principal investigator on the four research grants that funded the work. She led on the literature review and conceptualised the original version of the NASSS framework. SS took the overall lead on the empirical work and coordinated cross-case meetings and anlaysis. JW was the lead field worker on two empirical case studies; CP, JL, GH, CAC and SH each led or co-led one empirical case study. CP also provided theoretical input on complexity theory and provided analytic support in some case studies. RP provided specialist computer science and theoretical input. TG drafted the first version of this paper, drawing on detailed case summaries prepared by the case study leads. All authors helped revise drafts substantially. All authors read and approved the final manuscript.

Competing interests

The authors declare that they have no competing interests.

Author details

[1]Department of Primary Care Health Sciences, University of Oxford, Oxford OX2 6GG, UK. [2]School of Health and Social Work, University of Hertfordshire, Hatfield, UK. [3]RAFT Research consultancy, Clitheroe, UK. [4]Department of Computer Science, University of Warwick, Coventry, UK.

References

1. Garber S, Gates S, Keeler EB, Valana ME, Mulcahy AW, Lau C, Kellerman A. Redirecting Innovation in U.S. Health Care: options to decrease spending and increase value. Santa Monica: RAND Corporation; 2014. http://www.rand.org/pubs/research_reports/RR308.html. Accessed 27 Feb 2017.
2. Honeyman M, Dunn P, McKenna H. A Digital NHS? An introduction to the digital agenda and plans for implementation. London: King's Fund; 2014.
3. Wachter R. Making IT Work: harnessing the power of health information technology to improve care in England. Report to the National Advisory Group on Health Information Technology in England. London: The Stationery Office; 2016.
4. National Information Board. Personalised health and care 2020: using data andtechnology to transform outcomes for patients and citizens. London: The Stationery Office; 2014.
5. Department of Health. Digital strategy: leading the culture change in health and care. London: DH; 2012.
6. Lehoux P, Miller F, Daudelin G, Urbach D. How venture capitalists decide which new medical technologies come to exist. Sci Public Policy. 2016;43(3):375–85.
7. Greenhalgh T, Procter R, Wherton J, Sugarhood P, Hinder S, Rouncefield M. What is quality in assisted living technology? The ARCHIE framework for effective telehealth and telecare services. BMC Med. 2015;13:91.
8. Bentley CL, Powell LA, Orrell A, Mountain GA. Addressing design and suitability barriers to Telecare use: has anything changed? Technol Disabil. 2014;26(4):221–35.
9. Clark J, McGee-Lennon M. A stakeholder-centred exploration of the current barriers to the uptake of home care technology in the UK. J Assist Technol. 2011;5(1):12–25.
10. Wade VA, Eliott JA, Hiller JE. Clinician acceptance is the key factor for sustainable telehealth services. Qual Health Res. 2014; https://doi.org/10.1177/1049732314528809.
11. Harrison MI, Koppel R, Bar-Lev S. Unintended consequences of information technologies in health care—an interactive sociotechnical analysis. J Am Med Inform Assoc. 2007;14(5):542–9.
12. Symon G, Long K, Ellis J. The coordination of work activities: cooperation and conflict in a hospital context. Comput Supported Coop Work (CSCW). 1996;5(1):1–31.
13. Han YY, Carcillo JA, Venkataraman ST, Clark RS, Watson RS, Nguyen TC, Bayir H, Orr RA. Unexpected increased mortality after implementation of a commercially sold computerized physician order entry system. Pediatrics. 2005;116(6):1506–12.
14. van Limburg M, van Gemert-Pijnen JE, Nijland N, Ossebaard HC, Hendrix RM, Seydel ER. Why business modeling is crucial in the development of eHealth technologies. J Med Internet Res. 2011;13(4):e124.
15. Grin J, Rotmans J, Schot J. Transitions to sustainable development: new directions in the study of long term transformative change. New York: Routledge; 2010.
16. Greenhalgh T, Wherton J, Papoutsi C, Lynch J, Hughes G, A'Court C, Hinder S, Fahy N, Procter R, Shaw S. Beyond adoption: a new framework for theorizing and evaluating nonadoption, abandonment, and challenges to the scale-up, spread, and sustainability of health and care technologies. J Med Internet Res. 2017;19(11):e367.
17. Rogers EM. Diffusion of innovations. New York: Simon and Schuster; 2010.
18. Greenhalgh T, Robert G, Macfarlane F, Bate P, Kyriakidou O. Diffusion of innovations in service organizations: systematic review and recommendations. The Milbank quarterly. 2004;82(4):581–629.
19. Lehoux P, Miller FA, Daudelin G, Denis J-L. Providing value to new health technology: the early contribution of entrepreneurs, investors, and regulatory agencies. Int J Health Policy Manag. 2017;6(x):1–10.
20. May CR, Eton DT, Boehmer K, Gallacher K, Hunt K, MacDonald S, Mair FS, May CM, Montori VM, Richardson A. Rethinking the patient: using Burden of Treatment Theory to understand the changing dynamics of illness. BMC Health Serv Res. 2014;14(1):1.
21. Greenhalgh T, Swinglehurst D, Stones R. Rethinking 'resistance' to big IT: a sociological study of why and when healthcare staff do not use nationally mandated information and communication technologies. Health Services and Delivery Research. 2014;39(2):1–86.
22. May C, Finch T. Implementing, embedding, and integrating practices: an outline of normalization process theory. Sociology. 2009;43(3):535–54.
23. Weick KE. Technology as equivoque: sensemaking in new technologies. In: Goodman PS, Sproull LS, editors. Technology and organizations. San Francisco: Jossey-Bass; 1990. p. 1–44.
24. Cherns A. Principles of sociotechnical design revisted. Human relations. 1987;40(3):153–61.
25. Berg M. Patient care information systems and health care work: a sociotechnical approach. Int J Med Inform. 1999;55(2):87–101.
26. Nemeth C, Wears R, Woods D, Hollnagel E, Cook R: Minding the gaps: creating resilience in health care. In: Henriksen K, Battles JB, Keyes MA, Grady ML, Advances in patient safety: new directions and alternative approaches. Vol. 3. Rockville: Agency for Healthcare Research and Quality; 2008.
27. Chambers DA, Glasgow RE, Stange KC. The dynamic sustainability framework: addressing the paradox of sustainment amid ongoing change. Implement Sci. 2013;8(1):117.
28. Cho S, Mathiassen L, Robey D. The dialectics of resilience: a multilevel analysis of a telehealth innovation. The Transfer and Diffusion of Information Technology for Organizational Resilience; 2006. p. 339–57.
29. !!! INVALID CITATION !!! .
30. van Gemert-Pijnen JE, Nijland N, van Limburg M, Ossebaard HC, Kelders SM, Eysenbach G, Seydel ER. A holistic framework to improve the uptake and impact of eHealth technologies. J Med Internet Res. 2011;13(4):e111.
31. Greenhalgh T, Vijayaraghavan S, Wherton J, Shaw S, Byrne E, Campbell-Richards D, Bhattacharya S, Hanson P, Ramoutar S, Gutteridge C, et al. Virtual online consultations: advantages and limitations (VOCAL) study. BMJ Open. 2016;6(1):e009388.
32. Greenhalgh T, Shaw S, Wherton J, Hughes G, Lynch J, A'Court C, Hinder S, Fahy N, Byrne E, Finlayson A, et al. SCALS: a fourth-generation study of assisted living technologies in their organisational, social, political and policy context. BMJ Open. 2016;6(2):e010208.
33. Plsek PE, Greenhalgh T. Complexity science: the challenge of complexity in health care. BMJ. 2001;323(7313):625–8.
34. Cohn S, Clinch M, Bunn C, Stronge P. Entangled complexity: why complex interventions are just not complicated enough. J Health Serv Res Policy. 2013;18(1):40–3.
35. Tsoukas H. Don't simplify, complexify: from disjunctive to conjunctive theorizing in organization and management studies. J Manag Stud. 2017; 54(2):132–53.
36. Maylor H, Turner N. Understand, reduce, respond: project complexity management theory and practice. Int J Oper Prod Manag. 2017;37(8):1076–93.
37. Fitzgerald L, McDermott A. Challenging perspectives on organizational change in health care. London: Routledge; 2016.
38. Shaw S, Wherton J, Vijayaraghavan S, Morris J, Bhattacharya S, Hanson P, Campbell-Richards D, Ramoutar S, Collard A, Hodkinson I et al: Virtual online consultations: advantages and limitations (VOCAL). A mixed-method study at micro, meso and macro level. Health Serv Deliv Res. 2017. In press.
39. Greenhalgh T, Shaw S, Wherton J, Vijayaraghavan S, Morris J, Bhattacharya S, Hanson P, Campbell-Richards D, Ramoutar S, Collard A, et al. Video outpatient consultations: a case study of real-world implementation at macro, meso and micro level. J Med Internet Res. 2018; in press
40. Procter R, Wherton J, Greenhalgh T, Sugarhood P, Rouncefield M, Hinder S. Telecare call centre work and ageing in place. Comput Supported Coop Work (CSCW); 2016;25(1):79-105.
41. Procter R, Greenhalgh T, Wherton J, Sugarhood P, Rouncefield M, Hinder S. The day-to-day co-production of ageing in place. Comput Supported Coop Work. 2014;23(3):245–67.
42. Triantafyllidis A, Velardo C, Chantler T, Shah SA, Paton C, Khorshidi R, Tarassenko L, Rahimi K. A personalised mobile-based home monitoring system for heart failure: the SUPPORT-HF Study. Int J Med Inform. 2015; 84(10):743–53.
43. Department of Health. Supporting people with long term conditions. London: Stationery Office; 2005.
44. Stake RE. The art of case study research. Thousand Oaks: Sage; 1995.
45. Yin RK. Case study research: design and methods. Thousand Oaks: Sage Publications; 2013.
46. Greenhalgh T, Shaw S. Understanding heart failure; explaining telehealth–a hermeneutic systematic review. BMC Cardiovasc Disord. 2017;17(1):156.
47. Anonymous. Press release: New GP app could lead to patients being 'cherry picked' and create 'twin track' general practice, warns RCGP. London: Royal College of General Practitioners; 2017. http://www.rcgp.org.uk/news/2017/

Analysing the role of complexity in explaining the fortunes of technology programmes: empirical application...

15

november/new-gp-app-could-lead-to-patients-being-cherry-picked-and-create-twin-track-general-practice.aspx. Accessed 10 Nov 2017.

48. Finlayson A, Barry E, L Craven , Greenhalgh T: Primary healthcare, disruptive innovation, and the digital gold rush 2017. BMJ, Blog. http://blogs.bmj.com/bmj/2017/11/21/primary-healthcare-disruptive-innovation-and-the-digital-gold-rush/. Accessed 1 Dec 2017.

49. Taylor J, Coates E, Brewster L, Mountain G, Wessels B, Hawley MS. Examining the use of telehealth in community nursing: identifying the factors affecting frontline staff acceptance and telehealth adoption. J Adv Nurs. 2015;71(2):326–37.

50. Llewellyn S, Procter R, Harvey G, Maniatopoulos G, Boyd A: Facilitating technology adoption in the NHS: negotiating the organisational and policy context—a qualitative study. 2014.

51. Maniatopoulos G, Procter R, Llewellyn S, Harvey G, Boyd A. Moving beyond local practice: reconfiguring the adoption of a breast cancer diagnostic technology. Soc Sci Med. 2015;131:98–106.

52. Hollnagel E, Braithwaite J, Wears RL. Resilient health care. New York: Ashgate Publishing, Ltd.; 2013.

53. NHS England. Digital maturity assessment. London: NHS England; 2017. https://www.england.nhs.uk/digitaltechnology/info-revolution/maturity-index/. Accessed 4 Dec 2017.

54. ILX Group. WHat is PRINCE2? London: ILX; 2008. http://www.prince2.com/what-is-prince2.asp. Accessed 20 Nov 2017.

55. Hartswood M, Procter R, Rouchy P, Rouncefield M, Slack R, Voss A. Working IT out in medical practice: IT systems design and development as co-realisation. Methods Inf Med. 2003;42(4):392–7.

56. Williams R, Stewart J, Slack R. Social learning in technological innovation: experimenting with information and communication technologies. Northampton: Edward Elgar Publishing; 2005.

57. Procter R, Rouncefield M, Poschen M, Lin Y, Voss A. Agile project management: a case study of a virtual research environment development project. Comput Supported Coop Work (CSCW). 2011;20(3):197–225.

58. National Institute for Health and Clinical Excellence Health Technologies Adoption Programme. Health Technologies Adoption Programme: process guide for adoption support resources for health technologies. Processes and Methods Series PMG 23. London: NICE; 2015. https://www.nice.org.uk/process/pmg23/chapter/introduction#overview-of-adoption-support-resources. Accessed 4 Dec 2017.

59. Wittgenstein L. Philosophical investigations (Manuscript, 1945–1949). Transl. from Philosophische Untersuchungen. Transl. by GEM Anscombe. Oxford: Basil Blackwell Publishers; 1958.

60. Janssen M, Van Der Voort H, van Veenstra AF. Failure of large transformation projects from the viewpoint of complex adaptive systems: management principles for dealing with project dynamics. Inf Syst Front. 2015;17(1):15–29.

2

High-level artemisinin-resistance with quinine co-resistance emerges in *P. falciparum* malaria under in vivo artesunate pressure

Rajeev K. Tyagi[1,2,7†], Patrick J. Gleeson[1,2,8†], Ludovic Arnold[1,2†], Rachida Tahar[3,4], Eric Prieur[1,2], Laurent Decosterd[5], Jean-Louis Pérignon[1,2,9], Piero Olliaro[6] and Pierre Druilhe[1,2*]

Abstract

Background: Humanity has become largely dependent on artemisinin derivatives for both the treatment and control of malaria, with few alternatives available. A *Plasmodium falciparum* phenotype with delayed parasite clearance during artemisinin-based combination therapy has established in Southeast Asia, and is emerging elsewhere. Therefore, we must know how fast, and by how much, artemisinin-resistance can strengthen.

Methods: *P. falciparum* was subjected to discontinuous in vivo artemisinin drug pressure by capitalizing on a novel model that allows for long-lasting, high-parasite loads. Intravenous artesunate was administered, using either single flash-doses or a 2-day regimen, to *P. falciparum*-infected humanized NOD/SCID IL-2Rγ$^{-/-}$immunocompromised mice, with progressive dose increments as parasites recovered. The parasite's response to artemisinins and other available anti-malarial compounds was characterized in vivo and in vitro.

Results: Artemisinin resistance evolved very rapidly up to extreme, near-lethal doses of artesunate (240 mg/kg), an increase of > 3000-fold in the effective in vivo dose, far above resistance levels reported from the field. Artemisinin resistance selection was reproducible, occurring in 80% and 41% of mice treated with flash-dose and 2-day regimens, respectively, and the resistance phenotype was stable. Measuring in vitro sensitivity proved inappropriate as an early marker of resistance, as IC_{50} remained stable despite in vivo resistance up to 30 mg/kg (ART-S: 10.7 nM (95% CI 10.2–11.2) vs. ART-R$_{30}$: 11.5 nM (6.6–16.9), F = 0.525, $p = 0.47$). However, when in vivo resistance strengthened further, IC_{50} increased 10-fold (ART-R$_{240}$ 100.3 nM (92.9–118.4), F = 304.8, $p < 0.0001$), reaching a level much higher than ever seen in clinical samples. Artemisinin resistance in this African *P. falciparum* strain was not associated with mutations in *kelch-13*, casting doubt over the universality of this genetic marker for resistance screening. Remarkably, despite exclusive exposure to artesunate, full resistance to quinine, the only other drug sufficiently fast-acting to deal with severe malaria, evolved independently in two parasite lines exposed to different artesunate regimens in vivo, and was confirmed in vitro.

Conclusion: *P. falciparum* has the potential to evolve extreme artemisinin resistance and more complex patterns of multidrug resistance than anticipated. If resistance in the field continues to advance along this trajectory, we will be left with a limited choice of suboptimal treatments for acute malaria, and no satisfactory option for severe malaria.

Keywords: Malaria, *P. falciparum*, Artemisinin, Resistance, Artesunate, Quinine, NSG mice

---

* Correspondence: druilhe@vac4all.org
†Rajeev K. Tyagi, Patrick J. Gleeson and Ludovic Arnold contributed equally to this work.
[1]The Vac4All Initiative, 26 Rue Lecourbe, 75015 Paris, France
[2]Biomedical Parasitology Unit, Institut Pasteur, Paris, France
Full list of author information is available at the end of the article

Background

Artemisinin (ART) derivatives have become the keystone of malaria treatment and control [1]. ART has the advantage of killing all asexual blood stages of *Plasmodium falciparum* parasites, as well as affecting sexual development [2], resulting in rapid clinical and parasitological cure at an individual level, and a reduction in malaria transmission rates on a public health scale. All currently recommended first- and second-line treatments for uncomplicated malaria are a combination of ART with an unrelated antimalarial (artemisinin-based combination therapy, ACT) [1]. For severe malaria, artesunate (a type of ART; AS) is the first-line treatment, and quinine is the only available alternative [1]. Malaria control is thus highly reliant on ART, and adequate replacements are not forthcoming [3].

Historically, Southeast Asia has been the epicenter of malaria drug-resistance development – resistance to all major antimalarials has emerged there. *P. falciparum* resistance to ART (ART-R) given as part of ACT, was first reported from western Cambodia in 2008 [2, 4] and has already spread across the Greater Mekong subregion [5–11]. The ART-R phenotype is recognized clinically as a prolongation of parasitemia clearance as measured by peripheral blood smears (delayed parasite clearance time; DPCT) in patients with uncomplicated falciparum malaria. Unexplained slow parasite clearance times have been reported with high frequency among Ugandan children treated with intravenous AS for severe malaria [12] and in East Africa, where residual submicroscopic parasitemia after ACT has been reported [13].

Infections with DPCT still show some therapeutic response to ART. Frank ART-R, a situation where ART would fail to cause an appreciable reduction of parasite levels in patients' blood, has not yet been documented [5, 14]. Concerningly, reports are starting to emerge of multidrug-resistant malaria with treatment failures to ART and other key drugs, including quinine [15, 16].

Understanding ART-R has proved challenging both in the field and the laboratory [5, 6, 17–20]. In contrast to other antimalarials, no significant correlation between clinical response to ART and conventional in vitro determination of the 50% drug inhibitory concentration (IC_{50}) is seen [5, 6]. For in vivo studies, only non-human malaria parasites that infect rodents have been available [21, 22]. Recently, however, substantial progress has been made. A series of in vitro and clinical studies have characterized the variable susceptibility of different parasite blood-stages to ART [23] and identified *kelch-13* as an important *P. falciparum* gene associated with ART-R [10]. Besides *kelch-13*, these studies (including genome wide association studies; GWAS) [24], associated a number of other malaria parasite genes, such as *RAD5*

(which lies within 10 kb of *kelch-13*), *ferredoxin*, *tetratricopeptide*, and *nt1*, with ART-R. The altered regulation of many genes and metabolic pathways rather than a single gene polymorphism might be responsible for the ART-R phenotype [25–28]. The ring-stage survival (RSA) and trophozoite maturation inhibition assays have been developed following the observation of stage-specific susceptibility to ART, and are more sensitive at detecting decreased ART responsiveness than conventional laboratory methods [29, 30].

Despite the advances made, we have no way to foretell if *P. falciparum* can evolve beyond DPCT towards higher, more troublesome, levels of resistance. The successive loss of other antimalarial compounds to the rising tide of resistance, together with the remarkable potency of ART, has led to a worldwide switch to ACT. The consequences of this major shift in drug pressure on the *P. falciparum* genome, particularly the speed and strength with which ART-R might evolve, are difficult to gauge using available models.

Having developed a novel host that facilitates in vivo studies with *P. falciparum* [31, 32] – the *Pf*- NSG model grafted with human erythrocytes (huRBC), which allows high, long-lasting *P. falciparum* loads – we systematically assessed the resilience of *P. falciparum* in the face of defined ART exposure in vivo and characterized the resulting phenotype, particularly the drug-sensitivity profile, using both in vivo and in vitro methods concurrently.

We saw a remarkably rapid selection of very high-grade, stable resistance to ART with a delayed shift in IC_{50}. Remarkably, despite exclusive exposure of the parasite to AS, strong co-resistance to quinine also developed in the same strain. Once again, *P. falciparum* has demonstrated its adaptability and proven its rank as one of humanity's greatest challenges.

Methods
Mice

Four- to six-week-old male and female NOD/SCID IL-2Rγ$^{-/-}$ (NSG) mice (Charles River, France) were housed in sterile isolators and supplied autoclaved tap water with a γ-irradiated pelleted diet ad libitum. They were manipulated under pathogen-free conditions using a laminar-flux hood.

Human erythrocytes (huRBC)

HuRBC were used as host-cells for all in vitro and in vivo experiments. Packed huRBC were provided by the French Blood Bank (Etablissement Français du Sang, France) and taken from donors with no history of Malaria. HuRBC were suspended in SAGM (Saline, Adenine, Glucose, Mannitol solution) and kept at 4 °C for a maximum of 2 weeks. Before injection, huRBC were washed thrice in RPMI-1640 medium (Gibco-BRL, Grand Island, NY, USA) supplemented with 1 mg of hypoxanthine per liter (Sigma-Aldrich, St Louis, MO, USA) and warmed for 10 min to 37 °C.

P. falciparum parasites and culture

The *P. falciparum* Uganda Palo Alto Marburg strain (FUP/CB or PAM) was used for all experiments [33]. This pan-sensitive strain is used as a laboratory reference for antimalarial assays [34, 35]. Over time, strains with different levels of ART-R were cryopreserved using the glycerol/sorbitol method as described [36]. Parasites were cultured in vitro with 5% hematocrit, at 37 °C with 5% CO_2, using RPMI-1640 medium (Gibco-BRL) with 35 mM HEPES (Sigma-Aldrich), 24 mM $NaHCO_3$, 10% albumax (Gibco-BRL), and 1 mg/L of hypoxanthine (Sigma-Aldrich). When required, cultures were synchronized by either plasmagel (Roger Bellon, Neuilly-sur-Seine, France) flotation [37] or exposure to 5% sorbitol (Sigma-Aldrich) [38]. At regular intervals, cultures were tested for *Mycoplasma* contamination using PCR.

In vivo replication of P. falciparum in the NSG-IV model

P. falciparum was maintained in huRBC grafted in NSG immunocompromised mice undergoing additional modulation of innate defenses using clodronate-containing liposomes, as described previously [31, 32] ('*Pf*-NSG' model). The proportion of huRBC in mouse blood (chimerism) was measured during experiments every 6 ± 4.5 days (mean ± standard deviation (SD)) by flow cytometry (Facscalibur, BD Biosciences, Franklin Lakes, NJ, USA) using a FITC-labeled anti-human glycophorin monoclonal antibody (Dako, Denmark). Human erythrocytes were found to constitute 77.4% ± 19.9% (mean ± SD) of erythrocytes in mouse blood during periods of drug pressure. Mice were inoculated intravenously with 300 μL of 1% non-synchronized *P. falciparum*-infected huRBC. Follow-up of infection was performed by daily Giemsa-stained thin blood films drawn from the tail vein. In this paper, we report parasitemia as a percentage of all erythrocytes found in mouse peripheral blood; the true percentage of huRBC parasitized in the mice is higher, proportional to the level of chimerism, because murine erythrocytes cannot be infected but were included in counts.

Estimates of the total parasite biomass in each mouse were calculated based on the mean corpuscular volume of mouse erythrocytes (45 fL), the mean corpuscular volume of huRBC (86 fL), hematocrit in the mice of 0.7, weight of NSG mice (25 g), and a conservative estimate of 5.5 mL of blood per 100 g of mouse weight using the following equation:

$$\text{Number of infected RBC} = \frac{(0.055 \text{ mL/g})(25 \text{ g})(0.7)}{[86 \text{ fL} + (\text{mouse}_{\text{Chimerism}}/\text{human}_{\text{Chimerism}})45 \text{ fL}]} \times (\text{huRBC parasitemia})$$

In vivo induction of drug resistance

Mice were initially infected with drug-naïve parasites from in vitro culture of cryopreserved stabilates and subsequently put under discontinuous sub-therapeutic AS drug pressure. Sodium AS (a gift from Sigma-Tau, Italy) was dissolved in 10% dimethyl sulfoxide (DMSO) in RPMI-1640 (stock solution 30 mg/mL) each day of injection, then diluted 10-fold in RPMI-1640, sterilized through a 0.22 μm Millex filter (Millipore, MA, USA), further diluted in sterile RPMI-1640 as appropriate, and delivered intravenously via the retro-orbital sinus.

For the single-dose protocol, one dose of AS (ranging from 2.4 mg/kg to 240 mg/kg) was given, then parasitemia was monitored every 24 h and allowed to recover back to pre-treatment levels (AS pressure cycle; APC) before a further dose of AS was administered. For the 2-day protocol, two doses of AS (starting at 2.4 mg/kg/injection up to 80 mg/kg/injection) were delivered 24 h apart, then parasitemia was monitored every 24 h and was allowed to recover back to pre-treatment levels (APC) before a further two doses of AS were given (i.e., for a 2-day dose of 2.4 mg/kg, the mouse was injected with a total of 4.8 mg/kg AS per APC). The length of APC varied from case to case. When parasitemia failed to drop significantly (see below) after exposure to a given dose, the concentration was increased. The parasite strain used for the 2-day protocol had already developed resistance to a single dose of 30 mg/kg AS, and was then subjected to the 2-day regimen starting at 2.4 mg/kg/injection. Parasite strains were named ART-R_x, where x is the dose of AS (in mg/kg) to which resistance was established in that strain.

To determine what should be considered a significant drop in parasitemia, the normal day-to-day fluctuation of parasitemia was calculated from 13 non-drug-exposed NSG-IV mice (geometric mean of variability ± 18.3%, 95% confidence interval (CI) 12.5–27%). Taken from this, the parasite was deemed to be resistant to a given dose when parasitemia failed to drop more than 27% by the next day (all reported measures of parasite reduction are from the day after drug administration). We analyzed the drop in parasitemia seen among five mice infected with the PAM-sensitive strain the day after a single administration of intravenous AS to define a 'sensitive response' to AS in this model. The mean reduction was 78.4% with a SD of 18.2%. We conservatively chose a drop in parasitemia greater than 60.2%, corresponding to the mean (1 SD) as the definition of a sensitive response to guide decisions about dosing. For definitive statistical comparisons of parasitemia responses, a paired *t* test was used. Stability of resistance was determined when required by re-challenging the parasite strain in its new host with the dose of drug to which it had last shown resistance. The ART-R *P. falciparum* strain was continuously perpetuated in vivo by sub-inoculation directly from one mouse to another by the intravenous route, except where otherwise indicated.

In vitro drug sensitivity assays

The primary technique used to determine IC_{50} was the double-site enzyme-linked pLDH immunodetection assay, as previously described [39]. The ^{3}H-hypoxanthine isotopic method [40] was used as a secondary confirmatory assay. All in vitro results shown below come from the double-site enzyme-linked pLDH immunodetection assay.

For both methods, *P. falciparum* parasites at 0.05% parasitemia, synchronized at ring stage, were incubated at 2% hematocrit in 96-well microtiter plates (Nunc, Sigma-Aldrich) with serial dilutions of various anti-malarial drugs in 200 μL of complete culture medium at 37 °C and 5% CO_2 for 72 h. Non-drug-exposed wells were used as positive controls, and wells containing non-infected huRBC served as negative controls.

Stock solutions of the drugs (5 mL,1.5 mg/mL) were prepared by dissolving sodium AS (gift from Sigma-Tau), chloroquine sulphate (Rhone-Poulenc-Rorer, Vitry, France), dihydroartemisinin (DHA; Sigma-Tau), pyrimethamine (ICN Biochemicals, Aurora, Ohio), quinine hydrochloride (Sanofi, Montpellier, France), lumefantrine (Sigma-Aldrich), and mefloquine hydrochloride (Hoffman-La Roche, Basel, Switzerland) in 10% DMSO in RPMI-1640, whereas amodiaquine dihydrochloride and halofantrine hydrochloride were dissolved in 30% DMSO in RPMI-1640. Drug solutions were diluted 10-fold in RPMI-1640, sterilized by filtration through a 0.22 μM filter, and serially diluted in a 96-well incubation plate.

IC_{50} values were determined by performing a four-parameters, variable slope, non-linear regression analysis taking the least-squares fit without constraints, using Graph Pad Prism 6 software. Comparison of IC_{50} values and hillslopes was performed using the extra sum-of-squares F test (GraphPad, Inc., CA, USA).

In vivo co-resistance studies

Mice infected with the ART-R_{240} strain were given either single treatments or combinations of the following regimens: three doses of quinine hydrochloride 73 mg/kg every 8 h intravenously, four doses of halofantrine hydrochloride 1 mg/kg every 24 h intravenously, one dose of amodiaquine dihydrochloride 73 mg/kg orally (delivered by oro-gastric canula), one dose of chloroquine sulphate 73 mg/kg orally, or one dose of mefloquine hydrochloride

50 mg/kg intra-peritoneally, as previously described [41]. Stock solutions were made by dissolving 150 mg of quinine, chloroquine, and mefloquine in 5 mL of 10% DMSO, 150 mg of amodiaquine in 30% DMSO, and 60 mg of halofantrine in 30% DMSO, then dissolved 10-fold in RPMI-1640, and sterilized by filtration before being made up to the final concentration.

Determination of mouse plasma drug concentrations

Plasma concentrations of AS and DHA in blood samples (40–60 μL) collected from the retro-orbital sinus in four mice at 1, 2, and 4 h post intravenous drug administration were determined by reversed phase liquid chromatography coupled to tandem mass spectrometry (LC-MS/MS) using an adaptation of the previously described method [42]. Murine plasma was purified by protein precipitation with acetonitrile, evaporation, and reconstitution in 10 mM ammonium formate/methanol (1:1) adjusted to pH 3.9 with formic acid. Separations were done on a 2.1 mm × 50 mm Atlantis dC18 3 μm analytical column (Waters, Milford, MA, USA). The chromatographic system (CTC Analytics AG, Zwingen, Switzerland) was coupled to a triple stage quadrupole Thermo Quantum Discovery Max mass spectrometer equipped with an electrospray ionization interface (Thermo Fischer Scientific Inc., Waltham, MA, USA). The selected mass transitions were m/z 221.1 → 163.1, with a collision energy of 14 eV for AS and DHA, and m/z 226.2 → 168.1, with a collision energy of 20 eV for the stable isotope-labeled internal standard DHA-^{13}CD$_4$. Inter-assay precision obtained with plasma QC samples at 30, 300, and 3000 ng/mL of DHA and AS were 1.3, 2.1, 11.3%, and 7.3, 4.7, and 10.8%, respectively. Mean absolute deviation from nominal values of QC samples (30, 300, and 3000 ng/mL) during the analysis were 5.4, 5.9, and 1.3% and 3.8, 9.7, and 2.1%, for DHA and AS, respectively. The lower limit of quantification was 2 ng/mL. The laboratory participates in the External Quality Control program for anti-malarial drugs (http://www.wwarn.org/).

Restriction fragment length polymorphism

ART-R *P. falciparum* DNA was isolated from parasitized blood using QIAamp DNA mini kit (Qiagen, Limburg, Netherlands). A non-synonymous point mutation of *ubp1* in *P. chabaudi* (PCHAS020720) was reported by others [43] as being a marker of ART resistance in a rodent model. The orthologous gene in *P. falciparum* (PF3D7_0104300) is conserved and was amplified using the primers (500 nM) forward: 5'-TACAGGCTTTATAT AGTACAGTGTC-3', reverse: 5'-TTTTCGTTCGTACT TATAGGCACAGG-3', and AmpliTaq DNA Polymerase (1 U) (Hoffman-La Roche). The 451 bp PCR fragment was purified using the QIAquick PCR purification kit (Qiagen).

Polymorphisms in PF3D7_0104300 were assessed by digesting the PCR fragment with the restriction enzymes Mae III for V3275F and Rsa I for V3306F, corresponding to V2697F and V2728F in PCHAS 020720, respectively.

Genetic sequencing

Genes of interest in *P. falciparum* coding for the proteins RAD5, cNBP, RPB9, PK7, FP2A, Pfg27, Pfcrt, and Pfnhe, two fragments overlapping the kelch-13 propeller domain [44–46], and *Pfmdr1* gene were analyzed by PCR-sequencing. Primers used for *Pfmdr1* PCR and sequencing were previously described by Basco and Ringwald [47], and *Pfmdr1* gene copy analysis was performed as previously described [48]. For Pfnhe, two primer couples were designed for nested PCR on the basis of the 3D7 sequence. Control samples were taken from in vitro cultures of the *P. falciparum* 3D7 strain, and the sensitive progenitor PAM strain prior to any ART exposure (PAMwt); for the RAD5 experiment, additional control clinical isolates collected in the late 1990s were used from Brazil, Comoro Islands, Senegal, and Thailand. Experimental samples were recovered from *P. falciparum*-infected mice at various points during the ART resistance induction process (NSG415, 416, 424, 433, and 440). Genomic DNA was prepared using QIAamp DNA mini kit (Qiagen), according to the manufacturer's instructions, in 50 μL of Milli-Q water; 1 μL of DNA was PCR-amplified with 500 nM of the corresponding forward and reverse primers (Additional file 1), 0.8 mM dNTPs, 1.5 mM $MgCl_2$, 2.5 U *Taq* DNA polymerase (Hoffman-La Roche) in a volume of 50 μL with the following cycling program: 2 min at 94 °C, 30 cycles of 15 s at 94 °C, 30 s at 57 °C, 45 s at 72 °C, and a final extension of 2 min at 72 °C. The total contents of the reaction were electrophoresed on a 1% agarose gel and stained with ethidium bromide. The amplicons were extracted from the gel using the QIAquick° gel extraction kit (Qiagen). Concentration of the amplicons was measured by NanoDrop (Thermo Fischer Scientific Inc.) at 260 nm wavelength before sequencing of both strands was performed (Plateforme de séquençage, Institut Cochin, Paris/Eurofins MWG Operon). Sequences were analyzed with DNAstar software (DNAStar, Madison, WI, USA).

Results

Determination of the lowest effective dose (LED) for ART-sensitive progenitors

We infected seven mice with the PAM *P. falciparum* strain before any drug exposure to determine the LED. Single doses of 0.6, 0.3, and 0.15 mg/kg AS each caused a significant drop in parasitemia (> 27%, i.e., the upper 95% CI of normal fluctuation). Since 0.075 mg/kg AS failed to reduce parasitemia beyond normal day-to-day fluctuations, a single dose of 0.15 mg/kg AS (0.00375 mg AS/

mouse) was established as the LED in this model (Fig. 1). Effective doses of AS produced pyknotic parasites as seen in humans (Additional file 2).

Rapid induction of high level ART resistance in *P. falciparum*

We applied intense, discontinuous, sub-curative AS drug pressure in vivo to high *P. falciparum* parasitemia in NSG mice using the intravenous route. After each drug exposure, parasitemia was allowed to recuperate back to pre-treatment levels (APC) and, once resistance was established, the AS dose was increased (Fig. 2 and Additional file 3). For the single-dose regimen, the median APC length was 4 days (range 2–14 days).

During the single-dose regimen, after pre-conditioning of the drug-naïve parasites with 3 single doses of AS in one mouse, we passed the parasite line through 7 generations of mice by sub-inoculation, using 5, 9, 6, 1, 6, 10, and 6 mice in each generation, respectively (total 43).

In the first generation, we let parasites multiply to high parasitemias (25–35%) creating a pool of ~ 1.3×10^{10} *P. falciparum*-infected erythrocytes. We saw resistance to 2.4 mg/kg AS after 3 APC in 1 out of 4 mice exposed to that dose, then to 3.3 mg/kg AS after 2 APCs in 1 out of 3 mice, and to 4 mg/kg AS in 2 out of 2 mice exposed to a mean 1.5 APC.

In the second generation, resistance to 3.3 mg/kg was established in another mouse (1 APC), and to 4 mg/kg in 2 further mice (mean 1.5 APC, range 1–2). Later, we confirmed 4 mg/kg resistance in a new host. Seeing as resistance was so forthcoming, we increased drug pressure readily to 15 mg/kg AS, to which indeed 4 out of 5 mice exposed became resistant (mean 5 APC, range 2–9) (Additional file 4).

Resistance to 30 mg/kg AS then emerged in 2 out of 4 mice exposed to that dose (mean 1.5 APC, range 1–2). However, it was not stable and, in the third generation, an average of 3.6 APC (range 2–5) was required before it was re-established (ART-R_{30}). Subsequently, in 1 mouse, after applying variable-intensity drug pressure, resistance to 60 mg/kg AS was obtained (5 APC).

We confirmed the stability of resistance to 60 mg/kg AS (ART-R_{60}) immediately after sub-inoculation into the fourth generation, and after just three further exposures to 120 mg/kg AS, the strain showed the first signs of resistance to that dose.

In the fifth generation, we observed resistance to 120 mg/kg AS (ART-R_{120}) in all 4 mice exposed after an average of 3 APC (range 2–4). Then, in 1 mouse, the parasite went on to develop resistance against 240 mg/kg AS after 4 APC (78, 44, 60, and 13% reduction in parasitemia seen with each APC, respectively).

After sub-inoculation into the sixth generation, the parasite strain established resistance to 240 mg/kg AS in 4 out of 6 mice exposed to that dose (2.75 APC, 1–7).

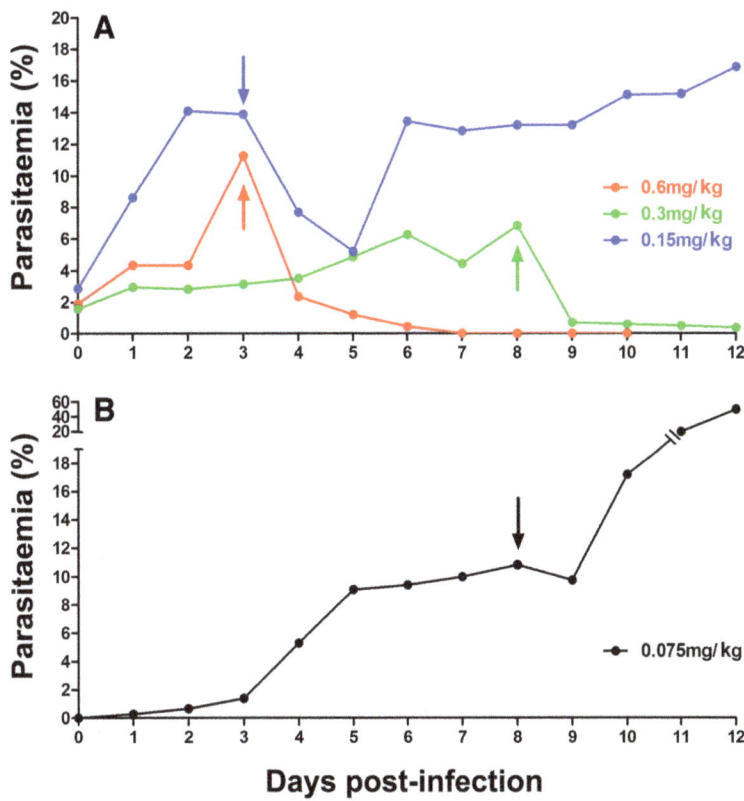

Fig. 1 Determination of the lowest effective dose (LED). Parasitemia trends from individual NSG mice that each received a unique dose of (**a**) 0.6 mg/kg, 0.3 mg/kg, 0.15 mg/kg, or (**b**) 0.075 mg/kg of artesunate (AS) are shown. We infected mice with the Uganda Palo Alto Marburg (FUP/ CB or PAM) progenitor strain before it was subjected to any drug pressure. Arrows indicate day of intravenous drug delivery. In panel **a**, day 0 represents the fourth day post-inoculation of mice. Results were reproducible in several mice treated at each dose

In the seventh generation, resistance was immediately stable, after sub-inoculation, to 240 mg/kg AS in all 6 mice (ART-R$_{240}$) (mean ± SD percentage drop in parasitemia of sensitive control 78.4% ± 18.2% vs. ART-R$_{240}$ 9.1% ± 6.3%; p = 0.0002).

Since further dose doubling would exceed the lethal dose for 50% of mice [41, 49], 240 mg/kg was the highest dose administered. We used NSG mice infected with the sensitive progenitor PAM strain as controls, and all treatments using the above doses were found effective. This represents a 3200-fold decrease in in vivo AS sensitivity, occurring within 51 APC over a 45-week period (Table 1, Additional file 2, Additional file 3, and Additional file 5). Further, we observed gametocytes in thin blood smears from mice infected with parasites expressing the ART-R phenotype (Additional file 6).

Induction of resistance to a 2-day regimen
Two doses of the same AS concentration administered 24 h apart – a double dose (DD) – caused a significant reduction in parasitemia in animals in which a single dose of the same concentration had failed.

We started with a concentration of 2.4 mg/kg/dose for the DD regimen using a parasite strain already resistant to a single dose of 30 mg/kg AS. The ART-R$_{30}$ strain became resistant to DD 2.4 mg/kg AS after just 1 APC. We passed the parasite line through four generations of mice with 6, 8, 3, and 4 mice in each generation, respectively. Once resistance was seen, we increased the dose concentration 2-fold, until reproducible resistance to DD 80 mg/kg AS (i.e., 160 mg/kg total) was achieved (ART-R$_{DD80}$) (Fig. 3, Additional file 7, and Additional file 8) (mean ± SD percentage drop parasitemia of sensitive control 95.9% ± 5.7% vs. ART-R$_{DD80}$ 25.7% ± 0.6%; p = 0.03).

It was possible to select for resistance to the highest dose used in 41% of the mice that survived the 2-day protocol, in contrast with 80% of mice that underwent the single-dose protocol (Table 2).

Verification of DHA concentration in mouse plasma
We measured levels of AS and DHA at 1 and 2 h post injection of 120 mg/kg AS in four ART-R$_{120}$-infected mice (Additional file 9). Serum concentrations of DHA at 1 h were 3159, 3219, 1573, and 2423 ng/mL in each

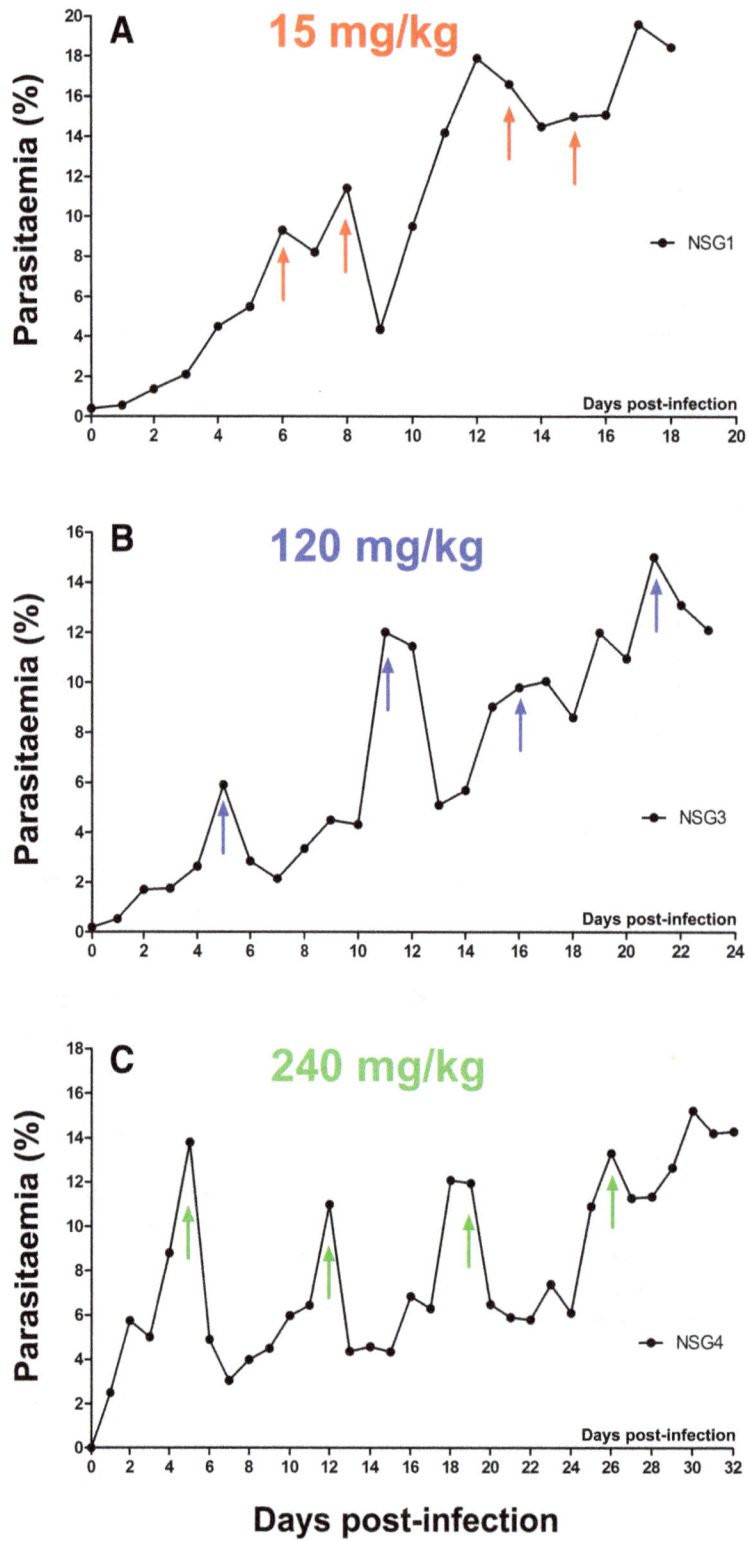

Fig. 2 Examples of selection for single-dose artemisinin resistance. Demonstrative parasitemia trends as seen at different time points during the resistance-selection process are shown from mice that received single flash doses of (**a**) 15 mg/kg, (**b**) 120 mg/kg, or (**c**) 240 mg/kg artesunate. Arrows indicate day of intravenous drug delivery. Results were reproduced in several mice as indicated in Table 1 and Table S2A

Table 1 Number of artesunate pressure cycles (APC) used to select for single-dose resistance in individual mice

Dose of Artesunate (mg/kg)	2.4	3.3	4	15	30	60	120	240
Number of APC required to reach resistance	3	2	2, 3, 1, 2, 1	3, 9, 6, 2	1, 2, 4, 5, 3, 4, 2	5, 1	3, 3, 4, 2, 3, 3, 2, 2, 2, 2, 2	4, 1, 7, 1, 2, 1, 2, 1, 1, 1, 1
Number of mice with resistance/total attempted	1/4	1/3	5/5	4/5	7/8	2/2	11/11	11/15

The number of artesunate pressure cycles (APC) after which resistance was seen to a given dose in individual mice is tabulated. The proportion of mice with parasites that evolved resistance can be seen to increase as the resistance strengthened, and as 'fitter' parasites were selected out by successive sub-inoculations, until the maximum dose was reached. A full account of the selection process and evolution of ART-R for the single and 2-day regimens can be found in the supplementary information (Additional files 1, 2, 5 and 8)

mouse, respectively, and we confirmed resistance to these levels on blood films drawn the following day. The mean $t_{1/2}$ of DHA in the infected NSG-IV model was 36 min (range 20.9–53.2 min).

Stability of the ART-resistant phenotype
Stability was assessed in three different manners:

Transmission to new animals: The parasite was found to maintain stable AS resistance after sub-inoculation into fresh mice for 60 mg/kg AS in 1 out of 1 mouse, 120 mg/kg AS in 5 out of 11 mice, and 240 mg/kg AS in 6 out of 6 mice (Additional file 3).
Cryopreservation and in vitro growth: At various points, parasites resistant to a given AS concentration were cryopreserved and stored for 1–6 months, thawed, and then cultured in vitro for 8 to 12 days. After inoculation of cultured parasites into new mice, the ART-R$_{30}$, ART-R$_{120}$, and ART-R$_{240}$ strains maintained their pre-freezing resistant phenotype (Fig. 4a, b).
Prolonged in vivo replication in the absence of drug pressure: We infected three mice with the ART-R$_{120}$ strain, and confirmed resistance by administration of 120 mg/kg AS. The parasites were then allowed to grow in vivo without any drug pressure for 1 month. Upon re-treatment of the two surviving mice with 120 mg/kg AS, they both showed the same resistant response as had been seen 1 month prior (mean ± SD percentage drop in parasitemia, start: 10% ± 14.1% vs. end: 8.4% ± 11.8%; $p = 0.94$). The in vitro response also remained unchanged (IC$_{50}$ AS: F = 0.03, $p = 0.87$; IC$_{50}$ DHA: F = 1.1, $p = 0.3$) (Fig. 4c, d).

In vitro drug sensitivity profiles of ART-R parasites show a two-step pattern
We monitored 50% IC$_{50}$ values over the course of resistance development for both single-dose and 2-day regimens, and compared them to the sensitive progenitor.

The initial IC$_{50}$ (95% CI) values for the sensitive strain to AS and DHA were 10.7 nM (10.2–11.2) and 13.8 nM (12.9–14.6), respectively. The ART-R$_{30}$ strain did not show any increase in IC$_{50}$ for AS (11.5 nM (6.6–16.9); F = 0.525, $p = 0.47$); however, there was a significant change in the slope of the curve compared to the sensitive control

(hillslope – 4.4 (–6 to –3.6) vs. – 1.9 (–6.4 to –0.8); F = 7.5, $p = 0.008$). It was not until the strain became resistant to 120 mg/kg AS in vivo that the IC$_{50}$ rose sharply for both AS (to 82.5 nM (69.5–95.8); F = 191.3, $p < 0.0001$) and DHA (to 54.6 nM (51.6–57.6); F = 300.3, $p < 0.0001$). The ART-R$_{240}$ strain reached an IC$_{50}$ of 100.3 nM (92.9–118.4) (F = 304.8, $p < 0.0001$) for AS.

In parasites submitted to a 2-day regimen, we saw the same pattern, with a delayed shift in IC$_{50}$ (Fig. 5 and Additional file 10).

ART-R parasites are also resistant to quinine, amodiaquine, and halofantrine both in vivo and in vitro
Despite exclusive exposure to AS, the ART-R$_{240}$ parasite strain showed markedly decreased responses to quinine, amodiaquine, and halofantrine. Indeed, the IC$_{50}$ increased by 4.6-fold to quinine (49.7 nM (46.6–52.8) vs. 226.9 nM (145.8–392.1); F = 23.12, $p < 0.0001$), 3.8-fold to halofantrine (7.9 nM (7.3–8.6) vs. 30.4 nM (25.9–34.9); F = 159.3, $p < 0.0001$), and 11.7-fold to amodiaquine (11.3 nM (10.6–12.1) vs. 132.4 nM (5.5–149.3); F = 243.7, $p < 0.0001$); similarly, the DD ART-R$_{DD80}$ strain increased its IC$_{50}$ 2.1-fold to quinine (F = 98.9, $p < 0.0001$) and 4.5-fold to amodiaquine (F = 152.5, $p < 0.0001$). Sensitivities to chloroquine (50.1 nM (46.5–53.7) vs. 53 nM (42.7–68.3); F = 0.39, $p = 0.54$), mefloquine (41.7 nM (39.1–44.4) vs. 39.1 nM (34.1–44.5); F = 0.82, $p = 0.37$), lumefantrine (7.5 nM (6.3–8.7) vs. 7.8 nM (6.2–9.8); F = 0.13, $p = 0.72$), and pyrimethamine (16.2 nM (13.8–18.8) vs. 19.9 nM (16.5–24.6); F = 4.75, $p = 0.05$) remained unchanged (Fig. 6 and Additional file 10).

Since the model accommodates simultaneous in vitro and in vivo studies with *P. falciparum*, this pattern of in vitro co-resistance to main-stream anti-malarial drugs could also be analyzed in vivo (Fig. 7). Therapeutic doses of 219 mg/kg quinine did not induce any decrease in parasitemia in vivo using ART-R$_{240}$ strain ($n = 4$, mean ± SD percentage drop in parasitemia 4.8% ± 6.8%); the same dose was effective for the sensitive strain ($n = 2$, mean ± SD percentage drop in parasitemia 92.2% ± 0.01%; $p = 0.03$). In addition, we confirmed in vivo resistance to amodiaquine in 4 mice (mean ± SD percentage drop in parasitemia sensitive control 76.6% ± 5.2% vs. ART-R$_{240}$ 9.3% ± 0.14%; $p = 0.03$), and halofantrine in 3

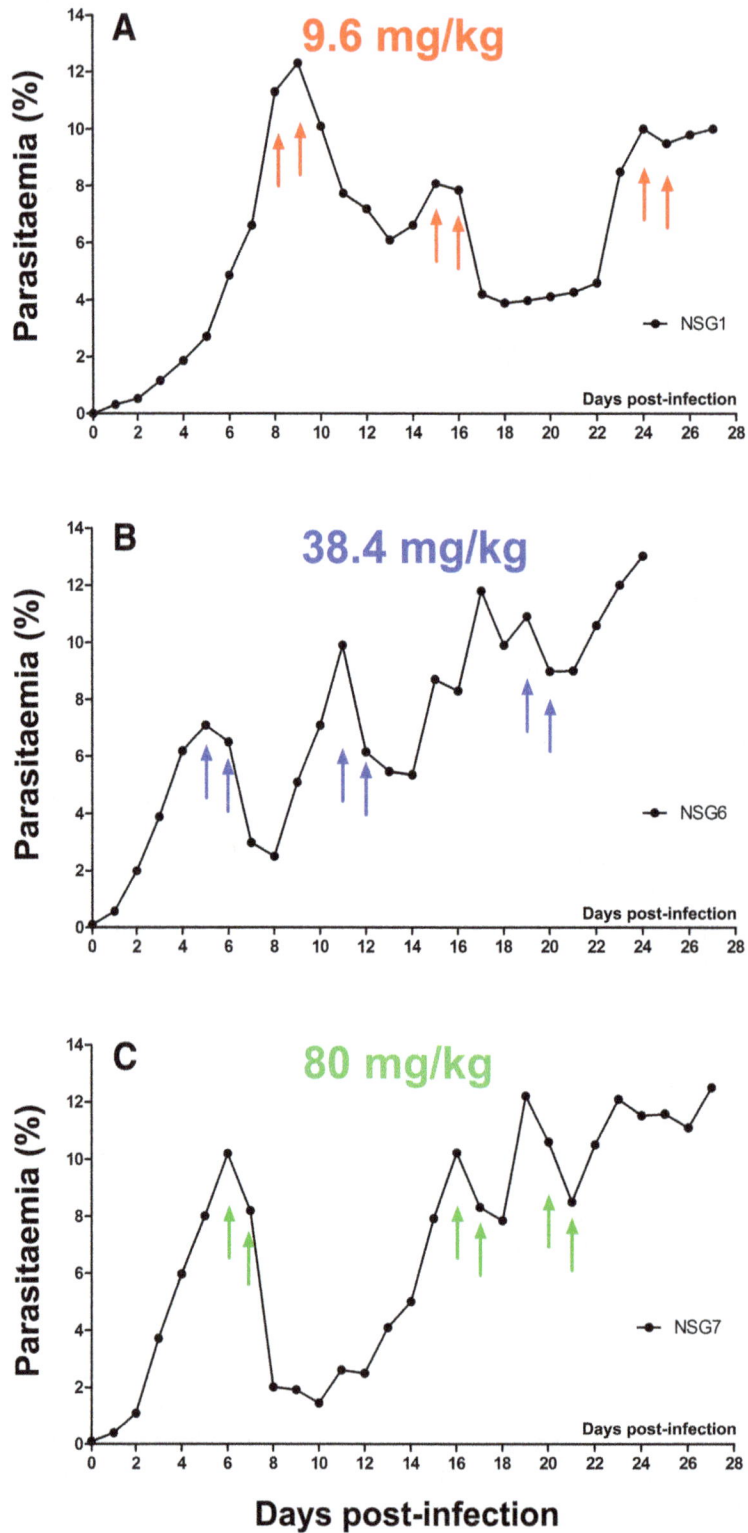

Fig. 3 Examples of selection for double-dose artemisinin resistance. Demonstrative parasitemia trends as seen at different time points during the resistance selection process are shown from mice that received a 2-day regimen comprising two doses 24 h apart of (**a**) 9.6 mg/kg, (**b**) 38.4 mg/kg, or (**c**) 80 mg/kg artesunate (i.e., total of 19.2 mg/kg, 86.8 mg/kg, or 160 mg/kg AS per APC). Arrows indicate day of intravenous drug delivery. Results were reproduced in several mice as indicated in Table S2B

Table 2 Number of mice used and outcome for both dosing regimens

	Total number of mice	Died before interpretable	Resistance seen against highest dose	Resistance not seen against highest dose
Single dose No.	43	8	28	7
%[a]			80%	20%
Double dose No.[b]	21	4	7	10
%[a]			41.2%	58.8%

[a]Percentages calculated excluding mice that died before significance
[b]Double dose regimen began using parasites resistant to single dose 30 mg/kg
The total number of mice used to select for resistance against both single and 2-day doses of artesunate across all dose concentrations, and the proportion of mice in which resistance emerged to the highest dose used, are tabulated. In instances where mice were sub-inoculated with the parasite strain but either died before receiving any drug treatment or died within 24 h of drug treatment (precluding meaningful measurement of their parasitemia), they were termed to have died before becoming experimentally interpretable. Parasites subjected to the 2-day regimen of artesunate were less likely to become resistant

mice (median, range percentage increase in parasitemia after 3 days of treatment 16.9%, 15.9–114.4%). Conversely, we observed in vivo susceptibility to treatment with mefloquine (2 mice, mean ± SD percentage drop in parasitemia 67.5% ± 7.8%; $p = 0.005$, compared to normal day-to-day fluctuation) and chloroquine (3 mice, mean ± SD percentage drop in parasitemia 73.3% ± 0.7%; $p < 0.001$, compared to normal day-to-day fluctuations).

We also addressed the in vivo response of ART-R$_{240}$ to two critical combinations in clinical use: AS plus amodiaquine was ineffective (mean ± SD percentage drop in parasitemia 13.1% ± 0.14% vs. 76.5% in the sensitive control), while AS plus mefloquine was effective (mean ± SD percentage drop in parasitemia 66.8% ± 33.6%; $p = 0.004$, compared to normal day-to-day fluctuations) (Fig. 7d, e).

Thus, in vivo findings mirrored the in vitro sensitivity profiles.

Molecular markers

Restriction fragment length polymorphism assessment of two putative polymorphisms, V3275F and V3306F, in the P. falciparum orthologue of the ubp1 gene revealed no such mutation in the ART-R$_{240}$, ART-R$_{DD38.4}$, or parent PAM strain.

Genetic sequencing of PF3D7_1343400 (RAD5 homolog) encoding a putative DNA-repair protein identified the non-synonymous a3392t SNP (MAL13–1718319) in all of the ART-R P. falciparum samples recovered from experimental mice, wherein they had shown resistance to single doses of 38.4 mg/kg, 120 mg/kg, and 240 mg/kg AS, and to a 2-day regimen of 80 mg/kg/day AS. This RAD5 mutation was not identified in the wild type progenitor PAM strain prior to undergoing ART exposure (PAMwt), nor in any of four control clinical P. falciparum isolates collected from Brazil, Senegal, Comoro Islands, and Thailand in the late 1990s. We did not identify any mutation of cNBP in the PAMwt control or ART-R parasites (Additional file 11).

Sequencing of the putative Kelch-13 propeller domain in PF3D7_1343700 (kelch-13) showed no difference between control (3D7, PAMwt) and ART-R strains; it revealed none of the 20 non-synonymous SNPs that have been reported from clinical isolates, nor the SNP identified in P. falciparum that evolved in vitro ART tolerance (M476I) after being cultured for 5 years under artemisinin pressure [45] (Additional file 11). None of the other non-synonymous SNPs in RPB9, PK7, FP2a, or Pfg27 reported in association with the in vitro ART tolerance seen in that strain were found either [45]. Sequencing of exon two of PfCRT revealed the rare CVIKT haplotype [50] linked to moderate resistance to chloroquine in agreement with the in vitro response (chloroquine IC$_{50}$ = 53 nM).

Pfmdr1 analysis showed a duplication of gene copy number from 1 to 2 copies, and acquisition of the N86Y mutation after in vivo artemisinin drug pressure. No sequence changes were found in the 611 bp PfNHE fragment gene, flanking the DNNND repeat, which is related to quinine resistance [51].

Discussion

Our results indicate that the P. falciparum human malaria parasite can evolve levels of resistance to ART that are much higher than the DPCT phenotype currently observed, and which could carry much graver consequences both for individual patients and global public health. The mechanisms of this stronger resistance are likely distinct from those underlying DPCT.

Progressive drug pressure in this model selected for high-level, stable resistance to ART in vivo rapidly and reproducibly. Parasites were characterized both in vivo and in vitro, yielding convergent data. The most concerning findings are (1) the degree of resistance selected for and (2) co-resistance to quinine, the only alternative for severe malaria. These results justify concerns about the potential of ART-R strengthening to insurmountable levels in patients, particularly if alternative treatments do not make it through the development pipeline fast enough to offset the prevailing ART drug pressure.

The Pf-NSG model – borne out of our malaria vaccine development project [31, 32] – includes a number of key

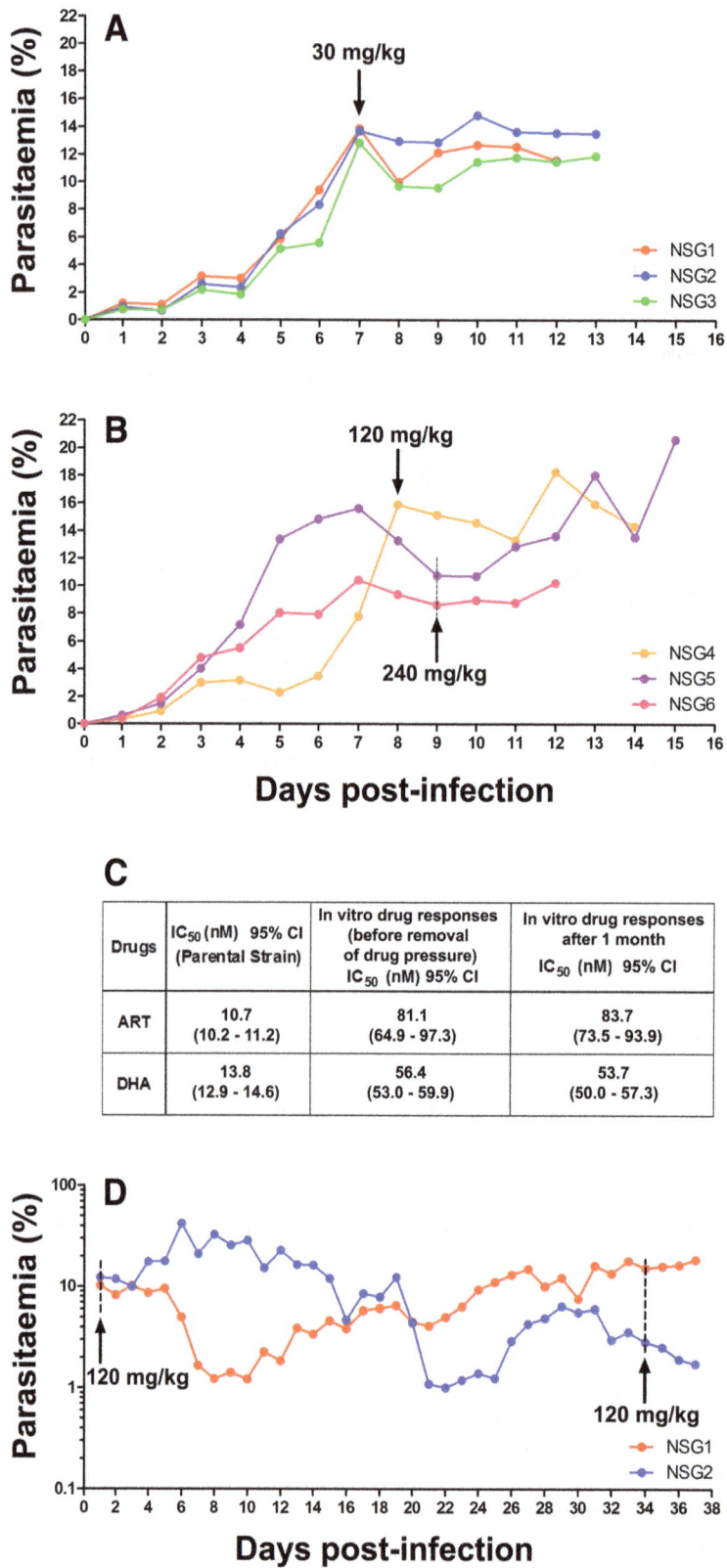

Fig. 4 (See legend on next page.)

(See figure on previous page.)

Fig. 4 Evidence for stability of artemisinin resistance. **a** Following cryopreservation of resistant parasites with unchanged IC_{50}: parasitemia trends from mice infected with the ART-R_{30} strain following cryopreservation and cultivation in vitro are shown. Arrows indicate day of re-challenge with 30 mg/kg AS. **b** Following cryopreservation of parasites with increased IC_{50}: parasitemia trends from animals infected with ART-R_{120} (orange) and ART-R_{240} (purple, pink) following cryopreservation and cultivation in vitro. Arrows indicate the day of re-challenge with either 120 or 240 mg/kg artesunate (AS). **c** In vitro response following in vivo replication without drug pressure: In vitro sensitivities for AS and dihydroartemisinin (DHA) measured for ART-R_{120} parasites grown ex vivo, that were sampled before and after 1 month of drug pressure-free in vivo replication (see **d**), are tabulated. **d** In vivo following drug free replication: We maintained the ART-R_{120} parasite in vivo for 4 weeks without drug pressure in three mice; parasitemia trends of the two mice that survived are shown (red, blue). Challenges performed before and after treatment with 120 mg/kg AS (arrows) show stability of the resistant phenotype. We employed a lower intensity huRBC grafting protocol for this experiment to increase mouse survival, which caused a drop in parasitemia in the interim

features that facilitated the selection of ART-R *P. falciparum*. Mice had parasite biomasses ranging from 2.5×10^9 to 3.8×10^9 per mouse, which is in the range seen in an uncomplicated human infection [52]. These parasites were exposed to AS and its bio-active metabolites (primarily DHA) under similar pharmacokinetics to human infection through metabolic factors that cannot be accounted for in vitro. Drug disposition in these mice (DHA $t_{\frac{1}{2}}$ of 36 min) is comparable to patients with malaria [53, 54]. While our drug administration protocol was designed to hasten the evolution of ART-R in vivo with single doses, it is not unrealistic to expect ART mono-therapy [55], poor treatment compliance [56, 57], and counterfeit products [58–60] to lead to similarly sub-therapeutic, resistance-selective dosing schedules in the field.

Notable differences between this model and human malaria are that both sexual recombination of parasite genes in the vector and effects of host immunity are by-passed through direct sub-inoculation between mice devoid of an adaptive immune system.

The model allowed us to exert progressive AS pressure, rapidly selecting for ART-R and to characterize resistant strains by their pattern of response to a range of antimalarial drugs in vivo and in vitro. Two stages could be distinguished during the evolution of ART-R. First, parasites showed substantial resistance to AS in vivo (up to absence of response to a single dose 30 mg/kg, i.e., 400-fold decrease in sensitivity) without an associated shift in IC_{50}. This discrepancy between early in vivo resistance and conventional in vitro assays fits with the DPCT pattern seen in humans [6, 7, 61–63], supporting the relevance of this model. It confirms that IC_{50} is not a reliable marker of ART-R.

The phenotype of the second stage of ART-R in this model is in stark contrast to the clinical manifestations of DPCT. This extreme phenotype is clearly different as (1) there is a complete absence of response to very high doses of intravenous AS (240 mg/kg, i.e., 3200-fold decrease in sensitivity), (2) a major shift in DHA-IC_{50} was demonstrated, and (3) the parasites demonstrated full co-resistance to quinine. The second stage was further characterized as having reproducible stability.

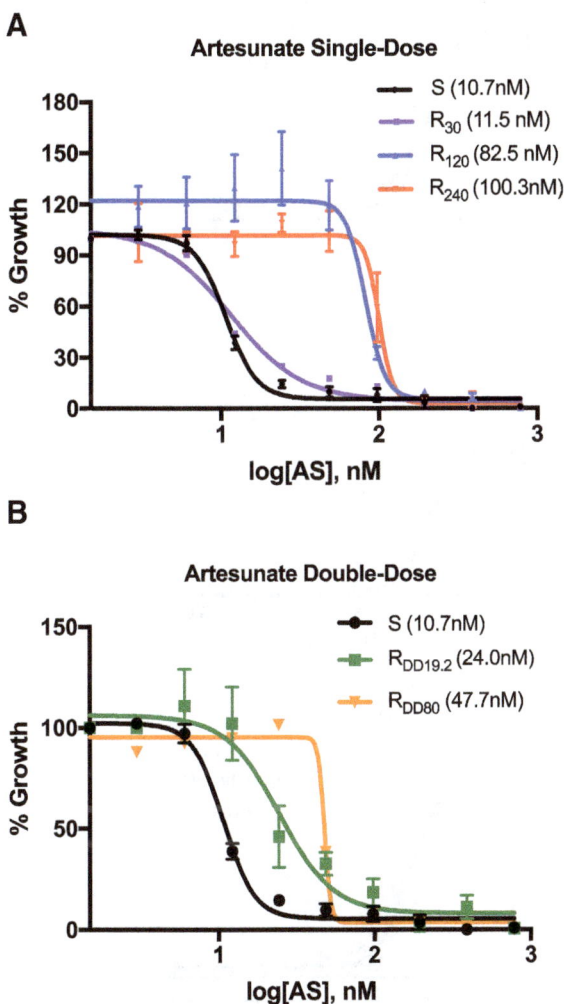

Fig. 5 In vitro artesunate sensitivities at different levels of in vivo resistance. In vitro artesunate (AS) dose–response curves, with SD error bars, are shown for parasites resistant in vivo to (**a**) single dose AS 30 mg/kg (purple), 120 mg/kg (blue), and 240 mg/kg (red) or (**b**) 2-day regimen AS 19.2 mg/kg/dose (green) and 80 mg/kg/dose (orange), and compared to the artemisinin-sensitive progenitor strain (black). Mean IC_{50} values (nM) are indicated in parentheses

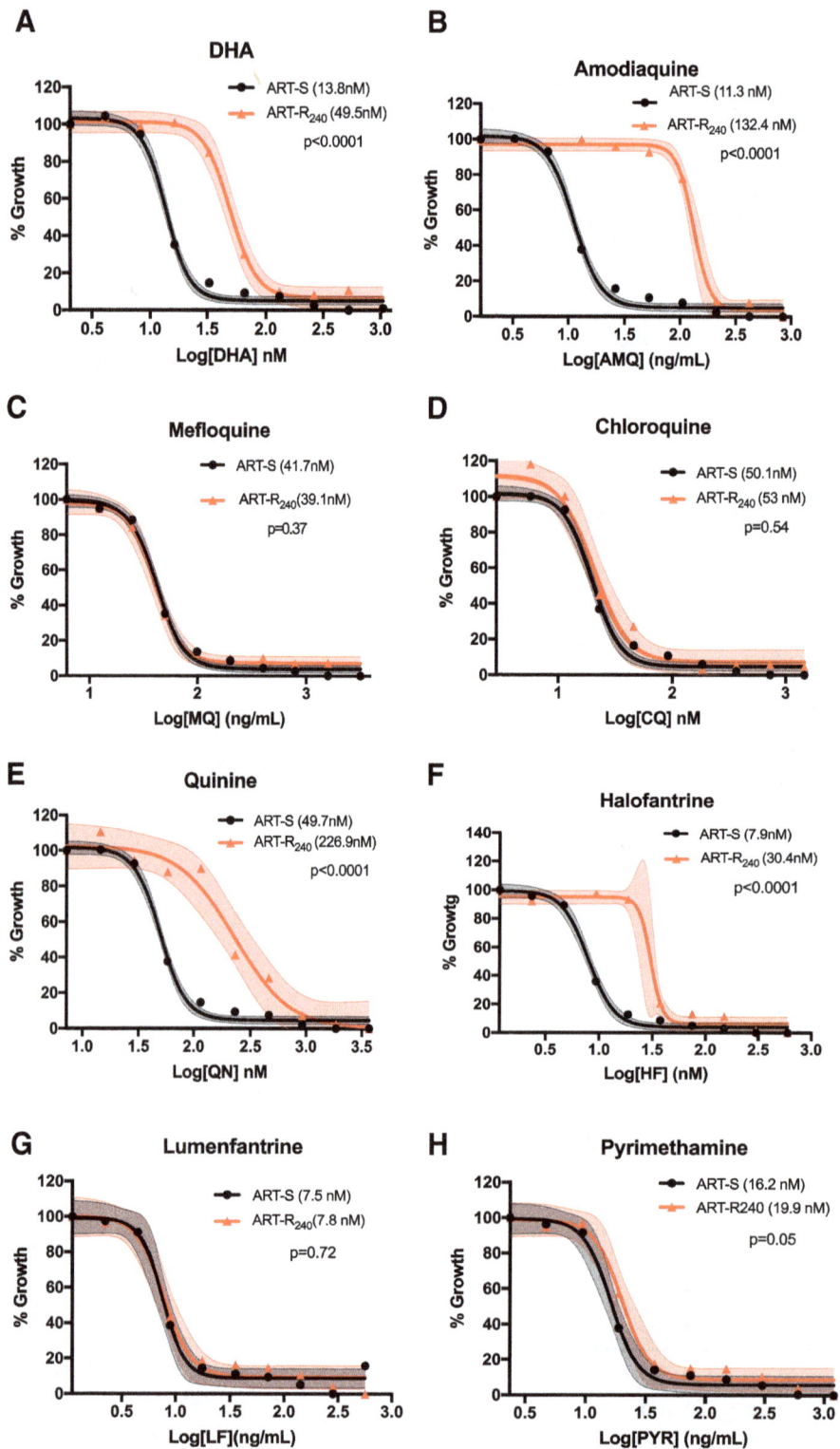

Fig. 6 In vitro drug sensitivity profile of the ART-R$_{240}$ strain. In vitro dose–response curves, with 95% CI error bands, of the ART-R$_{240}$ strain (red) to (**a**) dihydroartemisinin (DHA), (**b**) amodiaquine, (**c**) mefloquine, (**d**) chloroquine, (**e**) quinine, (**f**) halofantrine, (**g**) lumefantrine, and (**h**) pyrimethamine are shown and compared to the sensitive progenitor strain (ART-S) used as a control in each experiment (black). Results were reproducible in several independent experiments. Mean IC$_{50}$ values (nM) are indicated in parentheses. The probability (p) of these IC$_{50}$ values being from curves measured using the same strain of parasite, as determined by the extra sum-of-squares F test, are shown for each drug

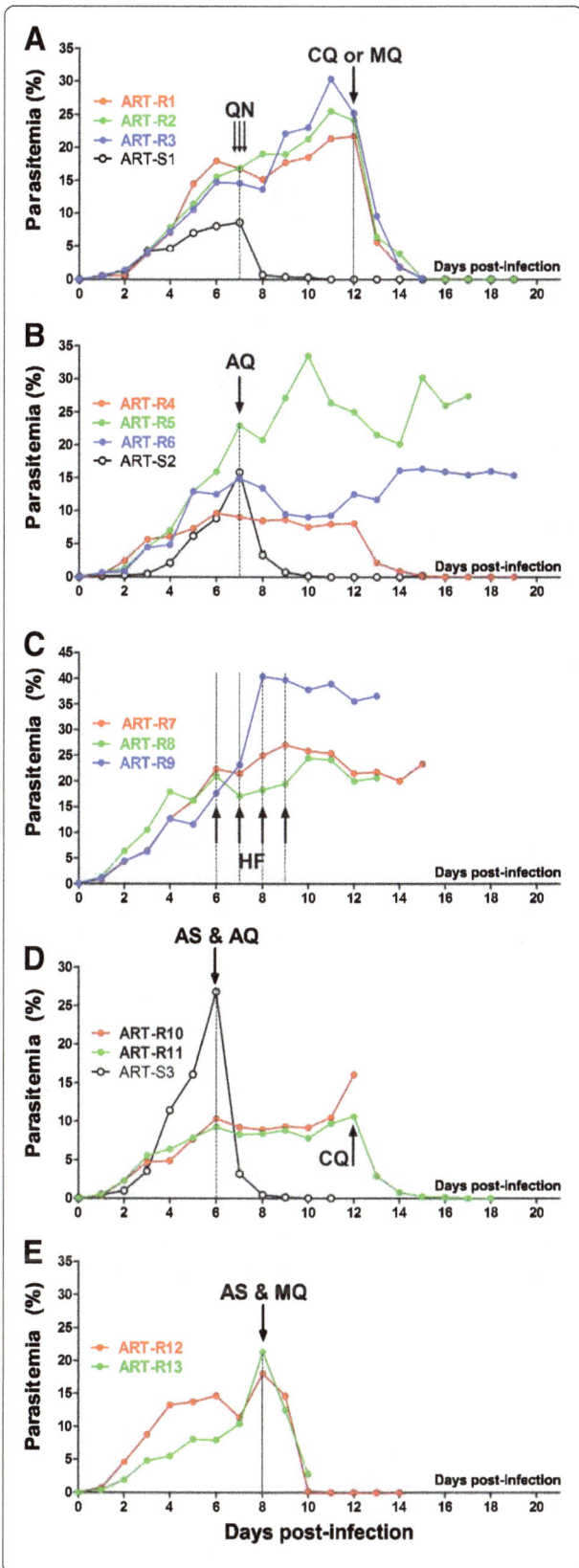

Fig. 7 In vivo co-resistance of ART-R$_{240}$ parasites to quinine, amodiaquine, and halofantrine. The ART-R$_{240}$ strain, which had shown various patterns of co-resistance to other anti-malarials in vitro, was assessed in vivo with the same compounds either alone or in combination with artesunate. **a** The ART-R$_{240}$ parasites showed full in vivo resistance to quinine (QN) 219 mg/kg (three doses of 73 mg/kg every 8 h IV). However, the same parasites in the same mice were sensitive to either chloroquine (CQ) (73 mg/kg PO) or mefloquine (MQ) (50 mg/kg i.p.). **b, c** In vivo resistance to amodiaquine (AQ) (73 mg/kg PO) and halofantrine (HF) (1 mg/kg IV per day, 4 consecutive days) confirmed in vitro indications. **d** As expected, resistance was seen to a combination of artesunate (AS) and amodiaquine (AQ), whereas parasites in the same animal remained susceptible to chloroquine. **e** Susceptibility to the artesunate-mefloquine combination was seen in keeping with in vitro results

Only two clinical cases of ART-R with increased DHA IC$_{50}$ (14.0 nM and 14.4 nM) have been reported [62]; the absolute increase of DHA IC$_{50}$ that we observed (99.9 nM) is far greater, confirming that it differs substantially from DPCT. We can expect that measuring conventional IC$_{50}$ in the field will continue to fail to unmask in vivo ART-R, even if resistance strengthens to considerably higher levels. The novel RSA could provide a more sensitive means for detecting the early emergence of ART-R, although it is technically challenging [29, 30]. As IC$_{50}$ did increase in our model, in contrast to the more moderately resistant parasites in the field, the need to perform RSA was less evident, although this could be of interest.

Not only is the degree of resistance achieved alarming, but also the ease with which ART-R selection occurred, specifically 80% of attempts with single-dose and 41% with 2-day treatments. The 2-day regimen was less efficient at inducing ART-R, the shift in IC$_{50}$ was lower, and co-resistance was less pronounced. This suggests that measures, such as intensified schedules, higher doses and improved compliance with anti-malarial therapy may retard the advancement of ART-R but, ultimately, are unlikely to be sufficient.

The most burning question that remains is, what point along the road to stable, high-level ART-R, as seen in this model, are we currently witnessing in humans? AS is administered at 4 mg/kg/day for uncomplicated malaria as part of a 3-day ACT course. In areas where ART-R has emerged in humans, the percentage parasite reduction rate after 24 h in patient's blood after drug treatment has decreased only modestly, from 99% to 85–91% [64]. We selected for a strain that showed no significant drop in parasitemia at 24 h (i.e., percentage parasite reduction rate after 24 h, 0–27%) after exposure to the human dose of 4 mg/kg AS. This full-resistance phenotype was maintained throughout a step-wise strengthening of the dose up to 240 mg/kg AS, leaving a frightening margin for increase in resistance in the field.

Thus, if wild parasites evolve along the same trajectory as observed in our *P. falciparum* experimental model, we are currently only seeing the tip of the iceberg in the clinic. The absence of adaptive immunity and reduced innate immunity in these mice makes it difficult to extrapolate our findings to human hosts, particularly the speed at which similar resistance may arise.

In the search for a molecular surveillance marker, genetic studies of well-defined clinical isolates from Southeast Asia have demonstrated an association between the DPCT phenotype and non-synonymous mutations of the propeller region in *kelch-13* [10, 11, 45, 46, 65, 66] and, to a lesser extent, an SNP in *RAD5*, which ranked first in one GWAS [44] and fourth in a meta-analysis of relevant GWAS [46]. In a recent GWAS from the China-Myanmar border, *RAD5* was significantly associated with ART-R, while *kelch-13* was not flagged at all [24]. In our highly ART-R strains we found no *kelch-13* mutation; conversely, we found selection of the exact same *RAD5* SNP identified in clinical samples [44, 46]. A limitation is that we refrained from performing whole genome sequencing, which would likely reveal numerous mutations, the roles of which would require lengthy investigation and could be the focus of future studies.

The significance of the many *kelch-13* mutations is not as straightforward as was once thought [67]. In the original Southeast Asia focus of ART-R, approximately 30 different SNPs have been found in *kelch-13*, circa 20 of which are in the paddle region. Mutations in this region have been confirmed by four distinct GWAS to be significantly associated with DPCT in Southeast Asian parasites [26, 44, 46, 68]. However, a substantial number of isolates with the same mutations (in the locations with high DPCT prevalence) showed no sign of delayed clearance and, perhaps more importantly, a number of isolates with the wild type genotype showed DPCT [10, 45]. Data from Africa are even more puzzling – in the absence of any clear DPCT phenotype, an unexpectedly large number of *kelch-13* propeller SNPs were found in parasites from 14 African sites, some at high frequency; 15 of these 24 SNPs were novel, but 3 have previously been associated with DPCT in Southeast Asia [69]. Thus, we are now faced with a number *of kelch-13* mutant alleles of uncertain clinical significance. On the other hand, SNPs in *RAD5* are extremely rare outside Asia [70], yet one was selected for in our parasites of African origin under ART pressure.

Our results add a further layer of complexity, showing that far stronger ART-R can exist in *P. falciparum* without *kelch-13* propeller domain mutations, implying that other ART-R genes or mechanisms exist and will need to be characterized. The two strains and the novel in vivo model we developed provide the tools to do so. In practical terms, ART-R should no longer be considered excluded just because there is an absence of *kelch-13* mutations. This has important consequences for ART-R surveillance in Africa.

Our results are in keeping with a recent study that relates ART-R to an interaction of dihydroartemisinin with phosphatidylinositol-3-phosphate kinase, and indicates that elevated phosphatidyl-inositol-3 phosphate can be associated with resistance in the absence of *kelch-13* mutations [71]. *kelch-13* is not a direct target of ART [27, 28]. Indirect effects of *kelch-13* mutations on phosphatidyl-inositol-3 phosphate and glutathione may counteract ART [28], but it is unlikely to be the only player. Whatever the mechanism, the suggestion that far stronger resistance might yet evolve stealthily in humans calls for urgent and radical measures to monitor and contain ART-R.

We did not run a control group in parallel. During our experience with *P. falciparum* in successive mouse models [32], using both drug-sensitive and drug-resistant parasites [41], and more recently in the NSG model [31], we never observed a spontaneous change in drug response. These models were developed for our vaccine development project; the many animals infected by *P. falciparum* either contributed to understanding innate defense against malaria [31, 72] or were passively immunized to screen vaccine candidates [32, 73]. In this context, the parasite employed for the present study had already been passaged in mice for 7 months and proved to have maintained sensitivity to ART derivatives and other drugs both in vivo (Figs. 1 and 7) and in vitro (Figs. 5 and 6), where it served as the sensitive reference. However, a control parasite line should have been maintained in mice, in parallel, without drug exposure – this is a limitation of the study.

We repeatedly find ourselves on the back-foot in the campaign against malaria as there is a lack of tools to help us anticipate how the parasite will adapt to policy changes. GWAS, which have been extensively used, have major limitations. They can only characterize resistant parasites after they have emerged and merely provide circumstantial, rather than causative, evidence. One practical suggestion could be the application of novel models, such as the one presented here, to study the evolution and analyze the phenotypic adaptation of malaria parasites to drug pressure in vivo. While clinical efficacy data should remain the gold standard, the model presented here could be used as a tool to assess the phenotype of isolates with given genotypes (e.g., novel *kelch-13* mutations identified in Africa). Patient isolates can readily grow in the *Pf*-NSG model [31], allowing in vitro and in vivo methods to be used concurrently on clinical isolates. The model may also be used to characterize in vivo responses to experimental molecules at a preclinical level, and to trial alternative drug combinations (including triple therapy) that might bridle the evolution of ART-R [3]. This will allow an estimation of the time to resistance evolution for each compound or combination, without the impractical delays seen using in vitro methods [23].

The concomitant development of full resistance to quinine, halofantrine, and amodiaquine in the ART-R$_{240}$ strain, despite exclusive exposure to AS, was unforeseen. However, it is not all too surprising as in vitro resistance to quinine has previously been reported after exclusive exposure to ART [74]. Resistance to structurally unrelated antimalarials has been linked to changes in the *Pfmdr1* gene, which encodes the P-glycoprotein pump essential for parasite detoxification [75]. In this study, the ART-R$_{120}$ strain and ART-R$_{240}$ had an amplified *pfmdr* gene, in agreement with the high level of resistance developed towards AS, quinine, halofantrine, and amodiaquine [48]. An association of AS-mefloquine treatment failure with increased *pfmdr* copy number has been reported in north-western Cambodia [76].

The phenomenon of multidrug resistance despite single drug exposure is well recognized in microbiology and, in some instances, is mediated by up-regulation of a pro-mutagenic DNA repair response [77]. Parasites from Cambodia have a pro-mutagenic phenotype, favoring acquisition of new mutations [78]. Intense oxidative stress caused by AS exposure could stimulate this process [79]. It remains to be seen if the mutation in *RAD5*, a gene encoding a DNA post-replication repair protein [80], contributes to a pro-mutagenic state and development of multidrug resistance, or if it improves DNA repair.

Co-resistance to IV quinine and to one of the most widely used ACTs (AS-amodiaquine) – two critical weapons in the anti-malaria armamentarium – was fully verified both in vivo and in vitro. Resistance to quinine also arose using the DD regimen, indicating it has unlikely occurred by chance. Though high quinine IC$_{50}$ values have occasionally been reported ex vivo (e.g., 829 nM and 1019 nM) [29, 41], to our knowledge, frank resistance to treatment with a 219 mg/kg dose, as seen here, has not been reported from the clinic. Given the widespread use of ACT worldwide, the suggestion that ART pressure might also favor quinine resistance is of major concern.

Conclusion

These results were obtained in vivo using *P. falciparum* maintained in huRBC. Should clinical resistance to ART and ACT evolve further along the trajectory seen here, with co-resistance to quinine and other antimalarials, we would be left abruptly with no satisfactory option for treating severe malaria and a compromised choice of treatments for uncomplicated malaria [3]. Indeed, the current dependence on ARTs for both uncomplicated and severe malaria, together with a lack of viable therapeutic alternatives, leaves decision-makers with very limited options. This would have dire consequences not only in the management of individual cases, but would cripple efforts to achieve malaria control globally.

Additional files

Additional file 1: Details of genes, regions and primers used in genetic sequencing of *P. falciparum* artemisinin-resistant and control strains. (PDF 83 kb)

Additional file 2: Morphological changes of artemisinin-resistant parasites under treatment. (PDF 181 kb)

Additional file 3: Selection schema for single-dose resistant strain. (PDF 160 kb)

Additional file 4: Schematic representation of use of drug pressure to select for single-dose resistance in one mouse. (PDF 204 kb)

Additional file 5: Number and intensity of artesunate drug pressure cycles required to select for artemisinin resistance using single doses of artesunate. (PDF 97 kb)

Additional file 6: Gametocytes developing from artemisinin resistant parasites. (PDF 108 kb)

Additional file 7: Selection schema for 2-day dose resistant strain. (PDF 140 kb)

Additional file 8: Number and intensity of artesunate drug pressure cycles required to select for artemisinin resistance using a 2-day artesunate regimen. (PDF 93 kb)

Additional file 9: Mouse plasma dihydroartemisinin (DHA) concentrations measured after intravenous administration of artesunate. (PDF 108 kb)

Additional file 10: In vitro IC$_{50}$ (95% CI) values at different stages of artemisinin resistance (ART-R). (PDF 69 kb)

Additional file 11: Genetic sequencing of *RAD5*, *cNBP*, and *K-13*. (PDF 1419 kb)

Abbreviations

ACT: artemisinin-based combination therapy; APC: artesunate pressure cycle; ART: artemisinin; ART-R: artemisinin resistance of any level; AS: artesunate; CI: confidence interval; DD: double dose; DHA: dihydroartemisinin; DMSO: dimethyl sulfoxide; DPCT: delayed parasite clearance time; GWAS: genome wide association study; huRBC : human erythrocytes; IC$_{50}$: 50% inhibitory concentration; LED: lowest effective dose; NSG: NOD/SCID IL-2Rγ$^{-/-}$ mice; PAM: Uganda Palo Alto Marburg strain of *P. falciparum*; RSA: ring-stage survival; SD: standard deviation

Acknowledgements

This work would not have been possible without the financial contributions received from the Vac4All Initiative. We are indebted to Nicolas Widmer for performing pharmacokinetic calculations. We thank Christian Roussilhon, Geneviève Milon, Karima Brahimi, and Edgar Badell for their advice and contributions. We are grateful to Dr. Nico van Rooijen, Antion Longo (Sigma-Tau), and Philippe Brasseur for their generous gifts of essential materials.

Funding

This work was funded by the Vac4All Initiative. The initial mouse model employed was developed by the Bio-Medical Parasitology Unit at Institut Pasteur. Vac4all thereafter covered the expenses of personnel, reagents, animals, molecular studies, rent, and sundries required to gather the results presented.

Authors' contributions

RKT performed in vivo and in vitro experiments. PJG performed in vitro experiments, analyzed data, and contributed to writing manuscript. LA performed in vivo experiments and designed methods. LD determined plasma DHA concentrations. RT performed molecular studies. EP performed molecular studies. JLP and PO analyzed data and contributed to writing the manuscript. PD designed experiments, analyzed results, and supervised writing manuscript. All authors read and approved the final manuscript.

Competing interests

The authors declare that they have no competing interests.

Author details

[1]The Vac4All Initiative, 26 Rue Lecourbe, 75015 Paris, France. [2]Biomedical Parasitology Unit, Institut Pasteur, Paris, France. [3]Faculté de Pharmacie, Université Paris Descartes, COMUE Sorbonne Paris Cité, Paris, France. [4]Institut de Recherche pour le Développement, UMR MERIT 216, Paris, France. [5]Division of Clinical Pharmacology, Centre Hospitalier Universitaire Vaudois, Lausanne, Switzerland. [6]Centre for Tropical Medicine and Global Health, Nuffield Department of Medicine, University of Oxford, Oxford, UK. [7]Present Address: Amity Institute of Microbial Technology, Amity University, Noida, Uttar Pradesh, India. [8]Present Address: Centre de Recherche sur l'Inflammation, INSERM U1149, Faculté de Médecine, Université Diderot-Site Bichat, 16 rue Henri Huchard, 75018 Paris, France. [9]Present Address: Laboratoire de Biochimie, Hôpital Necker-Enfants Malades, Paris, France.

References

1. Organisation WH. Guidelines for the Treatment of Malaria. In: 2nd edition: World Health Organisation; 2010; 2011.
2. White NJ. Qinghaosu (artemisinin): the price of success. Science. 2008; 320(5874):330–4.
3. Phyo AP, von Seidlein L. Challenges to replace ACT as first-line drug. Malar J. 2017;16(1):296.
4. Dondorp AM, Yeung S, White L, Nguon C, Day NP, Socheat D, von Seidlein L. Artemisinin resistance: current status and scenarios for containment. Nat Rev Microbiol. 2010;8(4):272–80.
5. Phyo AP, Nkhoma S, Stepniewska K, Ashley EA, Nair S. McGready R, ler Moo C, Al-Saai S, Dondorp AM, Lwin KM et al: Emergence of artemisinin-resistant malaria on the western border of Thailand: a longitudinal study. Lancet. 2012;379(9830):1960–6.
6. Dondorp AM, Nosten F, Yi P, Das D, Phyo AP, Tarning J, Lwin KM, Ariey F, Hanpithakpong W, Lee SJ, et al. Artemisinin resistance in Plasmodium falciparum malaria. N Engl J Med. 2009;361(5):455–67.
7. Noedl H, Se Y, Schaecher K, Smith BL, Socheat D, Fukuda MM. Evidence of artemisinin-resistant malaria in western Cambodia. N Engl J Med. 2008; 359(24):2619–20.
8. Hien TT, Thuy-Nhien NT, Phu NH, Boni MF, Thanh NV, Nha-Ca NT. Thai le H, Thai CQ, Toi PV, Thuan PD et al: In vivo susceptibility of Plasmodium falciparum to artesunate in Binh Phuoc Province, Vietnam. Malar J. 2012;11: 355.
9. Kyaw MP, Nyunt MH, Chit K, Aye MM, Aye KH, Aye MM, Lindegardh N, Tarning J, Imwong M, Jacob CG, et al. Reduced susceptibility of Plasmodium falciparum to artesunate in southern Myanmar. PLoS One. 2013;8(3):e57689.
10. Ashley EA, Dhorda M, Fairhurst RM, Amaratunga C, Lim P, Suon S, Sreng S, Anderson JM, Mao S, Sam B, et al. Spread of artemisinin resistance in Plasmodium falciparum malaria. N Engl J Med. 2014;371(5):411–23.
11. Menard D, Khim N, Beghain J, Adegnika AA, Shafiul-Alam M, Amodu O, Rahim-Awab G, Barnadas C, Berry A, Boum Y, et al. A Worldwide Map of Plasmodium falciparum K13-Propeller Polymorphisms. N Engl J Med. 2016; 374(25):2453–64.
12. Hawkes M, Conroy AL, Kain KC. Spread of artemisinin resistance in malaria. N Engl J Med. 2014;371(20):1944–5.
13. Beshir KB, Sutherland CJ, Sawa P, Drakeley CJ, Okell L, Mweresa CK, Omar SA, Shekalaghe SA, Kaur H, Ndaro A, et al. Residual Plasmodium falciparum parasitemia in Kenyan children after artemisinin-combination therapy is associated with increased transmission to mosquitoes and parasite recurrence. J Infect Dis. 2013;208(12):2017–24.
14. Dondorp AM, Fairhurst RM, Slutsker L, Macarthur JR, Breman JG, Guerin PJ, Wellems TE, Ringwald P, Newman RD, Plowe CV. The threat of artemisinin-resistant malaria. N Engl J Med. 2011;365(12):1073–5.
15. Dell'Acqua R, Fabrizio C, Di Gennaro F, Lo Caputo S, Saracino A, Menegon M, L'Episcopia M, Severini C, Monno L, Castelli F, et al. An intricate case of multidrug resistant Plasmodium falciparum isolate imported from Cambodia. Malar J. 2017;16(1):149.
16. Imwong M, Hien TT, Thuy-Nhien NT, Dondorp AM, White NJ. Spread of a single multidrug resistant malaria parasite lineage (PfPailin) to Vietnam. Lancet Infect Dis. 2017;17(10):1022–3.
17. Kwansa-Bentum B, Ayi I, Suzuki T, Otchere J, Kumagai T, Anyan WK, Osei JH, Asahi H, Ofori MF, Akao N, et al. Plasmodium falciparum isolates from southern Ghana exhibit polymorphisms in the SERCA-type PfATPase6 though sensitive to artesunate in vitro. Malar J. 2011;10:187.
18. Phompradit P, Wisedpanichkij R, Muhamad P, Chaijaroenkul W, Na-Bangchang K. Molecular analysis of pfatp6 and pfmdr1 polymorphisms and their association with in vitro sensitivity in Plasmodium falciparum isolates from the Thai-Myanmar border. Acta Trop. 2011;120(1-2):130–5.
19. Pillai DR, Lau R, Khairnar.K, Lepore R, Via A, Staines HM, Krishna S. Artemether resistance in vitro is linked to mutations in PfATP6 that also interact with mutations in PfMDR1 in travellers returning with Plasmodium falciparum infections. Malar J. 2012;11:131.
20. Jambou R, Legrand E, Niang M, Khim N, Lim P, Volney B, Ekala MT, Bouchier C, Esterre P, Fandeur T, et al. Resistance of Plasmodium falciparum field isolates to in-vitro artemether and point mutations of the SERCA-type PfATPase6. Lancet. 2005;366(9501):1960–3.
21. Afonso A, Hunt P, Cheesman S, Alves AC. Cunha CV, do Rosario V, Cravo P: Malaria parasites can develop stable resistance to artemisinin but lack mutations in candidate genes atp6 (encoding the sarcoplasmic and endoplasmic reticulum Ca2+ ATPase), tctp, mdr1, and cg10. Antimicrob Agents Chemother. 2006;50(2):480–9.
22. Puri SK, Chandra R. Plasmodium vinckei: selection of a strain exhibiting stable resistance to arteether. Exp Parasitol. 2006;114(2):129–32.
23. Witkowski B, Lelievre J, Barragan MJ, Laurent V, Su XZ, Berry A, Benoit-Vical F. Increased tolerance to artemisinin in Plasmodium falciparum is mediated by a quiescence mechanism. Antimicrob Agents Chemother. 2010;54(5): 1872–7.
24. Wang Z, Cabrera M, Yang J, Yuan L, Gupta B, Liang X, Kemirembe K, Shrestha S, Brashear A, Li X, et al. Genome-wide association analysis identifies genetic loci associated with resistance to multiple antimalarials in Plasmodium falciparum from China-Myanmar border. Sci Rep. 2016;6:33891.
25. Mok S, Ashley EA, Ferreira PE, Zhu L, Lin Z, Yeo T, Chotivanich K, Imwong M, Pukrittayakamee S, Dhorda M, et al. Population transcriptomics of human malaria parasites reveals the mechanism of artemisinin resistance. Science. 2014;47(6220):431–5.
26. Cheeseman IH, Miller BA, Nair S, Nkhoma S, Tan A, Tan JC, Al Saai S, Phyo AP, Moo CL, Lwin KM, et al. A major genome region underlying artemisinin resistance in malaria. Science. 2012;336(6077):79–82.
27. Wang J, Zhang CJ, Chia WN, Loh CC, Li Z, Lee YM, He Y, Yuan LX, Lim TK, Liu M, et al. Haem-activated promiscuous targeting of artemisinin in Plasmodium falciparum. Nat Commun. 2015;6:10111.
28. Siddiqui G, Srivastava A, Russell AS, Creek DJ. Multi-omics Based Identification of Specific Biochemical Changes Associated With PfKelch13-Mutant Artemisinin-Resistant Plasmodium falciparum. J Infect Dis. 2017; 215(9):1435–44.
29. Witkowski B, Amaratunga C, Khim N, Sreng S, Chim P, Kim S, Lim P, Mao S, Sopha C, Sam B, et al. Novel phenotypic assays for the detection of

artemisinin-resistant Plasmodium falciparum malaria in Cambodia: in-vitro and ex-vivo drug-response studies. Lancet Infect Dis. 2013;13(12):1043–9.

30. Chotivanich K, Tripura R, Das D, Yi P, Day NP, Pukrittayakamee S, Chuor CM, Socheat D, Dondorp AM, White NJ. Laboratory detection of artemisinin-resistant Plasmodium falciparum. Antimicrob Agents Chemother. 2014;58(6):3157–61.

31. Arnold L, Tyagi RK, Meija P, Swetman C, Gleeson J, Perignon JL, Druilhe P. Further improvements of the P. falciparum humanized mouse model. PLoS One. 2011;6(3):e18045.

32. Badell E, Oeuvray C, Moreno A, Soe S, van Rooijen N, Bouzidi A, Druilhe P. Human malaria in immunocompromised mice: an in vivo model to study defense mechanisms against Plasmodium falciparum. J Exp Med. 2000;192(11):1653–60.

33. Fandeur T, Bonnefoy S, Mercereau-Puijalon O. In vivo and in vitro derived Palo Alto lines of Plasmodium falciparum are genetically unrelated. Mol Biochem Parasitol. 1991;47(2):167–78.

34. Siddiqui WA, Schnell JV, Geiman QM. A model in vitro system to test the susceptibility of human malarial parasites to antimalarial drugs. The American journal of tropical medicine and hygiene. 1972;21(4):393–9.

35. De Lucia S, Tsamesidis I, Pau MC, Kesely KR, Pantaleo A, Turrini F. Induction of high tolerance to artemisinin by sub-lethal administration: A new in vitro model of P. falciparum. PloS One. 2018;13(1):e0191084.

36. Rowe AW, Eyster E, Kellner A. Liquid nitrogen preservation of red blood cells for transfusion; a low glycerol-rapid freeze procedure. Cryobiology. 1968;5(2):119–28.

37. Lambros C, Vanderberg JP. Synchronization of Plasmodium falciparum erythrocytic stages in culture. J Parasitol. 1979;65(3):418–20.

38. Reese RT, Langreth SG, Trager W. Isolation of stages of the human parasite Plasmodium falciparum from culture and from animal blood. Bull World Health Organ. 1979;57(Suppl 1):53–61.

39. Druilhe P, Moreno A, Blanc C, Brasseur PH, Jacquier P. A colorimetric in vitro drug sensitivity assay for Plasmodium falciparum based on a highly sensitive double-site lactate dehydrogenase antigen-capture enzyme-linked immunosorbent assay. The American journal of tropical medicine and hygiene. 2001;64(5-6):233–41.

40. Desjardins RE, Canfield CJ, Haynes JD, Chulay JD. Quantitative assessment of antimalarial activity in vitro by a semiautomated microdilution technique. Antimicrob Agents Chemother. 1979;16(6):710–8.

41. Moreno A, Badell E, Van Rooijen N, Druilhe P. Human malaria in immunocompromised mice: new in vivo model for chemotherapy studies. Antimicrob Agents Chemother. 2001;45(6):1847–53.

42. Hodel EM, Zanolari B, Mercier T, Biollaz J, Keiser J, Olliaro P, Genton B, Decosterd LA. A single LC-tandem mass spectrometry method for the simultaneous determination of 14 antimalarial drugs and their metabolites in human plasma. J Chromatogr B Anal Technol Biomed Life Sci. 2009;877(10):867–86.

43. Hunt P, Afonso A, Creasey A, Culleton R, Sidhu AB, Logan J, Valderramos SG, McNae I. Cheesman S, do Rosario V et al. Gene encoding a deubiquitinating enzyme is mutated in artesunate- and chloroquine-resistant rodent malaria parasites. Mol Microbiol. 2007;65(1):27–40.

44. Takala-Harrison S, Clark TG, Jacob CG, Cummings MP, Miotto O, Dondorp AM, Fukuda MM, Nosten F, Noedl H, Imwong M, et al. Genetic loci associated with delayed clearance of Plasmodium falciparum following artemisinin treatment in Southeast Asia. Proc Natl Acad Sci U S A. 2013;110(1):240–5.

45. Ariey F, Witkowski B, Amaratunga C, Beghain J, Langlois AC, Khim N, Kim S, Duru V, Bouchier C, Ma L, et al. A molecular marker of artemisinin-resistant Plasmodium falciparum malaria. Nature. 2014;505(7481):50–5.

46. Takala-Harrison S, Jacob CG, Arze C, Cummings MP, Silva JC, Dondorp AM, Fukuda MM, Hien TT, Mayxay M, Noedl H, et al. Independent emergence of artemisinin resistance mutations among Plasmodium falciparum in Southeast Asia. J Infect Dis. 2015;211(5):670–9.

47. Basco LK, Ringwald P. Molecular epidemiology of malaria in Yaounde, Cameroon. III. Analysis of chloroquine resistance and point mutations in the multidrug resistance 1 (pfmdr 1) gene of Plasmodium falciparum. The American journal of tropical medicine and hygiene. 1998;59(4):577–81.

48. Price RN, Uhlemann AC, Brockman A, McGready R, Ashley E, Phaipun L, Patel R, Laing K, Looareesuwan S, White NJ, et al. Mefloquine resistance in Plasmodium falciparum and increased pfmdr1 gene copy number. Lancet. 2004;364(9432):438–47.

49. Nontprasert A, Pukrittayakamee S, Nosten-Bertrand M, Vanijanonta S, White NJ. Studies of the neurotoxicity of oral artemisinin derivatives in mice. The American journal of tropical medicine and hygiene. 2000;62(3):409–12.

50. Nagesha HS, Casey GJ, Rieckmann KH, Fryauff DJ, Laksana BS, Reeder JC, Maguire JD, Baird JK. New haplotypes of the Plasmodium falciparum chloroquine resistance transporter (pfcrt) gene among chloroquine-resistant parasite isolates. The American journal of tropical medicine and hygiene. 2003;68(4):398–402.

51. Menard D, Andriantsoanirina V, Khim N, Ratsimbasoa A, Witkowski B, Benedet C, Canier L, Mercereau-Puijalon O, Durand R. Global analysis of Plasmodium falciparum Na(+)/H(+) exchanger (pfnhe-1) allele polymorphism and its usefulness as a marker of in vitro resistance to quinine. Int J Parasitol Drugs Drug Resist. 2013;3:8–19.

52. White NJ, Pongtavornpinyo W, Maude RJ, Saralamba S, Aguas R, Stepniewska K, Lee SJ, Dondorp AM, White LJ, Day NP. Hyperparasitaemia and low dosing are an important source of anti-malarial drug resistance. Malar J. 2009;8:253.

53. Melendez V. Metabolic profile of artesunate and DHA using human plasma, liver, and hepatocytes. In: Annual progress report. Pennsylvania. USA: Armed Forces Research Institute of Medical Sciences; 2003. p. 214.

54. Davis TM, Phuong HL, Ilett KF, Hung NC, Batty KT, Phuong VD, Powell SM, Thien HV, Binh TQ. Pharmacokinetics and pharmacodynamics of intravenous artesunate in severe falciparum malaria. Antimicrob Agents Chemother. 2001;45(1):181–6.

55. Yeung S, Van Damme W, Socheat D, White NJ, Mills A. Access to artemisinin combination therapy for malaria in remote areas of Cambodia. Malar J. 2008;7:96.

56. Cohen JL, Yavuz E, Morris A, Arkedis J, Sabot O. Do patients adhere to over-the-counter artemisinin combination therapy for malaria? evidence from an intervention study in Uganda. Malar J. 2012;11:83.

57. Lemma H, Lofgren C, San Sebastian M. Adherence to a six-dose regimen of artemether-lumefantrine among uncomplicated Plasmodium falciparum patients in the Tigray Region, Ethiopia. Malar J. 2011;10:349.

58. Newton PN, McGready R, Fernandez F, Green MD, Sunjio M, Bruneton C, Phanouvong S, Millet P, Whitty CJ, Talisuna AO, et al. Manslaughter by fake artesunate in Asia—will Africa be next? PLoS Med. 2006;3(6):e197.

59. Sengaloundeth S, Green MD, Fernandez FM, Manolin O, Phommavong K, Insixiengmay V, Hampton CY, Nyadong L, Mildenhall DC, Hostetler D, et al. A stratified random survey of the proportion of poor quality oral artesunate sold at medicine outlets in the Lao PDR - implications for therapeutic failure and drug resistance. Malar J. 2009;8:172.

60. El-Duah M, Ofori-Kwakye K. Substandard artemisinin-based antimalarial medicines in licensed retail pharmaceutical outlets in Ghana. Journal of vector borne diseases. 2012;49(3):131–9.

61. Amaratunga C, Sreng S, Suon S, Phelps ES, Stepniewska K, Lim P, Zhou C, Mao S, Anderson JM, Lindegardh N, et al. Artemisinin-resistant Plasmodium falciparum in Pursat province, western Cambodia: a parasite clearance rate study. Lancet Infect Dis. 2012;12(11):851–8.

62. Noedl H, Se Y, Sriwichai S, Schaecher K, Teja-Isavadharm P, Smith B, Rutvisuttinunt W, Bethell D, Surasri S, Fukuda MM, et al. Artemisinin resistance in Cambodia: a clinical trial designed to address an emerging problem in Southeast Asia. Clinical infectious diseases : an official publication of the Infectious Diseases Society of America. 2010;51(11):e82–9.

63. Leang R, Barrette A, Bouth DM, Menard D, Abdur R, Duong S, Ringwald P. Efficacy of dihydroartemisinin-piperaquine for treatment of uncomplicated Plasmodium falciparum and Plasmodium vivax in Cambodia, 2008 to 2010. Antimicrob Agents Chemother. 2013;57(2):818–26.

64. Das D, Tripura R, Phyo AP, Lwin KM, Tarning J, Lee SJ, Hanpithakpong W, Stepniewska K, Menard D, Ringwald P, et al. Effect of high-dose or split-dose artesunate on parasite clearance in artemisinin-resistant falciparum malaria. Clinical infectious diseases : an official publication of the Infectious Diseases Society of America. 2013;56(5):e48–58.

65. Ghorbal M, Gorman M, Macpherson CR, Martins RM, Scherf A, Lopez-Rubio JJ. Genome editing in the human malaria parasite Plasmodium falciparum using the CRISPR-Cas9 system. Nat Biotechnol. 2014;32(8):819–21.

66. Straimer J, Gnadig NF, Witkowski B, Amaratunga C, Duru V, Ramadani AP, Dacheux M, Khim N, Zhang L, Lam S, et al. Drug resistance. K13-propeller mutations confer artemisinin resistance in Plasmodium falciparum clinical isolates. Science. 2015;347(6220):428–31.

67. Sibley C. Artemisinin resistance: the more we know, the more complicated it appears. J Infect Dis. 2015;211(5):667–9.

68. Miotto O, Amato R, Ashley EA, MacInnis B, Almagro-Garcia J, Amaratunga C, Lim P, Mead D, Oyola SO, Dhorda M, et al. Genetic architecture of artemisinin-resistant Plasmodium falciparum. Nat Genet. 2015;47(3):226–34.
69. Taylor SM, Parobek CM, DeConti DK, Kayentao K, Coulibaly SO, Greenwood BM, Tagbor H, Williams J, Bojang K, Njie F, et al. Absence of putative artemisinin resistance mutations among Plasmodium falciparum in Sub-Saharan Africa: a molecular epidemiologic study. J Infect Dis. 2015; 211(5):680–8.
70. Murai K, Culleton R, Hisaoka T, Endo H, Mita T. Global distribution of polymorphisms associated with delayed Plasmodium falciparum parasite clearance following artemisinin treatment: genotyping of archive blood samples. Parasitol Int. 2015;64(3):267–73.
71. Mbengue A, Bhattacharjee S, Pandharkar T, Liu H, Estiu G, Stahelin RV, Rizk SS, Njimoh DL, Ryan Y, Chotivanich K, et al. A molecular mechanism of artemisinin resistance in Plasmodium falciparum malaria. Nature. 2015; 520(7549):683–7.
72. Arnold L, Tyagi RK, Mejia P, Van Rooijen N, Perignon JL, Druilhe P. Analysis of innate defences against Plasmodium falciparum in immunodeficient mice. Malar J. 2010;9:197.
73. Druilhe P, Spertini F, Soesoe D, Corradin G, Mejia P, Singh S, Audran R, Bouzidi A, Oeuvray C, Roussilhon C. A malaria vaccine that elicits in humans antibodies able to kill Plasmodium falciparum. PLoS Med. 2005;2(11):e344.
74. Chavchich M, Gerena L, Peters J, Chen N, Cheng Q, Kyle DE. Role of pfmdr1 amplification and expression in induction of resistance to artemisinin derivatives in Plasmodium falciparum. Antimicrob Agents Chemother. 2010;54(6):2455–64.
75. Reed MB, Saliba KJ, Caruana SR, Kirk K, Cowman AF. Pgh1 modulates sensitivity and resistance to multiple antimalarials in Plasmodium falciparum. Nature. 2000;403(6772):906–9.
76. Lim P, Alker AP, Khim N, Shah NK, Incardona S, Doung S, Yi P, Bouth DM, Bouchier C, Puijalon OM, et al. Pfmdr1 copy number and arteminisin derivatives combination therapy failure in falciparum malaria in Cambodia. Malar J. 2009;8:11.
77. Kohanski MA, DePristo MA, Collins JJ. Sublethal antibiotic treatment leads to multidrug resistance via radical-induced mutagenesis. Mol Cell. 2010;37(3):311–20.
78. Lee AH, Fidock DA. Evidence of a Mild Mutator Phenotype in Cambodian Plasmodium falciparum Malaria Parasites. PLoS One. 2016;11(4):e0154166.
79. Gupta DK, Patra AT, Zhu L, Gupta AP, Bozdech Z. DNA damage regulation and its role in drug-related phenotypes in the malaria parasites. Sci Rep. 2016;6:23603.
80. Ginsburg H. Progress in in silico functional genomics: the malaria Metabolic Pathways database. Trends Parasitol. 2006;22(6):238–40.

3

Optimising first- and second-line treatment strategies for untreated major depressive disorder — the SUN☺D study: a pragmatic, multi-centre, assessor-blinded randomised controlled trial

Tadashi Kato[1], Toshi A. Furukawa[2*], Akio Mantani[3], Ken'ichi Kurata[4], Hajime Kubouchi[5], Susumu Hirota[6], Hirotoshi Sato[7], Kazuyuki Sugishita[8], Bun Chino[9], Kahori Itoh[10], Yoshio Ikeda[11], Yoshihiro Shinagawa[12], Masaki Kondo[13], Yasumasa Okamoto[14], Hirokazu Fujita[15], Motomu Suga[16], Shingo Yasumoto[17], Naohisa Tsujino[18], Takeshi Inoue[19], Noboru Fujise[20], Tatsuo Akechi[13], Mitsuhiko Yamada[21], Shinji Shimodera[15], Norio Watanabe[2], Masatoshi Inagaki[22], Kazuhira Miki[23], Yusuke Ogawa[2], Nozomi Takeshima[2], Yu Hayasaka[2], Aran Tajika[2], Kiyomi Shinohara[2], Naohiro Yonemoto[24], Shiro Tanaka[25], Qi Zhou[26], Gordon H. Guyatt[26] and for the SUN☺D Investigators

Abstract

Background: For patients starting treatment for depression, current guidelines recommend titrating the antidepressant dosage to the maximum of the licenced range if tolerated. When patients do not achieve remission within several weeks, recommendations include adding or switching to another antidepressant. However, the relative merits of these guideline strategies remain unestablished.

Methods: This multi-centre, open-label, assessor-blinded, pragmatic trial involved two steps. Step 1 used open-cluster randomisation, allocating clinics into those titrating sertraline up to 50 mg/day or 100 mg/day by week 3. Step 2 used central randomisation to allocate patients who did not remit after 3 weeks of treatment to continue sertraline, to add mirtazapine or to switch to mirtazapine. The primary outcome was depression severity measured with the Patient Health Questionnaire-9 (PHQ-9) (scores between 0 and 27; higher scores, greater depression) at week 9. We applied mixed-model repeated-measures analysis adjusted for key baseline covariates.

Results: Between December 2010 and March 2015, we recruited 2011 participants with hitherto untreated major depression at 48 clinics in Japan. In step 1, 970 participants were allocated to the 50 mg/day and 1041 to the 100 mg/day arms; 1927 (95.8%) provided primary outcomes. There was no statistically significant difference in the adjusted PHQ-9 score at week 9 between the 50 mg/day arm and the 100 mg/day arm (0.25 point, 95% confidence interval (CI), − 0.58 to 1.07, $P = 0.55$). Other outcomes proved similar in the two groups.

In step 2, 1646 participants not remitted by week 3 were randomised to continue sertraline ($n = 551$), to add mirtazapine ($n = 537$) or to switch to mirtazapine ($n = 558$): 1613 (98.0%) provided primary outcomes. At week 9, adding mirtazapine
(Continued on next page)

* Correspondence: furukawa@kuhp.kyoto-u.ac.jp
[2]Department of Health Promotion of Human Behavior, Kyoto University
Graduate School of Medicine / School of Public Health, Yoshida Konoe-cho,
Sakyo-ku, Kyoto 606-8501, Japan
Full list of author information is available at the end of the article

(Continued from previous page)

achieved a reduction in PHQ-9 scores of 0.99 point (0.43 to 1.55, $P = 0.0012$); switching achieved a reduction of 1.01 points (0.46 to 1.56, $P = 0.0012$), both relative to continuing sertraline. Combination increased the percentage of remission by 12.4% (6.1 to 19.0%) and switching by 8.4% (2.5 to 14.8%). There were no differences in adverse effects.

Conclusions: In patients with new onset depression, we found no advantage of titrating sertraline to 100 mg vs 50 mg. Patients unremitted by week 3 gained a small benefit in reduction of depressive symptoms at week 9 by switching sertraline to mirtazapine or by adding mirtazapine.

Trial registration: ClinicalTrials.gov, NCT01109693. Registered on 23 April 2010.

Keywords: Major depressive disorder, Antidepressive agents: first-line treatment, Second-line treatment, Randomised controlled trial

Background

Every year, an estimated five million people in high-income countries alone start new antidepressants to treat their depression [1–3]. In the USA, the annual prevalence of prescribed antidepressant use exceeds 10% of the population, almost double that of 10 years before [2]. Antidepressant use is similarly high and increasing in European countries, ranging between 4 and 9% [1], with a 1-year incidence of new antidepressant prescription of approximately 1% [3]. Clinicians need specific, detailed and appropriate guidelines to guide their antidepressant pharmacotherapy.

To initiate antidepressant treatment, modern guidelines recommend new generation antidepressants and in particular selective serotonin reuptake inhibitors (SSRIs) [4]. A network meta-analysis of 12 new generation antidepressants suggested that the SSRI sertraline, because of its favourable balance of benefits, acceptability and cost, may be the best choice when starting treatment for major depression [5]. Sertraline has been the most widely prescribed antidepressant in the USA [6] and elsewhere [7].

Once they choose a first-line antidepressant, practitioners must optimise its dosage, considering the wide approved dose range for most drugs. Many guidelines only list such ranges and do not specify where within this range the initial treatment should aim [4, 8, 9]. The American Psychiatric Association guideline is more specific and recommends that the initial doses be incrementally raised and maximised, side effects permitting ([10], p. 43). However, systematic reviews of randomised controlled trials (RCTs) have provided conflicting results regarding the benefits and harms of lower vs higher doses of various antidepressants within their therapeutic ranges. One review synthesised results from 33 RCTs comparing two or more doses of the same antidepressants and found that a dose level of 100–200 mg imipramine equivalents (or 20–40 mg fluoxetine equivalents) showed the highest response rate, while lower doses showed a reduction in efficacy and higher doses were not accompanied by increased efficacy. Adverse events

increased monotonically with dose [11]. However, this study included both old and new generation antidepressants. The dose-response curves may be different for different classes of antidepressants. More recent reviews focussing on a single agent [12] or several agents [13] suggested that there was no dose-response relationship within the approved dose ranges for SSRIs.

Clinicians face another challenge because, after several weeks of the first-line treatment, only 50% of patients respond (i.e. achieve depression severity less than half that at pre-treatment), and only 30% remit (i.e. return to a euthymic state). Patients' failure to respond or remit requires consideration of alternative treatments. Guideline recommendations for second-line treatment include dose escalation, switching to a different antidepressant or adding a different drug [4, 10]. The last strategy may be divided into 'augmentation' when a non-antidepressant drug is added to an antidepressant and 'combination' when two antidepressants are used together [4]. Systematic reviews of RCTs agree that dose escalation confers no benefit beyond continuing the initial drug dose [14–17]; consistent with these results, the German National Guideline clearly states that dose escalation for SSRI does not work [8]. Two previous systematic reviews have found some support for the switching strategy [18], especially to an antidepressant from a different class [19]. However, a recent more rigorous meta-analysis found no high-level evidence that switching the antidepressant is effective when compared to simply continuing the initial antidepressant [20]. There are also reviews that support various augmentation strategies [21] and combination strategies [22]. However, most of the RCTs addressing patients who fail to respond to initial pharmacotherapy for depression compared new strategies against continuing preceding treatment; far less evidence exists comparing alternative second-line strategies against one another. For example, only two reports have directly compared switching vs combination strategies among patients who failed first-line treatment: one study compared combination vs switching vs continuing the prior treatment [23], while another compared dose escalation vs combination vs continuing the prior treatment [24]. Unfortunately, neither study was sufficiently powered (only 32–38 patients in each arm in the first study and 98–99 patients in the second study) to reach meaningful conclusions. The STAR*D trial randomised 1439 patients with major depression who had not remitted on citalopram to various switching strategies or augmentation/combination strategies. However, they used an equipoise-stratified design which gave patients choices in their treatment regimen: only 105 patients consented to randomisation to any of the drug switching or augmentation strategies, and consequently the analyses had to be conducted separately among the switching strategies or among the augmentation/combination strategies [25, 26]. A recently published study compared switching to bupropion against combining with bupropion or augmenting with an antipsychotic aripiprazole among 1522 patients with antidepressant-refractory major depression and found that aripiprazole augmentation significantly increased response over bupropion combination or switching [27]. Most patients in this trial were, however, chronically depressed and highly refractory (the mean duration of index episode was more than 85 months and the mean number of previous medication courses was 2.4). The trial does not, therefore, address the initial treatment of a new depressive episode.

Even less is known about when to institute second-line treatment. The American Psychiatric Association practice guideline recommends 4–8 weeks [10], the American College of Physicians 6–8 weeks [28] and the National Institute for Clinical Excellence (NICE) guideline 3–4 weeks at one place but 6–8 weeks at another [4].

Thus, in trying to optimise antidepressant pharmacotherapy for patients with major depression, clinicians face conflicting guidelines informed by low quality evidence. We therefore conducted a pragmatic RCT — an RCT that mimics the practice environment and thus maximises applicability — to examine the following two questions concerning the first- and second-line treatments for a hitherto untreated episode of major depression:

1. What is the relative effectiveness and safety of initially titrating to the lowest vs the highest value of the therapeutic dose range of an antidepressant? On the basis of the results of prior evidence [5] and existing practices [6, 7], we chose sertraline as the drug to be tested. Since the available evidence suggests that there may be differences between different classes of antidepressants with respect to dose-response relationship [15], the first hypothesis pertains to the choice of the initial target dose of an SSRI,

and of sertraline in particular, within its therapeutic range.

2. When patients do not remit on first-line treatment, what is the relative effectiveness and safety of continuing initial treatment, combining with mirtazapine or switching to mirtazapine? We set 3 weeks as this decision point as the earliest time point in guideline recommendations [4]. Our choice of mirtazapine is consistent with a systematic review reporting that combination of a reuptake inhibitor antidepressant such as an SSRI and a blocker of presynaptic alpha-2 autoreceptor (mirtazapine, mianserin, trazodone) was superior to other combinations [22]. In addition, mirtazapine poses a very low risk of drug interaction. Finally, in the recently updated network meta-analysis of 21 antidepressants, mirtazapine was the second most potent antidepressant after amitriptyline [29]; its less favourable acceptability profile renders it less suitable as first-line treatment, but when first-line treatment fails, mirtazapine represents a potentially appropriate second choice.

Methods
Study design and participants
The Strategic Use of New generation antidepressants for Depression (SUN☺D) is a multi-centre, open-label, assessor-blinded, pragmatic RCT that involved two randomisation steps to examine the first- and second-line treatment strategies for untreated unipolar major depressive episodes.

The study was conducted in the departments of psychiatry at 48 clinics and hospitals across Japan between December 2010 and September 2015. We recruited adult men and women between 25 and 75 years who had a primary diagnosis of a non-psychotic unipolar major depressive episode according to the Diagnostic and Statistical Manual of Mental Disorders, 4th Edition (DSM-IV) [30] within the past month as ascertained by the study psychiatrists administering the semi-structured interview using the major depression section of the Primary Care Evaluation of Mental Disorders (PRIME-MD) [31]. All recruited persons were also not allowed to be taking any antidepressant, antipsychotic or mood stabiliser. Other exclusion criteria included history of schizophrenia, schizoaffective disorder, bipolar disorder; current dementia, borderline personality disorder, eating disorder or substance dependence; and imminent high risk of suicide, as judged by the study psychiatrist. No severity threshold was required so long as the participant satisfied the diagnostic criteria for major depressive disorder in the past month. The protocol provides additional details of the eligibility criteria [32]. When the study psychiatrist decided that sertraline was indicated, the patient began taking 25 mg/day of sertraline; only those who tolerated sertraline for 3–16 days were eligible.

An institutional review board at each participating site approved the study. An independent data monitoring committee oversaw the trial. All participants provided written informed consent. The study protocol, its amendment and the statistical analysis plan have been published elsewhere [32, 33].

Randomisation and masking

Figure 1 presents the study flow. In step 1, using the minimisation method adjusting for expected recruitment, study sites were randomised to titrate sertraline up to the minimum or the maximum of the licenced dosage in Japan (50 mg/day or 100 mg/day) by week 3. The unit of randomisation was therefore by site. The cluster randomisation design was chosen to avoid any confusion and possible protocol violation that might have arisen had we asked study physicians, who often had their own preference for either the minimum or the maximum target doses, to use different titrating strategies for different patients. Further, we were concerned that requiring patients to undergo two individual randomisations within 3 weeks might decrease the feasibility of this large pragmatic trial.

In step 2, participants who had not reached remission, defined as scoring 4 or less on the Patient Health Questionnaire (PHQ-9) [34] at week 3, were randomised 1:1:1

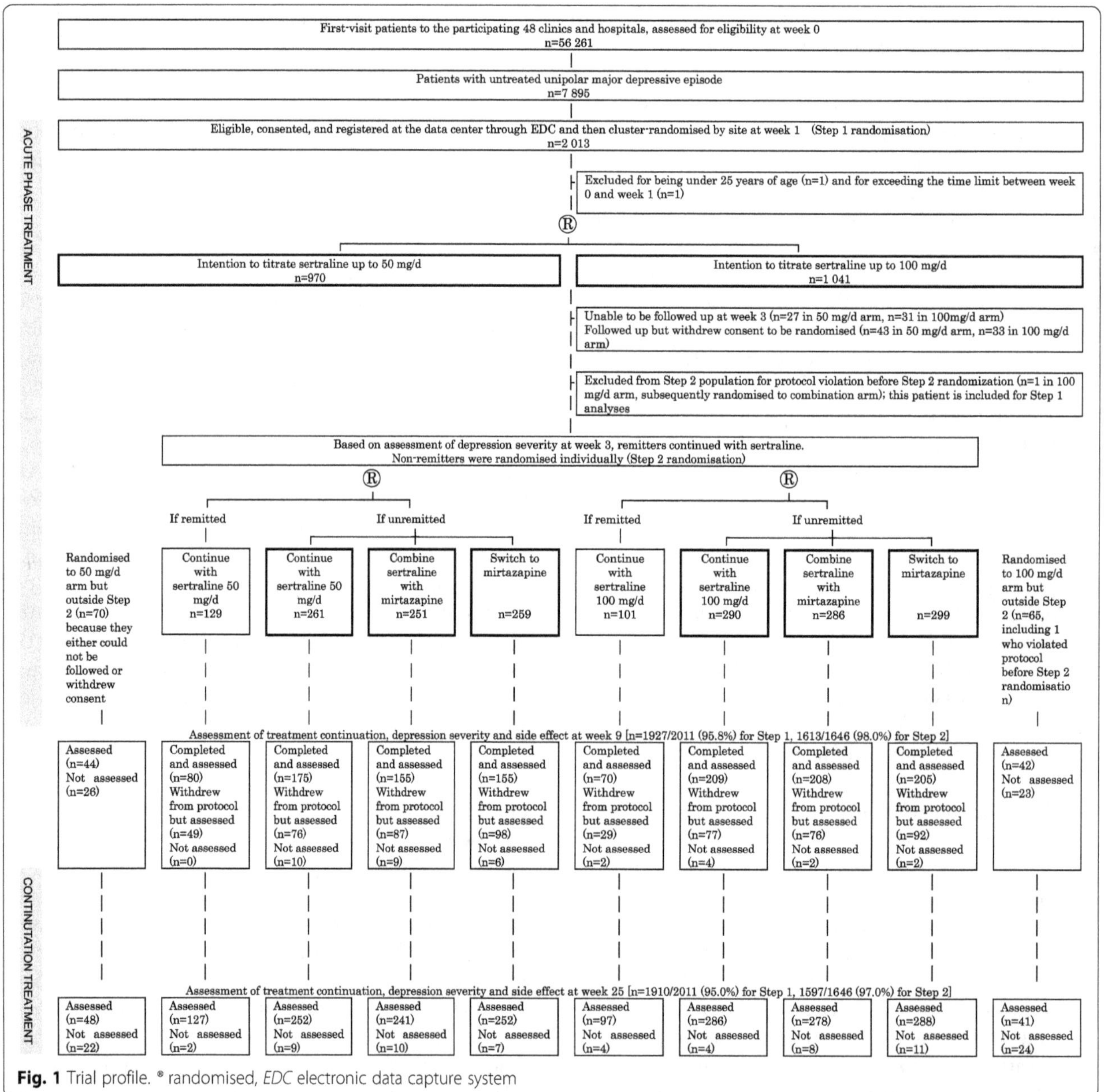

Fig. 1 Trial profile. ® randomised, *EDC* electronic data capture system

through the web-based central computer system to continue with sertraline, to combine sertraline with mirtazapine or to switch to mirtazapine. The step 2 randomisation used the minimisation method adjusting for site; whether 50% or greater reduction on PHQ-9 had been achieved; and whether patients reported moderate or greater impairment due to side effects.

Physicians and patients were aware of their treatments. Outcome assessors were blinded throughout. The statisticians conducting the analyses and the writing committee were masked to treatment allocation until they signed the agreed-upon interpretations of the results.

Procedures

In step 1, participants in the minimum dosage arm received 50 mg/day of sertraline at week 1 to be continued through week 3, and those in the maximum dosage arm received 50–75 mg/day at week 1 and 100 mg/day at week 2 to be continued through week 3. When these target dosages were not tolerated, lower dosages were accepted.

In step 2, in the continuing sertraline arm, sertraline was administered as 50 or 100 mg/day according to the initial randomisation. In the combination arm, sertraline was continued and mirtazapine was added between 7.5 and 45 mg/day at the discretion of the study psychiatrist. In the mirtazapine switch arm, mirtazapine between 7.5 mg and 45 mg/day was administered; sertraline was tapered and discontinued by week 7.

Co-administration of benzodiazepines, but not of another antidepressant, antipsychotic or mood stabiliser was allowed up to week 9. Neither was any depression-specific psychotherapy such as cognitive behavioural therapy (CBT) or interpersonal psychotherapy (IPT) allowed. Those who withdrew consent to the study treatments by week 9 but still participated in follow-up evaluations received treatment as negotiated with their physician. Between weeks 9 and 25, there were no restrictions on treatments, and the continuation therapy was at the physician's discretion.

Outcomes

For both the step 1 and step 2 randomisations, the primary outcome was depression severity as measured by masked assessors conducting semi-structured interviews using the PHQ-9 at week 9. The PHQ-9 consists of the nine diagnostic criteria items of major depression from the DSM-IV [35]. Each item is rated between 0 = 'Not at all' through 3 = 'Nearly every day', making the total score range 0–27, with higher ratings indicating increased depression severity. The instrument has demonstrated excellent reliability, validity and responsiveness [34].

Secondary outcomes included the Frequency, Intensity and Burden of Side Effects Rating (FIBSER) and the

Beck Depression Inventory 2nd edition (BDI-II). The FIBSER collects information regarding the frequency, intensity and burden of side effects, each on a 7-point scale with higher ratings indicating greater severity, and provides a total score between 3 and 21 [25]. The BDI-II is a self-report measure of depression severity addressing 21 symptoms of depression, each on a scale between 0 and 3, with the total score ranging between 0 and 63; higher scores indicate more severe depression [36]. In addition, the study psychiatrist recorded any incident of suicidality according to the Columbia Classification Algorithm of Suicide Assessment (C-CASA) [37] or of manic/hypomanic/mixed episodes at weeks 9 and 25, and reported any serious adverse events throughout the study. Response was defined as 50% or greater reduction from week 1 on PHQ-9, and remission as scoring 4 or less on PHQ-9 [34].

The PHQ-9 and the FIBSER were administered by telephone assessors [38], trained at and operating from the central office and blind to the treatment assignment and the timing of the assessment, at weeks 1, 3, 9 and 25. We had previously established the high inter-rater reliability of our telephone assessors [39]. The BDI-II was filled in by the participants at weeks 0, 1 and then every 2 weeks up to week 9, and every 4 weeks up to week 25.

Sample size

For step 1, we calculated that we would need 66 participants at each of 30 sites in order to ensure adequate power (beta level of 0.20) at a two-sided alpha level of 0.05 to detect a mean difference of 1 point on PHQ-9 with an estimated standard deviation (SD) of 5 or a standardised mean difference of 0.20 between the two arms, for the null hypothesis of no difference and an intracluster correlation coefficient of 0.05 [40]. We reasoned that an effect size of 0.20, corresponding with a small effect according to Cohen [41], would represent an important difference between active treatments. The required total sample size for step 1 was 1980.

For step 2, we calculated that 522 participants per group would ensure adequate power (beta level of 0.20) at a two-sided alpha level of 0.05 to detect a standardised mean difference of 0.20 among any two of the three treatment groups. Assuming a dropout rate of 10% and a remission rate of 10% at week 3, we needed 1934 participants entering step 1.

Statistical analysis

In order to examine the optimum initial target dose of sertraline, we analysed results from all those who were cluster-randomised at week 1 to titrate sertraline up to 50 mg/day or 100 mg/day and, had they followed the protocol, would have stayed on that sertraline dose up to week 9 — that is, those who had remitted and continued on sertraline; those who had not remitted and were randomised at week 3 to continue sertraline; and those who declined the second randomisation. We used a weighted mixed-model repeated-measures analysis to compare model-adjusted least squares means: the primary outcome was the PHQ-9 at week 9 as pre-specified in the study protocol. The model included random effects for subjects and sites and fixed effects of treatment, visit (as categorical) and treatment-by-visit interaction, adjusted for age, sex, education, marital status, number of previous depressive episodes and baseline scores at weeks 0 and 1. At the first blinded interpretation committee meeting, the statistician reported an imbalance in the baseline demographic and clinical variables. The writing committee therefore agreed, at that meeting, without knowledge of the identity of the arms and based on their prior knowledge regarding variables that may be associated with depression severity, on the following variables to be entered in the primary analysis as possible confounders: age, sex, education, marital status, number of previous depressive episodes and baseline PHQ-9 scores at weeks 0 and 1. Each observation was weighted by inverse probability of censoring (IPCW) to account for missing outcomes due to being allocated to the combination or switching arms at step 2 randomisation. The weight for IPCW was calculated by a logistic regression that included age, sex, education, marriage, number of episodes, PHQ-9 scores at weeks 0 and 1 and whether the participant was allocated to continue sertraline or otherwise at week 3 as predictors of missingness. We applied the same modelling approach to the continuous secondary outcomes. We used weighted generalised linear mixed models with the logit link and binomial distributions to account for clustering effects for the dichotomous secondary outcomes. For the time to discontinuation of the allocated or any treatment, we applied Cox regression with the same covariates and calculated the hazard ratio (HR) and its 95% confidence interval (CI). For step 1 analyses, we examined two subgroup hypotheses, pre-specified in the statistical analysis plan [33]: (1) whether the PHQ-9 score at week 1 was less than or greater than 15 and (2) whether the patient had shown improvement from week 0 to week 1 at or above the median of the sample. We also conducted four sensitivity analyses employing mixed models with different assumptions, described in the statistical analysis plan [33].

To compare the second-line strategies, we used the mixed-model repeated-measures analysis comparing model-adjusted least squares means of the PHQ-9 at week 9 among the three treatment arms. This model included the following: fixed effects of PHQ-9 at week 3, treatment, visit (as categorical), treatment-by-visit interaction, minimisation variables for step 2 randomisation. The model included individuals and sites as random effects. We applied the same modelling approach to the continuous secondary outcomes and the logistic regression model for the dichotomous secondary outcomes. In order to facilitate the clinical interpretation of the obtained odds ratio (OR), we calculated the risk difference (RD) and its CI by applying the model-adjusted OR and its CI to the event rate in the sertraline continuation arm. For the time to discontinuation, we applied Cox regression with the same covariates. We applied the Hochberg procedure for adjusting the multiple comparisons involved with three treatment arms in the primary comparison and reported adjusted P values. For step 2 analyses, we examined three pre-specified hypotheses regarding possible effect modifiers [33]: (1) whether patients had achieved a 50% or greater reduction on PHQ-9 from week 1 to week 3, (2) whether FIBSER results indicated 'moderate' or greater impairment due to side effects or (iii) whether step 1 was high or low dose.

All efficacy and safety analyses followed the intention-to-treat principle, and all patents were analysed in the groups to which they were randomised.

Blinded interpretation of the results
The writing committee reviewed a statistical report in which the treatments were masked, and developed interpretation of the results and associated conclusions under alternative scenarios for all possible permutations of treatments [42]. The treatments were revealed only after the writing committee signed off on the agreed-upon interpretations (See Additional file 1).

Role of the funding source
The funders of the study had no role in study design, data collection, data analysis, data interpretation or in writing of the report. The corresponding author had full access to all the data in the study and had final responsibility for the decision to submit for publication.

Changes from the original protocol
No major change was made since the original protocol and statistical analysis plan [32, 33]. Our published protocol [32] lists the several minor changes in the details since the original protocol.

Results
Figure 1 shows the screening, randomisation and follow-up of the study participants. Between December 2010 and March 2015, 56,261 first-visit patients to the participating 48 clinics and hospitals in Japan underwent eligibility assessment, of whom 7895 suffered from untreated unipolar major depressive episodes. Of these, 2011 patients satisfied eligibility criteria and were cluster

randomised to titrate sertraline up to the minimum or maximum of the licenced dosage within 3 weeks: 970 in 22 clinics and hospitals to the 50 mg/day arm and 1041 in 26 clinics and hospitals to the 100 mg/day arm. The participants' characteristics differed between the two arms, especially with regard to sex and PHQ-9 scores at weeks 0 and 1 (Table 1). Of those randomised at week 1, 1927 (95.8%) and 1910 (95.0%) were successfully followed up at week 9 and week 25, respectively.

Of these, 1647 had not remitted by week 3 and were individually randomised to continue sertraline ($n = 551$),

Table 1 Baseline characteristics of the participants at step 1 randomisation

	Titrate sertraline up to 50 mg/day by week 3 ($n = 970$)	Titrate sertraline up to 100 mg/day by week 3 ($n = 1041$)
Demographic characteristics		
Age, year mean (SD)	43.3 (12.2)	41.8 (12.3)
Female sex, n (%)	572 (59.0)	506 (48.6)
Education year, mean (SD)	13.8 (2.2)	14.1 (2.5)
Job status, n (%)		
Employed full-time	398 (41.1)	374 (36.0)
Employed part-time	103 (10.6)	76 (7.3)
On medical leave	206 (21.3)	328 (31.6)
Housewife	114 (11.8)	116 (11.9)
Student	5 (0.5)	14 (1.4)
Retired	18 (1.9)	5 (0.5)
Not employed	124 (12.8)	125 (12.0)
Missing	2	3
Marital status, n (%)		
Single, never married	262 (27.1)	355 (34.1)
Single, divorced or separated	148 (15.3)	124 (11.9)
Single, widowed	29 (3.0)	25 (2.4)
Married	528 (54.6)	537 (51.6)
Missing	3	0
Clinical characteristics		
Age of onset at first episode, years, mean (SD)	38.6 (13.3)	37.1 (13.5)
Number of previous depressive episodes, mean (SD)	2.3 (4.2)	2.2 (3.1)
Length of current episode, months, mean (SD)	6.6 (17.2)	5.3 (10.0)
Inpatient status at time of entry, n (%)	2 (0.2)	3 (0.3)
PHQ-9 at week 0	18.1 (4.1)	18.8 (3.7)
PHQ-9 at week 1	14.7 (5.5)	15.9 (4.9)
BDI-II at week 1	26.2 (10.9)	28.7 (10.6)

BDI-II Beck Depression Inventory 2nd edition, *PHQ-9* Patient Health Questionnaire-9

combine sertraline with mirtazapine ($n = 538$) or switch to mirtazapine ($n = 558$). Participants' characteristics proved similar across the three arms (Table 2). Of those randomised at week 3, 1613 (98.0%) and 1597 (97.0%) were successfully followed up at week 9 and week 25, respectively.

With regard to step 1 treatments, in the 50 mg/day arm, 91.7% (889/970) had been prescribed 50 mg/day, 0.1% (1/970) 37.5 mg/day, 1.3% (13/970) 25 mg/day and 0.1% (1/970) 75 mg/day by week 3; in the 100 mg/day arm, 82.0% (854/1041) had reached 100 mg/day, 5.3% (55/1041) 75 mg/day, 6.7% (70/1041) 50 mg/day and 0.9% (9/1041) 25 mg/day. In the 50 mg/day arm 6.8% (66/970) had stopped treatment as had 5.1% (53/1041) in the 100 mg/day arm. For step 2 randomised allocations at week 3, 99.5% (548/551), 96.1% (516/537) and 96.8% (540/558) of the randomised participants started their allocated treatment for the continuation, combination and switch arms, respectively; of the last group, 72.9% (407/558), 83.9% (468/558) and 87.8% (490/558) were successfully tapered off sertraline by weeks 5, 6 and 7, respectively.

In the following analyses, we ascertained the assumptions of normality and the homoscedasticity of the error in both the steps 1 and 2 mixed-effects models. We also ascertained the proportional hazards assumption by visual inspection of the log cumulative hazard curves and by testing the treatment*time interaction in Cox regression models.

Step 1: 50 mg/day vs 100 mg/day as initial target dose of sertraline

According to the adjusted and weighted mixed-model repeated-measures analyses, there was no statistically significant difference (0.25 point, 95% CI – 0.58 to 1.07, $P = 0.55$) between the 100 mg/day arm and the 50 mg/day arm in the PHQ-9 score at week 9 (Table 3). There were no statistically significant differences in the secondary efficacy outcomes at week 9. Neither were there any statistically significant differences in the global burden of side effects between the 50 mg/day and 100 mg/day arms.

At week 25, the 100 mg/day arm scored lower (– 2.28, 95% CI – 3.91 to – 0.66, $P = 0.0059$) on self-rated BDI-II than the 50 mg/day arm (Table 4). The two arms did not differ, however, in the other efficacy outcomes of PHQ-9, the proportion of remission or in the global burden of side effects.

The incidence of suicidality, manic switches or serious adverse events was very small, and there were no statistically significant differences between the two arms through 25 weeks (Additional file 2: Tables S1, S2).

Results were similar regardless of baseline depression severity or initial response (Additional file 2: Table S3).

Table 2 Baseline characteristics of the participants at step 2 randomisation

	Continue with sertraline ($n = 551$)	Combine sertraline with mirtazapine ($n = 537$)	Switch to mirtazapine ($n = 558$)
Demographic characteristics			
Age, year mean (SD)	41.5 (11.6)	42.0 (11.7)	41.4 (11.4)
Female sex, n (%)	289 (52.5)	284 (52.9)	281 (50.4)
Education year, mean (SD)	14.1 (2.4)	13.8 (2.2)	14.1 (2.3)
Job status, n (%)			
Employed full-time	213 (38.7)	218 (40.8)	215 (38.7)
Employed part-time	52 (9.4)	52 (9.7)	40 (7.2)
On medical leave	146 (26.5)	143 (26.7)	163 (29.3)
Housewife	47 (8.5)	62 (11.6)	53 (9.5)
Student	3 (0.5)	3 (0.6)	8 (1.4)
Retired	6 (1.1)	5 (0.9)	4 (0.7)
Not employed	84 (15.3)	52 (9.7)	73 (13.1)
Missing	0	2	2
Marital status, n (%)			
Single, never married	188 (34.2)	144 (26.9)	188 (33.7)
Single, divorced or separated	75 (13.6)	182 (15.3)	80 (14.3)
Single, widowed	10 (1.8)	17 (3.2)	9 (1.6)
Married	277 (50.4)	292 (54.6)	281 (50.4)
Missing	1	2	0
Clinical characteristics			
Age of onset at first episode, years, mean (SD)	37.0 (12.9)	37.0 (12.8)	36.4 (12.4)
Number of previous depressive episodes, mean (SD), range	2.4 (3.4), 1–30	2.1 (3.2), 1–50	2.4 (4.2), 1–50
Length of current episode, months, mean (SD), range	5.7 (10.6), 0.5–139	6.7 (16.9), 0.5–240	6.5 (16.3), 0.5–276
Inpatient status at baseline, n (%)	1 (0.2)	1 (0.2)	2 (0.4)
PHQ-9 at week 3, mean (SD)	12.8 (5.2)	12.6 (5.1)	12.8 (5.2)
BDI-II at week 3, mean (SD)	24.5 (10.7)	24.1 (10.7)	24.4 (10.9)
Sertraline at week 3, mean (SD), mg/day	72.2 (26.6)	71.4 (27.6)	72.6 (28.3)

BDI-II Beck Depression Inventory 2nd edition, *PHQ-9* Patient Health Questionnaire-9

All sensitivity analyses differed little from the primary findings (Additional file 2: Table S4).

Step 2: Continue sertraline vs combine with mirtazapine vs switch to mirtazapine at week 3

The adjusted mixed-model repeated-measures analysis revealed that the mirtazapine combination arm and the mirtazapine switch arm were both superior to the sertraline continuation arm; the combination arm by − 0.99 points (95% CI − 1.55 to − 0.43, $P = 0.0012$) and the switch arm by − 1.01 points (95% CI − 1.56 to − 0.46, $P = 0.0012$) on PHQ-9 after Hochberg adjustment for multiple comparison. Results were very similar between the combination and switch arms (0.02, 95% CI − 0.54 to 0.57, $P = 0.95$); see Table 5. Self-rated BDI-II scores and the dichotomised response and remission rates were consistent with the primary analysis. RDs for response and remission, respectively, were 9.1% (95% CI 2.8–15.4%) and 12.4% (6.1–19.0%) for the combination strategy, and 8.2% (1.7–14.3%) and 8.4% (2.5–14.8%) for the switching strategy, over the continuation strategy. They corresponded with numbers needed to treat (NNTs) of 11.0 (6.5–35.7) and 8.1 (5.3–16.4) for the combination and 12.2 (7.0–59) and 11.9 (6.8–40) for the switching strategies.

The proportion of continuation of the allocated treatment was significantly lower in the combination arm (RD 8.5%, 95% CI 2.9–14.9%) and the switching arm (6.4%, 95% CI 1.3–12.5%) than the continuation arm. The overall burden of side effects as measured with FIB-SER did not, however, differ among the three strategies (Table 5). Neither were there any material differences regarding incidence of suicidality, manic switches or serious adverse events (Additional file 2: Table S5).

At week 25, the treatment arms did not differ in any of the efficacy (PHQ-9, BDI-II, remission), acceptability

Table 3 Primary and secondary outcomes at week 9 for step 1 randomisation

	Titrate sertraline up to 50 mg/day by week 3	Titrate sertraline up to 100 mg/day by week 3	100 mg/day vs 50 mg/day
	Least squares mean (95% CI)	Least squares mean (95% CI)	Adjusted[a] difference (95% CI) P value
PHQ-9	7.90 (7.14 to 8.66)	8.15 (7.78 to 8.52)	0.25 (−0.58 to 1.07) P = 0.55
BDI-II	16.55 (15.43 to 17.67)	16.00 (14.88 to 17.13)	−0.55 (−2.09 to 1.00) P = 0.49
FIBSER	5.03 (4.81 to 5.26)	5.28 (4.96 to 5.61)	0.25 (− 0.15 to 0.65), P = 0.22
	Raw numbers	Raw numbers	Adjusted[b] OR (95% CI) P value
Proportion of response	216/424 (111 of 251 who were unremitted and allocated to continue sertraline, 91 of 129 who remitted and continued on sertraline and 14 out of 44 who withdrew from protocol)	229/425 (122 of 286 who were unremitted and allocated to continue sertraline, 84 of 99 who remitted and continued on sertraline and 23 out of 40 who withdrew from protocol)	1.23 (0.90 to 1.67), P = 0.19
Proportion of remission	185/424 (64 of 251 who were unremitted and allocated to continue sertraline, 110 of 129 who remitted and continued on sertraline and 11 out of 44 who withdrew from protocol)	170/426 (68 of 286 who were unremitted and allocated to continue sertraline, 86 of 99 who remitted and continued on sertraline and 16 out of 41 who withdrew from protocol)	1.09 (0.75 to 1.58), P = 0.64
Proportion of continuation of the allocated treatment up to week 9	302/460 (204 of 261 who were unremitted and allocated to continue sertraline, 96 of 129 who remitted and continued on sertraline and 2 out of 70 who withdrew from protocol)	330/455 (248 of 290 who were unremitted and allocated to continue sertraline, 80 of 101 who remitted and continued on sertraline and 2 out of 64 who withdrew from protocol)	1.17 (0.70 to 1.98) P = 0.53
	Mean (SD)	Mean (SD)	
Sertraline prescribed at week 9 (mg/day)	45.5 (19.8), n = 384	85.3 (32.1), n = 391	

[a]The linear mixed-effects repeated-measures model included fixed effects of treatment, visit (as categorical) and treatment-by-visit interaction, and random effects for subjects and sites, adjusted for age, sex, education, marital status, number of previous depressive episodes, baseline scores at weeks 0 and 1, and was weighted by inverse probability of censoring (IPCW) to account for missing outcomes due to being allocated to the combination or switching arms at step 2 randomisation
[b]We used weighted generalised linear mixed models with the logit link and binomial distributions to account for clustering effects for the dichotomous secondary outcomes, adjusted for age, sex, education, marital status, number of previous depressive episodes, baseline scores at weeks 0 and 1
BDI-II Beck Depression Inventory 2nd edition, *FIBSER* Frequency, Intensity and Burden of Side Effects Rating, *PHQ-9* Patient Health Questionnaire-9

(time to discontinuation of the allocated treatment or of any treatment) or harm outcomes (Table 6, Additional file 2: Table S6).

There was no evidence of effect modification in any of the three pre-planned subgroup analyses (Additional file 2: Table S7).

Discussion

The SUN☺D trial involved two randomisations to examine the first- and second-line antidepressant pharmacotherapies for the acute phase treatment of hitherto untreated major depressive disorder.

The step 1 randomisation examined the impact of titrating to the minimum or maximum of the licenced dose of sertraline by week 3. In patients starting treatment for major depressive disorder, there were no important differences in effectiveness or adverse effects

between these two starting sertraline doses. The results of the primary outcome at week 9 (0.25 point difference in adjusted PHQ-9 score, 95% CI – 0.58 to 1.07, P = 0.55) excluded an important difference in favour of the higher dose. Neither were there any important differences between the minimum vs the maximum target doses in side effects, burden or treatment acceptability up to either week 9 or week 25.

When patients do not remit after 3 weeks of sertraline treatment, however, adding mirtazapine or switching sertraline to mirtazapine resulted in approximately a one-point benefit in PHQ-9 at week 9, a standardised mean difference of around 0.16. This difference corresponded to RDs in response of 9.1% (95% CI 2.8–15.4%) for the combination and 8.2% (1.7–14.3%) for the switching strategy and, in remission, of 12.4% (6.1–19.0%) for the combination and 8.4% (2.5–14.8%) for the

Table 4 Secondary outcomes at week 25 for step 1 randomisation

	Titrate sertraline up to 50 mg/day by week 3	Titrate sertraline up to 100 mg/day by week 3	100 mg/day vs 50 mg/day
	Least squares mean (95%CI)	Least squares mean (95% CI)	Adjusted[a] difference (95% CI) P value
PHQ-9	6.00 (5.33 to 6.67)	5.52 (4.89 to 6.16)	−0.47 (− 1.39 to 0.44) P = 0.31
BDI-II	13.29 (12.11 to 14.46)	11.00 (9.82 to 12.19)	−2.28 (− 3.91 to − 0.66) P = 0.006
FIBSER	4.14 (3.86 to 4.42)	4.28 (4.04 to 4.51)	0.14 (−0.20 to 0.48) P = 0.43
	Raw numbers (%)	Raw numbers (%)	Adjusted[b] OR (95%CI) P value
Proportion of remission	240/427 (117 of 252 who were unremitted and allocated to continue sertraline, 110 of 127 who remitted and continued on sertraline and 13 out of 48 who withdrew from protocol)	226/423 (128 of 286 who were unremitted and allocated to continue sertraline, 84 of 97 who remitted and continued on sertraline and 14 out of 40 who withdrew from protocol)	0.99 (0.66 to 1.47), P = 0.94
	Mean (SE)	Mean (SE)	HR (95% CI) P value
Time to discontinuation of allocated treatment by week 25	14.68 (0.40)	13.82 (0.37)	0.88 (0.52 to 1.48) P = 0.63
Time to discontinuation of any treatment by week 25	17.55 (0.38)	15.55 (0.28)	1.37 (0.80 to 2.35) P = 0.25
	Mean (SD)	Mean (SD)	
Sertraline prescribed at week 25 (mg/day)	40.7 (29.1), n = 341	57.0 (45.0), n = 321	

[a]The linear mixed-effects repeated-measures model included fixed effects of treatment, visit (as categorical) and treatment-by-visit interaction, and random effects for subjects and sites, adjusted for age, sex, education, marital status, number of previous depressive episodes, baseline scores at weeks 0 and 1, and was weighted by inverse probability of censoring (IPCW) to account for missing outcomes due to being allocated to the combination or switching arms at step 2 randomisation
[b]We used weighted generalised linear mixed models with the logit link and binomial distributions to account for clustering effects for the dichotomous secondary outcomes, adjusted for age, sex, education, marital status, number of previous depressive episodes, baseline scores at weeks 0 and 1
BDI-II Beck Depression Inventory 2nd edition, *FIBSER* Frequency, Intensity and Burden of Side Effects Rating, *PHQ-9* Patient Health Questionnaire-9, *SE* Standard error

switching strategy. These values are slightly below or above the usually accepted clinically significant threshold of 10% RD, but they may be important to patients when one considers that they are differences between alternative active treatments and that RDs for antidepressants over placebo are approximately 20% only [29, 43]. In addition, these results were consistent with patients' self-reports by BDI-II. The benefits of combination and switching did not, however, persist after continuation treatment at the treating physician's discretion at week 25.

Combination or switching strategies resulted in 6–8% fewer patients continuing the allocated treatments up to week 9 than continuing on sertraline. However, given the greater improvement in depressive symptoms with the strategies that included mirtazapine; similar global ratings of side effects among the treatment arms at weeks 9 and 25; and similar time to discontinuation of allocated treatment or any treatment when considered up to 25 weeks; this finding does not raise concern regarding the use of combination and switching strategies.

The most recent comprehensive network meta-analysis of antidepressants found that mirtazapine may have a greater response rate than sertraline (OR = 1.15, 95% CI 0.93–1.43) when used as first-line monotherapy [29]. The current study findings are compatible with this network meta-analysis, and this superior efficacy of mirtazapine may be responsible for some of the benefits of switching or combination strategies over sertraline continuation found in the current study.

Some guidelines recommend dose increase within the approved range after non-response to a lower dose ([4], p. 356, [10], p.53). Two previous studies have tested this strategy for sertraline and found that there was no additional benefit: one study compared 50 mg vs 150 mg of sertraline for 5 weeks after an initial 3 weeks on 50 mg and reported no difference [44]. Another study compared 100 mg vs 200 mg of sertraline for 5 weeks after an initial 6 weeks in which patients received up to 100 mg and reported that the increase to 200 mg resulted in a lower response rate [24]. Although the current study did not specifically address this strategy,

Table 5 Primary and secondary outcomes at week 9 for step 2 randomisation

	Continue sertraline	Combine with mirtazapine	Switch to mirtazapine	Combine vs continue	Switch vs continue	Combine vs switch
	Least squares mean (95% CI)	Least squares mean (95% CI)	Least squares mean (95% CI)	Adjusted[a] difference (95% CI) P value	Adjusted[a] difference (95% CI) P value	Adjusted[a] difference (95% CI) P value
PHQ-9	9.26 (8.79 to 9.72)	8.27 (7.80 to 8.74)	8.25 (7.79 to 8.71)	−0.99 (−1.55 to −0.43) P=0.0006 P=0.0012[b]	−1.01 (−1.56 to −0.46) P=0.0004 P=0.0012[b]	0.02 (−0.54 to 0.58) P=0.94 P=0.94[b]
BDI-II	18.68 (17.87 to 19.49)	16.59 (15.77 to 17.40)	17.06 (16.25 to 17.86)	−2.10 (−3.12 to −1.07) P<0.0001	−1.62 (−2.63 to −0.61) P=0.0017	−0.47 (−1.49 to 0.55) P=0.36
FIBSER	5.34 (5.05 to 5.63)	5.43 (5.14 to 5.72)	5.59 (5.30 to 5.88)	0.09 (−0.32 to 0.50) P=0.66	0.25 (−0.16 to 0.66) P=0.22	−0.16 (−0.57 to 0.25) P=0.44
	Raw numbers (%)	Raw numbers (%)	Raw numbers (%)	Adjusted[c] OR (95% CI) P value	Adjusted[c] OR (95% CI) P value	Adjusted[c] OR (95% CI) P value
Proportion of response	233/537 (43.4%)	273/527 (51.8%)	275/550 (50.0%)	1.41 (1.11 to 1.85) P=0.0055	1.39 (1.08 to 1.78) P=0.0109	1.03 (0.81 to 1.33) P=0.79
Proportion of remission	132/537 (24.6%)	188/527 (35.7%)	174/550 (31.6%)	1.80 (1.36 to 2.38) P<0.0001	1.51 (1.14 to 1.99) P=0.0037	1.19 (0.92 to 1.55) P=0.19
Proportion of continuation of the allocated treatment up to week 9	452/551 (82.0%)	400/537 (74.5%)	427/558 (76.5%)	0.61 (0.45 to 0.83) P=0.0014	0.68 (0.50 to 0.92) P=0.0131	0.90 (0.67 to 1.19) P=0.46
	Mean (SD)	Mean (SD)	Mean (SD)			
Sertraline prescribed at week 9 (mg/day)	71.7 (30.0), n=520	71.1 (29.1), n=502	6.5 (19.0), n=524			
Mirtazapine prescribed at week 9 (mg/day)	0.6 (3.9), n=520	15.1 (11.8), n=501	18.4 (13.0), n=524			

[a]The linear mixed-effects repeated-measures model included fixed effects of PHQ-9 at week 3, treatment, visit (as categorical), treatment-by-visit interaction and minimisation variables for step 2 randomisation (step 1 treatment, 50% or greater reduction on PHQ-9 by week 3, moderate or greater impairment on FIBSER at week 3) and random effects for individuals and sites

[b]Hochberg method was used for adjustment of multiplicity for the primary outcome (italicised P values for PHQ-9) but not for secondary outcomes, as postulated in the statistical analysis plan [33]

[c]We used the logistic regression model adjusted for sites, step 1 treatment, 50% or greater reduction on PHQ-9 by week 3 and moderate or greater impairment on FIBSER at week 3

BDI-II Beck Depression Inventory 2nd edition, FIBSER Frequency, Intensity and Burden of Side Effects Rating, PHQ-9 Patient Health Questionnaire-9

Table 6 Secondary outcomes at week 25 for step 2 randomisation

	Continue sertraline	Combine with mirtazapine	Switch to mirtazapine	Combine vs continue	Switch vs continue	Combine vs switch
	Least squares mean (95% CI)	Least squares mean (95% CI)	Least squares mean (95% CI)	Adjusted[a] difference (95% CI) P value	Adjusted[a] difference (95% CI) P value	Adjusted[a] difference (95% CI) P value
PHQ-9	6.58 (6.09 to 7.07)	6.37 (5.88 to 6.87)	6.61 (6.12 to 7.10)	−0.20 (−0.80 to 0.40) P=0.51	0.03 (−0.56 to 0.63) P=0.91	−0.24 (−0.84 to 0.37) P=0.44
BDI-II	14.09 (13.15 to 15.03)	13.45 (12.49 to 14.41)	13.72 (12.78 to 14.67)	−0.64 (−1.88 to 0.60) P=0.31	−0.37 (−1.59 to 0.86) P=0.56	−0.27 (−1.51 0.96) P=0.66
FIBSER	4.34 (4.10 to 4.59)	4.46 (4.21 to 4.71)	4.48 (4.24 to 4.72)	0.12 (−0.23 to 0.47) P=0.51	0.14 (−0.21 to 0.48) P=0.44	−0.02 (−0.36 to 0.33) P=0.92
	Raw numbers (%)	Raw numbers (%)	Raw numbers (%)	Adjusted[b] OR (95% CI) P value	Adjusted[b] OR (95% CI) P value	Adjusted[b] OR (95% CI) P value
Proportion of remission	245/538 (45.5%)	263/520 (50.3%)	262/540 (48.5%)	1.24 (0.96 to 1.49) P=0.10	1.16 (0.90 to 1.48), P=0.25	1.07 (0.80 to 1.37) P=0.60
	Mean (SE)	Mean (SE)	Mean (SE)	HR (95% CI) P value	HR (95% CI) P value	HR (95% CI) P value
Time to discontinuation of allocated treatment by week 25	15.97 (0.30)	15.23 (0.32)	15.56 (0.31)	1.07 (0.92 to 1.25) P=0.40	1.04 (0.89 to 1.21) P=0.64	1.03 (0.88 to 1.20) P=0.70
Time to discontinuation of any treatment by week 25	17.32 (0.17)	20.47 (0.23)	20.22 (0.23)	0.89 (0.69 to 1.14) P=0.35	1.08 (0.85 to 1.38) P=0.51	0.82 (0.64 to 1.05) P=0.11
	Mean (SD)	Mean (SD)	Mean (SD)			
Sertraline prescribed at week 52 (mg/day)	51.6 (38.5), n=448	51.2 (38.3), n=440	10.3 (24.7), n=457			
Mirtazapine prescribed at week 52 (mg/day)	3.9 (10.6), n=448	12.3 (13.0), n=440	14.6 (13.8), n=456			

[a]The linear mixed-effects repeated-measures model included fixed effects of PHQ-9 at week 3, treatment, visit (as categorical), treatment-by-visit interaction, and minimisation variables for step 2 randomisation (step 1 treatment, 50% or greater reduction on PHQ-9 by week 3, moderate or greater impairment on FIBSER at week 3), and random effects for individuals and sites

[b]We used the logistic regression model adjusted for sites, step 1 treatment, 50% or greater reduction on PHQ-9 by week 3 and moderate or greater impairment on FIBSER at week 3

BDI-II Beck Depression Inventory 2nd edition, FIBSER Frequency, Intensity and Burden of Side Effects Rating, HR hazard ratio, PHQ-9 Patient Health Questionnaire-9, SE Standard error our results with regard to the initial target dose are consistent with these previous studies.

There are limitations of our study. First, the step 1 cluster randomisation by clinic was performed at the start of the study. As a result, there was no concealment at the level of randomisation of individual patients, which explains the differences in characteristics of patients enrolled in the two arms. Clinicians at study sites allocated to the lower dose were less inclined to enrol severe patients or male patients than were clinicians at sites allocated to the higher dose. We dealt with this prognostic imbalance by adjusting for key variables in the mixed-model repeated-measures analyses and confirmed robustness of the primary findings against model assumptions through sensitivity analyses. Unknown confounders may still, however, have biased our findings, limiting strength of inference in the step 1 findings.

Secondly, the open-label design may have created some undetected performance bias that may threaten the internal validity of both the step 1 and step 2 comparisons, such as differential administration of co-prescriptions or psychological support. Such bias is, however, likely to be minimal, because the protocol did not allow any depression-specific psychotherapies such as CBT or IPT or concomitant administration of antipsychotics or mood stabilisers up to week 9. Co-prescription of benzodiazepines was permitted, but they were prescribed very similarly in all arms (60–70% of the participants received either anxiolytics or hypnotics). Further, a differential placebo effect associated with adding or switching to mirtazapine vs continuing with sertraline could explain some of the apparent effect of the switching/adding arms in step 2. Blinded assessment of outcomes somewhat ameliorates this concern. Moreover, the open-label design was consonant with the pragmatic nature of the study, in which we made comparisons including such possible practice variability.

Thirdly, the tapering speed of sertraline in the switching arm was relatively slow and allowed some patients to take the combination of sertraline and mirtazapine for several weeks. The efficacy of the switching strategy might therefore be contaminated by that of the combination treatment. However, gradual tapering was appropriate for this pragmatic trial and allowed us to address the impact of interventions as clinicians would implement them in the real world.

Fourthly, one might question the generalisability of the current study findings beyond the specific drugs and dosages employed. As the initial target dose of the antidepressant, we compared the minimum and the maximum of the licenced dosage in Japan, 50 mg/day and 100 mg/day of sertraline. The maximum dosage for sertraline in the USA and in some other countries is 200 mg/day. The study specified dosing for mirtazapine

between 7.5 and 45 mg, which is also lower than the dosing sometimes used in other countries. These differences may reflect differences in body weights and other ethnically specific variations in the genetic as well as non-genetic mechanisms affecting the pharmacokinetics and dynamics of psychotropic drugs [45]. Up to now, however, inquiry has failed to identify ethnicity as a convincing modifier of antidepressant effect [46]. Had we compared 50 mg/day vs 200 mg/day, or had we required higher dose ranges for mirtazapine, the results might have differed. However, consistent with our step 1 findings, RCTs using other drugs have in most cases also suggested no additional benefit with higher doses [12, 47, 48]. It is also uncertain whether results would be similar had we chosen to begin with an antidepressant other than sertraline or chosen to combine or switch with a drug other than mirtazapine. Our step 2 findings for adding mirtazapine to sertraline are consistent with the previous systematic review examining various combination strategies [22]. One might consider our step 2 findings for switching to mirtazapine at odds with the recent meta-analysis on this topic that found no additional benefit in switching to various antidepressants [20]. However, the only study in this review specific to mirtazapine reported that using mirtazapine was more effective than continuing the prior medication [49].

A further limitation is that, although it provides evidence that changing therapy after failure to remit at an early point (in our study 3 weeks) may be preferable to waiting a longer period (e.g. the oft-recommended 6 to 8 weeks), the design did not specifically address the optimal timing of the decision to switch or combine. One RCT compared switching to duloxetine immediately after non-response to 4weeks of escitalopram against continuing 4 more weeks on escitalopram and then switching if non-responsive: the two arms did not differ in their primary outcome of time to response, while there was significant increase in a secondary outcome of remission in the early switch arm than in the later switch arm [50]. Another recent RCT examined the value of switching escitalopram to venlafaxine if patients have shown minimal improvement after 2 weeks; remission rates were 8% higher in the switched than in the continuation arm, but this difference did not reach statistical significance, possibly due to a small sample size ($n = 192$, $p = 0.21$) [51]. Thus, the optimal time to combine or switch remains uncertain.

Strengths of this pragmatic trial primarily relate to design features that enhance the real-world application of the results. We employed a large number of study sites using broad eligibility criteria, and thus enrolled sufficient patients to achieve high power to establish or refute differences between groups. Because Japan does not have a primary care system, patients with new onset depressive episodes usually consult office practice psychiatrists directly. Thus, in many other countries, primary care doctors would see and begin treatment of most participants entered in SUN☺D. In comparison to many multi-centre trials, we were able to enrol a large proportion (2011 of 7895) of potentially eligible patients. Enrolment of patients not yet treated for their current episode is another strength, eliminating a potential source of variability. For step 1 randomisation, we excluded patients who did not tolerate a low dose of sertraline, faithfully addressing the clinical question in which patients and clinicians are interested: In patients who tolerate an initial low dose of sertraline, should clinicians titrate to the maximum dose? For step 2 randomisation, we selected alternative interventions that are recommended in practice guidelines [4, 10] and are widely used [52].

We limited risk of bias through centralised, blinded, telephone assessments that allowed us to achieve more than 95% follow-up through 25 weeks, unique among large trials of psychiatric interventions. The centralised training of the raters enhanced the reliability and validity of the depression assessments [38]. A pre-published protocol [32], statistical analysis plan [33] and blinded interpretation of the results to minimise the researchers' interpretation bias further enhance the trustworthiness of this RCT.

Conclusions

The SUN☺D trial suggests that, for the initial antidepressant therapy for a new major depressive episode, titrating sertraline to the maximum over the minimum within the licenced dosage confers no additional benefit but increases cost. The confidence in this conclusion is limited by the failure of the cluster randomisation to achieve prognostic balance, and the possible residual confounding after our adjusted analysis. When patients fail to remit on this initial treatment, early combination or switching using mirtazapine resulted in a small benefit in reducing depression without an increase in adverse effects. Inferences apply to the strategies as implemented, which reflect clinical practice, including gradual tapering of sertraline in the switching arm. Factors bearing on the decision to combine or switch are likely to include costs (combination will be more costly), the current burden of side effects of the first-line treatment, the expected burden of combination or switching and the patient's readiness to change antidepressants.

The many drugs available allow clinicians considerable options in the selection of an initial antidepressant and of second-line antidepressants to switch to or combine with. Clinicians and patients may consider starting the treatment with a low dose of agents for which evidence suggests satisfactory efficacy and acceptability in the

current trial and in the comprehensive network meta-analysis [29]. Should they choose to combine antidepressants as the second-line strategy, the relative merits of potential combinations remain largely untested in RCTs, and it is implausible that RCTs will ultimately evaluate all such alternatives. A previous review suggested that a combination of a reuptake inhibitor antidepressant and an antagonist of presynaptic alpha-2 autoreceptor is more effective than other combinations [22], and the current findings were consistent with this suggestion. Those who place a high value in treatments that have been tested in large trials that both minimise risk of bias and mimic real-world conditions may prefer the specific strategies used in this trial.

Additional files

Additional file 1: Blinded data analyses statement of interpretation. (PDF 336 kb)

Additional file 2: Figure S1. Schedule of the assessments. **Table S1.** Incidence of suicidality, manic switches or any serious adverse events up to week 9 for step 1 randomisation. **Table S2.** Incidence of suicidality, manic switches or any serious adverse events up to week 25 for step 1 randomisation. **Table S3.** Two pre-specified subgroup analyses for step 1 randomisation. **Table S4.** Four pre-specified sensitivity analyses for step 1 randomisation. **Table S5.** Incidence of suicidality, manic switches or any serious adverse events up to week 9 for step 2 randomisation. **Table S6.** Incidence of suicidality, manic switches or any serious adverse events up to week 25 for step 2 randomisation. **Table S7.** Three pre-specified subgroup analyses for step 2 randomisation. (DOCX 32 kb)

Additional file 3: SUN☺D Investigators and committee members. (DOCX 17 kb)

Acknowledgements
Group information: A complete list of participating centres and investigators in the Strategic Use of New generation antidepressants for Depression (SUN☺D trial) is provided in Additional file 3.

Funding
The study was funded by the Ministry of Health, Labor and Welfare, Japan (H-22-Seishin-Ippan-008) from April 2010 through March 2012 to TAF (http://www.mhlw.go.jp/english/) and thereafter by the Japan Foundation for Neuroscience and Mental Health (JFNMH) to TAF (http://www.jfnm.or.jp/). The JFNMH received donations from Asahi Kasei, Eli Lilly, GlaxoSmithKline (GSK), Janssen, Merck Sharp & Dohme (MSD), Meiji, Mochida, Otsuka, Pfizer, Shionogi, Taisho and Mitsubishi-Tanabe. The funders of the study had no role in study design, data collection, data analysis, data interpretation or in writing of the report.

Authors' contributions
TAF is the principal investigator and had overall responsibility for the management of the study. TAF, NY, ST and QZ had full access to all the data in the study and take responsibility for the integrity of the data and the accuracy of the data analyses. TAF conceived the study. YOg, NTa, YH, AT and KSh performed data curation; NY, ST, QZ and TAF performed the formal

analysis. TAF and MY acquired the funding. TK, TAF, AM, KK, HK, SH, HS, KSu, BC, KI, YI, YS, MK, YOk, HF, MS, SY, NTs, TI, NF, TA, MY, SS, NW, MI, KM, YOg, NTa, YH, AT, KSh and GHG performed the investigation. TAF, TA, MY, SS, NW, MI, KM and NY developed the methodology.MK, YOk, HF, MS, SY, NTs, TI, NF, YOg, NTa, YH, AT and KSh administered the project. TAF and GHG supervised the project. TAF and GHG wrote the original draft. TK, AM, KK, HK, SH, HS, KSu, BC, KI, YI, YS, MK, YOk, HF, MS, SY, NTs, TI, NF, TA, MY, SS, NW, MI, KM, YOg, NTa, YH, AT, KSh, NY, ST and QZ reviewed and edited the manuscript. All authors read and approved the final manuscript.

Competing interests

TK has received lecture fees from Eli Lilly and Mitsubishi-Tanabe and has contracted research with GSK, MSD and Mitsubishi-Tanabe. He has received royalties from Kyowa Yakuhin. TAF has received lecture fees from Eli Lilly, Janssen, Meiji, MSD, Otsuka, Pfizer and Mitsubishi-Tanabe and consultancy fees from Takeda Science Foundation. He has received research support from Mochida and Mitsubishi-Tanabe. AM has received lecture fees from Mochida, Eli Lilly and Meiji. SH has received lecture fees from MSD, Pfizer, Meiji, Tanabe-Mitsubishi and Otsuka. HS has received lecture fees from Daiichi-Sankyo and Mochida. KSu has received lecture and/or consultant fees from Eli Lilly, Mochida, Eisai, Meiji and Daiichi-Sankyo. BC has received lecture fees from Eli Lilly, Meiji and Mitsubishi-Tanabe. KI has received lecture fees from Dainippon-Sumitomo, Eli Lilly, Otsuka, Takeda, Kyowa Yakuhin, Mitsubishi-Tanabe, Meiji and Shionogi. YI has received lecture fees from Meiji, Eli Lilly, Janssen and Otsuka. YS has received lecture fees from Janssen, Kyowa Yakuhin, Meiji, MSD, Otsuka and Mitsubishi-Tanabe. MK has received lecture fees from Yoshitomi and a research grant from Novartis. YOk has received lecture fees from Otsuka, Dainippon-Sumitomo, Astellas, Pfizer, Eli Lilly, Janssen, Meiji, Mochida, Yoshitomi, Eisai and GSK. HF has received lecture fees from Meiji, Mochida, MSD and Otsuka. SY has received lecture fees from Daiichi-Sankyo and Otsuka. NTs has received lecture fees from Astellas, Shionogi, Novartis, Fujifilm RI Pharma, Meiji, Mochida, Janssen, Eli Lilly and Dainippon-Sumitomo. TI has received lecture fees from GSK, Mochida, Asahi Kasei, Shionogi, Otsuka, Dainippon-Sumitomo, Eli Lilly, Eisai, Mitsubishi-Tanabe, Pfizer, AbbVie, MSD, Yoshitomi, Takeda and Meiji. He has received grants from Shionogi, Astellas, Otsuka, Dainippon-Sumitomo, Eli Lilly, Eisai, Mitsubishi-Tanabe, Pfizer, AbbVie, MSD, Yoshitomi, Takeda and Meiji. He is on advisor boards for GSK, Mochida, Otsuka, Eli Lilly, Mitsubishi-Tanabe, Pfizer and Takeda. NF has received lecture fees from Pfizer, Eisai, Mochida, Ono, Shionogi, MSD and Otsuka. TA has received lecture fees and/or research funds from Daiichi-Sankyo, Eisai, Hisamitsu, Eli Lilly, MSD, Meiji, Mochida, Otsuka, Pfizer, Novartis and Terumo. MY has received lecture fees from Meiji, MSD and Asahi Kasei and has contracted research with Nippon Chemiphar. SS has received lecture fees from Otsuka, MSD, Meiji, Eli Lilly, Mochida and Shionogi. MI has received a grant from Novartis Pharma. He has received lecture fees from Pfizer, Mochida, Shionogi, Sumitomo Dainippon Pharma, Daiichi-Sankyo, Meiji and Takeda. KM has received lecture fees from Eisai, GSK, Meiji, MSD, Otsuka, Pfizer, Eli Lilly, Mochida, Yoshitomi, Dainippon-Sumitomo, Takeda and Shionogi. YOg has received a lecture fee from Eli Lilly. NTa has received lecture fees from Otsuka and Meiji. YH has received a lecture fee from Yoshitomi. AT has received lecture fees from Eli Lilly and Mitsubishi-Tanabe. ST has received lecture fees from AstraZeneca, Taiho and Ono. He has received consultation fees from DeNA Life Science and CanBus. He has received outsourcing fees from Satt and Asahi Kasei Pharma. His wife has been engaged in a research project of Bayer. All these fees have been outside the submitted work. KK, HK, MS, NW, KSh, NY, QZ and GHG declare that they have no competing interests.

Author details

[1]Aratama Kokorono Clinic, Nagoya, Japan. [2]Department of Health Promotion of Human Behavior, Kyoto University Graduate School of Medicine / School of Public Health, Yoshida Konoe-cho, Sakyo-ku, Kyoto 606-8501, Japan. [3]Mantani Mental Clinic, Hiroshima, Japan. [4]Kabe Mental Health Clinic, Hiroshima, Japan. [5]Kokokara Clinic, Kochi, Japan. [6]Hirota Clinic, Kurume, Japan. [7]Harimayabashi Clinic, Kochi, Japan. [8]Oji Mental Clinic, Tokyo, Japan. [9]Ginza Taimei Clinic, Tokyo, Japan. [10]Sinsapporo Mental Clinic, Sapporo, Japan. [11]Narumi Himawari Clinic, Nagoya, Japan. [12]Shiki Clinic, Nagoya, Japan. [13]Department of Psychiatry and Cognitive-Behavioral Medicine, Nagoya City University Graduate School of Medical Sciences, Nagoya, Japan. [14]Department of Neuropsychiatry, Hiroshima University Graduate School of Biomedical & Health Sciences, Hiroshima, Japan. [15]Center to Promote Creativity in Medical Education, Kochi Medical School, Kochi University, Nankoku, Japan. [16]Department of Neuropsychiatry, University of Tokyo Hospital, Tokyo, Japan. [17]Department of Neuropsychiatry, Kurume University Medical School, Kurume, Japan. [18]Department of Psychiatry, Toho University School of Medicine, Tokyo, Japan. [19]Department of Neuropsychiatry, Tokyo Medical University, Tokyo, Japan. [20]Department of Neuropsychiatry, Kumamoto University Graduate School of Medicine, Kumamoto, Japan. [21]Department of Neuropsychopharmacology, National Center of Neurology and Psychiatry, Tokyo, Japan. [22]Department of Neuropsychiatry, Okayama University Hospital, Okayama, Japan. [23]Miki Mental Clinic, Yokohama, Japan. [24]Department of Biostatistics, Kyoto University Graduate School of Medicine / School of Public Health, Kyoto, Japan. [25]Department of Clinical Biostatistics, Kyoto University Graduate School of Medicine / School of Public Health, Kyoto, Japan. [26]Departments of Clinical Epidemiology and Biostatistics, and of Medicine, McMaster University, Hamilton, Canada.

References

1. Abbing-Karahagopian V, Huerta C, Souverein PC, de Abajo F, Leufkens HG, Slattery J, Alvarez Y, Miret M, Gil M, Oliva B, et al. Antidepressant prescribing in five European countries: application of common definitions to assess the prevalence, clinical observations, and methodological implications. Eur J Clin Pharmacol. 2014;70(7):849–57.
2. Kantor ED, Rehm CD, Haas JS, Chan AT, Giovannucci EL. Trends in prescription drug use among adults in the United States from 1999-2012. JAMA. 2015; 314(17):1818–31.
3. Kjosavik SR, Hunskaar S, Aarsland D, Ruths S. Initial prescription of antipsychotics and antidepressants in general practice and specialist care in Norway. Acta Psychiatr Scand. 2011;123(6):459–65.
4. NICE. Depression: the treatment and management of depression in adults (partial update of NICE clinical guideline 23). London: National Institute for Clinical Excellence; 2009.
5. Cipriani A, Furukawa TA, Salanti G, Geddes JR, Higgins JP, Churchill R, Watanabe N, Nakagawa A, Omori IM, McGuire H, et al. Comparative efficacy and acceptability of 12 new-generation antidepressants: a multiple-treatments meta-analysis. Lancet. 2009;373:746–58.
6. Medicines use and spending in the U.S. — a review of 2016 and outlook for 2021. https://www.iqvia.com/institute/reports/medicines-use-and-spending-in-the-us-a-review-of-2016. Accessed 20 June 2018.
7. Furukawa TA, Onishi Y, Hinotsu S, Tajika A, Takeshima N, Shinohara K, Ogawa Y, Hayasaka Y, Kawakami K. Prescription patterns following first-line new generation antidepressants for depression in Japan: a naturalistic cohort study based on a large claims database. J Affect Disord. 2013;150:916–22.
8. S3-Guideline/National Disease Management Guideline Unipolar Depression. Short version. https://www.leitlinien.de/nvl/depression. Accessed 20 June 2018.
9. Bauer M, Pfennig A, Severus E, Whybrow PC, Angst J, Moller HJ. World Federation of Societies of Biological Psychiatry (WFSBP) guidelines for biological treatment of unipolar depressive disorders, part 1: update 2013 on the acute and continuation treatment of unipolar depressive disorders. World J Biol Psychiatry. 2013;14(5):334–85.

50

Clinical and Translational Medicine

10. American Psychiatric Association. Practice guideline for the treatment of patients with major depressive disorder (third edition). Am J Psychiatry. 2010;167(Suppl):1–152.

11. Bollini P, Pampallona S, Tibaldi G, Kupelnick B, Munizza C. Effectiveness of antidepressants. Meta-analysis of dose-effect relationships in randomised clinical trials. Br J Psychiatry. 1999;174:297–303.

12. Purgato M, Gastaldon C, Papola D, Magni LR, Rossi G, Barbui C. Drug dose as mediator of treatment effect in antidepressant drug trials: the case of fluoxetine. Acta Psychiatr Scand. 2015;131(6):408–16.

13. Hieronymus F, Nilsson S, Eriksson E. A mega-analysis of fixed-dose trials reveals dose-dependency and a rapid onset of action for the antidepressant effect of three selective serotonin reuptake inhibitors. Transl Psychiatry. 2016;6(6):e834.

14. Corruble E, Guelfi JD. Does increasing dose improve efficacy in patients with poor antidepressant response: a review. Acta Psychiatr Scand. 2000;101(5):343–8.

15. Adli M, Baethge C, Heinz A, Langlitz N, Bauer M. Is dose escalation of antidepressants a rational strategy after a medium-dose treatment has failed? A systematic review. Eur Arch Psychiatry Clin Neurosci. 2005;255(6):387–400.

16. Ruhe HG, Huyser J, Swinkels JA, Schene AH. Dose escalation for insufficient response to standard dose selective serotonin reuptake inhibitors in major depressive disorder: systematic review. Br J Psychiatry. 2006;189:309–16.

17. Dold M, Bartova L, Rupprecht R, Kasper S. Dose escalation of antidepressants in unipolar depression: a meta-analysis of double-blind, randomized controlled trials. Psychother Psychosom. 2017;86(5):283–91.

18. Ruhe HG, Huyser J, Swinkels JA, Schene AH. Switching antidepressants after a first selective serotonin reuptake inhibitor in major depressive disorder: a systematic review. J Clin Psychiatry. 2006;67(12):1836–55.

19. Papakostas GI, Fava M, Thase ME. Treatment of SSRI-resistant depression: a meta-analysis comparing within- versus across-class switches. Biol Psychiatry. 2008;63(7):699–704.

20. Bschor T, Kern H, Henssler J, Baethge C. Switching the antidepressant after nonresponse in adults with major depression: a systematic literature search and meta-analysis. J Clin Psychiatry. 2018;79(1). https://doi.org/10.4088/JCP.16r10749.

21. Zhou X, Ravindran AV, Qin B, Del Giovane C, Li Q, Bauer M, Liu Y, Fang Y, da Silva T, Zhang Y, et al. Comparative efficacy, acceptability, and tolerability of augmentation agents in treatment-resistant depression: systematic review and network meta-analysis. J Clin Psychiatry. 2015;76(4):e487–98.

22. Henssler J, Bschor T, Baethge C. Combining antidepressants in acute treatment of depression: a meta-analysis of 38 studies including 4511 patients. Can J Psychiatr. 2016;61(1):29–43.

23. Ferreri M, Lavergne F, Berlin I, Payan C, Puech AJ. Benefits from mianserin augmentation of fluoxetine in patients with major depression non-responders to fluoxetine alone. Acta Psychiatr Scand. 2001;103(1):66–72.

24. Licht RW, Qvitzau S. Treatment strategies in patients with major depression not responding to first-line sertraline treatment. A randomised study of extended duration of treatment, dose increase or mianserin augmentation. Psychopharmacology. 2002;161(2):143–51.

25. Rush AJ, Trivedi MH, Wisniewski SR, Stewart JW, Nierenberg AA, Thase ME, Ritz L, Biggs MM, Warden D, Luther JF, et al. Bupropion-SR, sertraline, or venlafaxine-XR after failure of SSRIs for depression. N Engl J Med. 2006; 354(12):1231–42.

26. Trivedi MH, Fava M, Wisniewski SR, Thase ME, Quitkin F, Warden D, Ritz L, Nierenberg AA, Lebowitz BD, Biggs MM, et al. Medication augmentation after the failure of SSRIs for depression. N Engl J Med. 2006;354(12):1243–52.

27. Mohamed S, Johnson GR, Chen P, Hicks PB, Davis LL, Yoon J, Gleason TC, Vertrees JE, Weingart K, Tal I, et al. Effect of antidepressant switching vs augmentation on remission among patients with major depressive disorder unresponsive to antidepressant treatment: the VAST-D randomized clinical trial. JAMA. 2017;318(2):132–45.

28. Qaseem A, Snow V, Denberg TD, Forciea MA, Owens DK. Using second-generation antidepressants to treat depressive disorders: a clinical practice guideline from the American College of Physicians. Ann Intern Med. 2008; 149(10):725–33.

29. Cipriani A, Furukawa TA, Salanti G, Chaimani A, Atkinson LZ, Ogawa Y, Leucht S, Ruhe HG, Turner EH, Higgins JPT, et al. Comparative efficacy and acceptability of 21 antidepressant drugs for the acute treatment of adults with major depressive disorder: a systematic review and network meta-analysis. Lancet. 2018;391(10128):1357–66.

30. American Psychiatric Association. Diagnostic and statistical manual of mental disorders, 4th ed. Washington, DC: American Psychiatric Association; 1994.

31. Spitzer RL, Williams JB, Kroenke K, Linzer M, deGruy FV 3rd, Hahn SR, Brody D, Johnson JG. Utility of a new procedure for diagnosing mental disorders in primary care. The PRIME-MD 1000 study. JAMA. 1994;272(22):1749–56.

32. Furukawa TA, Akechi T, Shimodera S, Yamada M, Miki K, Watanabe N, Inagaki M, Yonemoto N. Strategic use of new generation antidepressants for depression: SUN☺D study protocol. Trials. 2011;12(1):116.

33. Yonemoto N, Tanaka S, Furukawa TA, Kato T, Mantani A, Ogawa Y, Tajika A, Takeshima N, Hayasaka Y, Shinohara A, et al. Strategic use of new generation antidepressants for depression: SUN☺D protocol update and statistical analysis plan. Trials. 2015;16:459.

34. Kroenke K, Spitzer RL, Williams JB. The PHQ-9: validity of a brief depression severity measure. J Gen Intern Med. 2001;16(9):606–13.

35. Spitzer RL, Kroenke K, Williams JB. Validation and utility of a self-report version of PRIME-MD: the PHQ primary care study. Primary Care Evaluation of Mental Disorders. Patient Health Questionnaire. JAMA. 1999;282(18):1737–44.

36. Beck AT, Steer RA, Brown GK. BDI-II: BeckDepression Inventory, second edition, manual. San Antonio: The Psychological Corporation; 1996.

37. Posner K, Oquendo MA, Gould M, Stanley B, Davies M. Columbia Classification Algorithm of Suicide Assessment (C-CASA): classification of suicidal events in the FDA's pediatric suicidal risk analysis of antidepressants. Am J Psychiatry. 2007;164(7):1035–43.

38. Pinto-Meza A, Serrano-Blanco A, Penarrubia MT, Blanco E, Haro JM. Assessing depression in primary care with the PHQ-9: can it be carried out over the telephone? J Gen Intern Med. 2005;20(8):738–42.

39. Shimodera S, Kato T, Sato H, Miki K, Shinagawa Y, Kondo M, Fujita H, Morokuma I, Ikeda Y, Akechi T, et al. The first 100 patients in the SUN☺D trial (strategic use of new generation antidepressants for depression): examination of feasibility and adherence during the pilot phase. Trials. 2012;13(1):80.

40. Wells KB, Sherbourne C, Schoenbaum M, Duan N, Meredith L, Unutzer J, Miranda J, Carney MF, Rubenstein LV. Impact of disseminating quality improvement programs for depression in managed primary care: a randomized controlled trial. JAMA. 2000;283(2):212–20.

41. Cohen J. Statistical power analysis in the behavioral sciences. Hillsdale: Erlbaum; 1988.

42. Jarvinen TL, Sihvonen R, Bhandari M, Sprague S, Malmivaara A, Paavola M, Schunemann HJ, Guyatt GH. Blinded interpretation of study results can feasibly and effectively diminish interpretation bias. J Clin Epidemiol. 2014; 67(7):769–72.

43. Turner EH, Matthews AM, Linardatos E, Tell RA, Rosenthal R. Selective publication of antidepressant trials and its influence on apparent efficacy. N Engl J Med. 2008;358:252–60.

44. Schweizer E, Rynn M, Mandos LA, Demartinis N, Garcia-Espana F, Rickels K. The antidepressant effect of sertraline is not enhanced by dose titration: results from an outpatient clinical trial. Int Clin Psychopharmacol. 2001;16(3):137–43.

45. Chaudhry I, Neelam K, Duddu V, Husain N. Ethnicity and psychopharmacology. J Psychopharmacol. 2008;22(6):673–80.

46. Kessler RC, van Loo HM, Wardenaar KJ, Bossarte RM, Brenner LA, Ebert DD, de Jonge P, Nierenberg AA, Rosellini AJ, Sampson NA, et al. Using patient self-reports to study heterogeneity of treatment effects in major depressive disorder. Epidemiol Psychiatr Sci. 2017;26(1):22–36.

47. Furukawa TA, McGuire H, Barbui C. Meta-analysis of effects and side effects of low dosage tricyclic antidepressants in depression: systematic review. BMJ. 2002;325(7371):991–5.

48. Meeker AS, Herink MC, Haxby DG, Hartung DM. The safety and efficacy of vortioxetine for acute treatment of major depressive disorder: a systematic review and meta-analysis. Syst Rev. 2015;4:21.

49. Zhu H, Jinlong Y, HOngbo Z. A study of switchig to mirtazapine for treatment-resistant depression. Shanghai Arch Psychiatry. 2003;15:355–7.

50. Romera I, Perez V, Menchon JM, Schacht A, Papen R, Neuhauser D, Abbar M, Svanborg P, Gilaberte I. Early switch strategy in patients with major depressive disorder: a double-blind, randomized study. J Clin Psychopharmacol. 2012;32(4):479–86.

51. Tadic A, Wachtlin D, Berger M, Braus DF, van Calker D, Dahmen N, Dreimuller N, Engel A, Gorbulev S, Helmreich I, et al. Randomized controlled study of early medication change for non-improvers to antidepressant therapy in major depression—the EMC trial. Eur Neuropsychopharmacol. 2016;26(4):705–16.

52. Kornbluh R, Papakostas GI, Petersen T, Neault NB, Nierenberg AA, Rosenbaum JF, Fava M. A survey of prescribing preferences in the treatment of refractory depression: recent trends. Psychopharmacol Bull. 2001;35(3):150–6.

4

Fast and expensive (PCR) or cheap and slow (culture)? A mathematical modelling study to explore screening for carbapenem resistance in UK hospitals

Gwenan M. Knight[1,2]* (iD), Eleonora Dyakova[3], Siddharth Mookerjee[3], Frances Davies[3], Eimear T. Brannigan[2,3], Jonathan A. Otter[1,3] and Alison H. Holmes[1,3]

Abstract

Background: Enterobacteriaceae are a common cause of hospital infections. Carbapenems are a clinically effective treatment of such infections. However, resistance is on the rise. In particular, carbapenemase-producing carbapenem-resistant Enterobacteriaceae (CP-CRE) are increasingly common. In order to limit spread in clinical settings, screening and isolation is being recommended, but many different screening methods are available. We aimed to compare the impact and costs of three algorithms for detecting CP-CRE carriage.

Methods: We developed an individual-based simulation model to compare three screening algorithms using data from a UK National Health Service (NHS) trust. The first algorithm, "Direct PCR", was highly sensitive/specific and quick (half a day), but expensive. The second, "Culture + PCR", was relatively sensitive/specific but slower, requiring 2.5 days. A third algorithm, "PHE", repeated the "Culture + PCR" three times with an additional PCR. Scenario analysis was used to compare several levels of CP-CRE prevalence and coverage of screening, different specialities as well as isolation strategies. Our outcomes were (1) days that a patient with CP-CRE was not detected and hence not isolated ("days at risk"), (2) isolation bed days, (3) total costs and (4) mean cost per CP-CRE risk day averted per year. We also explored limited isolation bed day capacity.

Results: We found that although a Direct PCR algorithm would reduce the number of CP-CRE days at risk, the mean cost per CP-CRE risk day averted per year was substantially higher than for a Culture + PCR algorithm. For example, in our model of an intensive care unit, during a year with a 1.6% CP-CRE prevalence and 63% screening coverage, there were 508 (standard deviation 15), 642 (14) and 655 (14) days at risk under screening algorithms Direct PCR, Culture + PCR and PHE respectively, with mean costs per risk day averted of £192, £61 and £79. These results were robust to sensitivity analyses.

Conclusions: Our results indicate that a Culture + PCR algorithm provides the optimal balance of cost and risk days averted, at varying isolation, prevalence and screening coverage scenarios. Findings from this study will help clinical organisations determine the optimal screening approach for CP-CRE, balancing risk and resources.

Keywords: Carbapenem resistance, Screening algorithms, Mathematical modelling, PCR, Culture

* Correspondence: gwen.knight@lshtm.ac.uk
[1]National Institute of Health Research Health Protection Research Unit in Healthcare Associated Infections and Antimicrobial Resistance, Imperial College London, Commonwealth Building, Hammersmith Campus, Imperial College London, Du Cane Road, London W12 0NN, UK
[2]Infectious Diseases and Immunity, Commonwealth Building, Hammersmith Campus, Imperial College London, Du Cane Road, London W12 0NN, UK
Full list of author information is available at the end of the article

Background

Carbapenem antibiotics are clinically effective and well tolerated for the treatment of antibiotic-resistant Gram-negative bacteria and hence extremely important for tackling life-threatening infections in UK hospitals [1]. The most common cause of blood stream infections in England is Gram-negative bacteria, specifically Enterobacteriaceae [2]. The number of infections with carbapenem-resistant Enterobacteriaceae (CRE) is on the rise [3]. These infections lead to increased morbidity, mortality and cost [4].

Carbapenemase-producing carbapenem-resistant Enterobacteriaceae (CP-CRE) are effectively a sub-population of CRE which represent a further threat, because the genes encoding the mechanisms of resistance (a carbapenemase) can be transferred between bacterial species and confer elevated levels of resistance compared with other mechanisms of carbapenem resistance [5, 6]. CP-CRE have shown a notable rise in the number of cases over the last decade in England [7]. They were close to absent in 2006 but have since increased to more than 2500 isolates being referred to the national reference laboratory in 2016 [8]. Outbreaks have also been detected in some centres [9], and others report endemic CP-CRE [10]. As a result, increasing numbers of patients have extremely limited therapy options; thus preventive infection control practices such as active screening and single room isolation play an even more important part in our clinical settings [11]. CP-CRE colonisation has been shown to correlate positively with the incidence of infection attributed to CP-CRE organisms, particularly in an intensive care unit (ICU) setting [12]. There are currently no accepted decolonisation protocols for CP-CRE organisms; hence early detection of asymptomatic carriage and isolation are key tools to prevent transmission. However, there is insufficient data on the effectiveness or cost-effectiveness of various CP-CRE screening algorithms.

US (Centers for Disease Control and Prevention, CDC), European (European Centre for Disease Prevention and Control, ECDC) and UK (Public Health England, PHE) organisations have published guidance highlighting the importance of patient screening for CP-CRE in order to identify the carriers and prevent subsequent infection and spread [13, 14]. The European Society of Clinical Microbiology and Infectious Diseases (ESCMID) recommended patient screening on admission in both endemic and epidemic settings as well as pre-emptive isolation in a single room in an epidemic setting [15]. However, there are a number of challenges associated with this, such as the high cost of patient screening on admission, which may not always be optimal due to the wide range of prevalence on admission in different areas [16, 17]. Moreover, some CP-CRE screening methods take up to 48 h to give a result. Hence, pre-emptive isolation may not be an option, as it could result in a high number of patients being

isolated unnecessarily for a prolonged period of time [18], nor may it be feasible given the limited availability of isolation facilities.

The most common existing CP-CRE screening methods include conventional culture-based approaches, which have good sensitivity and specificity but take several days to return a result [13], and molecular polymerase chain reaction (PCR)-based methods, which are much faster, at least as sensitive, but substantially more expensive [19]. Importantly, CRE is defined phenotypically, whereas CP-CRE is a genotypic phenomenon most commonly determined by means of a molecular-based test. Whilst PCR-based methods can only detect known carbapenemase-encoding genes that they are designed to detect [20], culture-based methods do not detect non-expressed genetic mechanisms [21]. This suggests that a combination of culture- and PCR-based tests should be used in order to detect all phenotypic resistance and also to confirm the underlying genetic mechanisms.

Mathematical models, often used in the field of infectious diseases, provide the ideal platform from which to simulate a range of laboratory screening options to detect CP-CRE. Their use in the field of healthcare-associated infections is well documented, with previous models of antibiotic-resistant Gram-negatives mostly focused on the ICU [22–24] to evaluate interventions and screening algorithms [25].

Our aim was to compare the impact of different currently used screening algorithms for CP-CRE using data from Imperial College Healthcare NHS Trust (ICHNT) using a newly designed mathematical model. By comparing different scenarios, parameterised by data from a group of London teaching hospitals, we were able to explore the predicted clinical impact and the comparative cost of different molecular- and culture-based screening tools. This will help to inform both ICHNT and other hospital trusts as to which screening methods to use in clinical settings to help combat this increasing threat.

Methods
Data

ICHNT implemented a combination of universal screening for all admissions to certain high-risk specialities and risk factor-based screening for all other admissions in June 2015. Universal screening was implemented in the ICU, renal, vascular and haematology in-patient wards. This group of patients accounts for nearly half of all trust admissions. We used this universal admission screening data over a 9-month period (June 2015–March 2016) to calculate the prevalence of CP-CRE carriage at admission and screening coverage levels (Table 1). For the purpose of the prevalence calculation, each patient was only included once, despite the fact that most patients were screened multiple times during their hospital stay. Length of stay

Table 1 Parameter table. All parameters were estimated using ICHNT data

Parameter	Description		Value	References and notes
CP-CRE prevalence at admission	ICU		1.6% (16/1007)	Calculated from universal screening data of a total of 2870 patients, over a 9-month period
	Renal		1.9% (16/858)	
	Vascular		0.4% (2/541)	
	Haematology		1.3% (6/464)	
Coverage of initial admission screening	ICU		63.0%	
	Renal		67.0%	
	Vascular		48.0%	
	Haematology		68.0%	
Number of speciality beds	ICU		112	Sum of all wards in each speciality as in March 2016
	Renal		71	
	Vascular		65	
	Haematology		66	
Length of stay (mean/median)	ICU	S	7.9/4.0	Taken from speciality data and based on initial screening result
		CRE	15.9/10.0	
	Renal	S	7.8/5.0	
		CRE	15.5/12.0	
	Vascular	S	6.2/4.0	
		CRE	12.4/7.0	
	Haematology	S	9.6/5.0	
		CRE	19.6/9.0	
Time to result (days)	Culture		2	For single component test
	PHE PCR		7[a]	
	PCR		0.5	
	(A) Direct PCR		0.5	For complete algorithm
	(B) Culture + PCR		2.5	
	(C) PHE		13	

S patient was carrying no Enterobacteriaceae or Enterobacteriaceae susceptible to carbapenems, CRE patient was carrying Enterobacteriaceae resistant to carbapenems. These data come from the patients identified as carriers using the current ICHNT screening procedure
[a]Accounts for the PHE workload and specimen transportation

(LoS) distributions by CRE status (no carriage vs. carriage) were gathered for each speciality separately (Table 1 and Additional file 1: Table S1). We assumed that those patients with colonisation due to CRE-producing carbapenemases (CP-CRE) or non-carbapenemase-producing CRE (NCP-CRE) could be grouped as having the same LoS distribution.

We used data from ICHNT to parameterise the costs of our screening tools (Additional file 1: Table S2). We performed an economic evaluation from the hospital perspective, following the Consolidated Health Economic Evaluation Reporting Standards (CHEERS) guidelines [26]. Over the time period investigated here, no charge was applied for additional diagnostic work performed at PHE. The cost of one isolation bed day was composed of a daily cost of £20.33 (£20 for gloves and aprons, £0.33 for infectious waste stream) and a one-off cost from stock disposal of £113 (£385 for the ICU) incurred at the time of patient discharge [9]. The time horizon was 1 year with no discount rate.

Diagnostic algorithms

Three diagnostic algorithms to detect CP-CRE were compared. The first (A) is a PCR test direct from a sample swab, the second (B) represents culture followed by carbapenemase confirmation by PCR (the current ICHNT hospital-based protocol), and the third (C) repeats (B) three times, with an additional PCR performed at the PHE national reference laboratory to confirm a lack of CRE. All sensitivity and specificity values are provided in Table 2. The details of the first two algorithms are shown in Fig. 1 (all algorithms are detailed in Additional file 1: Figure S1).

In detail, (A) "Direct PCR", is a single, in-house PCR direct from a screening sample. It is a quick test, which would dramatically reduce detection time by giving results within half a day. We used estimates from the literature [27] to give a sensitivity and specificity of this test (Table 2).

The second algorithm (B) represents the current ICHNT protocol of "Culture + PCR". The culture part has

Table 2 Details of tests used in the algorithms

Test	Negative result	Sensitivity	Specificity	References and notes	Screening algorithm		
					(A) Direct PCR	(B) Culture + PCR	(C) PHE
PCR from swab	S	96%	99%	Tato et al., 2016 [27]	x		
ICHNT PCR	NCP-CRE[a]	98%	99%	ICHNT data		x	x
Culture (1)	S	89%	91%	ICHNT data		x	x
Culture (2)	NCP-CRE	100%	85%	ICHNT data		x	x
PHE PCR	NCP-CRE[a]	100%	100%	Assumed optimal			x

Sensitivity is the probability that the test detects resistance given that the patient carries resistant Enterobacteriaceae. Specificity is the probability of a negative test for resistance given that the patient does not carry resistant bacteria
[a]As both of these PCR tests are on samples that have shown to be culture positive for CRE, they are classified as NCP-CRE if the PCR test for CPE is negative

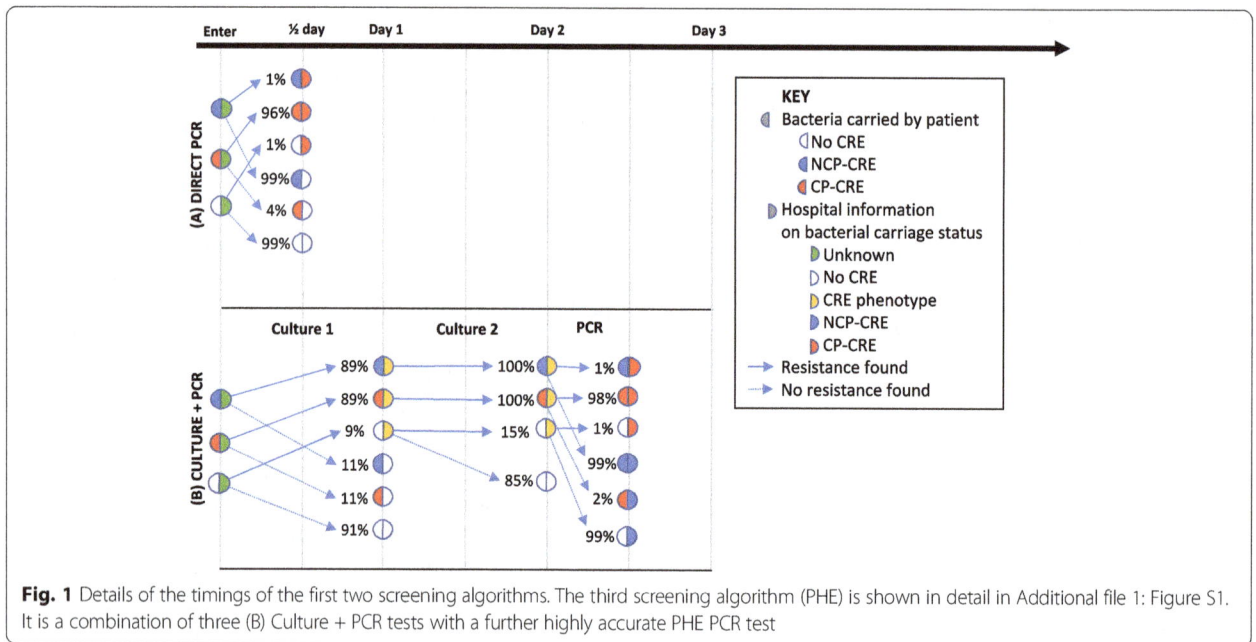

Fig. 1 Details of the timings of the first two screening algorithms. The third screening algorithm (PHE) is shown in detail in Additional file 1: Figure S1. It is a combination of three (B) Culture + PCR tests with a further highly accurate PHE PCR test

two stages: a screening swab plated onto chromogenic media (Colorex™ mSuperCARBA™, E&O Laboratories, Bonnybridge, UK), followed by suspicious colonies being tested for antimicrobial susceptibility (EUCAST disc diffusion). Those colonies with defined antimicrobial resistance profiles are tested using the ICHNT in-house PCR for carbapenemase gene detection (Xpert® Carba-R, Cepheid Inc., Sunnyvale, CA, USA). The genes targeted in this kit are *KPC, NDM, VIM, OXA-48* and *IMP* [28]. Sensitivity and specificity values were estimated from ICHNT data (Table 2). Each culture stage takes a day, whilst the PCR takes half a day (Table 1, Fig. 1).

The third algorithm (C) "PHE", is aligned with the PHE recommendation of three sequential screens, each separated by 48 h to test for CRE carriage. Three culture tests, paired with ICHNT PCR, are performed across the whole population. In addition, a confirmatory PHE PCR test is performed for any suspicious colonies from culture. The PHE PCR was assumed to have a higher sensitivity than the ICHNT PCR. As above, sensitivity and specificity values were estimated from ICHNT data where possible (Table 2), and algorithm C takes 6.5 days to perform the three within-hospital screening tests, with a further 7 days for a PCR result from PHE (Table 1). This latter PCR test is unlikely to have an impact on our results, but it is included to reflect the current recommended algorithm and, due to the increased sensitivity, it may detect further colonisation.

Scenarios

We considered four main scenarios including a baseline scenario parameterised to represent the ICHNT ICU with 100% screening coverage. This baseline scenario was then modified to include (1) an ICHNT ICU with screening coverage at < 100% (63%, the screening coverage in 2015–2016), (2) 63% screening coverage and high CP-CRE prevalence (20%) and (3) high (20%) CP-CRE prevalence. The high CP-CRE prevalence (20%) was used to represent a potentially catastrophic though not unrealistic scenario, as 2014 European average CRE prevalence levels were already 7.3% [29]. The corresponding prevalence of NCP-CRE was set at 5%, making overall CRE prevalence 25% in the high prevalence scenarios. In Additional file 1, we also provide results for the three other high-risk specialities (renal, vascular and haematology).

Isolation strategies

We considered one main isolation strategy: (1) only those with confirmed CP-CRE were isolated (matching current ICHNT practice). In Additional file 1, we also provide results for (2) isolating no one and (3) isolating all patients with confirmed CRE (NCP- and CP-CRE). We did not consider any pre-emptive isolation strategies. In our main analysis, we report the number of isolation days required, making no assumptions about adherence to isolation policy or availability of isolation beds.

Mathematical model

We constructed a stochastic (random) individual-based model of patients with or without CP-CRE carriage in hospital specialities (Fig. 2). This model captured four key parameters: (1) the rates at which patients exit the hospital (based on ICHNT LoS data and independent of screening status), (2) incoming CP-CRE prevalence rates, (3) time taken for a finalised result and (4) the efficacy of the screening tests (see screening algorithms in Table 2). The

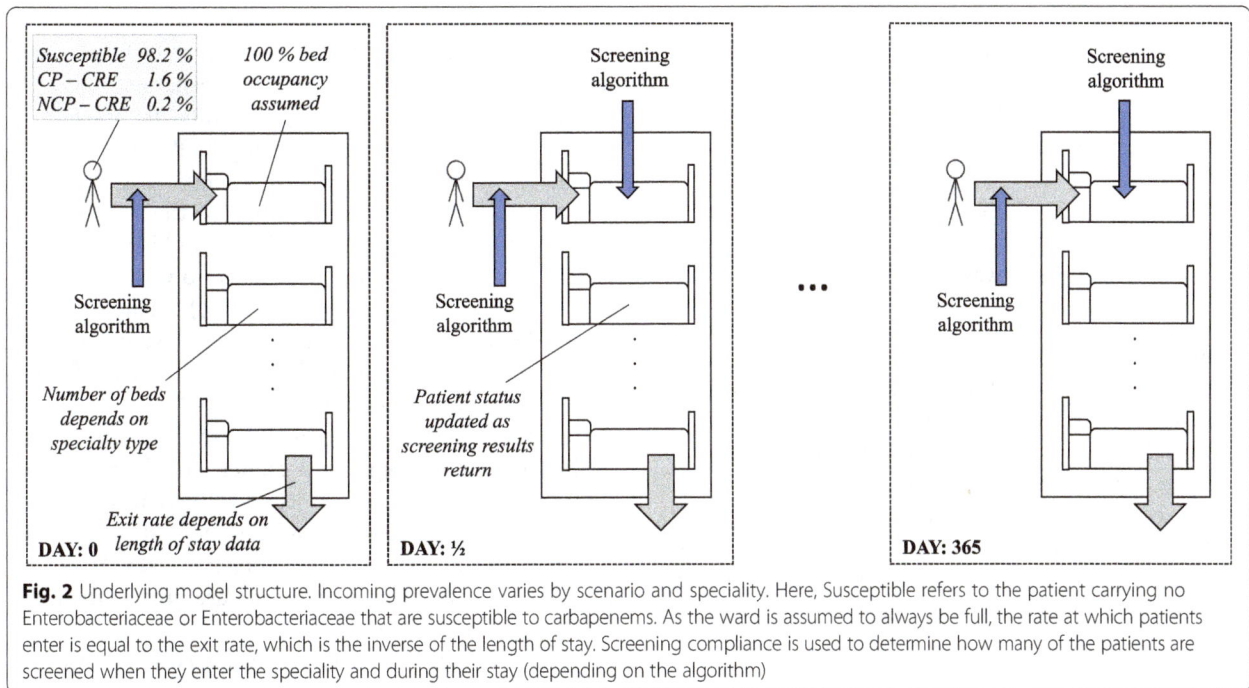

Fig. 2 Underlying model structure. Incoming prevalence varies by scenario and speciality. Here, Susceptible refers to the patient carrying no Enterobacteriaceae or Enterobacteriaceae that are susceptible to carbapenems. As the ward is assumed to always be full, the rate at which patients enter is equal to the exit rate, which is the inverse of the length of stay. Screening compliance is used to determine how many of the patients are screened when they enter the speciality and during their stay (depending on the algorithm)

model was built to consider each speciality separately, allowing for patients to stay for an appropriate LoS and then replacing those who exit with new patients, screened on entry at a certain compliance level, making the speciality full at all times (Fig. 2).

The model was parameterised using data from ICHNT (Table 1). A stochastic model formulation was used to account for the small population sizes. The stochastic parameters included within the model were (1) the chance of being colonised with CRE (CP-CRE, NCP-CRE or no CRE) on entry, (2) the chance of being tested (based on screening coverage levels), (3) the chance of being detected (using the efficacy values as a probability) and (4) the LoS (selected with replacement from the data distribution).

We did not include secondary transmission in this model, as there is insufficient evidence on the levels of transmission of Enterobacteriaceae in a clinical setting and on the impact of isolation interventions on this transmission. Instead, the number of "days at risk" is a proxy for transmission level.

Simulation

All simulations were performed in R [30]. All results are calculated from 100 runs, where one run captures the scenario for 1 year, with a time step of half a day. Error bars represent the standard error taken over the 100 runs. The single cost estimates were used to multiply the mean, minimum and maximum values from the 100 model outputs to give a range.

Outcomes

Our primary outcome was the number of days at risk: the number of days that a patient with CP-CRE is not detected and hence not isolated.

Our secondary outcome was the total number of isolation days and the number of days those without CP-CRE were isolated (inappropriate isolation). These values were presented as totals, which we compared to the number of side rooms suitable for isolation at ICHNT in 2015, which totalled 60 [18, 25]. This results in a total number of isolation bed days available a year of 3650, 6205, 9125 and 2920 for ICU, renal, haematology and vascular specialities respectively.

Our third outcome was the total cost evaluation of each algorithm. The fourth outcome was the mean cost per risk day averted for patients with CP-CRE. This was obtained by dividing the mean total direct costs of each scenario (screening and isolation bed day costs) by the mean number of averted risk days (i.e. number of days that a patient with CP-CRE was isolated). At ICHNT, as screening algorithm (B) is the current protocol, we also calculated the average incremental cost associated with 1 additional averted risk day for screening algorithms (A) and (C) to inform direct decision making in our setting.

Isolation bed day capacity effects

As previously outlined, there are currently a limited number of isolation beds at ICHNT. To account for this potential implementation barrier, we also calculated a "days at risk (adjusted for isolation capacity)" value. In this analysis, the isolation days that exceeded isolation capacity were added to the number of days at risk, so "days at risk (adjusted for isolation capacity)" included CP-CRE non-isolation because of (1) non-detection and (2) detection but a lack of available isolation bed. For this we assumed that isolation beds would only be used for CP-CRE.

We also recalculated the costs per risk day averted for patients with CP-CRE assuming that a risk day could only be averted if there was an isolation bed available.

Sensitivity analysis

The four main scenarios (baseline ICU speciality with four different screening coverage and CRE prevalence levels) comprised our main sensitivity analysis. We also explored the impact of dramatically reducing the sensitivity of PCR to 60% to account for a change in the circulating genetic marker encoding the carbapenemase, such as the appearance of a novel or unusual carbapenemase, within the ICU ICHNT scenario (with 63% screening coverage).

Results
Outcomes

Our primary outcome, the number of CP-CRE days at risk in a year, was lowest for the (A) Direct PCR screening algorithm under all scenarios (Table 3, Fig. 3a). Under the high prevalence scenario, with 63% screening coverage, there were 5080 (standard deviation, SD of 36), 6664 (42) and 5194 (31) days at risk under the screening algorithms (A) Direct PCR, (B) Culture + PCR and (C) PHE respectively (Table 3, Fig. 3a). These high levels were reduced considerably by increasing the screening coverage to 100% (Table 3, Fig. 3a).

Our secondary outcome, the total number of isolation bed days, was highest for the (A) Direct PCR screening algorithm (991–11,834 across the scenarios, Table 3), many of which were inappropriate (due to isolation of patients without CP-CRE, i.e. many PCR false positives) (Table 3, Fig. 3c). In the high prevalence, high screening scenario, between 254% and 324% of the 3650 annual ICU isolation bed days at ICHNT would be required, simply for CP-CRE. In the ICU scenario with low prevalence and low screening coverage (63%), changing to (A) Direct PCR (from (B) Culture + PCR) would increase the percentage of the annual isolation bed days for the ICU required for CP-CRE from 16% to 27%.

Our third outcome, the total costs associated with each algorithm, highlights the higher cost, from the hospital perspective, of (A) Direct PCR screening (Fig. 3d, Additional file 1: Table S3) and the increasing contribution of isolation costs as prevalence increases. Note that for (A) Direct PCR screening costs are greater than isolation costs at low prevalence.

For our fourth outcome, the mean cost per risk day averted for patients with CP-CRE per year, the pattern was reversed (Fig. 3b). The lowest value was for our (B) Culture + PCR algorithm (range across the four scenarios of £48–£63) and highest for (A) Direct PCR (£59–£198) (Table 3), despite a reduced total number of days at risk under the latter (Fig. 3a). The main driver of changes in this outcome was the prevalence, with the two low prevalence scenarios resulting in high costs per CP-CRE carrier risk day averted, i.e. one to three times higher than in the high prevalence (20%) scenario.

The average incremental cost associated with 1 additional averted risk day for algorithms (A) and (C)

Table 3 Results table

Screening algorithm	Scenario			Outcomes				
	Speciality	Screening coverage	CP-CRE prevalence	Number of "days at risk"	Total isolation bed days	Total isolation bed days of patients without CP-CRE	Cost per risk day averted (£)	Average incremental cost per additional averted risk day (£)
(A) Direct PCR	ICU	100%	1.6%	90 (4.39)	1500 (19.25)	368 (94.96)	198.45	743.56
		63%	1.6%	508 (14.83)	991 (17.98)	244 (72.30)	192.18	712.38
		63%	20%	5080 (36.20)	**7649** (50.40)	173 (58.47)	58.18	97.10
		100%	20%	918 (14.39)	**11,834** (49.99)	263 (85.91)	58.69	99.57
(B) Culture +PCR		100%	1.6%	335 (9.31)	910 (17.59)	3 (5.55)	63.05	–
		63%	1.6%	642 (14.06)	600 (15.84)	4 (10.01)	61.38	–
		63%	20%	6664 (42.32)	**5955** (38.82)	17 (20.84)	48.09	–
		100%	20%	3308 (24.68)	**9282** (53.2)	29 (38.32)	48.44	–
(C) PHE		100%	1.6%	221 (3.74)	1024 (19.37)	28 (31.95)	83.18	288.63
		63%	1.6%	655 (14.00)	623 (17.57)	13 (18.32)	78.69	819.56
		63%	20%	5194 (31.49)	**7465** (45.2)	17 (21.47)	48.05	47.90
		100%	20%	2309 (11.15)	**10,287** (51.71)	41 (38.09)	49.68	61.23

The outcomes are given as the mean (standard deviation) from 100 simulations. The cost per risk day averted is the mean total cost divided by the mean number of "days at risk". Total isolation bed days shown in bold text are greater than the existing total number of isolation bed days available to the ICU at ICHNT

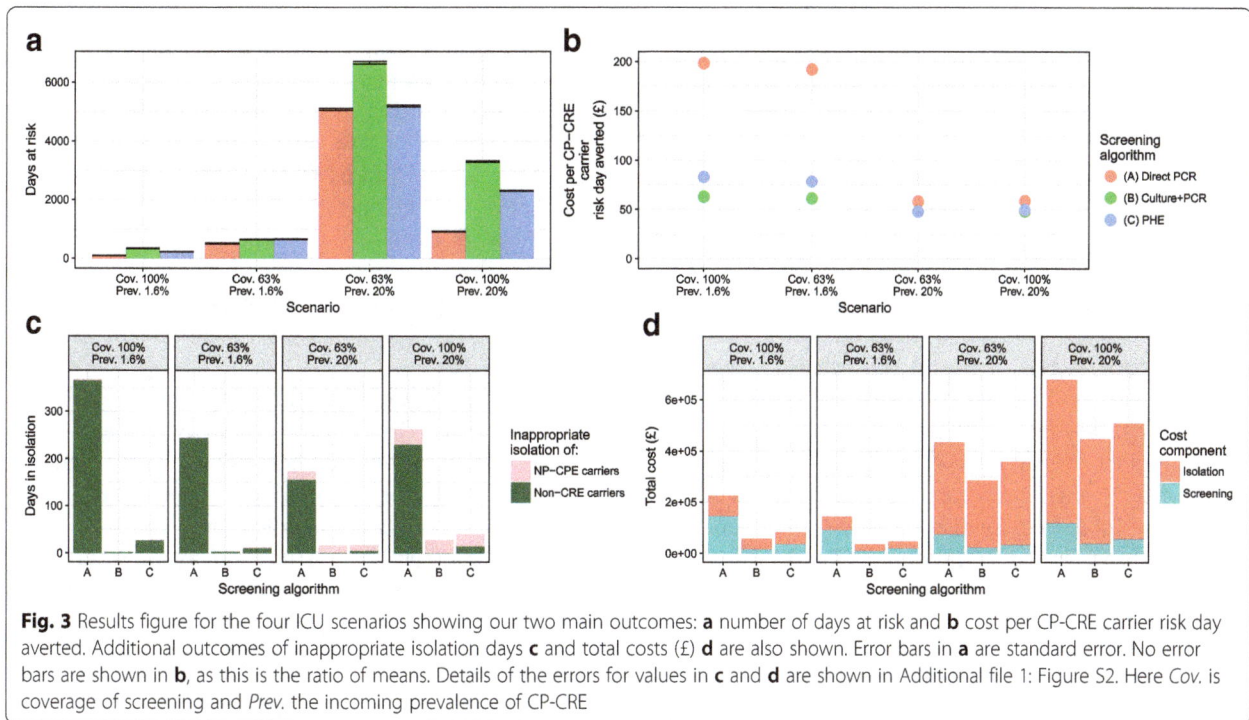

Fig. 3 Results figure for the four ICU scenarios showing our two main outcomes: **a** number of days at risk and **b** cost per CP-CRE carrier risk day averted. Additional outcomes of inappropriate isolation days **c** and total costs (£) **d** are also shown. Error bars in **a** are standard error. No error bars are shown in **b**, as this is the ratio of means. Details of the errors for values in **c** and **d** are shown in Additional file 1: Figure S2. Here *Cov.* is coverage of screening and *Prev.* the incoming prevalence of CP-CRE

against the comparison algorithm (B) was between £97 and £744 and £48 and £820 respectively (Table 3).

Isolation bed day capacity effects
The "days at risk (adjusted for isolation capacity)" value was higher than our primary outcome only for the high prevalence scenarios (Additional file 1: Table S4) at ~ 8900. In particular, for the high prevalence, high screening coverage scenario, taking into account the isolation bed day capacity limits results in a 9.6 times increase in the number of days at risk.

Using this new "days at risk (adjusted for isolation capacity)" value, the new costs per risk day averted were higher for the high prevalence scenarios, with no difference in the relative comparison between the scenarios ((B) < (C) < (A)), although the relative difference between (B) and (C) became greater (Additional file 1: Table S4).

Other specialities
The results for the other specialities highlight the importance of variance in coverage and prevalence (Additional file 1: Figure S2 and Tables S5–S8). The vascular speciality was associated with substantially lower numbers of risk days, due to the low CP-CRE prevalence (0.4%), whilst renal and haematology specialities showed substantially higher numbers of days at risk than the ICU (base case) due to higher prevalence and longer average lengths of stay respectively. The low prevalence of CP-CRE in the vascular speciality also had increased costs per averted CP-CRE risk day compared to the ICU,

whilst the other specialities had similar values to those from the ICU. The patterns of relative algorithm performance, described for the ICU above, were robust across these specialities.

Other isolation strategies
Isolation of all patients confirmed to carry a CRE would result in many inappropriate isolation days (i.e. isolation of someone without CP-CRE) under the (C) PHE algorithm due to the high false positive rate resulting from the multiple tests (Additional file 1: Figures S3–S5), about five times higher than under the other algorithms. With a no isolation strategy, it can be seen that there would be approximately 1200 and 15,000 CP-CRE "at risk" patient days under existing or high CP-CRE prevalence respectively (Additional file 1: Figure S5).

Sensitivity analysis
Reducing the sensitivity of our PCR to 60% to account for a change in genetic marker results in a substantially higher primary outcome (from ~ 500 to ~ 750 days at risk) and increased final outcome (~ £200 vs. ~ £250) for the (A) Direct PCR algorithm (Additional file 1: Figure S6).

Fit to data
Our model accurately recreated the LoS distributions from the data, providing assurance that the model was functioning as anticipated (Additional file 1: Figures S7–S10). For the ICU, there were between 4000 and 5200 patients in

the speciality over the year. An example of how the model captures the changing status of a patient over time is shown in Fig. 4, matching the algorithm given in Fig. 1.

Discussion

We estimated the number of CP-CRE days at risk to be lowest when using our (A) Direct PCR algorithm, owing to the rapidity of result confirmation by PCR. This applied to all scenarios, but was most pronounced in the scenarios with 100% screening coverage levels. However, the false positive rate of the (A) Direct PCR algorithm (a direct false positive rate of 1% vs. an effective false positive of 0.01% for (B) Culture + PCR) resulted in a higher number of inappropriate isolation days and hence substantially higher costs per CP-CRE carrier risk day averted and total costs for the (A) Direct PCR algorithm. This meant that, in terms of cost per CP-CRE carrier risk day averted, the (B) Culture + PCR algorithm performed best.

The differences between algorithms were reduced under scenarios with high prevalence, when the cost per CP-CRE carrier risk day averted was similar for all three algorithms, independently of screening prevalence. This highlights the importance of local epidemiology on determining the impact of screening algorithms. At ICHNT, the screening coverage has risen considerably since the study was performed (now at 96% for the ICU) due to quality improvement work in the trust. This suggests that for the ICHNT ICU setting, where CP-CRE prevalence is low but near 100% coverage (similar to our baseline scenario), the (A) Direct PCR algorithm would

give the smallest number of days at risk. However, the (B) Culture + PCR algorithm would be substantially better in terms of cost per CP-CRE carrier risk day averted. The (C) PHE algorithm, which is basically three repeats of the (B) Culture + PCR algorithm with an additional high-performance PCR, performs slightly better in terms of risk days averted than (B) Culture + PCR; however, the cumulative costs of these repeats result in a higher cost per CP-CRE carrier risk day averted. This is reflected in substantial average incremental costs, suggesting that the ICHNT should continue to use (B) Culture + PCR.

The same pattern of algorithm performance is seen in the three other ICHNT specialities considered, which have CP-CRE prevalence on admission ranging from 0.4 to 1.9%, but different bed numbers and lengths of stay. Data on CP-CRE admission prevalence across England (0.1% from another London hospital in 2015 [21]) and Europe (1.1% in a Spanish hospital in 2006–2010 [31]) are scarce, but the level is likely to lie within the range considered here (< 8%) [29]. Thus, the cost per CP-CRE carrier risk day averted is likely to be lowest for (B) Culture + PCR in other English settings. Only as prevalence increases will the false positive rate of Direct PCR algorithms be counterbalanced, and the use of multiple screens or a direct-from-swab PCR have decreasing cost per CP-CRE carrier risk day averted. This is similar to cost-effectiveness results from the USA, where culture-based algorithms were found to be cost-effective, whilst PCR gave much higher costs [32].

The impact of these screening algorithms on the demand for isolation bed days rapidly increases with both

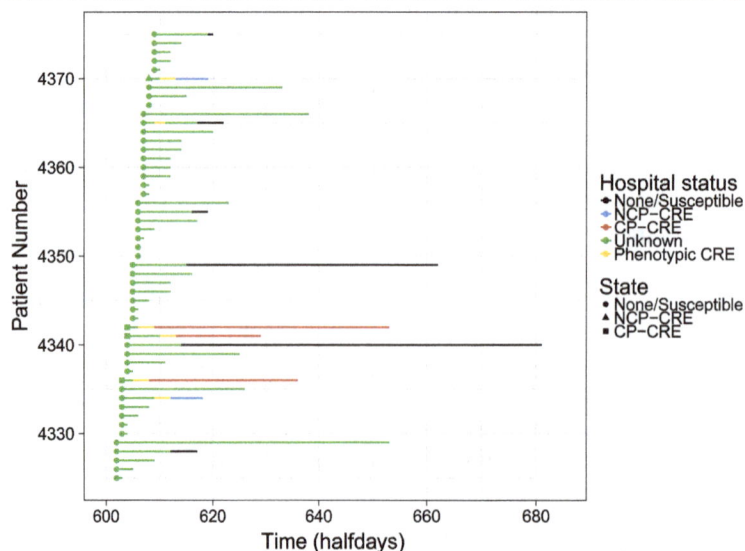

Fig. 4 Example model output showing how hospital status changes over a year for patients 4225 to 4375 in one run for the ICU speciality with the (C) PHE screening algorithm. Here each *line* represents a single patient, with *colours* showing how their hospital status changed over time. See Additional file 1: Figure S11 for all patients

screening coverage and CP-CRE prevalence. Isolation beds (side rooms) are in demand for other uses than CP-CRE, and thus even before the > 100% demand under all the high CP-CRE (20%) prevalence scenarios is seen, such requirements may not be available. However, increasing screening coverage is very important in reducing the number of days at risk (and hence the potential for onward transmission). In our case, increasing screening coverage from 63 to 100% reduced the number of days at risk by more than 50%. This, however, was only true when we ignored the limits of the existing isolation bed day capacity. When we included this, the number of days at risk was similar, as the limit on the days at risk was not screening coverage but isolation bed availability. Thus, pairing increased screening coverage with concurrent isolation bed day availability should be a focus of hospitals [25], especially as CP-CRE prevalence on admission rises. Alternatives such as nurse cohorting or increased contact precautions for certain patients, instead of speciality isolation beds, could also be employed. Laboratory capacity should also be considered under increased prevalence demands, as well as screening outside of only high-risk areas, neither of which we included here.

The rapidity of direct PCR tests or equivalent "point-of-care" rapid diagnostic tests makes them an attractive option for hospitals. However, their cost and the impact on isolation bed day capacity cannot be ignored. As CP-CRE prevalence increases, this cost would be reduced due to the lower proportion of false positives and the rapidity of detection. Our costings include the extra cost generated from a patient isolated following a false positive test. We considered only existing technology; however, future diagnostic tests for CP-CRE including "lab on a chip" mechanisms would be rapid and highly specific. As shown here, if these tests can improve on the false positive detection rate of PCR, potentially by combining phenotypic and genotypic output, then at a low cost, these could be greatly improved algorithms, reducing dramatically the number of days at risk.

The clinical impact of our results is to provide evidence for hospitals to decide between screening strategies for detection and isolation of CP-CRE carriers to prevent ongoing transmission. One aspect of the screening algorithms modelled in this paper that is not captured in the outcomes that we evaluated is that the Direct PCR algorithm would result in more rapid identification of the specific carbapenemase involved: this has value for the rapid identification of potential clusters and understanding short-term local epidemiological trends. In addition, these screening results, in the identification of CP-CRE carriage, can aid in the design of antimicrobial treatment if subsequent infection occurs (or is present already at admission). Whilst the greatest

clinical impact would be achieved by the most rapid test, clinical settings operate with strict budgets, and thus a comparison such as those presented here must be made for on-the-ground decision making.

This study's main strength is its direct linkage to a "real" hospital setting. This leading London teaching hospital group, with 15,000 admissions a month and 1300 beds, provided screening coverage data, CP-CRE prevalence by speciality and LoS data, making the modelling outputs based on "real" data, rather than hypothesised parameters. This makes the applicability of the model better and supports the reliability of the results.

The main weakness of this study was that transmission was not explicitly included in the model due to a lack of reliable estimates for CP-CRE transmission rates. Therefore, the effects of isolation on CPE prevalence could not be explored, and we do not capture the indirect impact of these screening algorithms. However, the number of CP-CRE days at risk is a proxy for heightened levels of transmission, and our comparison of screening tests would be similar with the addition of indirect transmission effects, although the likely impact may change, potentially non-linearly, with increasing resistance prevalence. There is likely to be considerable uncertainty in the transmission rate from individual patients (those isolated and not) and between settings, making the addition of this complexity unlikely to clarify or improve on our results. Such "colonisation" burden proxies of transmission risk have been proposed before [33], with analysis showing that they link directly to acquisition rates of other resistant pathogens [34, 35]. Other weaknesses, in terms of modelling assumptions, come from our assumption that those with CP-CRE and NCP-CRE could be grouped as having the same LoS distribution, i.e. that those with CRE have the same LoS. Apart from CRE status, other bacterial and all host heterogeneities were missing, such as risk factors for carriage. We also did not undertake a cost-effectiveness analysis, instead looking at the overall effect of different variables on the impact of screening algorithms. In addition, although we explored implementation through exploring the impact of limited numbers of isolation bed days, we did not include further financial or technical constraints.

There are also limitations to our cost calculations, in particular, the specific nature of our parameterisation, which makes the costing results specific to our setting and does not include the variation that may be seen. This limits the generalisability to broad conclusions about the comparative nature of the algorithms. We also decided to use "cost per CP-CRE carrier risk day averted" as the main cost comparison method. As we did not include transmission, we could not include the cost of CP-CRE outbreaks, and instead only the proxy of "risk days". In terms of clinical impact, time to detection of CP-CRE may override this cumulative "risk day" calculation (if we believe that transmission from a patient could saturate), but we believe that this is unlikely due to rapid patient movement and therefore the same ongoing transmission risk from every "risk day". Thus rapidity of test result may not be optimal when making difficult value-based decisions for infection control.

The key next step for this work depends on an improved understanding of the transmission routes and pathways that lead to patients being carriers of CP-CRE, as well as the length of time patients are carriers. Once this is available, adding in transmission, and the effect of isolation on transmission, would allow for estimation of the impact on the additional indirect effects of screening. Similarly, with information on the quantitative impact of different risk factors on CP-CRE carriage (e.g. by what relative increase are those who travel abroad more likely to carry CP-CRE) and the prevalence of these risk factors, more heterogeneity in the patient host population could be included.

Conclusions
In conclusion, in English settings, where CP-CPE prevalence is still low, we would recommend continuation of Culture + PCR-based algorithms, despite the reduction in days at risk if a Direct PCR algorithm were introduced. The latter suffers from a higher false positivity rate, which results in an unacceptably high cost per risk day averted whilst CP-CRE prevalence remains low.

Abbreviations
CDC: Centers for Disease Control and Prevention; CP-CRE: Carbapenemase-producing carbapenem-resistant Enterobacteriaceae; CRE: Carbapenem-resistant Enterobacteriaceae; ECDC: European Centre for Disease Prevention and Control; ESCMID: European Society of Clinical Microbiology and Infectious Diseases; ICHNT: Imperial College Healthcare NHS Trust; ICU: Intensive care unit; LoS: Length of stay; NCP-CRE: Non-carbapenemase-producing carbapenem-resistant Enterobacteriaceae; PCR: Polymerase chain reaction; PHE: Public Health England

Acknowledgements
We would like to thank the ICHNT laboratory staff, Preetha Shibu and Jyothsna Dronavalli, for their help with the test data.

Funding
The research was funded by the National Institute for Health Research Health Protection Research Unit (NIHR HPRU) in Healthcare Associated Infections and Antimicrobial Resistance at Imperial College London in partnership with Public Health England (PHE). The views expressed are those of the author(s) and not necessarily those of the NHS, the NIHR, the Department of Health or PHE.

Authors' contributions
The study design was formulated by GMK, AH, JAO and ED. GMK led the modelling design and coding, with support from ED. Data collection and analysis was performed by ED, SM, FD, EB and JAO. Results analysis was conducted by all authors. Manuscript writing was led by GMK and ED, with support in interpretation and application from all co-authors. All authors read and approved the final manuscript.

Competing interests
JAO was previously employed part-time by Bioquell (ceased April 2015) and is now a consultant to Gama Healthcare and Pfizer outside the submitted work; AH was awarded an honorarium for presenting at a conference entitled South African Antibiotic Stewardship Programme Annual Workshop, sponsored by Merck (MSD Hoddesdon). All other authors decare that they have no competing interests.

Author details
[1]National Institute of Health Research Health Protection Research Unit in Healthcare Associated Infections and Antimicrobial Resistance, Imperial College London, Commonwealth Building, Hammersmith Campus, Imperial College London, Du Cane Road, London W12 0NN, UK. [2]Infectious Diseases and Immunity, Commonwealth Building, Hammersmith Campus, Imperial College London, Du Cane Road, London W12 0NN, UK. [3]Imperial College Healthcare NHS Trust, London, UK.

References
1. World Health Organization: Antimicrobial resistance global report on surveillance. 2014.
2. Public Health England: English surveillance programme for antimicrobial utilisation and resistance (ESPAUR), ESPAUR annual report. 2017.
3. European Antimicrobial Resistance Surveillance Network (EARS-Net): Annual Report: Antimicrobial resistance surveillance in Europe. 2009.
4. Falagas ME, Tansarli GS, Karageorgopoulos DE, Vardakas KZ. Deaths attributable to carbapenem-resistant Enterobacteriaceae infections. Emerg Infect Dis. 2014;20(7):1170–5.
5. Nordmann P, Naas T, Poirel L. Global spread of carbapenemase-producing Enterobacteriaceae. Emerg Infect Dis. 2011;17(10):1791–8.
6. Karah N, Sundsfjord A, Towner K, Samuelsen O. Insights into the global molecular epidemiology of carbapenem non-susceptible clones of Acinetobacter baumannii. Drug Resist Updat. 2012;15(4):237–47.
7. Donker T, Henderson KL, Hopkins KL, Dodgson AR, Thomas S, Crook DW, Peto TEA, Johnson AP, Woodford N, Walker AS, et al. The relative importance of large problems far away versus small problems closer to home: insights into limiting the spread of antimicrobial resistance in England. BMC Med. 2017;15(1):86.
8. Public Health England. English surveillance programme for antimicrobial utilisation and resistance (ESPAUR). London: Public Health England; 2017.
9. Otter JA, Burgess P, Davies F, Mookerjee S, Singleton J, Gilchrist M, Parsons D, Brannigan ET, Robotham J, Holmes AH. Counting the cost of an outbreak of carbapenemase-producing Enterobacteriaceae: an economic evaluation from a hospital perspective. Clin Microbiol Infect. 2017;23(3):188–96.
10. Poole K, George R, Decraene V, Shankar K, Cawthorne J, Savage N, Welfare W, Dodgson A. Active case finding for carbapenemase-producing Enterobacteriaceae in a teaching hospital: prevalence and risk factors for colonization. J Hosp Infect. 2016;94(2):125–9.
11. Schwaber MJ, Lev B, Israeli A, Solter E, Smollan G, Rubinovitch B, Shalit I, Carmeli Y, Israel Carbapenem-Resistant Enterobacteriaceae Working Group. Containment of a country-wide outbreak of carbapenem-resistant Klebsiella pneumoniae in Israeli hospitals via a nationally implemented intervention. Clin Infect Dis. 2011;52(7):848–55.

12. Dautzenberg MJ, Wekesa AN, Gniadkowski M, Antoniadou A, Giamarellou H, Petrikkos GL, Skiada A, Brun-Buisson C, Bonten MJ, Derde LP, et al. The association between colonization with carbapenemase-producing enterobacteriaceae and overall ICU mortality: an observational cohort study. Crit Care Med. 2015;43(6):1170–7.

13. Viau R, Frank KM, Jacobs MR, Wilson B, Kaye K, Donskey CJ, Perez F, Endimiani A, Bonomo RA. Intestinal carriage of carbapenemase-producing organisms: current status of surveillance methods. Clin Microbiol Rev. 2016; 29(1):1–27.

14. Otter JA, Mutters NT, Tacconelli E, Gikas A, Holmes AH. Controversies in guidelines for the control of multidrug-resistant Gram-negative bacteria in EU countries. Clin Microbiol Infect. 2015;21(12):1057–66.

15. Tacconelli E, Cataldo MA, Dancer SJ, De Angelis G, Falcone M, Frank U, Kahlmeter G, Pan A, Petrosillo N, Rodriguez-Bano J, et al. ESCMID guidelines for the management of the infection control measures to reduce transmission of multidrug-resistant Gram-negative bacteria in hospitalized patients. Clin Microbiol Infect. 2014;20(Suppl 1):1–55.

16. Munoz-Price LS, Hayden MK, Lolans K, Won S, Calvert K, Lin M, Stemer A, Weinstein RA. Successful control of an outbreak of Klebsiella pneumoniae carbapenemase-producing K. pneumoniae at a long-term acute care hospital. Infect Control Hosp Epidemiol. 2010;31(4):341–7.

17. Birgand G, Armand-Lefevre L, Lepainteur M, Lolom I, Neulier C, Reibel F, Yazdanpanah Y, Andremont A, Lucet JC. Introduction of highly resistant bacteria into a hospital via patients repatriated or recently hospitalized in a foreign country. Clin Microbiol Infect. 2014;20(11):O887–90.

18. Vella V, Gharbi M, Moore LS, Robotham J, Davies F, Brannigan E, Galletly T, Holmes AH. Screening suspected cases for carbapenemase-producing Enterobacteriaceae, inclusion criteria and demand. J Inf Secur. 2015;71(4):493–5.

19. Huang TD, Bogaerts P, Ghilani E, Heinrichs A, Gavage P, Roisin S, Willems E, Verbruggen AM, Francart H, Denis O, et al. Multicentre evaluation of the Check-Direct CPE(R) assay for direct screening of carbapenemase-producing Enterobacteriaceae from rectal swabs. J Antimicrob Chemother. 2015;70(6): 1669–73.

20. Okoche D, Asiimwe BB, Katabazi FA, Kato L, Najjuka CF. Prevalence and characterization of carbapenem-resistant Enterobacteriaceae isolated from Mulago National Referral Hospital, Uganda. PLoS One. 2015;10(8):e0135745.

21. Otter JA, Dyakova E, Bisnauthsing KN, Querol-Rubiera A, Patel A, Ahanonu C, Tosas Auguet O, Edgeworth JD, Goldenberg SD. Universal hospital admission screening for carbapenemase-producing organisms in a low-prevalence setting. J Antimicrob Chemother. 2016;71(12):3556–61.

22. Pelat C, Kardas-Sloma L, Birgand G, Ruppe E, Schwarzinger M, Andremont A, Lucet JC, Yazdanpanah Y. Hand hygiene, cohorting, or antibiotic restriction to control outbreaks of multidrug-resistant Enterobacteriaceae. Infect Control Hosp Epidemiol. 2016;37(3):272–80.

23. Sypsa V, Psichogiou M, Bouzala GA, Hadjihannas L, Hatzakis A, Daikos GL. Transmission dynamics of carbapenemase-producing Klebsiella pneumoniae and anticipated impact of infection control strategies in a surgical unit. PLoS One. 2012;7(7):e41068.

24. Ho KW, Ng WT, Ip M, You JH. Active surveillance of carbapenem-resistant Enterobacteriaceae in intensive care units: is it cost-effective in a nonendemic region? Am J Infect Control. 2016;44(4):394–9.

25. Vella V, Moore LS, Robotham JV, Davies F, Birgand GJ, Otter JA, Brannigan E, Dyakova E, Knight GM, Mookerjee S, et al. Isolation demand from carbapenemase-producing Enterobacteriaceae screening strategies based on a West London hospital network. J Hosp Infect. 2016;94(2):118–24.

26. Husereau D, Drummond M, Petrou S, Carswell C, Moher D, Greenberg D, Augustovski F, Briggs AH, Mauskopf J, Loder E, et al. Consolidated Health Economic Evaluation Reporting Standards (CHEERS)—explanation and elaboration: a report of the ISPOR Health Economic Evaluation Publication Guidelines Good Reporting Practices Task Force. Value Health. 2013;16(2):231–50.

27. Tato M, Ruiz-Garbajosa P, Traczewski M, Dodgson A, McEwan A, Humphries R, Hindler J, Veltman J, Wang H, Canton R. Multisite evaluation of Cepheid Xpert Carba-R assay for detection of carbapenemase-producing organisms in rectal swabs. J Clin Microbiol. 2016;54(7):1814–9.

28. Xpert Carba-R. http://www.cepheid.com/us/cepheid-solutions/clinical-ivd-tests/healthcare-associated-infections/xpert-carba-r. Accessed July 2018.

29. ECDC Database. https://ecdc.europa.eu/en. Accessed July 2018.

30. R Core Team: R: A language and environment. 2005.

31. Gijon D, Curiao T, Baquero F, Coque TM, Canton R. Fecal carriage of carbapenemase-producing Enterobacteriaceae: a hidden reservoir in hospitalized and nonhospitalized patients. J Clin Microbiol. 2012;50(5):1558–63.

32. Lapointe-Shaw L, Voruganti T, Kohler P, Thein HH, Sander B, McGeer A. Cost-effectiveness analysis of universal screening for carbapenemase-producing Enterobacteriaceae in hospital inpatients. Eur J Clin Microbiol Infect Dis. 2017;36(6):1047–55.

33. Kono K. A formula for infection control using colonization pressure and compliance rates. Infect Control Hosp Epidemiol. 2014;35(9):1200–1.

34. Bonten MJ, Slaughter S, Ambergen AW, Hayden MK, van Voorhis J, Nathan C, Weinstein RA. The role of "colonization pressure" in the spread of vancomycin-resistant enterococci: an important infection control variable. Arch Intern Med. 1998;158(10):1127–32.

35. Arvaniti K, Lathyris D, Ruimy R, Haidich AB, Koulourida V, Nikolaidis P, Matamis D, Miyakis S. The importance of colonization pressure in multiresistant Acinetobacter baumannii acquisition in a Greek intensive care unit. Crit Care. 2012;16(3):R102.

5

Impact of preventive primary care on children's unplanned hospital admissions: a population-based birth cohort study of UK children 2000–2013

Elizabeth Cecil[1*], Alex Bottle[1], Richard Ma[1], Dougal S. Hargreaves[2], Ingrid Wolfe[3], Arch G. Mainous III[4] and Sonia Saxena[1]

Abstract

Background: Universal health coverage (UHC) aims to improve child health through preventive primary care and vaccine coverage. Yet, in many developed countries with UHC, unplanned and ambulatory care sensitive (ACS) hospital admissions in childhood continue to rise. We investigated the relation between preventive primary care and risk of unplanned and ACS admission in children in a high-income country with UHC.

Methods: We followed 319,780 children registered from birth with 363 English practices in Clinical Practice Research Datalink linked to Hospital Episodes Statistics, born between January 2000 and March 2013. We used Cox regression estimating adjusted hazard ratios (HR) to examine subsequent risk of unplanned and ACS hospital admissions in children who received preventive primary care (development checks and vaccinations), compared with those who did not.

Results: Overall, 98% of children had complete vaccinations and 87% had development checks. Unplanned admission rates were 259, 105 and 42 per 1000 child-years in infants (aged < 1 year), preschool (1–4 years) and primary school (5–9 years) children, respectively.
Lack of preventive care was associated with more unplanned admissions. Infants with incomplete vaccination had increased risk for all unplanned admissions (HR 1.89, 1.79–2.00) and vaccine-preventable admissions (HR 4.41, 2.59–7.49). Infants lacking development checks had higher risk for unplanned admission (HR 4.63, 4.55–4.71). These associations persisted across childhood. Children who had higher consulting rates with primary care providers also had higher risk of unplanned admission (preschool children: HR 1.17, 1.17–1.17). One third of all unplanned admissions (62,154/183,530) were for ACS infectious illness. Children with chronic ACS conditions, asthma, diabetes or epilepsy had increased risk of unplanned admission (HR 1.90, 1.77–2.04, HR 11.43, 8.48–15.39, and HR 4.82, 3.93–5.91, respectively). These associations were modified in children who consulted more in primary care.

Conclusions: A high uptake of preventive primary care from birth is associated with fewer unplanned and ACS admissions in children. However, the clustering of poor health, a lack of preventive care uptake, and social deprivation puts some children with comorbid conditions at very high risk of admission. Strengthening immunisation coverage and preventive primary care in countries with poor UHC could potentially significantly reduce the health burden from hospital admission in children.

Keywords: Universal health coverage, Child health, Unplanned hospital admissions, Ambulatory care sensitive conditions, Preventive primary care

* Correspondence: e.cecil@imperial.ac.uk
[1]Department of Primary Care and Public Health, Imperial College London
Charing Cross Campus, London W6 8RP, UK
Full list of author information is available at the end of the article

Background

Achieving universal health care (UHC) coverage is a Sustainable Development Goal (SDG3.8.1) [1] to improve global health without exposing individuals to financial hardship. Indicators of UHC, such as child immunisation, access to preventive primary care and service capacity [2], are particularly relevant for improving children's health [3, 4], contributing to substantial progress in reducing under five mortality in children [5].

Yet, even in high-income countries such as the United Kingdom (UK), which has high UHC coverage and where 98% of children are registered with a general practitioner (GP) from birth, children's health lags behind other Western European nations and unplanned hospital admissions have steadily increased [6, 7]. Rising admissions have been ascribed partly to health system failures to adapt to a growing chronic disease burden in children [6] and primary care policies that have impeded children's access to high quality primary care [8].

Cross sectional and ecological trend studies using aggregate data have reported correlations between access to primary care and lower hospitalisation rates for ambulatory care sensitive (ACS) conditions in children [7, 8]. ACS conditions in children include common infectious conditions but also chronic conditions commonly seen in primary care (asthma, diabetes and epilepsy) [9, 10].

However, previous studies have been unable to demonstrate how specific UHC interventions such as child immunisation and preventive care around the time of birth may mitigate a child's risk of admission to hospital, partly due to a previous lack of linked data records between primary care and hospital.

We hypothesised that preventive primary care use, including timely vaccination and development checks, is associated with fewer childhood illness consultations and unplanned and ACS admissions to hospital in a high-income country with a high UHC index.

Methods

Study design and data sources

We undertook a birth cohort study using prospectively collected data from the UK Clinical Practice Research Datalink (CPRD), the largest and best validated primary care research database within the UK [11]. It contains longitudinal, patient-level, anonymised computerised health records from 674 general practices and is broadly representative of approximately 7% of the UK population. Clinicians use codes to record diagnoses, prescriptions and procedures, including vaccination. Three quarters (75%) of all English CPRD practices are now linked with Hospital Episode Statistics (HES) [11], which contains International Classification of Diseases version 10 (ICD-10) coded records for the main reason for admission for all National Health Service (NHS) hospitals in England.

Cohort construction

Our target population was children born between January 1, 2000, and March 31, 2013. A delivery date is provided in the CPRD mother-baby link but also in HES. HES records a child's birth as an admission method as '82' for a birth of a baby within the hospital or '83' for a baby born outside the hospital [12]. Babies born at home 'as intended' will not have a HES birth record. Therefore, to establish a birth cohort we took the child's date of birth from hospital record and when missing (potentially due to home birth) from the primary care records.

To ensure our cohort included children's full consulting history in primary care from the time of a child's birth, we included children born to mothers who were registered at an 'up to standard' CPRD-participating practice at the time of their birth (Fig. 1). This is because many children are not registered with a GP until their first visit for vaccination and development checks. We assumed that a child would not visit another practice prior to their registration at their mother's practice.

Children were followed up from birth to the end of the study period (December 31, 2013), the date a child left a practice (deregistered) or the last practice data collection date (whichever came first). During follow-up, children were assigned to one of four developmental age groups, defined as infants (when aged < 1 year), pre-school (1–4 years) and primary school (5–9 years). We restricted our cohort to children aged less than 10 years because older children (10–15 years) in CPRD would have had insufficient follow-up time (Fig. 1). We created three sub-cohorts of children aged 5–9 years with ACS conditions as those who had a diagnosis code for asthma, diabetes or epilepsy in their consulting history (Additional file 1: Table S1); this age group was chosen as asthma and epilepsy cannot be reliably diagnosed in young children.

Exposure to preventive care and illness consultations

In the UK, all children are invited for a development check at 6–8 weeks old (recommended by Healthy Child Programme) and to receive vaccinations at 8, 12 and 16 weeks, and again at 1 and 3 years of age as an integral part of a child's health and immunisation programme during their early years [13]. At each visit, vaccinations are given both orally and by injection. We determined the dates of vaccinations and also identified children who had incomplete infant vaccinations defined as those with fewer than three consultations for vaccination in their first year and identified children with delayed vaccination if their first vaccine was given after 5 months of age [2].

We defined an infant development check or vaccination as 'preventive' consultations (Additional file 1: Table S1) and an illness consultation as any face-to-face clinical contact with a GP excluding those for preventive care [14].

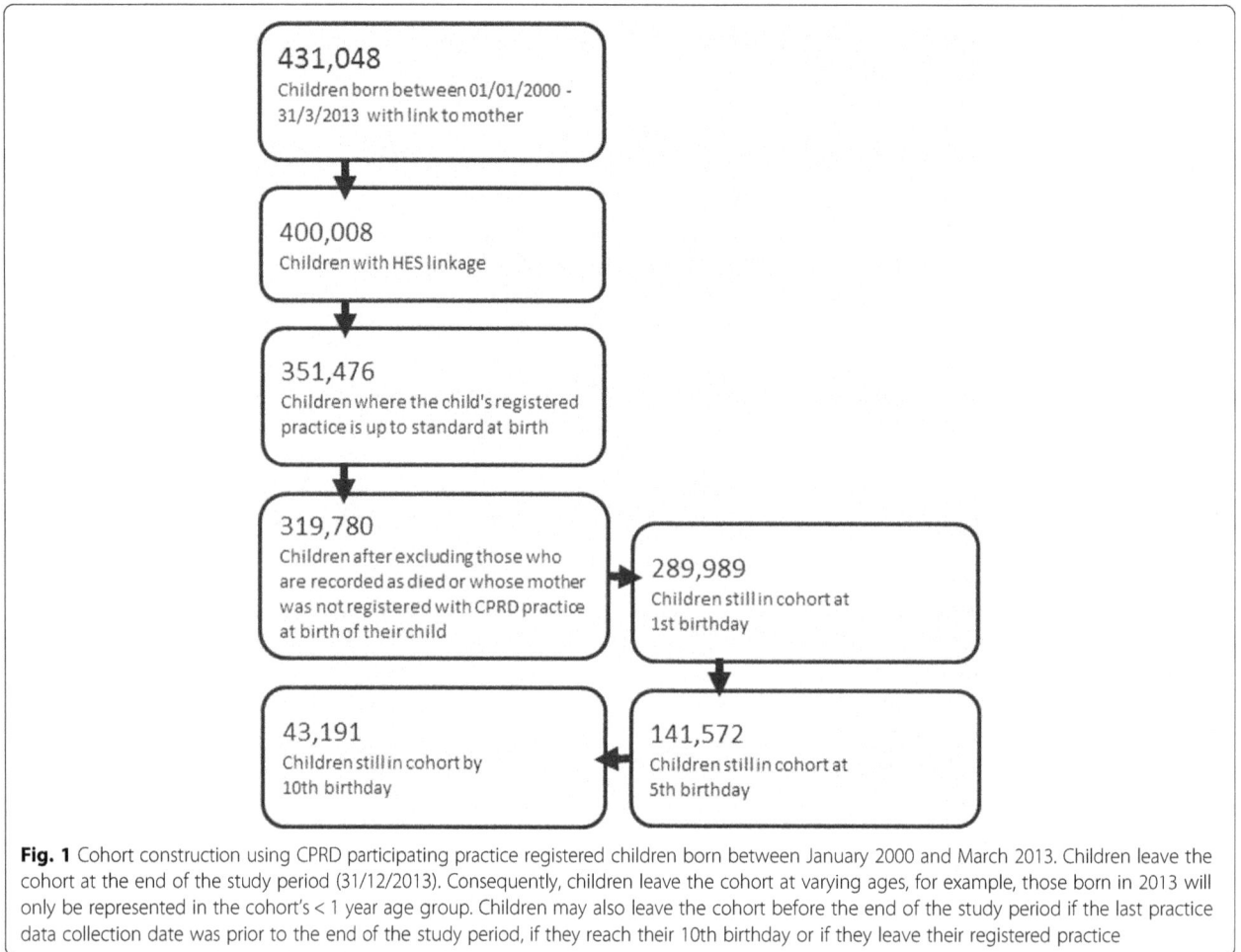

Fig. 1 Cohort construction using CPRD participating practice registered children born between January 2000 and March 2013. Children leave the cohort at the end of the study period (31/12/2013). Consequently, children leave the cohort at varying ages, for example, those born in 2013 will only be represented in the cohort's < 1 year age group. Children may also leave the cohort before the end of the study period if the last practice data collection date was prior to the end of the study period, if they reach their 10th birthday or if they leave their registered practice

Details of this process are provided in Additional file 2. We explored illness consultations primarily as an explanatory variable for unplanned and ACS admissions.

Outcomes

The primary outcome was the first record of an unplanned (rather than elective) or ACS admission [7]. We defined admissions for ACS conditions using ICD-10 codes (Additional file 1: Table S2) [9, 10, 15]. ACS infectious illnesses were defined as vaccine-preventable conditions, gastroenteritis, lower and upper respiratory tract infection, and urinary tract infection in all children. We calculated risk for admission with chronic ACS conditions in sub-cohorts of children aged 5–9 years.

Secondary outcomes were illness consultation and unplanned admission rates.

Covariates: social factors, parenting experience and co-morbid conditions

We examined the relation between several covariates identified from previous studies known to increase admission risk, including social factors and the presence of

co-morbid conditions diagnosed in the child's HES records [16–18].

We identified children who had preterm birth recorded in any diagnosis field of their HES birth record [12] (Additional file 1: Table S3). We also identified children with congenital conditions such as immunodeficiency, cystic fibrosis, chronic lung disease, congenital heart disease, nervous system congenital anomalies, other congenital anomalies (including Down's syndrome), other perinatal conditions and cerebral palsy (Additional file 1: Table S4) [19].

We assigned each child to one of five population weighted deprivation groups using English Indices of Multiple Deprivation quintiles [20] based on the child's post code; < 1% of children were missing these data. We identified children of first time mothers to indicate a relative lack of parenting experience compared with mothers who had a previous child, and used maternal age at birth of the child to identify teenage mothers aged < 20 years, who are known to have high consulting rates in primary care, comparing them with mothers aged 20–39 years and older mothers aged 40+ years.

Statistical analysis

We calculated illness consultation rates by summing consultations for each child divided by their follow-up time in each of the three developmental age bands. We calculated unplanned admission rates as the total number of admissions divided by total follow-up time within each developmental age band. Since unplanned admission rates change with the age of a child, we used Cox proportional hazard model to estimate hazard ratios (HR) for admission. One strength of this methodology is that it does not assume a baseline rate allowing admission rates to change over time. We carried out bivariate and multivariable analyses adjusting (where relevant) for sex, deprivation level, whether the child was a firstborn, maternal age band at birth, child's prior illness consultation rate (an age band-specific measure: GP consultations prior to admission or, if no admission, within an age band divided by follow-up time), the presence of comorbid health conditions (prematurity and congenital disease), vaccination status and development checks (as preventive care in infants is at 8 weeks old vaccinations and development checks were included as time updating variables when modelling in infants). Covariates were added sequentially to the models based on bivariate association and we considered an association of $p < 0.05$ as statistically significant (model Wald test).

We assessed for interactions between illness consultation and ACS chronic condition status on admission risk. We calculated population attributable risks and, using previously published admission numbers [7], estimated how many preschool children in 2011 could have avoided an admission if fully vaccinated.

We checked Cox proportional hazard assumptions of proportionality, using Nelson–Aalen cumulative hazard plots and non-informative censoring as a sensitivity analysis stratifying by censored versus non-censored children. As sensitivity analyses, we investigated multilevel (random intercept) Cox models, clustering by GP practice. This method models within practice variability allowing GP practice factors such as access to be ignored. We used Stata version 14 (StataCorp, College Station, Texas, USA) for the analyses.

Results

Our birth cohort consisted of 319,780 children born and registered with 363 English practices between January 2000 and March 2013. One in three of these children (97,836) left their practices during the study period. There were a total of 4,801,171 illness consultations and 183,530 unplanned admissions, with 1,540,977 child-years of follow-up. The median follow-up time (interquartile range) in infants, preschool and primary school children

was 1.0 (1.0–1.0), 3.0 (1.1–4.0) and 3.4 (1.5–5.0) years, respectively.

Twenty-three percent (74,233/319,780) of children lived in the most affluent areas compared with 18% (57,440/319,780) of children living in the most deprived areas. Four percent (12,814/319,780) of children were born to teenage mothers (Table 1). One in five infants in the cohort had a record of a congenital condition (18.2%) or were born prematurely (6.0%). Nine percent of primary school children (13,484/141,519) had a diagnosis of an ACS chronic condition (asthma, diabetes mellitus or epilepsy).

Uptake of preventive care was high; 98% (5417/289,989) of preschool children had complete vaccinations, of whom 1% (1736/289,989) had delayed vaccination, and 87% (253,408/289,989) of preschool children had development checks.

Infants had, on average, four illness consultations in their first year; while preschool had 2.9 and primary school aged children had 1.3 illness consultations per year, respectively (Table 2). Primary school children with ACS chronic conditions consulted GPs more frequently than children without, on average, twice per year (Table 2).

Table 1 Sociodemographic characteristics and comorbid conditions in birth cohort[a]

Number of children	$N = 319,780$
Characteristics	Number (%)
Boys	163,713 (51.2)
Deprivation[b]	
Least deprived fifth	74,233 (23.2)
Most deprived fifth	57,440 (18.0)
Maternal age at birth of child (years)	
< 20	12,814 (4.0)
20–39	291,846 (91.3)
40+	15,120 (4.7)
Mother's first child	234,781 (73.6)
Prematurity for constisency	19,275 (6.0)
Congenital condition	57,937 (18.2)
Diagnosed with ACS[c] chronic condition in children aged 5–9 years ($N = 141,519$)	
Asthma	12,654 (8.9)
Diabetes	268 (0.2)
Epilepsy	670 (0.5)
More than one ACS chronic condition	123 (0.1)

[a]Born between 01/01/2000 and 31/03/2013 registered with 363 practices partnered with the Clinical Practice Research Datalink in England and followed up until 31/12/2013
[b]Index of multiple deprivation fifths (5 the most deprived, 1 least deprived)
[c]Ambulatory care sensitive

Table 2 Annual illness consultation in primary care and unplanned and ambulatory care sensitive (ACS) hospital admission rates[a]

Number of children in cohort	Infant (age < 1 year)	Preschool (age 1–4 years)	Primary school (age 5–9 years)		Asthma diagnosis (age 5–9 years)	Diabetes diagnosis (age 5–9 years)	Epilepsy diagnosis (age 5–9 years)
	$N = 319,780$	$N = 289,989$	$N = 141,572$		$N = 12,654$	$N = 268$	$N = 670$
Rate per child/year (95% confidence interval)							
Illness consultation[b]	4.01 (4.00–4.03)	2.91 (2.90–2.92)	1.33 (1.32–1.34)		2.18 (2.15–2.22)	2.02 (1.81–2.23)	2.22 (2.06–2.39)
Rate per 1000 child-years (95% confidence interval)							
Unplanned admissions	259 (256–261)	105 (104–107)	42 (40–44)		84 (77–91)	342 (279–405)	461 (365–558)
Infectious ACS admissions							
URTI	26.6 (25.9–27.2)	19.7 (19.3–20.1)	6.5 (6.2–6.8)				
LRTI	36.1 (35.3–36.9)	4.6 (4.4–4.8)	1.0 (0.9–1.1)				
Gastroenteritis	23.3 (22.7–23.9)	10.5 (10.2–10.7)	2.2 (2.0–2.4)		Not measured	Not measured	Not measured
Urinary tract infection	6.5 (6.1–6.8)	1.9 (1.7–2.0)	0.9 (0.8–1.0)				
Vaccine-preventable infections	0.7 (0.6–0.8)	0.07 (0.06–0.10)	(number too small to compute rate)				
Chronic ACS admissions[c]	N/A	N/A	N/A		26.0 (23.5–28.8)	193 (168–223)	178 (147–216)

[a]Cohort of 319,780 children born between 01/01/2000 and 31/03/2013 registered with 363 Clinical Practice Research Datalink practices linked to Hospital Episode Statistics in England, and followed up until 31/12/2013
[b]Illness consultation: face-to-face consultation with a GP excluding preventive care
[c]ACS chronic admission rates (primary diagnosis at admission) in children aged 5–9 years diagnosed with ACS condition. We chose to analyse the age group alone because asthma cannot reliably be diagnosed in children aged less than 5 years
ACS ambulatory care sensitive, LRTI lower respiratory tract infection, URTI upper respiratory tract infection

Risk of unplanned hospital admissions

Unplanned admission rates were 259 per 1000 child-years among infants, 105/1000 among preschool children and 42/1000 among primary school children (Table 2). The subset of primary school-aged children diagnosed with an ACS chronic condition (asthma, diabetes and epilepsy) had higher unplanned admission rates compared to all primary school children (84/1000, 342/1000 and 461/1000 child-years for children with ACS chronic conditions).

Lack of preventive care was associated with a higher risk for unplanned admission, after adjusting for deprivation, maternal age and firstborn indicators (Table 3). In preschool children, the adjusted HR for incomplete vaccination was 1.89 (1.79–2.00) and the population attributable risk was 0.0115 (95% CI 0.0101–0.0130). We estimated that, annually, approximately 2000 (0.0115 × 207,573) unplanned admissions in England could be avoided if all preschool children had the same admission rate as those who were fully immunised. In preschool children, those who had delayed vaccinations had an increased risk of unplanned admissions compared to those who had timely vaccinations (HR 1.15, 1.04–1.27). Infants who had no development checks had over four times the risk for unplanned admission than those who had development checks (HR 4.63, 4.55–4.71); this was observed to a lesser extent for preschool and primary school children (HR 1.19 and 1.09, respectively).

Illness consultations were associated with a higher risk for unplanned admission, with the risk increasing across childhood; an additional consultation per year increased the average admission rate by 0.5% (HR 1.005, 1.005–1.005) in infants and by 23% (HR 1.23, 1.23–1.24) in primary school children.

The presence of comorbid conditions and social factors, such as material deprivation, were also strongly associated with unplanned admission. Children born prematurely or with a congenital condition had a greater risk of unplanned admission across all age groups (HR 1.21, 1.18–1.25 in preterm infants; HR 2.40, 2.36–2.45 in infants with congenital conditions). Children living in the most deprived quintile had a 22% higher risk of an unplanned admission from infancy. This increased risk of admission doubled to 44% in primary school years (HR 1.22, 1.20–1.25) and in infants (HR 1.44, 1.37–1.51) (Table 3). Infants of teenage mothers had a 33% increased risk of an unplanned admission compared with older mothers aged 20–39 years HR 1.33 (1.28–1.38).

Risk factors for ACS infectious admissions (Table 4)

One-third of all unplanned admissions (62,154/183,530) in the birth cohort were for ACS infectious illness, of which only 271 were for vaccine-preventable conditions. Overall, the risk factors for ACS infectious admissions were similar to the risks for all unplanned admissions (Table 4); however, the magnitude of the association between deprivation and ACS infectious illness tended to

Table 3 Association of preventive primary care, comorbidity and social factors on risk of unplanned hospital admission[a]

Adjusted hazard ratio[b] (95% confidence interval)		Infant (age < 1 year)	Preschool (age 1–4 years)	Primary school (age 5–9 years)
Incomplete vaccinations[c]		1.20 (1.16–1.25)	1.89 (1.79–2.00)	1.27 (1.07–1.51)
No development check[d]		4.63 (4.55–4.71)	1.19 (1.16–1.22)	1.09 (1.03–1.14)
Illness consultation rate[e]		1.00 (1.00–1.00)	1.17 (1.17–1.17)	1.23 (1.23–1.24)
Prematurity		1.21 (1.18–1.25)	1.26 (1.22–1.30)	1.12 (1.04–1.21)
Congenital conditions		2.40 (2.36–2.45)	1.17 (1.15–1.20)	1.15 (1.10–1.21)
Deprivation[f]	5 vs. 1	1.22 (1.20–1.25)	1.38 (1.34–1.41)	1.44 (1.37–1.51)
Maternal age	< 20 vs. 20–39 years	1.33 (1.28–1.38)	1.35 (1.30–1.40)	1.28 (1.18–1.39)
	40+ vs. 20–39 years	0.86 (0.83–0.90)	0.93 (0.89–0.97)	0.96 (0.88–1.05)
Being the firstborn child		0.88 (0.86–0.90)	0.97 (0.95–0.99)	No association
Sex		0.83 (0.81–0.84)	0.87 (0.86–0.89)	0.80 (0.77–0.83)

[a]Cohort of children born between 01/01/2000 and 31/03/2013 registered with 363 practices partnered with the Clinical Practice Research Datalink practices linked to Hospital Episode Statistics in England and followed up until 31/12/2013
[b]Hazard ratios have been adjusted for listed covariates. Covariates were added sequentially to the models, p values of < 0.05 were considered statistically significant
[c]In modelling admissions in infants, incomplete vaccination is a time-updated variable. In children aged 1 and over, incomplete vaccination is less than three infant vaccinations
[d]Did not complete infant development checks within primary care
[e]An illness consultation is a face-to-face consultation with a GP which is not for preventive care
[f]Index of multiple deprivation fifths (5 the most deprived, 1 least deprived)

be greater than for all admissions. Infants with incomplete vaccination were over four times more likely to be admitted for a vaccine-preventable condition (HR 4.41, 2.59–7.49), with the risk persisting, and increasing in magnitude, across childhood.

Risk factors for ACS chronic admissions
Primary school-aged children diagnosed with an ACS chronic condition, compared with children without an ACS chronic condition, had an increased risk of unplanned admission (for any admission diagnosis) of 1.90 (1.77–2.04), 11.43 (8.48–15.39) and 4.82 (3.93–5.91) for asthma, diabetes and epilepsy. There was no evidence that deprivation was a stronger risk factor for children with an ACS chronic condition (Table 5).

Illness consultation rates modified the association of unplanned admissions for ACS chronic conditions, with interaction factors of 0.92 (0.91–0.93), 0.88 (0.82–0.95) and 0.95 (0.92–0.98) in asthma, diabetes or epilepsy, respectively. For example, a child with asthma has, on average, 90% greater risk of an unplanned admission compared with children without an ACS chronic condition (holding consultation rate constant); this reduced to 74% with a single additional illness consultation per year.

Of the primary school children diagnosed with an ACS chronic condition, 19% (2597/13,484) had an unplanned admission (any diagnoses), while only 5% (729/13,484) had an unplanned admission for an ACS chronic condition.

Sensitivity analyses
Sensitivity analyses showed that our findings were robust to age and duration of registration. Unplanned admission HRs for variables of interest were similar when children were followed up from 8 weeks of age compared with follow-up from birth. HRs were similar but more extreme in those who were censored due to leaving their registered practice compared with those who remained until the end of the study period (December 2013) or the practice's last data collection date (if earlier) (Additional file 1: Tables S5 and S6).

Unplanned admission HRs for variables of interest were higher in infants when we applied a multilevel model (Additional file 1: Table S7), but were similar in older age groups.

Discussion
Main findings
To our knowledge, this is the largest study of its kind to assess the impact of preventive primary care on the risk of unplanned and ACS hospital admissions across childhood. In our birth cohort of 319,780 children registered with UK primary care and followed over 1,540,977 child-years, there was a high uptake of preventive care, with 98% of children having complete vaccinations and 87% having development checks in infancy and high contact rates with GP (four times in infancy for illness). A lack of preventive primary care, including vaccination and development checks, was strongly associated with a higher risk of unplanned and ACS admission in children. For example, there was a four-fold increased risk of

Table 4 Association of preventive primary care, comorbidity and social factors on risk of ambulatory care sensitive infectious admissions[a]

	Infant (aged < 1 year) HR[b] (95% CI)	Preschool (aged 1–4 years) HR[b] (95% CI)	Primary school (aged 5–9 years) HR[b] (95% CI)
Vaccine preventable admissions			
Incomplete vaccinations[c]	4.41 (2.59–7.49)	6.62 (2.80 to 15.66)	19.98 (2.40–166.25)
No development check[d]	3.56 (2.64–4.81)	1.95 (3.66–1.04)	No association
Illness consultation rate[e]	1.00 (1.00–1.00)	1.15 (1.10–1.20)	1.26 (1.11–1.43)
Prematurity	No association	No association	No association
Congenital conditions	1.74 (1.26–2.40)	No association	No association
Deprivation[f] 5 vs. 1	2.11 (1.37–3.25)	2.27 (1.08–4.76)	No association
Upper respiratory tract infection			
Incomplete vaccinations[c]	1.62 (1.40–1.88)	1.58 (1.41–1.77)	No association
No development check[d]	2.16 (2.05–2.27)	1.18 (1.12 to1.24)	1.15 (1.03–1.28)
Illness consultation rate[e]	1.00 (1.00–1.00)	1.16 (1.16–1.17)	1.24 (1.23–1.25)
Prematurity	1.62 (1.50–1.76)	1.32 (1.24–1.40)	1.41 (1.21–1.64)
Congenital conditions	1.39 (1.32–1.48)	1.22 (1.17–1.27)	1.15 (1.03–1.28)
Deprivation[f] 5 vs. 1	1.54 (1.44–1.65)	1.48 (1.41–1.56)	1.79 (1.60–2.00)
Lower respiratory tract infection			
Incomplete vaccinations[c]	1.53 (1.40–1.68)	2.16 (1.77–2.64)	No association
No development check[d]	2.60 (2.49–2.71)	1.29 (1.17–1.43)	No association
Illness consultation rate[e]	1.00 (1.00–1.00)	1.15 (1.15–1.16)	No association
Prematurity	2.24 (2.11–2.39)	1.87 (1.67–2.10)	1.82 (1.29–2.57)
Congenital conditions	1.36 (1.30–1.43)	1.36 (1.25–1.48)	1.25 (1.23–1.28)
Deprivation[f] 5 vs. 1	1.50 (1.42–1.60)	1.26 (1.15–1.39)	No association
Gastroenteritis admissions			
Incomplete vaccinations[c]	1.16 (0.99–1.35)	1.82 (1.58–2.09)	No association
No development check[d]	2.02 (1.92–2.13)	1.29 (1.21–1.37)	No association
Illness consultation rate[e]	1.00 (1.00–1.00)	1.15 (1.15–1.16)	1.24 (1.23–1.26)
Prematurity	1.28 (1.17–1.41)	1.19 (1.10–1.30)	1.35 (1.04–1.74)
Congenital conditions	1.40 (1.32–1.49)	1.23 (1.16–1.30)	No association
Deprivation[f] 5 vs. 1	1.69 (1.58–1.82)	1.67 (1.57–1.78)	1.63 (1.34–1.98)
Urinary tract infection			
Incomplete vaccinations[c]	No association	2.01 (1.43–2.82)	No association
No development check[d]	2.41 (2.17–2.68)	1.28 (1.09–1.50)	No association
Illness consultation rate[e]	1.00 (1.00–1.00)	1.15 (1.14–1.17)	1.27 (1.24–1.30)
Prematurity	1.44 (1.21–1.71)	No association	No association
Congenital conditions	1.35 (1.19–1.52)	1.42 (1.24–1.62)	No association
Deprivation[f] 5 vs. 1	No association	1.59 (1.35–1.87)	1.42 (1.04–1.95)

[a]Data is from a cohort of 319,780 children born between 01/01/2000 and 31/03/2013, registered with 363 Clinical Practice Research Datalink practices in England, with Hospital Episode Statistics linkage, and followed up until 31/12/2013
[b]Adjusted hazard ratio and 95% confidence interval; hazard ratios have been adjusted for listed covariates as well as sex, maternal age and whether first child; covariates were added sequentially to the models, p values of < 0.05 were considered statistically significant
[c]In modelling admissions in infants, incomplete vaccination is a time updated variable; in children aged 1 and over, incomplete vaccination is less than three infant vaccinations
[d]Did not complete infant development checks within primary care
[e]An illness consultation is a face-to-face consultation with a GP that is not for preventive care
[f]Index of multiple deprivation fifths (5 most deprived, 1 least deprived)

Table 5 Association of preventive primary care, comorbidity and social factors on risk of ambulatory care sensitive chronic admissions in primary school-aged children

	Primary school (aged 5–9 years) HR[a] (95% CI)
Asthma	
Incomplete vaccinations[b]	2.24 (1.11–4.50)
No development check[c]	No association
Illness consultation rate[d]	1.14 (1.11–1.16)
Prematurity	No association
Congenital conditions	No association
Deprivation[e] 5 vs. 1	1.38 (1.10–1.72)
Diabetes	No Associations
Epilepsy	
Incomplete vaccinations[d]	3.83 (1.21–12.07)
No development check[e]	No association
Illness consultation rate[c]	1.09 (1.05–1.12)
Prematurity	No association
Congenital conditions	No association
Deprivation[e] 5 vs. 1	No association

[a]Adjusted hazard ratio and 95% confidence interval; hazard ratios have been adjusted for listed covariates as well as sex, maternal age and whether first child; covariates were added sequentially to the models, p values of < 0.05 were considered statistically significant
[b]In modelling admissions in infants, incomplete vaccination is a time updated variable; in children aged 1 and over, incomplete vaccination is less than three infant vaccinations
[c]Did not complete infant development checks within primary care
[d]An illness consultation is a face-to-face consultation with a GP that is not for preventive care
[e]Index of multiple deprivation fifths (5 the most deprived, 1 least deprived)

vaccine-preventable hospital admissions that increased across childhood. We estimate that, in the UK, 2000 preschool children are admitted annually to hospital for problems that are potentially attributable to a lack of basic vaccinations. One-third of all unplanned admissions, in our cohort, were for ACS infectious illness. One in five primary school age children who had a chronic ACS condition (asthma, diabetes or epilepsy) were admitted to hospital. We also found comorbidity and social deprivation to be associated with unplanned admission.

Comparison with past research

We found no previous studies specifically investigating the impact of preventive primary care on children's admission risk over time. However, our findings are consistent with systematic reviews and numerous other studies that have demonstrated a relation between various features of primary care in adults and avoidable admission [3, 21].

We, and others, have previously reported that emergency department visits and admissions for ACS chronic conditions are associated with poor access to primary care, highlighting the importance of primary care in preventing adverse outcomes for children with chronic conditions [7, 8]. Our study further supports this evidence, which is especially important since the number of children with chronic conditions is increasing. In recent years, adult admission rates for ACS chronic diseases, including asthma, diabetes and epilepsy, are reported to have fallen following major financial incentives in primary care to improve chronic disease management [22], suggesting scope for a similar policy intervention for children.

The age, sex and sociodemographic profile of our sample was representative of the national population [23] and other variable characteristics, such as the proportion of children born to teenage mothers, were comparable over the study period. A similar proportion of our birth cohort was born prematurely compared with national and international estimates [24]. We could not find comparable studies giving estimates of congenital anomalies. One study investigating child mortality found that only 3% of children who died had a congenital anomaly [25]. However, our study purposefully took a much broader definition of congenital conditions, which included comorbid conditions diagnosed within infancy as well as suspected conditions affected by birth.

In England, since 2007/2008, the combined vaccine coverage in infants for diphtheria, tetanus, polio, pertussis and haemophilus influenza B and for pneumonia vaccine has reached 93-95%. Our cohort may have achieved a higher uptake rate firstly because the national picture is likely to include some children who do not engage with primary care, but also because CPRD participating practices may perform better. We found illness consultation rates in the community and rates of unplanned admission in children were comparable to recent studies [7, 14, 26].

Implications for research and policy

Our findings support a body of evidence in favour of UHC of primary care to add to efforts to reduce the burden of disease in the population and alleviate strain on hospital services from unplanned admissions [3, 8, 27]. The high level of infant immunisation coverage across all four nations in the UK in recent years is a success story that other nations have yet to achieve [28]. UHC is an important means of improving health equity, especially essential in lower-income settings. However, even in high-income countries, we found a significantly higher risk for hospital admission for children living below the poorest quintile, demonstrating additional room for improvement in countries with UCH and that service provision alone is not enough. Our findings suggest preventive primary care may help to reduce unplanned admissions, particularly in infants who have the highest contact rates with primary care. Nevertheless, health services beyond infancy tend to be responsive rather than anticipatory, which may disadvantage children with chronic illness.

The UK health system currently lacks a clear framework for the health and wellbeing of children beyond infant immunisation. The healthcare needs of children differ in important ways from those of adults; with greater dependency on parents, education remains an important component of families' ability to care. In the United States, potentially preventable admissions among children have been decreasing [29]. Future work could explore cost effectiveness of new models of care such as GP-led urgent care centres and impact of certain core features of primary care such as access, structured preventive care, continuity of care and case management of children with chronic conditions [30]. We need to better understand how primary care can serve the needs of children with long-term or complex conditions.

Limitations

Data quality and extensive coverage of the CPRD database [11] reduces the possibility that our findings are due to chance but, as with any observational cohort study, there are several important biases relating to coding accuracy, completeness and losses to follow-up [31]. A main source of bias in our findings likely arises due to losses to follow-up across the period; however, these were minimised by the way our cohort was constructed such that children contributed time in the cohort according to their age band. We excluded children registered at practices without HES and mother and baby linkage. We found children living in deprived areas were more likely to deregister than children from affluent groups; therefore, our findings are not likely to be generalisable to these children, who may represent a more mobile population and may require a different policy response [32]. However, our sensitivity analysis suggests findings are similar for these families although effect sizes of associations are diluted by their loss to follow-up over the period. We did not obtain health records for the mother, restricting our ability to investigate further health maternal factors or those arising from birth.

Our analysis was highly powered and all reported associations in the full cohort had a significance level greater than 99%. However, in the ACS cohorts, numbers were much smaller, for example, only 268 (0.2%) children aged 5–9 years had a diagnosis of diabetes. As a result, we lacked power to identify association between preventive care and unplanned admissions in children with diabetes.

Our measure of incomplete vaccination may be an underestimate. Determining whether children in birth cohorts, born over several birth years, have received all their primary immunisations is complex given the relatively frequent changes to the detail of the nationally recommended immunisation schedule. In some years, catch up immunisations took place, increasing the basic number [33, 34].

There is residual confounding in our study comparing children with delayed or incomplete vaccination with those who engage with the immunisation programme. These groups are likely to differ in important ways relating to their underlying health, health seeking behaviour and health beliefs, which could also impact on their risk for admission to hospital.

Although most routine preventive care occurs in the community, our data sources would not capture preventive care such as developmental check-ups and vaccinations received in specialist settings. This may be the case in a small minority of children, for example, those with preterm birth or congenital conditions.

Our methodologies, calculating within practice variation and marginal means, reduce the impact of practice level confounding and our sensitivity analyses suggest that practice level confounding may exist in infants but has little effect in older children. Differentiating between health status and illness severity is challenging given a lack of reliable indicators in routine data. In a UHC system, consultations with GPs are not a good proxy for poor health status since preventive advice or disease management for ACS chronic conditions can be given during a consultation; this is highlighted by the fact that illness consultations modify the effect of having an ACS chronic condition on unplanned hospital admissions [35]. Hence, this is among a number of sources of residual confounding that we were unable to account for.

Conclusions

A high uptake of preventive primary care, including vaccination and development checks, is associated with fewer unplanned and ACS admissions from birth and through childhood. However, the clustering of poor health, a lack of preventive care uptake, and social deprivation puts some children with comorbid conditions at very high risk of admission. Countries with poor immunisation coverage and preventive primary care could significantly reduce the health burden from hospital admission in children, especially those with ACS conditions, through strengthening UHC and primary care.

Additional files

Additional file 1: Table S1. Read codes identifying preventive care consultations and children with a coded diagnosis of an ambulatory care sensitive condition. **Table S2.** Ambulatory care sensitive admission ICD-10 codes. **Table S3.** International Classification of Disease version 10 (ICD-10) diagnoses for prematurity/low birth weight. **Table S4.** ICD-10 diagnoses for congenital disease. **Table S5.** Covariates and outcomes in children with full versus censored follow-up. **Table S6.** Adjusted hazard ratios for unplanned admission stratified by full versus censored follow-up in infants. **Table S7.** Association of preventive primary care, comorbidity and social factors on risk of unplanned hospital admission in using a random intercept model clustering by GP practice. (DOCX 107 kb)

Additional file 2: A supplementary file detailing the methodology used for creating the birth cohort; the preventive care consultations and illness consultations. (DOCX 24 kb)

Abbreviations

ACS: ambulatory care sensitive; CPRD: Clinical Practice Research Datalink; GP: general practitioner; HES: Hospital Episode Statistics; ICD-10: International Classification of Diseases version 10; NHS: National Health Service; UHC: universal health care; UK: United Kingdom

Funding

Elizabeth Cecil and Sonia Saxena were funded by a National Institute for Health Research (NIHR) Career Development Fellowship (CDF-2011-04-048). Richard Ma was funded by NIHR for In-Practice Fellowship (NIHR-IPF-2014-08-11). This article presents independent research commissioned by the NIHR. The views expressed in this publication are those of the authors and not necessarily those of the NHS, the NIHR or the Department of Health.

Authors' contributions

EC contributed to the conception and design of the study, carried out the analysis, took part in interpreting the data, drafted the initial manuscript and wrote the final manuscript as submitted. AB contributed to the conception and design of the study, provided statistical advice, took part in interpreting the data and helped to revise drafts of the manuscript. SS and RM contributed to the conception and design of this study, took part in interpreting the data and helped to revise drafts of the manuscript. DSH, IW and AGM took part in interpreting the data and helped to revise drafts of the manuscript. All authors approved the final manuscript as submitted and agree to be accountable for all aspects of the work.

Competing interests

The authors declare that they have no competing interests.

Author details

[1]Department of Primary Care and Public Health, Imperial College London Charing Cross Campus, London W6 8RP, UK. [2]Institute of Child Health, University College London, London, England. [3]Department of Primary Care and Public Health Sciences, King's College London, London, England. [4]Department of Health Services Research, Management and Policy, University of Florida, Gainesville, FL, USA.

References

1. United Nations. Report of the Secretary-General: Progress Towards the Sustainable Development Goals. New York, NY: UN; 2017.
2. Hogan DR, Stevens GA, Hosseinpoor AR, Boerma T. Monitoring universal health coverage within the sustainable development goals: development and baseline data for an index of essential health services. Lancet Glob Health. 2017;6(2):e152–e68.
3. Starfield B, Shi L, Macinko J. Contribution of primary care to health systems and health. Milbank Q. 2005;83(3):457–502.
4. Guttmann A, Shipman SA, Lam K, Goodman DC, Stukel TA. Primary care physician supply and Children's health care use, access, and outcomes: findings from Canada. Pediatrics. 2010;125(6):1119–26.
5. Global, regional, and national under-5 mortality, adult mortality, age-specific mortality, and life expectancy, 1970–2016: a systematic analysis for the Global Burden of Disease Study 2016. Lancet. 2017;390(10100):1084–150.
6. Wolfe I, Thompson M, Gill P, Tamburlini G, Blair M, van den Bruel A, et al. Health services for children in western Europe. Lancet. 2013; 381(9873):1224–34.
7. Cecil E, Bottle A, Sharland M, Saxena S. Impact of UK primary care policy reforms on short stay unplanned hospital admissions for children with primary care sensitive conditions: interrupted time series analysis. Ann Fam Med. 2015;13(3):214–20.
8. Cecil E, Bottle A, Cowling TE, Majeed A, Wolfe I, Saxena S. Primary care access, emergency department visits, and unplanned short hospitalizations in the UK. Pediatrics. 2016;137(2):e20151492.
9. AHRQ. Pediatric Quality Indicators 2006. http://www.qualityindicators.ahrq.gov/Downloads/Modules/PDI/V30/2006-Feb-PediatricQualityIndicators.pdf. Accessed 12 Aug 2018.
10. NHS Digital. NHS Outcomes Framework Indicators. https://digital.nhs.uk/data-and-information/publications/clinical-indicators/nhs-outcomes-framework/archive/nhs-outcomes-framework-indicators---february-2018-release. Accessed 12 Aug 2018.
11. Herrett E, Gallagher AM, Bhaskaran K, Forbes H, Mathur R, van Staa T, et al. Data resource profile: clinical practice research datalink (CPRD). Int J Epidemiol. 2015;44(3):827–36.
12. NHS Digital. HES Data Dictionary. https://digital.nhs.uk/binaries/content/assets/legacy/pdf/1/c/hes_data_dictionary_-_admitted_patient_care.pdf. Accessed 12 Aug 2018.
13. Public Health England. UK Immunisation Schedule: The Green Book, Chapter 11. 2013. https://www.gov.uk/government/publications/immunisation-schedule-the-green-book-chapter-11.
14. Hippisley-Cox J, Fenty J, Heaps M. Trends in consultation rates in general practice 1995 to 2006: analysis of the QRESEARCH database. QRESEARCH research highlights. Leeds: The Information Centre; 2007. p. 29.
15. Gill PJ, Goldacre MJ, Mant D, Heneghan C, Thomson A, Seagroatt V, et al. Increase in emergency admissions to hospital for children aged under 15 in England, 1999–2010: national database analysis. Arch Dis Child. 2013;98(5):328–34.
16. Saxena S, Eliahoo J, Majeed A. Socioeconomic and ethnic group differences in self reported health status and use of health services by children and young people in England: cross sectional study. BMJ. 2002;325(7363):520.
17. Harrington KF, Zhang B, Magruder T, Bailey WC, Gerald LB. The impact of Parent's health literacy on pediatric asthma outcomes. Pediatr Allergy Immunol Pulmonol. 2015;28(1):20–6.
18. Paranjothy S, Broughton H, Adappa R, Fone D. Teenage pregnancy: who suffers? Arch Dis Child. 2009;94(3):239–45.
19. Murray J, Bottle A, Sharland M, Modi N, Aylin P, Majeed A, et al. Risk factors for hospital admission with RSV bronchiolitis in England: a population-based birth cohort study. PLoS One. 2014;9(2):e89186.
20. Department for Communities and Local Government. English Index of Multiple Deprivation 2010 [updated 2012/11/22/17:35:29]. www.gov.uk/government/statistics/english-indices-of-deprivation-2010. Accessed 12 Aug 2018.
21. Rosano A, Loha CA, Falvo R, van der Zee J, Ricciardi W, Guasticchi G, et al. The relationship between avoidable hospitalization and accessibility to primary care: a systematic review. Eur J Public Health. 2013;23(3):356–60.
22. Harrison MJ, Dusheiko M, Sutton M, Gravelle H, Doran T, Roland M. Effect of a national primary care pay for performance scheme on emergency hospital admissions for ambulatory care sensitive conditions: controlled longitudinal study. BMJ. 2014;349:g6423.
23. Office for National Statistics. Birth Summary Tables. http://www.ons.gov.uk/peoplepopulationandcommunity/birthsdeathsandmarriages/livebirths/datasets/birthsummarytables. Accessed 12 Aug 2018.
24. Morken N-H, Vogel I, Kallen K, Skjærven R, Langhoff-Roos J, Kesmodel US, et al. Reference population for international comparisons and time trend surveillance of preterm delivery proportions in three countries. BMC Womens Health. 2008;8(1):16.

25. Zylbersztejn A, Gilbert R, Hjern A, Hardelid P. How can we make international comparisons of infant mortality in high income countries based on aggregate data more relevant to policy? BMC Pregnancy Childbirth. 2017;17(1):430.

26. Hobbs FDR, Bankhead C, Mukhtar T, Stevens S, Perera-Salazar R, Holt T, et al. Clinical workload in UK primary care: a retrospective analysis of 100 million consultations in England, 2007-14. Lancet. 2016;387(10035):2323–30.

27. Baker R, Honeyford K, Levene LS, Mainous AG, Jones DR, Bankart MJ, et al. Population characteristics, mechanisms of primary care and premature mortality in England: a cross-sectional study. BMJ Open. 2016;6:e009981.

28. de Figueiredo A, Johnston IG, Smith DMD, Agarwal S, Larson HJ, Jones NS. Forecasted trends in vaccination coverage and correlations with socioeconomic factors: a global time-series analysis over 30 years. Lancet Glob Health. 2016;4(10):e726–35.

29. Torio CM, Elixhauser A, Andrews RM. Trends in Potentially Preventable Hospital Admissions among Adults and Children, 2005–2010: Statistical Brief #151. Rockville: Agency for Health Care Policy and Research (US); 2013.

30. Gnani S, Ramzan F, Ladbrooke T, Millington H, Islam S, Car J, et al. Evaluation of a general practitioner-led urgent care centre in an urban setting: description of service model and plan of analysis. JRSM Short Rep. 2013;4(6):2042533313486263.

31. Khan NF, Harrison SE, Rose PW. Validity of diagnostic coding within the general practice research database: a systematic review. Br J Gen Pract. 2010;60(572):e128–36.

32. Howe LD, Tilling K, Galobardes B, Lawlor DA. Loss to follow-up in cohort studies: bias in estimates of socioeconomic inequalities. Epidemiology. 2013;24(1):1–9.

33. Koshy E, Murray J, Bottle A, Sharland M, Saxena S. Impact of the seven-valent pneumococcal conjugate vaccination (PCV7) programme on childhood hospital admissions for bacterial pneumonia and empyema in England: national time-trends study, 1997–2008. Thorax. 2010;65(9):770–4.

34. Ladhani SN. Two decades of experience with the Haemophilus influenzae serotype b conjugate vaccine in the United Kingdom. Clin Ther. 2012;34(2):385–99.

35. Wijlaars LP, Hardelid P, Woodman J, Allister J, Cheung R, Gilbert R. Contribution of recurrent admissions in children and young people to emergency hospital admissions: retrospective cohort analysis of hospital episode statistics. Arch Dis Child. 2015;100(9):845–9.

6

Efficacy and safety of ascending doses of praziquantel against *Schistosoma haematobium* infection in preschool-aged and school-aged children: a single-blind randomised controlled trial

Jean T. Coulibaly[1,2,3], Gordana Panic[1,2], Richard B. Yapi[4], Jana Kovač[1,2], Beatrice Barda[1,2], Yves K. N'Gbesso[5], Jan Hattendorf[2,6] and Jennifer Keiser[1,2*]

Abstract

Background: Despite decades of experience with praziquantel treatment in school-aged children (SAC) and adults, we still face considerable knowledge gaps relevant to the successful treatment of preschool-aged children (PSAC). This study aimed to assess the efficacy and safety of escalating praziquantel dosages in PSAC infected with *Schistosoma haematobium*.

Methods: We conducted a randomised, dose-finding trial in PSAC (2–5 years) and as comparator a cohort of SAC (6–15 years) infected with *S. haematobium* in Côte d'Ivoire. A total of 186 PSAC and 195 SAC were randomly assigned to 20, 40 or 60 mg/kg praziquantel or placebo. The nature of the dose-response relationship in terms of cure rate (CR) was the primary objective. Egg reduction rate (ERR) and tolerability were secondary outcomes. CRs and ERRs were assessed using triplicate urine filtration over 3 consecutive days. Available-case analysis was performed including all participants with primary endpoint data.

Results: A total of 170 PSAC and 174 SAC received treatment. Almost 90% of PSAC and three quarters of SAC were lightly infected with *S. haematobium*. Follow-up data were available for 157 PSAC and 166 SAC. In PSAC, CRs of praziquantel were 85.7% (30/35), 78.0% (32/41) and 68.3% (28/41) at 20, 40 and 60 mg/kg and 47.5% (19/40) for placebo. In SAC, CRs were 10.8% for placebo (4/37), 55.6% for 20 mg/kg (25/45), 68.3% for 40 mg/kg (28/41) and 60.5% for 60 mg/kg (26/43). ERRs based on geometric means ranged between 96.5% (60 mg/kg) and 98.3% (20 mg/kg) in PSAC and between 97.6% (20 mg/kg and 60 mg/kg) and 98.6% (40 mg/kg) in SAC. Adverse events were mild and transient.

Conclusions: Praziquantel revealed dose-independent efficacy against light infections of *S. haematobium*. Over the dose range tested, praziquantel displayed a ceiling effect with the highest response for 20 mg/kg in PSAC. In SAC maximum efficacy was obtained with 40 mg/kg praziquantel. Further investigations are required in children with moderate to heavy infections.

Trial registration: This trial is registered with International Standard Randomised Controlled Trial Number ISRCTN15280205.

Keywords: Efficacy, Praziquantel, Preschool-aged children, *Schistosoma haematobium*, School-aged children

* Correspondence: jennifer.keiser@swisstph.ch
[1]Department of Medical Parasitology and Infection Biology, Swiss Tropical and Public Health Institute, P.O. Box, CH-4002, Basel, Switzerland
[2]University of Basel, Basel, Switzerland
Full list of author information is available at the end of the article

Background

Schistosomiasis is a major public health problem with an estimated 779 million people at risk of infection [1]. The disease is caused by trematode worms of the genus *Schistosoma*, where infection with *Schistosoma japonicum* and *S. mansoni* causes mostly intestinal schistosomiasis, while *S. haematobium* is responsible for genitourinary schistosomiasis [2–6]. Cumulative schistosome infections over years, due to rapid reinfection, result in morbid sequelae, including haematuria, nutritional deficiencies, anaemia, hepatic peri-portal fibrosis and consequent portal hypertension and delayed physical and cognitive development [7–9]. Moreover, genitourinary schistosomiasis can lead to obstruction and carcinomas of urogenital organs and impairment to female reproductive health [6, 10]. To control schistosomiasis morbidity, health authorities rely on mass administration (preventive chemotherapy) of praziquantel in school-aged children (SAC), the population most affected [11–13]. In 2010, the World Health Organization (WHO) endorsed the inclusion of preschool-aged children (PSAC) in preventative chemotherapy programmes, since there is increasing evidence that they are also affected by schistosomiasis and could suffer from morbidity [14–17]. In the absence of an appropriate paediatric formulation, broken or crushed praziquantel tablets are commonly used in PSAC using the standard 40 mg/kg dose [18]. A range of studies showed that this dose was well tolerated and efficacious [15, 19, 20]. However, the heterogeneity of methodology and reporting on praziquantel efficacy and safety assessment make decision-making difficult [21].

In the paediatric population, growth and maturation of organs are dynamic. Changes in body proportion and metabolism occur throughout infancy and childhood that affect how drugs are metabolised [22, 23]. Well-designed paediatric drug trials are therefore warranted in order to guide the proper usage of drug treatments to avoid underdosing, overdosing, ineffectiveness and safety problems.

We recently conducted a randomised, controlled dose-finding study assessing the safety and efficacy of praziquantel in PSAC and SAC infected with *S. mansoni*. Considerable differences were observed between these two age groups with regard to efficacy. For example, while treatment of SAC with 40 or 60 mg/kg met the WHO standards of clinical efficacy of ≥ 90% egg reduction rate (ERR) based on arithmetic mean (AM), none of the doses administered could reach this threshold in PSAC [24].

This study was designed to support the ongoing efforts to successfully control schistosome infections in PSAC by assessing the efficacy and safety of escalating praziquantel dosages in PSAC compared to SAC infected with *S. haematobium*. The clinical evidence for praziquantel obtained for both *S. haematobium* and *S. mansoni* in PSAC will facilitate the clinical decision-making

process, resulting in successful control of schistosome infection and disease.

Methods
Study design and participants

We conducted a randomised, parallel-group, single-blind, placebo-controlled, dose-ranging trial between November 2015 and February 2016. PSAC (aged 2–5 years) and SAC (6–15 years) were surveyed in five villages of the health district of Adzopé, southern Côte d'Ivoire. In total, 740 PSAC and 444 SAC were registered during the census and were invited to participate in the study.

Randomisation and masking

Eligibility of children was based on the presence of *S. haematobium* eggs in their urine. In addition, a clinical examination and an oral medical history by active questioning were implemented in order to exclude children with abnormal medical conditions (i.e. clinical malaria or hepato-splenic schistosomiasis) or those who received an antimalarial or anthelmintic drug in the past 4 weeks.

S. haematobium egg-positive PSAC and SAC, eligible for the study, were stratified according to baseline infection intensity into light (< 50 eggs/10 mL of urine) or heavy (≥ 50 eggs/10 mL of urine) infection intensities [25]. Children were then randomly assigned to placebo or 20, 40 or 60 mg/kg praziquantel treatment arms using computer-generated stratified block randomisation codes provided by an independent statistician based on the aforementioned infection intensity (block size of 8). Only the investigator dealing with drug administration was aware of the treatment assignments. The physician and laboratory technicians were blinded to the treatment. SAC might have recognised the treatment dose due to the number of tablets administered; however, the crushing of tablets for PSAC was prepared in advance. Masking was maintained throughout the trial. Randomisation codes were released after the database was unlocked.

Field and laboratory procedures

During the baseline survey, three urine samples over 3 consecutive days and a single stool sample from the first collection day were collected between 10:00 and 14:00 am from each participating child. Urine and stool samples were transferred to a nearby laboratory in Azaguié town and examined on the day of collection. *S. haematobium* was detected using the urine filtration method (syringe filtration of 10 mL of urine followed by microscopic examination of the filter) [26]. A subsequent independent quality control of sample results (approximately 10%) was conducted. If a difference in presence/absence of *S. haematobium* eggs was observed or egg counts exceeded +/−10 eggs for light infections or +/−20 eggs for heavy infections, all the slides were read once again by the senior technician. *S. mansoni* infection was assessed through duplicate Kato-Katz thick smears (standard template of 41.7 mg) [27]. Eggs of soil-transmitted helminths, i.e. *Ascaris lumbricoides*, hookworm and *Trichuris trichiura*, were also assessed and recorded for each parasite species separately. Moreover, finger prick blood samples were taken to assess *Plasmodium* infections and haemoglobin amount using, respectively, thick and thin blood smears [24] and a calibrated HemoCue device (HemoCue 301 system, HemoCue, Ängelholm, Sweden).

To assess treatment efficacy, another three urine samples and a single stool sample were collected between 21 and 25 days post-treatment and subjected to the same diagnostic approaches applied at baseline. At the end of the study, all children enrolled in the study were offered albendazole (400 mg) and praziquantel (40 mg/kg) for the treatment of helminth infections according to local guidelines.

Treatment
Prior to treatment, each child received breakfast. In both study groups (SAC and PSAC), treatment was done based on the child's body weight (graduated increments of 0.1 kg). Praziquantel (600 mg Cesol®) (used in quarter-tablet increments) and placebo were obtained from Merck KGaA, Darmstadt, Germany and Fagron, Barsbüttel, Germany, respectively. For PSAC, tablets were crushed using a mortar and pestle and dissolved in a small volume of syrup-flavoured water to mask the taste. SAC and the mothers/guardians of PSAC were interviewed 3, 24, 48 and 72 h after treatment for adverse events and the intensities graded by the study physician as mild, moderate, severe or intolerable [24].

Outcomes and sample size determination
The cure rate (CR) (primary outcome) was expressed as the proportion of children positive for *S. haematobium* eggs at baseline survey who became negative at follow-up. The secondary outcomes were ERR and the safety of different doses of praziquantel.

Simulations showed that with 40 children enrolled per treatment arm (0, 20, 40 and 60 mg/kg), the dose-response prediction model should have a median precision—defined as one half length of the 95% confidence interval (CI)—of 10% points, assuming associated cure rates of 2.5%, 50%, 75% [28] and 90%.

Statistical analysis
All data were first double entered into an Excel spreadsheet, then transferred into Epi Info version 3.5.2 (Centers for Disease Control and Prevention, Atlanta, GA, USA) and cross-checked. R version 3.4.0 was used for all statistical analyses. Available-case analysis was

implemented including all treated participants (regardless of whether they could swallow the drug or not or were wrongly dosed) who had at least one urine sample examined with the urine filtration method at follow-up and were not excluded due to a medical condition.

In order to calculate ERR, the AM and geometric mean (GM) of eggs per 10 mL of urine before and after treatment were assessed. Geometric mean egg counts were calculated as follows: $e^{1/n \; \Sigma \; \log(x+1)}$ -1, and the corresponding ERR ([1 – geometric mean egg output after treatment/geometric mean egg output at baseline] × 100) was assessed. A bootstrap resampling method with 5000 replicates was used to estimate 95% CIs for ERRs.

E_{max} models using the DoseFinding package (version 0.9–14) of the statistical software environment R (v3.3.0) were implemented to predict the dose-response curves in terms of CRs and ERRs. Logistic regression was used to predict CR by infection intensity at baseline.

Results
Study flow and baseline characteristics
Overall, 1184 children were invited to participate in the study (Fig. 1). At baseline, 628 PSAC and 356 SAC were screened for *S. haematobium* infection. Of these, 186 (29.6%) PSAC and 195 (45.7%) SAC had a detectable *S. haematobium* infection and were randomised for treatment. On the treatment day, 16 PSAC and 21 SAC were absent. PSAC received 20 mg/kg (*n* = 40), 40 mg/kg (*n* = 44) or 60 mg/kg (*n* = 44) praziquantel or placebo (*n* = 42). SAC were likewise allocated to 20 mg/kg (*n* = 46), 40 mg/kg (*n* = 46) or 60 mg/kg praziquantel (*n* = 44) or placebo (*n* = 38). Two PSAC and one SAC were not able to swallow the drug. One PSAC and one SAC were wrongly dosed (62.5 mg/kg instead of 40 mg/kg and 75 mg/kg instead of 40 mg/kg, respectively).

At follow-up, data were available for 157 PSAC and 166 SAC. One PSAC and 12 SAC provided only two urine samples, while one SAC provided only one urine sample.

The median age, weight, height and sex of PSAC and SAC were balanced among the treatment groups (Table 1). Three quarters of PSAC and SAC were lightly infected with *S. haematobium*. No infection with *A. lumbricoides*, *T. trichiura* or hookworm was recorded. Co-infections among *S. haematobium*-infected children with *S. mansoni* and *P. falciparum* were very low (less than 9%) in PSAC and SAC. Median haemoglobin values ranged between 10.5 and 11.0 g/dL in PSAC and between 11.0 and 11.7 g/dL in SAC.

Efficacy of praziquantel
The nature of the dose response based on CRs is depicted in Fig. 2. Praziquantel revealed dose-independent efficacy

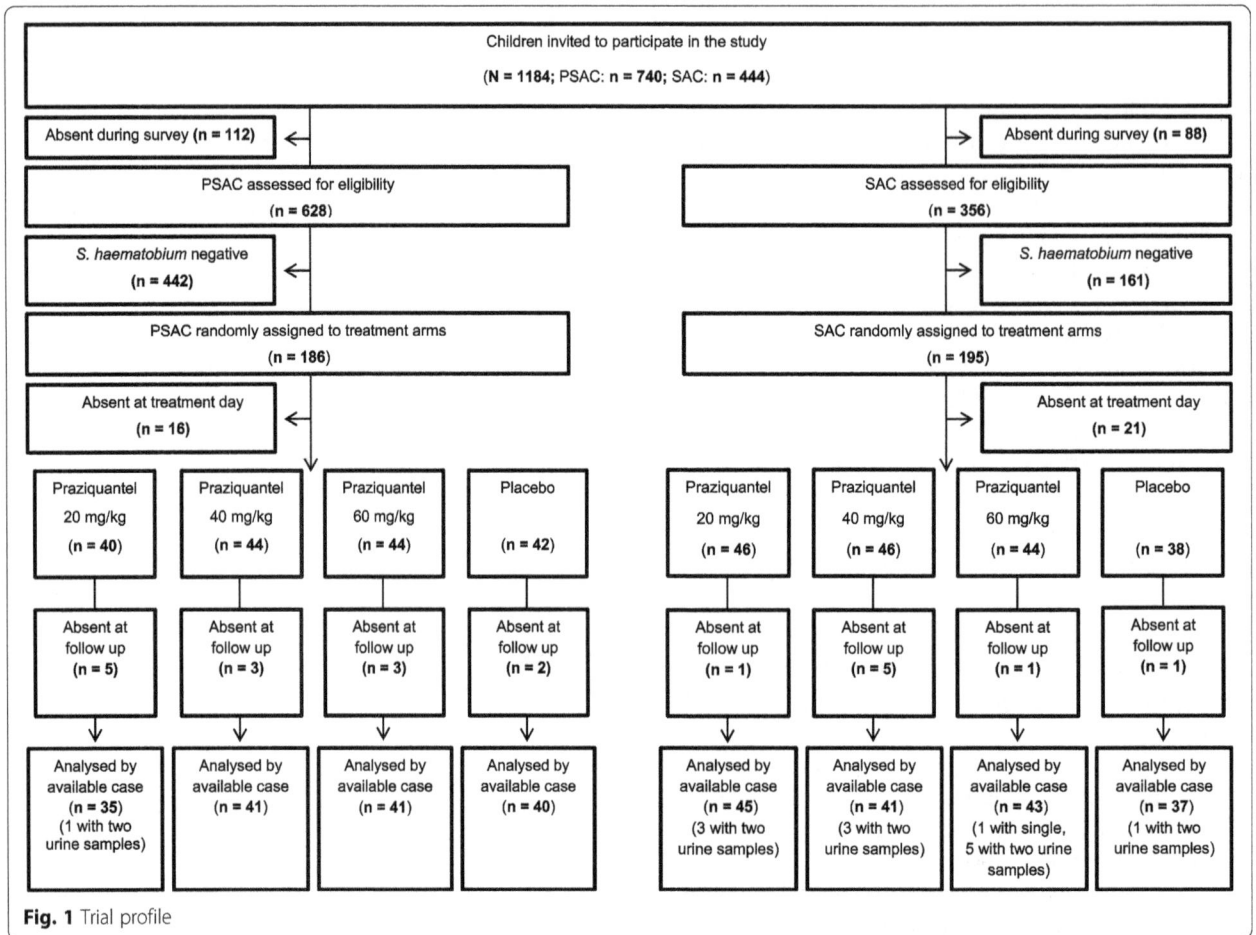

Fig. 1 Trial profile

with the highest cure rates observed at 20 and 40 mg/kg in PSAC and SAC, respectively. The E_{max} model based on actual doses on the per protocol population is presented in Additional file 1: Figure S1 and shows a similar trend. Additional file 1: Figure S2 presents the predicted probability of being cured by baseline infection intensity. For all treatments, including placebo, there was a high probability of being cured at low infection intensities.

CRs in PSAC for 20 mg/kg, 40 mg/kg and 60 mg/kg were 85.7 (95% CI 69.7–95.2), 78.0% (95% CI 62.4–89.4) and 68.3% (95% CI 51.9–81.9), respectively, whereas in SAC the respective CRs were 55.6% (95% CI 40.0–70.4), 68.3% (95% CI 51.9–81.9) and 60.5% (95% CI 44.4–75.0). In the placebo groups, *S. haematobium* eggs were not detected in the urine samples of 47.5% (19/40) and 10.8% (4/37) in PSAC and SAC, respectively (Table 2). Imputation of missing data with treatment failure or success in the intention-to-treat analysis did not change the observed outcomes (Additional file 1: Table S1).

ERRs are summarized in Table 2 and depicted in Fig. 3. ERRs in PSAC were 98.3% for 20 mg/kg, 97.6% for 40 mg/kg and 96.5% for 60 mg/kg. In SAC ERRs of

97.6%, 98.6% and 97.6% were observed with increasing dosages. ERRs based on AMs had similar profiles to those based on GMs and are presented in Table 2. Table 2 also presents an exploratory subgroup analysis on CRs according to *S. haematobium* infection intensity. The CR in PSAC ranged from 73.0% (60 mg/kg) to 87.9% (20 mg/kg) in light infections and from 25.0% (60 mg/kg) to 66.7% (40 mg/kg) in heavy infections. In SAC, CRs were 70.6% (20 mg/kg) to 78.8% (40 mg/kg) for light *S. haematobium* infections and between 9.1% (20 mg/kg) and 27.3% (60 mg/kg) for heavy infections.

Safety of praziquantel
Adverse events data were available for 168 PSAC and 173 SAC (Table 3). In both groups, more children reported signs and symptoms at pre-treatment compared to 3 and 24 h post-treatment. No serious adverse events were reported. Overall, adverse events were mild with fewer adverse events observed at 3 h post-treatment compared to pre-treatment in PSAC (52 episodes versus 88 episodes) and in SAC (88 episodes versus 92 episodes), respectively. Mild events mainly included fever,

Table 1 Baseline characteristics

	Preschool-aged children (PSAC)				School-aged children (SAC)			
	Treatment arm				Treatment arm			
Characteristics	Placebo	20 mg/kg	40 mg/kg	60 mg/kg	Placebo	20 mg/kg	40 mg/kg	60 mg/kg
	42	40	44	44	38	46	46	44
Female N (%)	23 (54.8)	21 (52.5)	20 (45.5)	27 (61.4)	23 (60.5)	25 (54.3)	25 (54.3)	25 (56.8)
Age, years; median	4	4	4	4	9	8	8	9
[IQR]	[2–5]	[2–5]	[2–5]	[2–5]	[6–13]	[6–13]	[6–14]	[6–13]
Weight, kg; median	15	15	15	15	22	22	24	22
[IQR]	[10–21]	[11–19]	[11–19]	[11–18]	[18–35]	[18–33]	[18–38]	[18–40]
Height, cm; median	97	98	101	100	125	125	125	124
[IQR]	[80–117]	[83–115]	[84–116]	[83–114]	[109–141]	[114–139]	[113–149]	[112–150]
Haemoglobin (g/dL); median	10.5	11.0	10.9	10.9	11.4	11.2	11.7	11.6
[IQR]	[9.1–13.2]	[9.1–12.8]	[8.8–12.5]	[8.5–12.9]	[9.7–13.7]	[9.9–12.4]	[9.7–12.8]	[10.1–13.5]
Infection intensity N (%)								
Light	36 (85.7)	38 (95.0)	38 (86.4)	40 (90.9)	27 (71.1)	35 (76.1)	36 (78.3)	33 (75.0)
Heavy	6 (14.3)	2 (5.0)	6 (13.6)	4 (9.1)	11 (28.9)	11 (23.9)	10 (21.7)	11 (25.0)
Co-infections N (%)								
S. mansoni	0 (0.0)	0 (0.0)	1 (2.3)	1 (2.3)	0 (0.0)	1 (2.2)	1 (2.2)	0 (0.0)
Plasmodium falciparum	1 (2.4)	0 (0.0)	1 (2.3)	0 (0.0)	1 (2.6)	4 (8.7)	2 (4.3)	3 (6.8)
(based on thin/thick smear)								

IQR interquartile range

headache, nausea, diarrhoea, vomiting, dizziness and stomach ache. Few moderate cases were reported at 3 h after treatment in PSAC (only one with moderate diarrhoea) and in SAC (n = 12). At 24 h post-treatment, 25 (14.9%) and 47 (27.2%) adverse events were recorded in PSAC and SAC, respectively. For both age groups the number of adverse events was similar among the three praziquantel treatment arms,

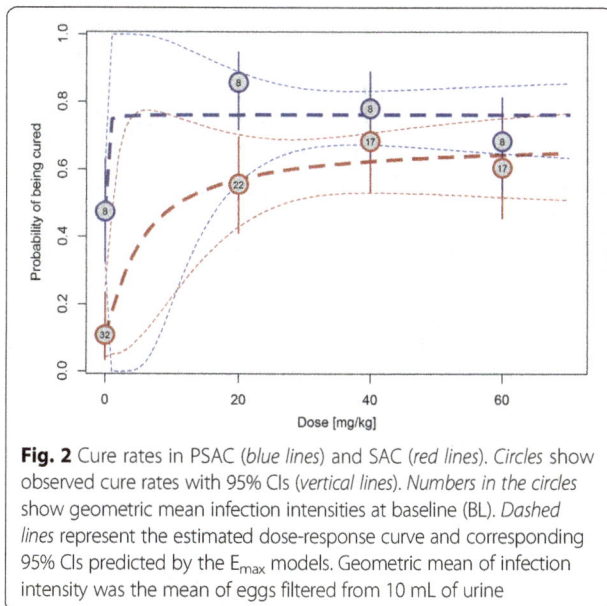

Fig. 2 Cure rates in PSAC (*blue lines*) and SAC (*red lines*). *Circles* show observed cure rates with 95% CIs (*vertical lines*). *Numbers in the circles* show geometric mean infection intensities at baseline (BL). *Dashed lines* represent the estimated dose-response curve and corresponding 95% CIs predicted by the E_{max} models. Geometric mean of infection intensity was the mean of eggs filtered from 10 mL of urine

with fewer adverse events observed in the placebo-treated groups. The most common adverse events in PSAC and SAC 24 h post-treatment were diarrhoea (4.8 and 3.5%), stomach ache (3.6 and 9.8%), fever (6.0 and 13.3%), headache (3.0 and 15.6%) and nausea (2.4 and 6.9%).

Discussion

Over the past decade, preventive chemotherapy programmes for the control of schistosomiasis targeting SAC have scaled up across many countries in tropical and subtropical areas. Great progress has been made in decreasing the burden of this disease [29–31]. However, recent modelling and health economic studies found that expanded community-wide preventive chemotherapy that includes adolescents, adults and PSAC would better reduce the overall disease burden, rates of transmission and reinfection [32].

It was recommended in 2010 that PSAC should be included in preventive chemotherapy programmes [33] using an adequate dose, though this age group is still lacking a suitable formulation. A paediatric formulation of praziquantel (small, orally dispersible tablets) is under development (https://www.pediatricpraziquantelconsortium.org/node/28), but it will take several more years until the drug is marketed and available to all PSAC. To be able to treat preschoolers safely and effectively, we studied ascending doses of praziquantel in PSAC and SAC infected

Table 2 Available-case analysis of cure and egg reduction rates of 20, 40 and 60 mg/kg praziquantel versus placebo against urogenital schistosomiasis in PSAC and SAC based on the urine filtration method

	Preschool-aged children (PSAC)				School-aged children (SAC)			
	Placebo	20 mg/kg	40 mg/kg	60 mg/kg	Placebo	20 mg/kg	40 mg/kg	60 mg/kg
Infected children before treatment (N)	40	35	41	41	37	45	41	43
Actual dose administered (range; mg/kg)	–	13.6–25	34.6–62.5[a]	50–70	–	16.7–23.7	36.4–75[b]	56.3–65.6
Cured children after treatment N (%)	19 (47.5)	30 (85.7)	32 (78.0)	28 (68.3)	4 (10.8)	25 (55.6)	28 (68.3)	26 (60.5)
95% CI	32.5–63.9	69.7–95.2	62.4–89.4	51.9–81.9	3.0–25.4	40.0–70.4	51.9–81.9	44.4–75.0
Cured children according to sex								
Male	6 (31.6)	14 (46.7)	19 (59.4)	10 (35.7)	1 (25.0)	9 (36.0)	13 (46.4)	9 (34.6)
95% CI	12.5–56.6	28.3–65.7	40.6–76.3	18.6–55.9	0.6–80.6	18.0–57.5	27.5–66.1	17.2–55.7
Female	13 (68.4)	16 (53.3)	13 (40.6)	18 (64.3)	3 (75.0)	16 (64.0)	15 (53.6)	17 (65.4)
95% CI	43.4–87.4	34.3–71.7	23.7–59.4	44.1–81.4	19.4–99.4	42.5–82.0	33.9–72.5	44.3–82.8
Cured children with light infection	19/40 (47.5)	29/33 (87.9)	28/35 (80.0)	27/37 (73.0)	4/26 (15.4)	24/34 (70.6)	26/33 (78.8)	23/32 (71.9)
Cured children with heavy infections (%)	0/6 (0)	1/2 (50.0)	4/6 (66.7)	1/4 (25.0)	0/11 (0.0)	1/11 (9.1)	2/8 (25.0)	3/11 (27.3)
Geometric mean eggs/10 mL of urine								
Before treatment	7.8	7.5	8.4	8.3	31.5	21.6	16.6	17.2
After treatment	2.4	0.1	0.2	0.3	13.1	0.5	0.2	0.4
Egg reduction rate	68.9	98.3	97.6	96.5	58.5	97.6	98.6	97.6
(95% CI)	46.6–83.6	95.4–99.8	94.9–99.2	93.1–98.7	38.7–71.4	96.4–98.6	97.7–99.3	95.3–98.9
Arithmetic mean eggs/10 mL of urine								
Before treatment	22.7	14.3	21.7	16.9	94.4	89.5	31.0	34.4
After treatment	11.5	0.3	0.4	0.9	49.0	1.2	0.4	1.0
Egg reduction rate	49.5	97.8	98.2	94.5	46.9	98.7	98.8	97.0
(95% CI)	0.2–77.3	93.6–99.9	96.1–99.5	85.7–99.1	36.4–77.6	96.7–99.3	97.7–99.5	92.9–99.2

[a]Range 34.6–44.1 excluding the wrongly dosed child
[b]Range 36.4–42.9 excluding the wrongly dosed child

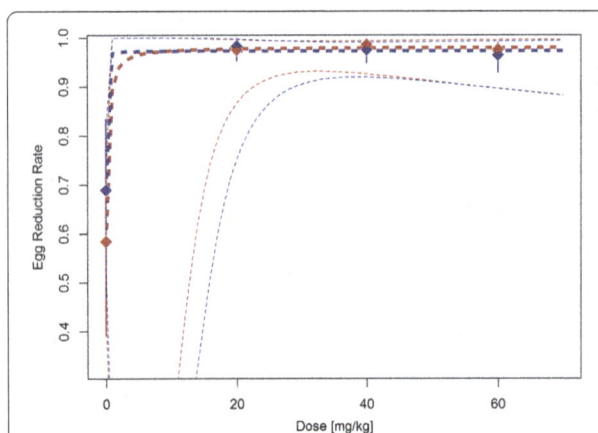

Fig. 3 Egg reduction rates in PSAC (*blue lines*) and SAC (*red lines*). *Diamonds* show observed cure rates with 95% CIs (*vertical lines*). *Dashed lines* represent the estimated dose-response curve and corresponding 95% CI predicted by the E_{max} model

with *S. haematobium*. Our results build on an earlier dose-finding study in *S. mansoni*-infected children [24].

Several findings of our study are worth highlighting. First, the highest overall CRs among PSAC (85.7%) and SAC (68.3%) were obtained with 20 mg/kg and 40 mg/kg praziquantel, respectively and not with the highest dose administered, 60 mg/kg. For both age groups, CRs revealed even a slight inverse dose-rate effect. Similarly, ERRs increased very fast up to 98% and did not increase further regardless of the praziquantel dose administered. Interestingly, 60 mg/kg praziquantel also showed lower CRs in PSAC with moderate/high *S. haematobium* infection intensities compared to the two lower doses. For example, the CR in PSAC characterised by heavy infection intensities treated with 60 mg/kg praziquantel was as low as 25%. However, only a handful of PSAC suffered from moderate and high infection intensities; hence, no clear picture can be drawn for this age group. In SAC similar CRs were observed in children harbouring heavy infection intensities treated with 40 and 60 mg/kg. In summary, a high dose of praziquantel seems to have no additional benefit in the treatment of *S. haematobium* infections. This result is in contrast with our recent

Table 3 Main type of clinical symptoms (number and percentage) before treatment and adverse events 3 and 24 h after praziquantel administration in *Schistosoma haematobium*-infected preschool-aged children (*n* = 168) and school-aged children (*n* = 173)

Symptoms	Preschool-aged children (PSAC)[a]					School-aged children (SAC)[b]				
	Placebo	20 mg/kg	40 mg/kg	60 mg/kg	Overall	Placebo	20 mg/kg	40 mg/kg	60 mg/kg	Overall
	(*n* = 41)	(*n* = 40)	(*n* = 44)	(*n* = 43)	(*n* = 168)	(*n* = 38)	(*n* = 45)	(*n* = 46)	(*n* = 44)	(*n* = 173)
Before treatment										
Moderate	0 (0.0)	0 (0.0)	0 (0.0)	0 (0.0)	0 (0.0)	0 (0.0)	0 (0.0)	0 (0.0)	0 (0.0)	0 (0.0)
Mild	24 (58.5)	19 (47.5)	26 (59.1)	19 (44.2)	88 (52.4)	20 (52.6)	26 (57.8)	25 (54.3)	21 (47.7)	92 (53.2)
None	17 (41.5)	21 (52.5)	18 (40.9)	24 (55.8)	80 (47.6)	18 (47.4)	19 (42.2)	21 (45.7)	23 (52.3)	81 (46.8)
Fever	6 (14.1)	3 (7.5)	7 (15.9)	5 (11.6)	21 (12.5)	5 (13.2)	7 (15.6)	5 (10.9)	6 (13.6)	23 (13.3)
Headache	8 (19.5)	6 (15.0)	13 (29.5)	10 (23.3)	37 (22.0)	3 (7.9)	7 (15.6)	10 (21.7)	7 (15.9)	27 (15.6)
Nausea	3 (7.3)	4 (10.0)	3 (6.8)	1 (2.3)	11 (6.5)	2 (5.3)	1 (2.2)	4 (8.7)	5 (11.4)	12 (6.9)
Vomiting	1 (2.4)	1 (2.5)	1 (2.3)	2 (4.7)	5 (3.0)	0 (0.0)	0 (0.0)	1 (2.2)	0 (0.0)	1 (0.6)
Diarrhoea	4 (9.6)	4 (10.0)	4 (9.1)	5 (11.6)	17 (10.1)	0 (0.0)	1 (2.2)	3 (6.5)	2 (4.5)	6 (3.5)
Dizziness	2 (4.9)	0 (0.0)	0 (0.0)	0 (0.0)	2 (1.2)	0 (0.0)	0 (0.0)	0 (0.0)	0 (0.0)	0 (0.0)
Stomach ache	2 (4.9)	5 (12.5)	8 (18.2)	4 (9.3)	19 (11.3)	1 (2.6)	6 (13.3)	6 (13.0)	4 (9.1)	17 (9.8)
3 h post-treatment										
Moderate	0 (0.0)	0 (0.0)	0 (0.0)	1 (2.3)	1 (0.6)	1 (2.6)	2 (4.4)	4 (8.7)	5 (11.4)	12 (6.9)
Mild	6 (14.6)	8 (20.0)	15 (34.1)	23 (53.5)	52 (31.0)	18 (47.4)	23 (51.1)	21 (45.7)	26 (59.1)	88 (50.9)
None	35 (85.4)	32 (80.0)	29 (65.9)	19 (44.2)	115 (68.5)	19 (50.0)	20 (44.4)	21 (45.7)	13 (29.5)	73 (42.2)
Fever	3 (7.3)	3 (7.5)	2 (4.5)	4 (9.3)	12 (7.1)	6 (15.8)	4 (8.9)	8 (17.4)	12 (27.3)	30 (17.3)
Headache	1 (2.4)	2 (5.0)	1 (2.3)	7 (16.3)	11 (6.5)	8 (21.1)	10 (22.2)	6 (13.0)	6 (13.6)	30 (17.3)
Nausea	1 (2.4)	1 (2.5)	4 (9.1)	5 (11.6)	11 (6.5)	4 (10.5)	3 (6.7)	9 (19.6)	14 (31.8)	30 (17.3)
Vomiting	0 (0.0)	1 (2.5)	3 (6.8)	9 (20.9)	13 (7.7)	1 (2.6)	3 (6.7)	8 (17.4)	10 (22.7)	22 (12.7)
Diarrhoea	0 (0.0)	1 (2.5)	1 (2.3)	3 (7.0)	5 (3.0)	3 (7.9)	3 (6.7)	2 (4.3)	0 (0.0)	8 (4.6)
Dizziness	1 (2.4)	1 (2.5)	2 (4.5)	4 (9.3)	8 (4.8)	5 (13.2)	4 (8.9)	8 (17.4)	5 (11.4)	22 (12.7)
Stomach ache	3 (7.3)	4 (10.0)	4 (9.1)	2 (4.7)	13 (7.7)	5 (13.2)	11 (24.4)	9 (19.6)	12 (27.3)	37 (21.4)
24 h post-treatment										
Moderate	0 (0.0)	0 (0.0)	0 (0.0)	0 (0.0)	0 (0.0)	0 (0.0)	0 (0.0)	0 (0.0)	0 (0.0)	0 (0.0)
Mild	4 (9.6)	7 (17.5)	8 (18.2)	6 (14.0)	25 (14.9)	12 (31.6)	12 (26.7)	12 (26.1)	11 (25.0)	47 (27.2)
None	37 (90.2)	33 (82.5)	36 (81.8)	37 (86.0)	143 (85.1)	26 (68.4)	33 (73.3)	34 (73.9)	33 (75.0)	126 (72.8)
Fever	2 (4.9)	4 (10.0)	2 (4.5)	2 (4.7)	10 (6.0)	5 (13.2)	7 (15.6)	5 (10.9)	6 (13.6)	23 (13.3)
Headache	1 (2.4)	1 (2.5)	1 (2.3)	2 (4.7)	5 (3.0)	3 (7.9)	7 (15.6)	10 (21.7)	7 (15.9)	27 (15.6)
Nausea	1 (2.4)	0 (0.0)	0 (0.0)	3 (7.0)	4 (2.4)	2 (5.3)	1 (2.2)	4 (8.7)	5 (11.4)	12 (6.9)
Vomiting	0 (0.0)	0 (0.0)	0 (0.0)	3 (7.0)	3 (1.8)	0 (0.0)	0 (0.0)	1 (2.2)	0 (0.0)	1 (0.6)
Diarrhoea	1 (2.4)	2 (5.0)	5 (11.4)	0 (0.0)	8 (4.8)	0 (0.0)	1 (2.2)	3 (6.5)	2 (4.5)	6 (3.5)
Dizziness	1 (2.4)	0 (0.0)	0 (0.0)	1 (2.3)	1 (0.6)	0 (0.0)	0 (0.0)	0 (0.0)	0 (0.0)	0 (0.0)
Stomach ache	2 (4.9)	0 (0.0)	2 (4.5)	2 (4.7)	6 (3.6)	1 (2.6)	6 (13.3)	6 (13.0)	4 (9.1)	17 (9.8)

[a]2 children were absent (placebo (*n* = 1) and 60 mg/kg (*n* = 1)) following treatment and were not assessed for adverse events
[b]1 child was absent (20 mg/kg treatment arm) following treatment and was not assessed for adverse events

study, where we reported that in SAC infected with *S. mansoni*, CRs increased with higher doses of praziquantel [24], while only moderate CRs were observed in PSAC at all doses administered.

Overall higher CRs were observed in PSAC (68–86%) when compared to SAC (56–68%), which mirrors a recent meta-analysis by Zwang et al., where 40 mg/kg praziquantel cured 87.3% of *S. haematobium*-infected PSAC compared to 71.4% of SAC [34]. Nonetheless, our finding can most likely be explained with the lower infection intensities present in PSAC, as CRs in children characterised by heavy infection intensities were low. Hence, our results confirm the relationship between CRs and infection intensity observed in previous studies [35, 36]. Overall, the results emphasise the need for rigorous treatment programmes in settings with heavy infection of *S. haematobium*, since reductions in egg output significantly correlated with decreased morbidity [37, 38].

No dose-response relationship was observed for ERRs in both age groups above 20 mg/kg. This finding is in line with an earlier meta-analysis by Zwang et al. [34] which found no significant relationship for dose and ERR for any of the *Schistosoma* species. However, our dose-finding study in *S. mansoni*-infected children showed that higher ERRs (based on GMs) were observed in children treated with 40 and 60 mg/kg compared to 20 mg/kg [24]. Recent WHO Standard Operating Procedures have set a threshold of a 90% ERR based on AM for clinical efficacy and recommend that control programmes should investigate drug performance in populations where the ERR is lower [39]. Regardless of age group and whether GM or AM was used to determine ERRs, we found that all praziquantel doses used against *S. haematobium*, in contrast to preschoolers infected with *S. mansoni* [24], yielded ERRs above 90%. Despite the excellent efficacy of 20 mg/kg of praziquantel against light *S. haematobium* infections in this study, the use of two different doses, namely 20 mg/kg for *S. haematobium* and 40 mg/kg for *S. mansoni* in settings where *Schistosoma* species are overlapping, would raise logistical and operational challenges since control programmes are acting at large-scale levels such as district or country levels. Therefore, rigorous cost-effectiveness studies need to be implemented before a change of treatment guidelines could be considered. However, at a point-of-care level, using a test-and-treat approach, 20 mg/kg and 40 mg/kg could be recommended to treat PSAC for *S. haematobium* and *S. mansoni* infections, respectively.

In PSAC we observed a high CR in the placebo arm similar to what was observed in our *S. mansoni* study [24]. The probability of being cured for placebo-treated children was particularly high in children with low egg loads despite using a relatively strong diagnostic approach at baseline and follow-up by collecting per child three consecutive urine samples for each time point (baseline and follow-up). On the other hand, no cured individual was observed in placebo-treated children with heavy infection intensity at baseline. The high CR observed in the placebo treatment arm among PSAC was thus likely reflective of the low sensitivity of the urine filtration method for light infections [40, 41]. Our findings underscore the value of adding a placebo group in *Schistosoma* drug efficacy trials—the overestimation of CRs due to potential false negatives in light infections is visible. More importantly, our observations emphasise the need for *Schistosoma* species-related standard operating procedures including reliable diagnostic tools, suitable for drug efficacy assessment for low infection intensities [40–42].

With regard to safety outcomes, the main adverse events observed in both PSAC and SAC are in line with the adverse events reported in previous studies [16, 24, 34]. We observed an increase of adverse events severity that was proportional to praziquantel dose in SAC, while only one child showed moderate diarrhoea at the 60 mg/kg treatment dose in PSAC. However, as mentioned earlier, the accuracy of the adverse event severity assessment in PSAC is questionable, in particular for the less visible mild adverse events, since the reporting is done by the children's mothers.

Conclusions

Praziquantel showed a high response rate in PSAC and SAC infected with *S. haematobium*, with high efficacy observed already at 20 mg/kg, particularly in light infections. No benefit was observed using higher praziquantel doses in the current study. However, to be able to provide ultimate dosing recommendations of praziquantel for PSAC, additional studies might be required to support our conclusions, including pharmacokinetic studies and studies in PSAC suffering from moderate and heavy *S. haematobium* infections.

Abbreviations
AM: Arithmetic mean; CR: Cure rate; ERR: Egg reduction rate; GM: Geometric mean; PSAC: Preschool-aged children; SAC: School-aged children; WHO: World Health Organization

Acknowledgements
We are grateful to all participating children and their parents. We thank the mothers of the PSAC from the study of all five villages and the teachers from Mopé and Nyan for their support. Moreover, we are thankful to our staff of doctors, nurses, technicians, volunteers and drivers, whose expertise and dedication were indispensable. We are grateful to the European Research Council for financial support. This work was supported by the donation of Cesol® tablets provided by Merck KGaA, Darmstadt, Germany.

Funding
This work was supported by the European Research Council (grant number ERC-2013-CoG 614739-A_HERO).

Authors' contributions
JTC, JH and JK designed the study; JTC, GP, RBY, YKN, BB, JK and JKo conducted the study; JTC, JH and JK analysed and interpreted the data; JTC and JK wrote the first draft of the manuscript; GP, RBY, BB, YKN and JH revised the manuscript. All authors read and approved the final version of the manuscript. Merck KGaA, Darmstadt, Germany reviewed the manuscript for medical accuracy only before journal submission. The authors are fully responsible for the content of this manuscript, and the views and opinions described in the publication reflect solely those of the authors.

Competing interests
The authors declare that they have no competing interests.

Author details
[1]Department of Medical Parasitology and Infection Biology, Swiss Tropical and Public Health Institute, P.O. Box, CH-4002, Basel, Switzerland. [2]University of Basel, Basel, Switzerland. [3]Unité de Formation et de Recherche Biosciences, Université Félix Houphouët-Boigny, Abidjan, Côte d'Ivoire. [4]Centre Suisse de Recherches Scientifiques, Abidjan, Côte d'Ivoire. [5]Departement d'Agboville, Centre de Santé Urbain d'Azaguié, Azaguié, Côte d'Ivoire. [6]Department of Epidemiology and Public Health, Swiss Tropical and Public Health Institute, Basel, Switzerland.

References
1. Steinmann P, Keiser J, Bos R, Tanner M, Utzinger J. Schistosomiasis and water resources development: systematic review, meta-analysis, and estimates of people at risk. Lancet Infect Dis. 2006;6:411–25.
2. King CH. Parasites and poverty: the case of schistosomiasis. Acta Trop. 2010; 113:95–104.
3. Gryseels B, Polman K, Clerinx J, Kestens L. Human schistosomiasis. Lancet. 2006;368:1106–18.
4. Colley DG, Bustinduy AL, Secor WE, King CH. Human schistosomiasis. Lancet. 2014 ;383(9936):2253–64.
5. Utzinger J, Raso G, Brooker S, De Savigny D, Tanner M, Ornbjerg N, Singer BH, N'Goran EK. Schistosomiasis and neglected tropical diseases: towards integrated and sustainable control and a word of caution. Parasitology. 2009;136:1859–74.
6. Gray DJ, Ross AG, Li YS, McManus DP. Diagnosis and management of schistosomiasis. BMJ. 2011;342:d2651.
7. King CH, Dickman K, Tisch DJ. Reassessment of the cost of chronic helmintic infection: a meta-analysis of disability-related outcomes in endemic schistosomiasis. Lancet. 2005;365:1561–9.
8. Jukes MC, Nokes CA, Alcock KJ, Lambo JK, Kihamia C, Ngorosho N, Mbise A, Lorri W, Yona E, Mwanri L, et al. Heavy schistosomiasis associated with poor short-term memory and slower reaction times in Tanzanian schoolchildren. Tropical Med Int Health. 2002;7:104–17.
9. Bhargava A, Jukes M, Lambo J, Kihamia CM, Lorri W, Nokes C, Drake L, Bundy D. Anthelmintic treatment improves the hemoglobin and serum ferritin concentrations of Tanzanian schoolchildren. Food Nutr Bull. 2003;24: 332–42.
10. Hotez PJ, Bundy DAP, Beegle K, Brooker S, Drake L, de Silva N, Montresor A, Engels D, Jukes M, Chitsulo L, et al. Helminth infections: soil-transmitted helminth infections and schistosomiasis. In: Jamison DT, Breman JG, Measham AR, Alleyne G, Claeson M, Evans DB, Jha P, Mills A, Musgrove P, e, editors. Disease control priorities in developing countries. 2nd ed. Washington, DC:The World Bank; 2006.
11. World Health Organization. Preventive chemotherapy in human helminthiasis: coordinated use of anthelminthic drugs in control interventions: a manual for health professionals and programme managers. Geneva: WHO; 2006.
12. Lelo AE, Mburu DN, Magoma GN, Mungai BN, Kihara JH, Mwangi IN, Maina GM, Kinuthia JM, Mutuku MW, Loker ES, et al. No apparent reduction in schistosome burden or genetic diversity following four years of school-based mass drug administration in Mwea, Central Kenya, a heavy transmission area. PLoS Negl Trop Dis. 2014;8:e3221.
13. Leenstra T, Coutinho HM, Acosta LP, Langdon GC, Su L, Olveda RM, McGarvey ST, Kurtis JD, Friedman JF. Schistosoma japonicum reinfection after praziquantel treatment causes anemia associated with inflammation. Infect Immun. 2006;74:6398–407.
14. Stothard JR, Gabrielli AF. Schistosomiasis in African infants and preschool children: to treat or not to treat? Trends Parasitol. 2007;23:83–6.
15. Stothard JR, Sousa-Figueiredo JC, Betson M, Bustinduy A, Reinhard-Rupp J. Schistosomiasis in African infants and preschool children: let them now be treated! Trends Parasitol. 2013;29:197–205.
16. Coulibaly JT, N'Gbesso YK, Knopp S, Keiser J, N'Goran EK, Utzinger J. Efficacy and safety of praziquantel in preschool-aged children in an area co-endemic for Schistosoma mansoni and S. haematobium. PLoS Negl Trop Dis. 2012;6:e1917.
17. Coulibaly JT, N'Gbesso YK, N'Guessan NA, Winkler MS, Utzinger J, N'Goran EK. Epidemiology of schistosomiasis in two high-risk communities of south Cote d'Ivoire with particular emphasis on pre-school-aged children. Am J Trop Med Hyg. 2013;89:32 41.
18. World Health Organization: Report of a meeting to review the results of studies on the treatment of schistosomiasis in pre-school-age children. 13–14 September 2010. Geneva, World Health Organization. 2010.
19. Garba A, Barkire N, Djibo A, Lamine MS, Sofo B, Gouvras AN, Bosque-Oliva E, Webster JP, Stothard JR, Utzinger J, Fenwick A. Schistosomiasis in infants and preschool-aged children: infection in a single Schistosoma haematobium and a mixed S. haematobium-S. mansoni foci of Niger. Acta Trop. 2010;115:212–9.
20. Olliaro PL, Vaillant M, Hayes DJ, Montresor A, Chitsulo L. Practical dosing of praziquantel for schistosomiasis in preschool-aged children. Tropical Med Int Health. 2013;18:1085–9.
21. Jule AM, Vaillant M, Lang TA, Guerin PJ, Olliaro PL. The schistosomiasis clinical trials landscape: a systematic review of antischistosomal treatment efficacy studies and a case for sharing individual participant-level data (IPD). PLoS Negl Trop Dis. 2016;10:e0004784.
22. Kearns GL, Abdel-Rahman SM, Alander SW, Blowey DL, Leeder JS, Kauffman RE. Developmental pharmacology—drug disposition, action, and therapy in infants and children. N Engl J Med. 2003;349:1157–67.
23. Fernandez E, Perez R, Hernandez A, Tejada P, Arteta M, Ramos JT. Factors and mechanisms for pharmacokinetic differences between pediatric population and adults. Pharmaceutics. 2011;3:53–72.
24. Coulibaly JT, Panic G, Silue KD, Kovac J, Hattendorf J, Keiser J. Efficacy and safety of praziquantel in preschool-aged and school-aged children infected with Schistosoma mansoni: a randomised controlled, parallel-group, dose-ranging, phase 2 trial. Lancet Glob Health. 2017;5:e688–98.
25. World Health Organisation. Prevention and control of schistosomiasis and soil-transmitted helminthiasis: report of a WHO expert committee. WHO Tech Rep Ser. 2002;912:1–57.
26. Plouvier S, Leroy J-C, Colette J. A propos d'une technique simple de filtration des urines dans le diagnostic de la bilharziose urinaire en enquête de masse. Med Trop (Mars) 1975; 35:229–230.
27. Katz N, Chaves A, Pellegrino J. A simple device for quantitative stool thick-smear technique in schistosomiasis mansoni. Rev Inst Med Trop Sao Paulo. 1972;14:397–400.
28. Olliaro PL, Vaillant MT, Belizario VJ, Lwambo NJ, Ouldabdallahi M, Pieri OS, Amarillo ML, Kaatano GM, Diaw M, Domingues AC, et al. A multicentre randomized controlled trial of the efficacy and safety of single-dose praziquantel at 40 mg/kg vs. 60 mg/kg for treating intestinal schistosomiasis in the Philippines, Mauritania, Tanzania and Brazil. PLoS Negl Trop Dis. 2011; 5:e1165.
29. Rollinson D, Knopp S, Levitz S, Stothard JR, Tchuem Tchuente LA, Garba A, Mohammed KA, Schur N, Person B, Colley DG, Utzinger J. Time to set the agenda for schistosomiasis elimination. Acta Trop. 2013;128:423–40.
30. World Health Organisation. Schistosomiasis: number of people treated worldwide in 2013. Wkly Epidemiol Rec. 2015;90:25–32.
31. Savioli L, Gabrielli AF, Montresor A, Chitsulo L, Engels D. Schistosomiasis control in Africa: 8 years after World Health Assembly Resolution 54.19. Parasitology. 2009;136:1677–81.
32. Lo NC, Addiss DG, Hotez PJ, King CH, Stothard JR, Evans DS, Colley DG, Lin W, Coulibaly JT, Bustinduy AL, et al. A call to strengthen the global strategy against schistosomiasis and soil-transmitted helminthiasis: the time is now. Lancet Infect Dis. 2017;17:e64–9.
33. World Health Organisation. Report of a meeting to review the results of studies on the treatment of schistosomiasis in preschool-age children. Geneva: World Health Organization; 2011.
34. Zwang J, Olliaro PL. Clinical efficacy and tolerability of praziquantel for intestinal and urinary schistosomiasis-a meta-analysis of comparative and non-comparative clinical trials. PLoS Negl Trop Dis. 2014;8:e3286.
35. Midzi N, Sangweme D, Zinyowera S, Mapingure MP, Brouwer KC, Kumar N, Mutapi F, Woelk G, Mduluza T. Efficacy and side effects of praziquantel treatment against Schistosoma haematobium infection among primary school children in Zimbabwe. Trans R Soc Trop Med Hyg. 2008;102:759–66.
36. Utzinger J, N'Goran EK, N'Dri A, Lengeler C, Tanner M. Efficacy of praziquantel against Schistosoma mansoni with particular consideration for intensity of infection. Tropical Med Int Health. 2000;5:771–8.
37. Andrade G, Bertsch DJ, Gazzinelli A, King CH. Decline in infection-related morbidities following drug-mediated reductions in the intensity of Schistosoma infection: a systematic review and meta-analysis. PLoS Negl Trop Dis. 2017;11:e0005372.

38.   Barda B, Coulibaly JT, Hatz C, Keiser J. Ultrasonographic evaluation of urinary tract morbidity in school-aged and preschool-aged children infected with *Schistosoma haematobium* and its evolution after praziquantel treatment: A randomized controlled trial. PLoS Negl Trop Dis. 2017;11(2):e0005400.

39.   WHO. Assessing the efficacy of anthelminthic drugs against schistosomiasis and soil-transmitted helminthiases. Geneva: World Health Organization; 2013.

40.   McCarthy JS, Lustigman S, Yang GJ, Barakat RM, Garcia HH, Sripa B, Willingham AL, Prichard RK, Basanez MG. A research agenda for helminth diseases of humans: diagnostics for control and elimination programmes. PLoS Negl Trop Dis. 2012;6:e1601.

41.   Solomon AW, Engels D, Bailey RL, Blake IM, Brooker S, Chen JX, Chen JH, Churcher TS, Drakeley CJ, Edwards T, et al. A diagnostics platform for the integrated mapping, monitoring, and surveillance of neglected tropical diseases: rationale and target product profiles. PLoS Negl Trop Dis. 2012;6:e1746.

42.   Saathoff E, Olsen A, Magnussen P, Kvalsvig JD, Becker W, Appleton CC. Patterns of *Schistosoma haematobium* infection, impact of praziquantel treatment and re-infection after treatment in a cohort of schoolchildren from rural KwaZulu-Natal/South Africa. BMC Infect Dis. 2004;4:40.

7

Designs of trials assessing interventions to improve the peer review process: a vignette-based survey

Amytis Heim[1,2], Philippe Ravaud[1,2,3], Gabriel Baron[1,2,3] and Isabelle Boutron[1,2,3*]

Abstract

Background: We aimed to determine the best study designs for assessing interventions to improve the peer review process according to experts' opinions. Furthermore, for interventions previously evaluated, we determined whether the study designs actually used were rated as the best study designs.

Methods: Study design: A series of six vignette-based surveys exploring the best study designs for six different interventions (training peer reviewers, adding an expert to the peer review process, use of reporting guidelines checklists, blinding peer reviewers to the results (i.e., results-free peer review), giving incentives to peer reviewers, and post-publication peer review).
Vignette construction: Vignettes were case scenarios of trials assessing interventions aimed at improving the quality of peer review. For each intervention, the vignette included the study type (e.g., randomized controlled trial [RCT]), setting (e.g., single biomedical journal), and type of manuscript assessed (e.g., actual manuscripts received by the journal); each of these three features varied between vignettes.
Participants: Researchers with expertise in peer review or methodology of clinical trials.
Outcome: Participants were proposed two vignettes describing two different study designs to assess the same intervention and had to indicate which study design they preferred on a scale, from − 5 (preference for study A) to 5 (preference for study B), 0 indicating no preference between the suggested designs (primary outcome). Secondary outcomes were trust in the results and feasibility of the designs.

Results: A total of 204 experts assessed 1044 paired comparisons. The preferred study type was RCTs with randomization of manuscripts for four interventions (adding an expert, use of reporting guidelines checklist, results-free peer review, post-publication peer review) and RCTs with randomization of peer reviewers for two interventions (training peer reviewers and using incentives). The preferred setting was mainly several biomedical journals from different publishers, and the preferred type of manuscript was actual manuscripts submitted to journals. However, the most feasible designs were often cluster RCTs and interrupted time series analysis set in a single biomedical journal, with the assessment of a fabricated manuscript. Three interventions were previously assessed: none used the design rated first in preference by experts.

Conclusion: The vignette-based survey allowed us to identify the best study designs for assessing different interventions to improve peer review according to experts' opinion. There is gap between the preferred study designs and the designs actually used.

Keywords: Peer review, Randomized controlled trials, Design, Quality, Validity

* Correspondence: isabelle.boutron@aphp.fr
[1]INSERM, U1153 Epidemiology and Biostatistics Sorbonne Paris Cité Research Center (CRESS), Methods of Therapeutic Evaluation of Chronic Diseases Team (METHODS), Paris, France
[2]Paris Descartes University, Sorbonne Paris Cité, Paris, France
Full list of author information is available at the end of the article

Background

The peer review process is the cornerstone of research [1–3]. This process aims to provide a method for rational, fair, and objective decision-making and to raise the quality of publications. However, this process is increasingly being questioned [4]. Primary functions of peer reviewers are poorly defined, and often expectations of manuscripts differ between editors and peer reviewers [5]. Peer review frequently fails to be objective, rational, and free of prejudice [6]. Flawed and misleading articles are still being published [7]. Less than half of biomedical academics think that the peer review process is fair, scientific, or transparent [8]. Studies have highlighted some limitations of peer review [9–11], including limitations in detecting errors and fraud, improving the completeness of reporting [12], or decreasing the distortion of study results [13].

Some interventions developed and implemented by editors to improve the quality of peer review include blinding the peer reviewer to the author's identity, using open peer review, or training peer reviewers [14]. However, research evaluating these interventions with an experimental design is scarce [15]. Furthermore, assessing these interventions can raise important methodological issues related to the choice of study type, setting, and type of manuscript being evaluated [15].

Here, we used a vignette-based survey of experts to determine the best study designs for assessing interventions to improve the peer review process according to experts' opinions. Furthermore, for interventions that were previously evaluated [15], we determined whether the study designs actually used were the study designs experts preferred.

Methods

Study design

We performed a series of vignette-based surveys. A vignette can be defined as a hypothetical situation for which research participants are asked a set of directed questions to reveal their values and perceptions. The vignette-based survey has been found useful in different biomedical fields. It is frequently used to examine judgments and decision-making processes and to evaluate clinical practices [16, 17]. The method has also been used to identify the best trial designs for methodological questions [18, 19]. In this study, vignettes were case scenarios of trials assessing different interventions aimed at improving the quality of peer review.

Vignettes' conception

To build the vignettes, we performed a methodological review to identify a variety of interventions for improving peer review.

Methodological review

We searched MEDLINE (via PubMed), with no restriction on language or date of publication. Our search strategy relied on the search terms "peer review," "peer reviews," "peer reviewer," or "peer reviewers" in the title. We included all types of experimental designs evaluating any intervention aiming to improve the quality of the peer review process in biomedical journals. We also included all articles (including editorials, comments) highlighting an intervention to improve the peer review process. The title and abstract of papers were screened by one researcher (AH) for eligibility.

A total of 12 interventions were identified. Interventions were classified according to their goal (Fig. 1): (1) to improve the accuracy of peer review (i.e., training; adding a specialist to peer review; using checklists); (2) to avoid bias and increase transparency (i.e., blinding; open peer review); (3) to reduce the duration of the peer review process (i.e., using communication media; early screening; use of incentives such as payment), and (4) to make peer review a team effort (i.e., using the wisdom of the crowd such as post publication peer review and expert collaboration).

Six different interventions were selected: training peer reviewers, adding an expert to the peer review process, use of reporting guidelines checklists, blinding peer reviewers to the results (i.e., results-free peer review), giving incentives to peer reviewers, and post-publication peer review. These interventions are described in Table 1.

The choice of these interventions took into account the following factors: having at least one intervention within each group and making sure that the interventions' assessment raised different methodological issues and consequently required different types of study design. For this purpose, we selected interventions that targeted the peer reviewers (e.g., training, incentives) or the manuscript (e.g., adding a specialist) or involved important changes in the process (e.g., post-publication peer review). Furthermore, we favored interventions that we believed were important in terms of their goal (improving the accuracy of peer review and avoiding bias), were implemented but never tested (blinding peer reviewers to results; post-publication peer review), or were frequently suggested (use of incentives).

More specifically, we decided to consider three interventions aimed at improving the accuracy of peer review (i.e., training, adding a specialist to peer review, using checklists), which we believe is a very important goal of the peer review. The intervention "results-free peer review" was selected because of clear evidence of outcome bias in the peer review process [20], and some editors (e.g., *BMC Psychology*) have implemented this new form of review. Nevertheless, the intervention has never been evaluated. Use of incentives is regularly highlighted as being essential to improve the peer review process, and some initiatives

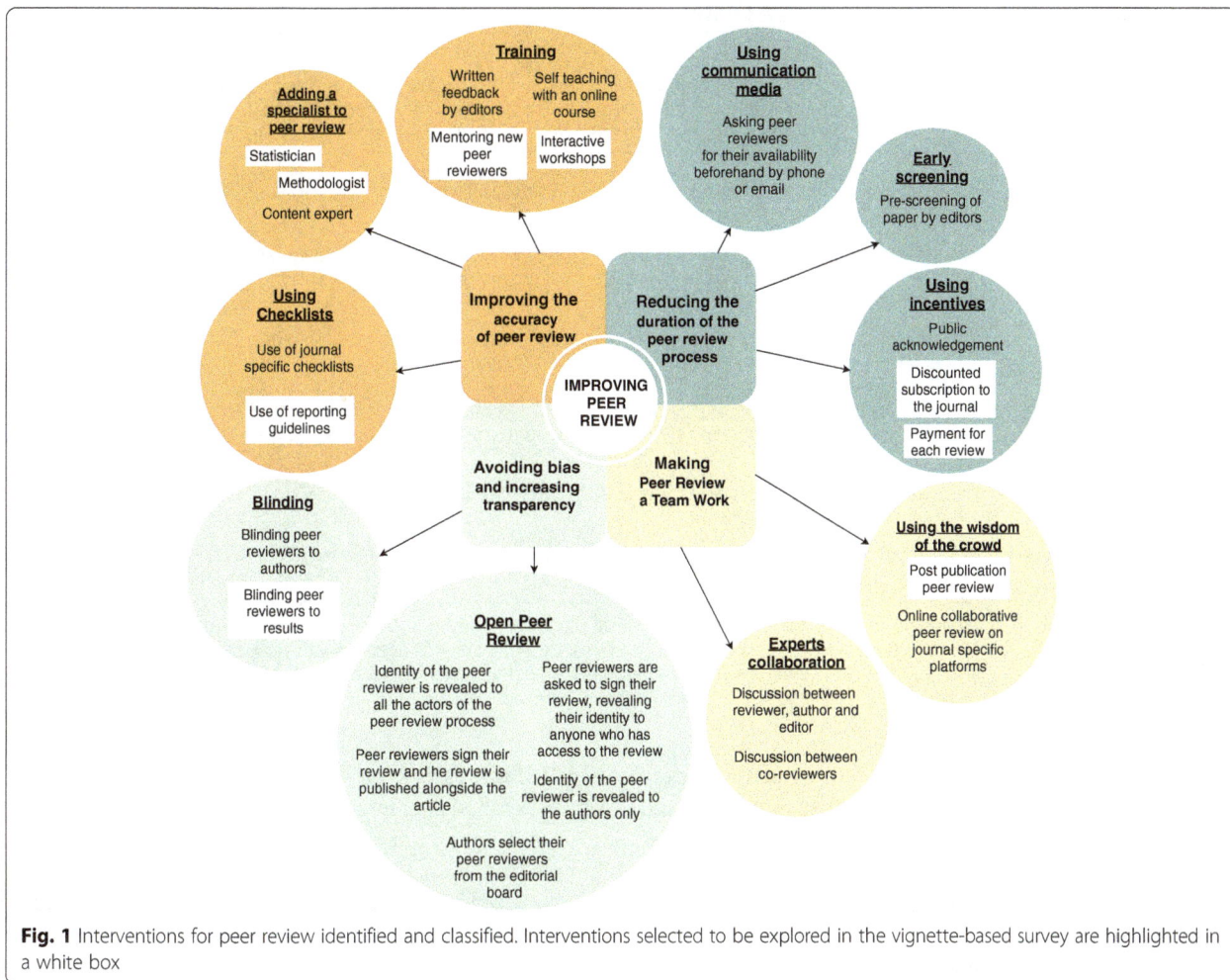

Fig. 1 Interventions for peer review identified and classified. Interventions selected to be explored in the vignette-based survey are highlighted in a white box

such as Publon are being implemented. Finally, post-publication peer review is widely implemented in some fields and is increasingly been used in biomedical research with specific publishers such as F1000. However, this new process has never been evaluated.

Vignettes' content

The vignettes were structured in two parts as shown in Fig. 2. The first part described the study objective. It included the description of the intervention, the comparator (i.e., usual process of peer review), and the main outcome measure (i.e., quality of the peer review report or quality of the manuscript revised by the authors according to the type of intervention assessed) and remained unchanged for all vignettes.

The second part of the vignette described the study design considering three different features: the study type, setting, and type of manuscript assessed by the peer reviewer when appropriate; each of these three features varied among the vignettes (Fig. 2). The study type could be an RCT randomizing manuscripts, an RCT randomizing peer reviewers, a cluster RCT randomizing journals, an

interrupted time series analysis, a pairwise comparison, or a stepped wedge cluster RCT with randomization of journals (Table 2). The setting could be a single biomedical journal, several biomedical journals from a single publisher, or several biomedical journals from several publishers. The type of manuscript assessed by the peer reviewer could be the actual manuscripts received by the journal(s) or a fabricated manuscript that purposely included methodological issues, errors, and poorly reported items.

All possible combinations of designs were generated, and two methodologists assessed each design to exclude implausible and contradictory ones. Particularly, we considered a single type of manuscript (i.e., actual manuscripts received by the journal[s]) for the following interventions: adding an expert to the peer review process, use of reporting guidelines checklists, use of incentives, and post-publication peer review.

Participants

Our target population consisted of researchers with an expertise in the field of peer review or methodology of clinical trials. To recruit such participants, we searched

Table 1 Interventions included in the vignette-based survey

Intervention	Description
Training	Peer reviewers are asked to attend an online training program, with lessons on how to evaluate the methodology, the reporting of data and results, the ethical issues, and how to address them in a review. The course will also inform peer reviewers on what journals want from them from an editor's perspective. Peer reviewers are then supervised for three articles specifically selected for the course.
Adding an expert to the peer review process	An expert is asked to peer review the manuscript in addition to the usual peer review process. The expert should be a statistician or a methodologist.
Use of reporting guidelines checklist	Peer reviewers are asked to complete a checklist based on guidelines (such as CONSORT or STARD, depending on the nature of their manuscript), in addition to their usual review. The checklist is then sent to the authors so they can revise their manuscript.
Results-free peer review	Peer reviewers are blinded to the results of the study. The peer review process unfolds in 2 steps: 1. Peer reviewers receive the manuscript without the abstract, results or discussion. They write a first review and make a recommendation for publication. This first review is sent to the editor. 2. Peer reviewers then receive the full manuscript to comment on the results, discussion and abstract by answering two simple questions on the completeness of the reporting and on the validity of the interpretation. The review is sent to the editor and combined with the first one.
Use of incentives	Reviewers are told they will receive an incentive (payment or discounted subscription to the journal) when they are asked to peer review the manuscript.
Post-publication peer review	Manuscripts are posted online on an open access platform where researchers from all around the world with any background can peer review the study. Chosen researchers are also actively invited by the author and the editor to peer review the online publication. The peer review is entirely transparent: the reviewers' names and affiliation, their report and the approval status they choose are published along with the article. Peer review reports are posted as soon as they are received and the peer review status of the article is updated with every published report. Once an article has passed peer review (i.e., it has received at least two "Approved" statuses from independent peer reviewers), it will be indexed in PubMed, PubMed Central, Scopus, and Embase.

for the email addresses for all the authors of the papers of our review. We also identified and searched for the email addresses of participants of the 2013 Peer Review Congress, members of the Editorial Boards of the five journals with the highest impact factor, the Journal of Clinical Epidemiology and Public Library of Science Medicine (PLOS); members of the Enhancing the QUAlity and Transparency Of health Research (EQUATOR) network, the REduce research Waste and Reward DIligance (REWARD) Alliance, the METHODS Cochrane Group, the Methods in Research on Research (MiRoR) project, Trial Forge and Meta-Research Innovation Center at Stanford (METRICS). The full list is available in Additional file 1: Appendix 1.

Surveys

A total of 94 vignettes were included in the study: 24 for training, 24 for results-free peer review, 13 for the use of reporting guidelines checklist, 10 for adding an expert to the process, 13 for the use of incentives, and 10 for post-publication peer review. Participants received an invitation via email with a personalized link to the survey. On the home page of the website, participants were informed that the data collected was anonymous and were asked to give their informed consent before starting the questionnaire. A maximum of three reminders were sent to participants, and no incentive was used to maximize the response rate. Participants were proposed two vignettes describing two different study designs to assess a same intervention, and had to indicate which study design they preferred

(Fig. 2). Each participant was invited to evaluate six pairs of vignettes for a given intervention.

Sample size

From a pragmatic point of view, we wanted each pair of vignettes to be assessed by participants at least once. For the interventions with fewer than 20 vignettes, we planned for each pair of vignettes to be assessed twice, to increase the number of evaluations per vignette. Therefore, to assess all pairs of vignettes ($n = 1044$ in total: 276 each for training and results-free peer review, 156 each for the use of reporting guidelines checklist and the use of incentives, and 90 each for adding an expert to the process and for post-publication peer review), and assuming each participant would assess six pairs of vignettes, we needed a minimum of 174 participants. If participants could not evaluate six pairs of vignettes, other participants were recruited.

Ranking of the study designs actually implemented

Using the results of our methodological review, we determined how the study designs actually used were ranked in our survey. For this purpose, we extracted the study type, setting, and type of manuscript used to assess these interventions in the review.

Outcomes

Our main outcome was the overall preference for a study design. Participants had to answer the following

Fixed for each intervention

Does the use of reporting guidelines by the peer reviewer improve the quality of the final manuscript, compared to the usual process?

Intervention
Peer reviewers are asked to fill in a checklist based on guidelines (such as CONSORT or STARD, depending on the nature of their manuscript) in addition to their usual review. The checklist is then sent to the authors so they can revise their manuscript.

Comparator
Peer reviewers are not asked to fill in a guidelines checklist. They follow the usual process of peer review.

Main outcome measure
Quality of the revised manuscript updated by the authors
• Measured with a manuscript quality assessment tool: a 5 point Likert scale from 1 (low) to 5 (high) , with 34 items regarding the originality of the paper, the strengths and weaknesses of the method, the presentation, the constructiveness of comments, the substantiation of comments and the interpretation of results
• By a blinded independent outcome assessor

Varied within a same intervention

	DESIGN A		DESIGN B
Study type	**Randomized controlled trial with randomization of manuscripts** Each manuscript is randomized to be peer reviewed by either : • A peer reviewer asked to fill in the reporting guidelines checklist in addition to the usual process, if allocated to the intervention group. • A peer reviewer following the usual process, if allocated to the control group.	Study type	**Interrupted time series analysis** In interrupted time series studies, data are collected at multiple time points before and after an intervention in order to detect whether or not the intervention had a significantly greater effect than any underlying secular trend. • **Period 1: usual peer-review process.** In the first part of the study, peer reviewers follow the usual process of peer review. • **Period 2: addition of an expert to the usual peer review process.** An assessment by an expert is systematically added to the usual peer review process.
Setting	A single biomedical journal	Setting	A single biomedical journal
Type of manuscript assessed by the peer reviewer	The manuscript(s) used in the study are the **actual manuscripts submitted to the journal(s)** and selected for peer-review during the time of the study (i.e. 2 years follow-up).	Type of manuscript assessed by the peer reviewer	The manuscript(s) used in the study are the **actual manuscripts submitted to the journal(s)** and selected for peer-review during the time of the study (i.e. 2 years follow-up).

Which design would you choose?
Design A   5 4 3 2 1 0 1 2 3 4 5   Design B
Design A ←   No difference between design A and design B   → Design B

Which design would you trust the most?
Design A   5 4 3 2 1 0 1 2 3 4 5   Design B
Design A ←   No difference between design A and design B   → Design B

Which design is logistically simpler to set up?
Design A   5 4 3 2 1 0 1 2 3 4 5   Design B
Design A ←   No difference between design A and design B   → Design B

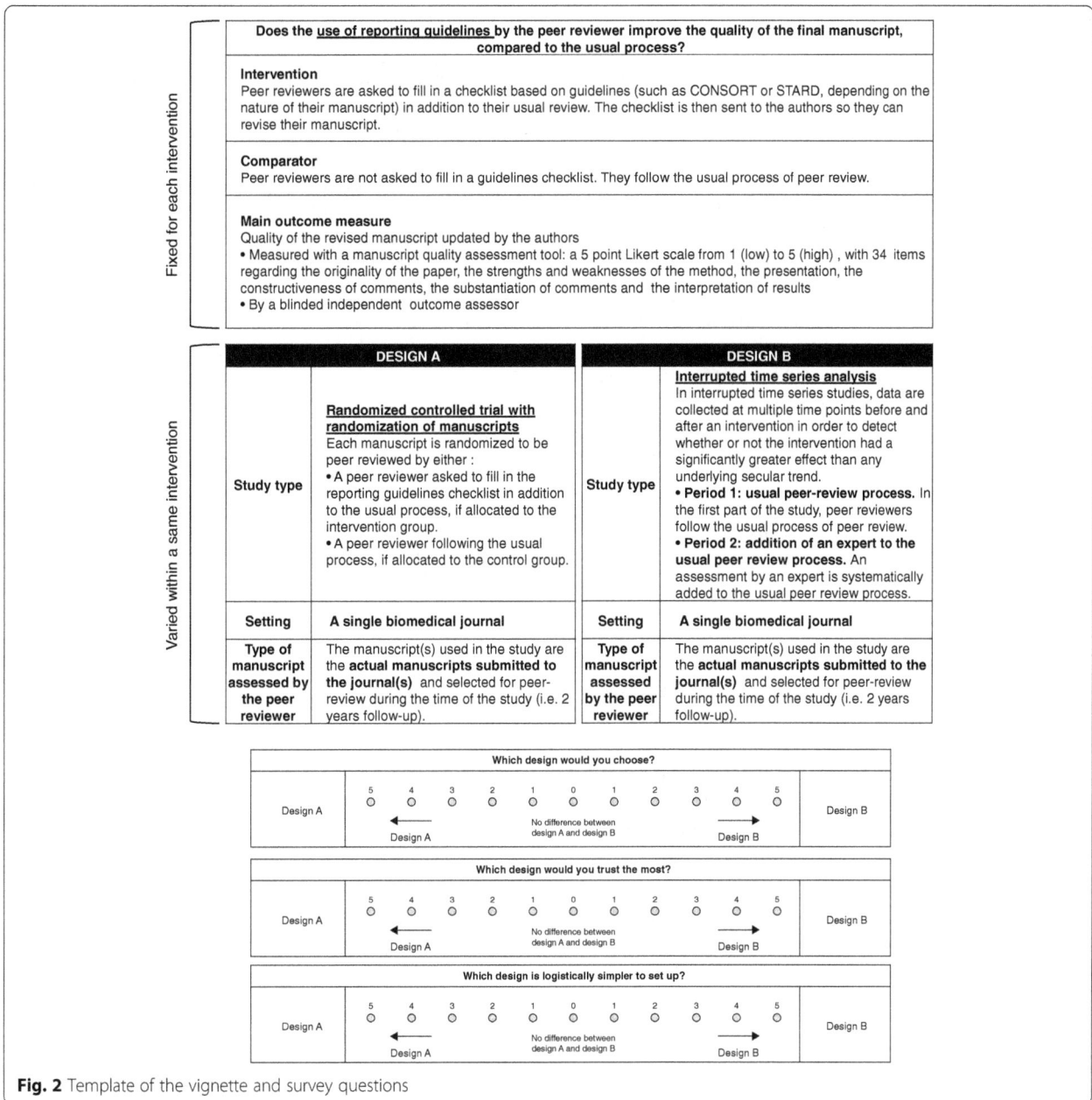

Fig. 2 Template of the vignette and survey questions

question: "If you had to conduct this trial, which study would you choose?" on a semantic differential scale rated from – 5 (preference for study A) to 5 (preference for study B), 0 indicating no preference between the suggested designs.

Other outcomes were the rankings for trust in the results and feasibility, measured by using the same scale. The questions asked were as follows:

• "If you read the results of this study, which study would you trust most?"
• "Which protocol is logistically simpler to set up?"

Participants had the opportunity to leave comments if they wished to.

Statistical analysis
Answers for the online questionnaire were collected through the website. The results were recorded in a .csv file and analyzed with R v3.2.2 (http://www.R-project.org, the R Foundation for Statistical Computing, Vienna, Austria) and SAS 9.4 (SAS Institute Inc., Cary, NC). For each intervention and each outcome (overall preference, trust in results, and feasibility), the mean score for each vignette was calculated for each combination of designs in

Table 2 Study types

Study type	
RCT with randomization of manuscripts	Each manuscript is randomized to be peer reviewed by a peer reviewer in the intervention group or a peer reviewer in the control group.
RCT with randomization of peer reviewers	Peer reviewers are randomized to the intervention group or the control group.
Cluster RCT with randomization of journals	Journals are randomized to the intervention group or the control group. All peer reviewers from a journal follow the same peer review process.
Interrupted time series analysis	Data are collected at multiple time points before and after an intervention to detect whether the intervention had a significantly greater effect than any underlying secular trend. • Period 1: Peer reviewers follow the usual process of peer review. • Intervention: All peer reviewers follow the process of the intervention. • Period 2: Manuscripts are evaluated after the peer review process.
Pairwise comparison	Each manuscript is sent to be reviewed by both a peer reviewer from the intervention group AND a peer reviewer from the control group.
Stepped wedge cluster RCT with randomization of journals	The intervention is rolled out sequentially to the journals over a number of time periods. • During the first period, none of the journals follow the intervention. • During the second period, one journal is randomized to invite its peer reviewers to participate in the intervention peer review process. The other journals continue the usual process. • During the third period, an extra journal is randomized to participate in the intervention peer review process, and the other journals continue with the usual process. Therefore, two journals are undergoing the intervention during this period. This process of randomization is repeated at each period until the last journal finally joins the intervention group.

order to have a ranking. For each intervention, we used a linear mixed model to assess the association between each outcome and the following three fixed effects: study type, setting, and type of manuscript. The reading order of the two vignettes of a pair was added as a fourth fixed effect. To account for correlation between vignettes, an intercept term that randomly varied at the level of the vignette effect was included in the model. To account for correlation within vignette pairs (at each comparison, two vignettes have exactly opposite scores), we bootstrapped pairs with 1000 replications of the original sample to estimate the parameters (and 95% confidence intervals) of the model. Correlation due do respondents was found to be null, so it was not modeled.

Results

Participants
Between May 11, 2017, and July 31, 2017, 1037 people were contacted in waves until all pairs of vignettes were evaluated. Of the 331 participants who clicked on the link, 210 gave their consent, and 204 completed the survey (Table 3). Participants were located mainly in Europe (n = 114, 56%) and North America (n = 72, 35%). More than half worked as a methodologist (n = 135, 66%) and about half were trialists (n = 99, 49%) or editors (n = 102, 50%).

Vignette-based surveys
Additional file 1: Appendix 2 summarizes the results in a spider diagram of mean vignette scores per intervention in terms of overall preference, trust in the results, and feasibility.

Table 3 Baseline demographics and other characteristics of participants (n = 204)

	No. of participants (%)
Age, years	
< 40	65 (32)
40–50	52 (25)
51–60	45 (22)
60	42 (21)
Sex	
Male	117 (57)
Female	87 (43)
Location	
Europe	114 (56)
North America	72 (35)
South America	0 (0)
Asia	4 (2)
Africa	2 (1)
Oceania	12 (6)
Occupation*	
Methodologist	135 (66)
Trialist	99 (49)
Editor	102 (50)
Other	22 (11)

*Many participants had combined occupations (methodologist and/or trialist and/or editor)

Preferred study designs

Additional file 1: Appendix 3 provides the mean score for each vignette for each combination of features (i.e., study type, setting, manuscript type). Table 4 reports the factors associated with overall preference for each study design feature (study type, setting, type of manuscript). For each feature, we arbitrarily identified a reference (*stepped wedge cluster RCT with randomization of journals* for the study type, *several biomedical journals from different publishers* for the setting, and *one fabricated manuscript* for the type of manuscript). The parameter reported is the mean difference in overall preference associated with each category of independent variable as compared with the reference (after adjusting for all other variables).

Overall, the preferred study type was RCTs with randomization of manuscripts for four interventions (adding an expert, use of reporting guidelines checklist, results-free peer review, post-publication peer review) and RCTs with randomization of peer reviewers for two interventions (training peer reviewers and using incentives), with adjustment for all other variables. The preferred setting was mainly several biomedical journals from different publishers, and the preferred type of manuscript was actual manuscripts submitted to journals.

Table 4 Results—factors associated with overall preference for each study design feature: parameter estimates [and 95% confidence intervals]. For each independent variable, parameter estimates represent mean difference in overall preference associated with each category of independent variable as compared with the reference (after adjusting for all other variables in the table and after taking into account the reading order of the 2 vignettes of the pair)

	Training peer reviewers (24 vignettes, 276 pairs)	Adding an expert to the peer review process (10 vignettes, 90 pairs*)	Use of reporting guidelines checklist (13 vignettes, 156 pairs*)	Results free peer review (24 vignettes, 276 pairs)	Using incentives (13 vignettes, 156 pairs*)	Post-publication peer review (10 vignettes, 90 pairs*)
	Estimate [95% CI]	Estimate [95% CI]	Estimate [95% CI]	Estimate [95% CI]	Estimate [95% CI]	Estimate [95% CI]
Study type						
RCT with randomization of manuscripts	0.92 [-0.50 ; 2.41]	**2.03 [0.51 ; 3.49]**	**2.69 [1.39 ; 3.95]**	**2.53 [1.27 ; 3.76]**	1.00 [-0.21 ; 2.16]	**2.55 [1.13 ; 4.09]**
RCT with randomization of peer reviewers	**1.45 [0.14 ; 2.78]**	N/A	1.99 [0.69 ; 3.37]	2.24 [0.98 ; 3.50]	**2.25 [0.94 ; 3.49]**	N/A
Cluster RCT with randomization of journals	0.30 [-1.12 ; 1.63]	0.76 [-0.90 ; 2.43]	0.34 [-1.25 ; 1.93]	0.63 [-0.56 ; 1.88]	-0.16 [-1.49 ; 1.18]	1.73 [0.13 ; 3.51]
Interrupted time series analysis	-0.10 [-1.48 ; 1.38]	-0.19 [-1.74; 1.39]	0.10 [-1.21 ; 1.44]	0.07 [-1.28 ; 1.40]	0.73 [-0.51 ; 2.02]	1.58 [0.13; 3.15]
Pairwise comparison	0.83 [-0.49 ; 2.18]	N/A	N/A	1.61 [0.35 ; 2.86]	N/A	N/A
Stepped wedge cluster RCT with randomization of journals***	0.00 [-]	0.00 [-]	0.00 [-]	0.00 [-]	0.00 [-]	0.00 [-]
Setting						
Single biomedical journal	-1.02 [-1.82 ; -0.27]	-2.62 [-4.23 ; -0.80]	-2.50 [-3.51 ; 1.50]	-0.20 [-1.03 ; 0.62]	-1.51 [-2.59 ; -0.43]	-3.13 [-4.09 ; -1.53]
Several biomedical journals from a single publisher	-0.21 [-0.84 ; 0.44]	-1.10 [-2.32 ; 0.06]	-0.12 [-1.06 ; 0.80]	**0.18 [-0.52 ; 0.83]**	-0.01 [-0.82 ; 0.83]	-0.92 [-1.95 ; 0.22]
Several biomedical journals from different publishers***	**0.00 [-]**	**0.00 [-]**	**0.00 [-]**	0.00 [-]	**0.00 [-]**	**0.00 [-]**
Type of manuscript						
Actual manuscripts submitted to the journal(s)	**1.04 [0.37 ; 1.79]**	N/A	N/A	**0.57 [-0.15 ; 1.26]**	N/A	N/A
One fabricated manuscript***	0.00 [-]	N/A	N/A	0.00 [-]	N/A	N/A

N/A, not applicable

Results in bold indicate the most preferred study design features for each intervention

*Indicates the pairs of vignettes for these interventions were assessed twice each

***Indicates reference category for each independent variable

Other designs, such as the cluster stepped wedge of journals or the interrupted time series, scored low.

Trust and feasibility

Additional file 1: Appendices 4 and 5 provide the mean score for each vignette for each combination of features (i.e., study type, setting, manuscript type) for trust and feasibility. After adjustment for all other variables, the most trusted study designs were consistent with the preferred study designs for all interventions (Additional file 1: Appendix 6). In contrast, the study designs rated first in terms of feasibility were not the preferred study designs (Additional file 1: Appendix 7). The preferred study types in terms of feasibility were a pairwise comparison for training peer reviewers (rated as third preferred study type), a cluster RCT with randomization of journals for results-free peer review and use of reporting guidelines checklists (rated fourth and third preferred study type, respectively), and interrupted time series analysis for adding an expert to the peer review process, using incentives and post-publication peer review (rated last, third and third preferred study types, respectively). The setting and type of manuscript were mainly a single biomedical journal and use of a fabricated manuscript.

Ranking of the study designs actually implemented

The ranking of the study design actually implemented is reported in Table 5. Our review identified no studies assessing results-free peer review, use of incentives, and post-publication peer review; five RCTs and one cross-sectional study assessing training; two RCTs assessing use of reporting guidelines checklists and two RCTs assessing adding an expert. None used the designs rated first by experts in terms of preference. None were ranked in the first quarter. This ranking is mainly related to the choice of setting.

Discussion

The peer review process is central to the publication of scientific articles. Our series of vignette-based surveys attempted to surpass the methodological problems of performing research on research by assembling a panel of experts on this research question and using their collective wisdom to identify the best designs. We created 94 vignettes of different study designs for 6 different interventions. Overall, 204 experts in peer review or methodology of clinical trials assessed 1044 paired comparisons of designs, which allowed participants to select their answers in terms of overall preference, trust in the results, and feasibility of the study. We identified the study design that was preferred by experts. We did not specify what is considered the "best" study design because we wanted to give full freedom to the experts and let them balance the different features of the design in terms of internal validity, external validity, and feasibility.

Our study has important strengths. We performed a methodological review to identify interventions for evaluating peer review and to classify them according to their effect on the peer review process. Participants, with expertise as a methodologist, an editor, a trialist or involved in research on peer review, were well suited to compare and score the vignettes. The vignette-based survey we used is an innovative study design [18], which, to our knowledge, has never been used in the context of peer review. This method also allowed experts to discuss the pros and cons of each designs. Table 6 provides the notable characteristics of the preferred study designs for each intervention.

Our results revealed that the preferred designs were often very similar to the most trusted designs but very different from the most feasible ones. Preferred settings were generally in several biomedical journals from one or more publishers, and the preferred type of manuscript assessed by the peer reviewer was always an actual manuscript submitted to the journal. In contrast, the most feasible designs were often set in a single biomedical journal, with assessment of a fabricated manuscript. Some designs, such

Table 5 Ranking of the study designs of the RCTs identified in the methodological review of interventions to improve the peer review process according experts

	Studies identified				Ranking according to experts*		
	No. of studies	Study type	Setting	Type of manuscript	Preference	Trust	Feasibility
Training	6	- 5 randomized controlled trial of peer reviewers - 1 cross-sectional study	Single journal	- Real manuscripts - 1 RCT with fabricated manuscript	8/24 (4 RCTs) 21/24 (1 RCT)	11/24 (4 RCTs) 22/24 (1 RCT)	9/24 (4 RCTs) 6/24 (1 RCT)
Use of reporting guidelines checklist	2	Randomized controlled trial of manuscripts	Single journal	Real manuscripts	5/13	5/13	2/13
Adding an expert	2	Randomized controlled trial of manuscripts	Single journal	Real manuscripts	8/10	8/10	1/10

*The cross-sectional design was not included in the vignette study

Table 6 Notable characteristics of the preferred designs for each intervention

Intervention	Comments on the best study design according to experts
Training intervention	The design recommended by the experts was an RCT with randomization of peer reviewers, set in several biomedical journals from different publishers, using actual manuscripts submitted to the journal. The choice of an RCT with randomization of peer reviewers has the advantage of being close to the real-life procedures of the peer review process, with the benefit of using randomization. The issue with the training intervention is its length in time. This raises issues related to poor adherence and missing outcome when peer reviewers randomized never assess a manuscript. The pairwise comparison was the second-ranked design. This design has the advantage of addressing the issue of manuscript variability, thus increasing statistical power, and avoiding the loss to follow-up problem, because no long-term follow up is needed. Such design has never been used to our knowledge. The cluster RCT and stepped wedge cluster RCT were not often chosen by the participants because of the risk of contamination, because peers can review for more than one journal at a time.
Addition of an expert (methodologist or statistician)	The addition of an expert to the peer review process was preferably assessed with an RCT of manuscripts, set in several journals from different publishers, using the actual manuscripts submitted to the journal. The cluster RCT was the second preferred design for all three of the outcomes. This design has the advantage of including a large variety of reviewers and manuscripts, and it is logistically easy for the editors who do not have to change process for each manuscript. It is nevertheless a difficult design to put in place, as shown by its systematically low score in the feasibility rankings, and a very large number of clusters would be needed to compensate for the high variability between journals (publisher, editorial policies, subject area, quality of reviewers etc.). The interrupted time series set in a single journal was the preferred design in terms of feasibility. This study type is not randomized, which could potentially create bias.
Use of reporting guidelines checklist	The favored designs to assess the use of reporting guidelines checklist was an RCT of manuscripts, set in several biomedical journals from several or a single publisher, using actual manuscripts. The choice to randomize manuscripts rather than peer reviewers is interesting in terms of logistics, because manuscripts receiving the intervention can be sent directly with the checklist. The preferred settings give a good external validity to the study.
Results-free peer review	Our analysis suggests the factor influencing the most participant's decision in their overall preference was the type of study. The favorite type of studies overall were the RCT of peer reviewers and the RCT of manuscripts. The choice of an RCT randomizing manuscripts for the results-free peer review seems appropriate because the intervention is held directly on the manuscript. The issue with the randomization of manuscripts in this situation is the possibility for peer reviewers to perform both with-results and results-free reviews. With the intervention having a potential learning effect, it would artificially increase the quality of reviews in the control group. This intervention has—to our knowledge—never been assessed, which is notable as it could help reduce the important bias towards positive results.
Use of incentives	The use of incentives raised interesting comments from participants. Particularly, they highlighted that the existence of an incentive may encourage reviewers to accept invitations even if not fully qualified. In a similar way, reviewers in the incentive arm are likely to accept more reviews than the control arm, which raises some issues for the design.
Post-publication peer review	It was one of the most innovative intervention we included in our study. Although this system has already been in place in several journals, such as F1000, it has, to our knowledge, never been assessed. This intervention is interesting because it changes the entire peer review process, not just the way peer reviews assess the manuscripts. The preferred type of study for this intervention was the randomization of manuscripts. Being randomized, this design would indeed lower the risk of bias of the study; however, it may be hard to implement such an intervention, because journals would have to manage two completely different peer review systems at the same time.

as RCTs with randomization of manuscripts or peer reviewers, were usually high-ranked. Other designs, such as the cluster stepped wedge of journals or the interrupted time series, regularly scored low.

This preference for trust in the results of the study rather than feasibility could be explained by the fact that the most trusted study designs does not raise important feasibility issues and should be easy to implement. Indeed, there are no major barriers to the randomization of manuscripts or peer reviewer. Opt-out consent procedures and blinding procedures are usually easy to implement; authors and reviewers are informed that studies of peer review are being conducted within a journal but are not informed of the studies to avoid any change in behavior. Outcome assessment (quality of the peer review report or quality of the manuscript) can be assessed by blinded outcome assessors. However, the ability to coordinate between journals and publishers and achieve a required sample size could be considered a major barrier.

Our results also highlighted that the designs actually implemented was never the preferred study design. Particularly, all studies performed involved a single journal, whereas the preferred study designs were set in several medical journals from different publishers, which provides high external validity because it is close to the real-world situation, including many types of journals, manuscripts, and reviewers. This inconsistency between implemented studies and preferred study designs may be due to these trials being the first performed in this field and that investigators, who were pioneers in these fields, favored ensuring feasibility. Furthermore, investigators and researchers in this field must have learned a lot from these trials and would probably improve the design of future trials taking into account these previous experiences.

The following limitations should be acknowledged. We focused on 6 interventions of the 12 identified and on the assessment of a single intervention per study, even though the synergistic use of interventions could improve the quality of peer review. Because of the restrictive format of the vignettes, not all elements of study designs could be addressed. No indication of the sample size was included, which could have an effect on both feasibility and trust in the results. The number of vignettes we included in the questionnaire was also limited, which restricted the number of interventions, comparators, and outcomes. Our study focused solely on the interventions improving the quality of peer review and thus of manuscripts, but other innovations such as re-review opt out and portable or cascade peer review were not included [21]. Participation level was about 20%, which could have biased our results. However, the level of expertise of participants was appropriate. Finally, we cannot exclude that participants could have been influenced by ideological or other preferences for a study design for a given intervention.

Conclusion

Well-performed trials are needed to assess interventions proposed to improve the peer review process. We encourage editors and other investigators to pursue the research on peer review and plan their studies in light of the findings of this vignette-based survey. We hope the evaluation of study designs with a vignette-based survey, based on international expertise, will help to develop a standardization of practices. This standardization will help improve the comparison and ensure the quality of future studies.

Abbreviations
95% CI: 95% confidence intervals; RCT: Randomized controlled trials

Acknowledgements
We thank Elise Diard for designing and managing the survey website. We thank Iosief Abraha, Sabina Alam, Loai Albarqouni, Doug Altman, Joseph Ana, Jose Anglez, Liz Bal, Vicki Barber, Ginny Barbour, Adrian Barnett, Beatriz Barros, Hilda Bastian, Jesse Berlin, Theodora Bloom, Charles Boachie, Peter Bower, Matthias Briel, William Cameron, Patrice Capers, Viswas Chhapola, Anna Chiumento, Oriana Ciani, Anna Clark, Mike Clarke, Erik Cobo, Peter Craig, Rafael Dal-Ré, Simon Day, Diana Elbourne, Caitlyn Ellerbe, Zen Faulkes, Padhrag Fleming, Robert H. Fletcher, Rachael Frost, Marcelo Gama de Abreu, Chantelle Garritty, Julie Glanville, Robert Goldberg, Robert Golub, Ole Haagen Nielse, Gergö Hadlaczky, Barbara Hawkins, Brian Haynes, Jerome Richard Hoffman, Virginia Howard, Haley Hutchings, Philip Jones, Roger Jones, Kathryn Kaiser, Veronique Kiermer, Maria Kowalczuk, Yannick Lemanach, Alex Levis, Dandan Liu, Andreas Lundh, Herve Maisonneuve, Mario Malicki, Maura Marcucci, Evan Mayo-Wilson, Lawrence Mbuagbaw, Elaine McColl, Joanne McKenzie, Bahar Mehmani, John Moran, Tim Morris, Elizabeth Moylan, Cynthia Mulrow, Christelle Nguyen, Leslie Nicoll, John Norrie, David Ofori-Adjei, Matthew Page, Nikolaos Pandis, Spyridon N. Papageorgiou, Nathalie Percie du Sert, Morten Petersen, Patrick Phillips, Dawid Pieper, Raphael Porcher, Jonas Ranstam, Jean Raymond, Barney Reeves, Melissa Rethlefsen, Ludovic Reveiz, Daniel Riddle, Yves Rosenberg, Timothy Rowe, Roberta W. Scherer, David Schoenfeld, David L. Schriger, Sara Schroter, Larissa Shamseer, Richard Smith, Ines Steffens, Philipp Storz-Pfennig, Caroline Struthers, Brett D. Thombs, Shaun Treweek, Margaret Twinker, Cornelis H. Van Werkhoven, Roderick P. Venekamp, Alexandre Vivot, Sunita Vohra, Liz Wager, Ellen Weber, Wim Weber, Matthew Westmore, Ian White, Sankey Williams for their participation in our vignette-based questionnaire.

Funding
This study required no particular funding.

Authors' contributions
AH, PR, GB, and IB made substantial contributions to conception and design, acquisition of data, analysis, and interpretation of data. AH, PR, GB and IB have been involved in drafting the manuscript or revising it critically for important intellectual content. AH, PR, GB, and IB gave the final approval of the version to be published. Each author have participated sufficiently in the work to take public responsibility for appropriate portions of the content and agreed to be accountable for all aspects of the work in ensuring that questions related to the accuracy or integrity of any part of the work are appropriately investigated and resolved.

Competing interests
The authors declare that they have no competing interests.

Author details
[1]INSERM, U1153 Epidemiology and Biostatistics Sorbonne Paris Cité Research Center (CRESS), Methods of Therapeutic Evaluation of Chronic Diseases Team (METHODS), Paris, France. [2]Paris Descartes University, Sorbonne Paris Cité, Paris, France. [3]Centre d'Epidémiologie Clinique, Hôpital Hôtel-Dieu, Assistance Publique des Hôpitaux de Paris, Paris, France.

References
1. Smith R. Peer review: reform or revolution? BMJ. 1997;315(7111):759–60.
2. Rennie D. Suspended judgment. Editorial peer review: let us put it on trial. Control Clin Trials. 1992;13(6):443–5.
3. Kronick DA. Peer review in 18th-century scientific journalism. JAMA. 1990; 263(10):1321–2.
4. Jefferson T, Rudin M, Brodney Folse S, Davidoff F. Editorial peer review for improving the quality of reports of biomedical studies. Cochrane Database Syst Rev. 2007;2:MR000016.
5. Chauvin A, Ravaud P, Baron G, Barnes C, Boutron I. The most important tasks for peer reviewers evaluating a randomized controlled trial are not congruent with the tasks most often requested by journal editors. BMC Med. 2015;13:158.
6. Mahoney MJ. Publication prejudices: an experimental study of confirmatory bias in the peer review system. Cogn Ther Res. 1977;1(2):161–75.
7. The Editors of The L. Retraction—Ileal-lymphoid-nodular hyperplasia, non-specific colitis, and pervasive developmental disorder in children. Lancet. 2010;375(9713):445.
8. Ho RC, Mak KK, Tao R, Lu Y, Day JR, Pan F. Views on the peer review system of biomedical journals: an online survey of academics from high-ranking universities. BMC Med Res Methodol. 2013;13:74.
9. Wager E, Jefferson T. Shortcomings of peer review in biomedical journals. Learned Publishing. 2001;14(4):257–63.
10. Rennie D (ed.): Misconduct and journal peer review; 1999.
11. Henderson M. Problems with peer review. BMJ. 2010;340:c1409.

12. Hopewell S, Collins GS, Boutron I, Yu LM, Cook J, Shanyinde M, Wharton R, Shamseer L, Altman DG. Impact of peer review on reports of randomised trials published in open peer review journals: retrospective before and after study. BMJ. 2014;349:g4145.

13. Lazarus C, Haneef R, Ravaud P, Boutron I. Classification and prevalence of spin in abstracts of non-randomized studies evaluating an intervention. BMC Med Res Methodol. 2015;15:85.

14. Galipeau J, Moher D, Skidmore B, Campbell C, Hendry P, Cameron DW, Hebert PC, Palepu A. Systematic review of the effectiveness of training programs in writing for scholarly publication, journal editing, and manuscript peer review (protocol). Syst Rev. 2013;2:41.

15. Bruce R, Chauvin A, Trinquart L, Ravaud P, Boutron I. Impact of interventions to improve the quality of peer review of biomedical journals: a systematic review and meta-analysis. BMC Med. 2016;14(1):85.

16. Hughes R, Huby M. The application of vignettes in social and nursing research. J Adv Nurs. 2002;37(4):382–6.

17. Bachmann LM, Mühleisen A, Bock A, ter Riet G, Held U, Kessels AG. Vignette studies of medical choice and judgement to study caregivers' medical decision behaviour: systematic review. BMC Med Res Methodol. 2008;8(1):50.

18. Do-Pham G, Le Cleach L, Giraudeau B, Maruani A, Chosidow O, Ravaud P. Designing randomized-controlled trials to improve head-louse treatment: systematic review using a vignette-based method. J Invest Dermatol. 2014; 134(3):628–34.

19. Gould D. Using vignettes to collect data for nursing research studies: how valid are the findings? J Clin Nurs. 1996;5(4):207–12.

20. Emerson GB, Warme WJ, Wolf FM, Heckman JD, Brand RA, Leopold SS. Testing for the presence of positive-outcome bias in peer review: a randomized controlled trial. Arch Intern Med. 2010;170(21):1934–9.

21. Kovanis M, Trinquart L, Ravaud P, Porcher R. Evaluating alternative systems of peer review: a large-scale agent-based modelling approach to scientific publication. Scientometrics. 2017;113(1):651–671.

8

Simultaneously characterizing the comparative economics of routine female adolescent nonavalent human papillomavirus (HPV) vaccination and assortativity of sexual mixing in Hong Kong Chinese: a modeling analysis

Horace C. W. Choi[1,2,3†], Mark Jit[1,4,5], Gabriel M. Leung[1], Kwok-Leung Tsui[2] and Joseph T. Wu[1*†]

Abstract

Background: Although routine vaccination of females before sexual debut against human papillomavirus (HPV) has been found to be cost-effective around the world, its cost-benefit has rarely been examined. We evaluate both the cost-effectiveness and cost-benefit of routine female adolescent nonavalent HPV vaccination in Hong Kong to guide its policy, and by extension that of mainland China, on HPV vaccination. One major obstacle is the lack of data on assortativity of sexual mixing. Such difficulty could be overcome by inferring sexual mixing parameters from HPV epidemiologic data.

Methods: We use an age-structured transmission model coupled with stochastic individual-based simulations to estimate the health and economic impact of routine nonavalent HPV vaccination for girls at age 12 on cervical cancer burden and consider vaccine uptake at 25%, 50%, and 75% with at least 20 years of vaccine protection. Bayesian inference was employed to parameterize the model using local data on HPV prevalence and cervical cancer incidence. We use the human capital approach in the cost-benefit analysis (CBA) and GDP per capita as the indicative willingness-to-pay threshold in the cost-effectiveness analysis (CEA). Finally, we estimate the threshold vaccine cost (TVC), which is the maximum cost for fully vaccinating one girl at which routine female adolescent nonavalent HPV vaccination is cost-beneficial or cost-effective.

Results: As vaccine uptake increased, TVC decreased (i.e., economically more stringent) in the CBA but increased in the CEA. When vaccine uptake was 75% and the vaccine provided only 20 years of protection, the TVC was US$444 ($373–506) and $689 ($646–734) in the CBA and CEA, respectively, increasing by approximately 2–4% if vaccine protection was assumed lifelong. TVC is likely to be far higher when non-cervical diseases are included. The inferred sexual mixing parameters suggest that sexual mixing in Hong Kong is highly assortative by both age and sexual activity level.

(Continued on next page)

* Correspondence: joewu@hku.hk
†Horace C. W. Choi and Joseph T. Wu contributed equally to this work.
[1]WHO Collaborating Centre for Infectious Disease Epidemiology and Control, School of Public Health, Li Ka Shing Faculty of Medicine, The University of Hong Kong, 1/F North Wing, Patrick Manson Building, 7 Sassoon Road, Pok Fu Lam, Hong Kong
Full list of author information is available at the end of the article

(Continued from previous page)

Conclusions: Routine HPV vaccination of 12-year-old females is highly likely to be cost-beneficial and cost-effective in Hong Kong. Inference of sexual mixing parameters from epidemiologic data of prevalent sexually transmitted diseases (i.e., HPV, chlamydia, etc.) is a potentially fruitful but largely untapped methodology for understanding sexual behaviors in the population.

Keywords: Human papillomavirus, Vaccination, Cervical cancer, Hong Kong, Cost-benefit analysis, Cost-effectiveness analysis, Mathematical model, Sexual mixing

Background

The cost-effectiveness of routine female adolescent human papillomavirus (HPV) vaccination and other strategies (e.g., vaccinating males as well) has been extensively studied for many high-income countries (e.g., the UK, Australia, Canada) as well as middle- and low-income countries (e.g., Malaysia, Brazil, Peru) [1]. The consensus among these studies is that routine female adolescent HPV vaccination is cost-effective. In contrast, very few studies have examined the corresponding cost-benefit, which is an important alternative criterion for health technology assessment because (1) in some jurisdictions, such as Hong Kong, health policymaking is based on cost-benefit instead of cost-effectiveness; (2) economists have suggested that cost-benefit analysis (CBA) is able to capture a wider range of the benefits of vaccination compared to cost-effectiveness analysis (CEA) [2]; and (3) CBA and CEA may lead to discordant conclusions regarding the economic favorability of health interventions due to different but equally sound methodologies and assumptions [3].

Despite the recent advent of a second-generation HPV vaccine (which targets nine HPV types that account for approximately 90% of cervical cancer worldwide [4]), Hong Kong and mainland China have not yet decided whether to include HPV vaccines in their routine immunization programs. The primary objective of this study is to provide a robust evidence base for HPV vaccination policy in the sentinel Chinese population of Hong Kong by performing both CBA and CEA of routine female adolescent nonavalent HPV vaccination for reducing cervical cancer burden using methodology that conforms with health technology assessments in this city. The health technology assessments framework for HPV vaccination in Hong Kong can serve as a reference for mainland China's public health policy on prevention of cervical cancer, which is the second-most common cancer in women aged below 45 in the country [5].

A key challenge in a rigorous evaluation of HPV vaccination programs is to adequately parameterize the HPV transmission model. To robustly evaluate the health impact of HPV vaccination, evidence-based HPV transmission models are needed to estimate the herd immunity effect [6]. Extensive research in recent years has identified assortativity of sexual mixing and the duration of naturally acquired immunity as two major sources of uncertainty in our understanding of HPV transmission dynamics [7–9]. Regarding sexual mixing, models for heterosexual transmission of HPV require specification on (1) heterogeneity in sexual activity levels (e.g., the number of sexual partners over the past year) within each age group and (2) assortativity of sexual mixing by age and sexual activity level (i.e., how differences in age and sexual activity level between two individuals affect their probability of forming a sexual partnership). Most populations, including Hong Kong, lack empirical data on point (2), in which case assortativity of sexual mixing is modeled by either extrapolating from the few populations with such data (e.g., a study for Austria used the sexual mixing data from the UK [10]) or by making hypothetical assumptions (e.g., [11]). Regarding natural immunity, although a recent meta-analysis suggested that natural recovery from HPV infection provides modest short-term protection against re-infection among females [9], the longevity of this effect remains unknown. To account for the uncertainty in assortativity of sexual mixing and natural immunity, we adopt the novel approach of Korostil et al. [8], who suggested that the underlying parameters could be inferred from HPV epidemiologic data during model parameterization. Consequently, as we evaluate the cost-benefit and cost-effectiveness of routine female adolescent nonavalent HPV vaccination for Hong Kong, we will also be simultaneously characterizing the underlying assortativity of heterosexual mixing, which in itself is an important knowledge gap on sexually transmitted infections.

Methods

Herein, we briefly describe the model structure. Please see the Additional file 1 for more details on the model.

Model overview

Our model comprises (1) a deterministic age-structured compartmental dynamic model for simulating heterosexual transmission of high-risk HPV (HR-HPV) and (2) a stochastic individual-based cohort model for simulating the development of cervical cancer over the lifetime of each female. This hybrid approach has been used in previous studies of HPV vaccination (e.g., [11]). We group HR-HPV into four classes: (1) HPV-16; (2) HPV-18; (3) HPV-OV (for 'other vaccine types'), which comprises the other five HR-HPV targeted by the nonavalent vaccine, namely HPV-31, 33, 45, 52, and 58; and (4) HPV-NV, which comprises all the non-vaccine HR-HPV. The dynamic model is used to estimate the model parameters and the herd immunity effect after routine female adolescent HPV vaccination has begun. The age-specific force of infection from the dynamic model is fed into the stochastic individual-based model to simulate cervical cancer incidence for each birth cohort. The cohort model explicitly simulates cervical screening, which cannot be accurately and easily performed with compartmental models because of the history-dependent nature of screening and treatment per the guidelines issued by the Hong Kong College of Obstetricians and Gynecologists [12]. The time step is 1 month in all simulations. The maximum age is 85 years for all individuals.

Natural history

Each individual enters the model at age 10 without any HPV infection (Additional file 1: Figure S1). After a female has been infected, she remains free of lesions for some time and then either clears the infection or progresses to cervical intraepithelial neoplasia (CIN1, 2, or 3). We assume that individuals with CIN3 do not recover naturally and will eventually progress to cervical cancer if untreated. The mean duration of natural immunity for HPV-16 and HPV-18 from HPV epidemiologic data are inferred during model parameterization (see below). HPV-OV and HPV-NV each comprise multiple HR-HPV that are unlikely to have significant cross-immunity [13]. As such, we assume no natural immunity for HPV-NV (i.e., individuals remain fully susceptible after clearance of infection). In contrast, to avoid overestimating the herd immunity effect conferred by vaccination [8], we allow natural immunity for HPV-OV and infer its mean duration during model parameterization. We assume that natural immunity provides 100% protection against reinfection of the same HPV class and that its duration is exponentially distributed. We model co-infections among the four HPV classes by assuming that disease progression of a given co-infection follows the progression rate of the most aggressive class therein, whereas class-specific clearance is unaffected by co-infections. We assume that the duration of HPV infection is the same among males and females [11]. When estimating the health burden associated with HPV, we consider only cervical cancer because Hong Kong does not have robust age-specific data on incidence of genital warts (more than 90% of which are caused by HPV-6 and HPV-11, against which the nonavalent vaccine is more than 90% efficacious) and other

forms of HPV-associated cancers (e.g., vulvar, penile). As such, our study will tend to underestimate the health and economic benefits of nonavalent HPV vaccination.

Sexual mixing

We stratify the population into two sexes ($g \in \{f, m\}$), 76 1-year age groups ($a = 10,11,12,...,85$), and three sexual activity levels ($s \in \{none, low, high\}$ that denote no, one, and multiple sexual partners during the past 6 months, respectively). Let $N_{g,a,u}(t)$ be the number of individuals in stratum (g, a, u) at time t, and $c_{g,a,u}$ be the rate at which these individuals form new sexual partnerships. The age-specific distribution of individuals with different sexual activity levels are based on the sexuality study results published by the Family Planning Association of Hong Kong (FPAHK) [14]; see Additional file 1 for details. We model assortativity of sexual mixing by age and sexual activity based on the formulation in Walker et al. [15]. Specifically, given that an individual in stratum (g, a, u) forms a sexual partnership at time t, the probability that their partner belongs to stratum (g', b, v), $g \neq g'$, is

$$\rho_{g,a,u,b,v}(t) = \varepsilon_A \varepsilon_S \, \Phi\left(\frac{a-b}{\sigma_g}\right) \delta_{uv}$$

$$\underbrace{}$$
assortative mixing for both
age and sexual activity level

$$+ \varepsilon_A(1-\varepsilon_S) \, \Phi\left(\frac{a-b}{\sigma_g}\right) \frac{c_{g',b,v} N_{g',b,v}(t)}{\sum_l c_{g',b,l} N_{g',b,l}(t)}$$

$$\underbrace{}$$
assortative mixing for age
proportionate mixing for sexual activity level

$$+ (1-\varepsilon_A)\varepsilon_S \, \frac{c_{g',b,v} N_{g',b,v}(t)}{\sum_k c_{g',b,k,v} N_{g',k,v}(t)} \delta_{uv}$$

$$\underbrace{}$$
proportionate mixing for age
assortative mixing for sexual activity level

$$+ (1-\varepsilon_A)(1-\varepsilon_S) \, \frac{c_{g',b,v} N_{g',b,v}(t)}{\sum_k \sum_l c_{g',k,l} N_{g',k,l}(t)}$$

$$\underbrace{}$$
proportionate mixing for both
age and sexual activity level

where δ_{uv} has value 1 when $u = v$ and 0 otherwise, and $\Phi(\cdot)$ is the Gaussian kernel. We use the Gaussian kernel to model age assortativity because its shape conforms with intuition as well as the patterns empirically observed in sexual activity surveys from the UK, Australia, and the US [16–18]. In this formulation, age assortativity is controlled by ε_A and σ_g whereas risk assortativity is controlled by ε_S. For simplicity, we assume that σ_g is the same for males and females.

Let $I_{g,a,u,h}(t)$ be the prevalence of HPV class h among individuals in stratum (g,a,u) at time t. The force of infection from HPV class h for individuals in stratum (g,a,u) at time t is

$$\lambda_{g,a,u,h}(t) = \sum_b \sum_v \left[\alpha_a \alpha_b \beta_h c^*_{g,a,u,b,v}(t) \rho_{g,a,u,b,v}(t) \frac{I_{g',b,v,h}(t)}{N_{g',b,v}(t)} \right]$$

where β_h is the class-specific baseline probability of transmission per sexual partnership, $c^*_{g,a,u,b,v}(t)$ is the adjusted contact rate between stratum (g,a,u) and (g',b,v) (see Additional file 1 for details), and

$$\alpha_a = \begin{cases} 1 & \text{if } a < W_1 \\ 1 + \dfrac{\mu-1}{W_2-W_1}(a-W_1) & \text{if } W_1 \le a \le W_2 \\ \mu & \text{if } a > W_2 \end{cases}$$

for modeling the effect of age on susceptibility and infectiousness (e.g., to reflect the age dependence of condom use, which increased from 26% in the 15–19 age group to 70% in the 18–27 age group according to the Youth Sexuality Study 2011 by the FPAHK [19]). The model assumes that susceptibility and infectiousness is (1) highest $(\alpha_a = 1)$ for individuals aged below W_1; (2) linearly decreases from 1 to μ as individuals age from W_1 to W_2; and (3) remains at $\alpha_a = \mu$ for individuals aged above W_2. The parameters μ, W_1, and W_2 are inferred during model parameterization.

Model parameterization
The following epidemiologic data were used to parameterize the model:

1. Age-specific prevalence of HR-HPV in Hong Kong as reported in two previous studies [20, 21].
2. Age-specific cervical cancer incidence in 1980–1984 as recorded by the Hong Kong Cancer Registry [22]. We choose this period to minimize the confounding effect of screening on cervical cancer incidence (there are no data on screening coverage in Hong Kong before 2000).
3. HR-HPV distribution among cervical cancer cases in Hong Kong hospitals during 1972–1973 and 1984–1986 [23].
4. The cumulative proportion of cases with disease progression and recovery for different stages of HPV infection from two overseas studies [24, 25]. Analogous data are not available in Hong Kong.

We infer the following model parameters by fitting the model to these data using Markov chain Monte Carlo methods with non-informative flat priors [7]: (1) class-specific progression and clearance rates for different stages of HPV infection; (2) the mean duration of

natural immunity for HPV-16, HPV-18, and HPV-OV; (3) baseline class-specific transmission probability per sexual partnership (β_h); (4) assortativity of sexual mixing $(\varepsilon_A, \sigma_g, \text{ and } \varepsilon_S)$; and (5) age-specific susceptibility and infectiousness $(\mu, W_1, \text{ and } W_2)$.

Routine HPV vaccination
We compare routine vaccination for girls at age 12 to opportunistic vaccination with status quo vaccine uptake (12% [26]). We assume that the nonavalent HPV vaccines are used in both routine HPV vaccination and status quo opportunistic vaccination and that full vaccination is provided by the two-dose regime recommended for individuals aged 9–14 years in Hong Kong [27]. Our previous survey suggested that approximately 40–50% of mothers in Hong Kong would consent to HPV vaccination for their adolescent daughters [28]. On the other hand, the uptake in the UK and Australia is 70–80%, which is the highest around the world [29, 30]. As such, we consider three scenarios of vaccine uptake for routine vaccination, namely 25%, 50%, and 75%. The class-specific vaccine efficacy is as follows [4, 31]: (1) 95.5% (95% confidence interval 90.0%–98.4%) for HPV-16; (2) 95.8% (84.1%–99.5%) for HPV-18; (3) 96.0% (94.4%–97.2%) for HPV-OV; and (4) 0% for HPV-NV. The latest clinical trial results showed that individuals who were vaccinated at age 9–15 years while they were still sexually naive remained seropositive (against vaccine-type HPV) after 10 years [32]. A modeling study used immunogenicity data to estimate that vaccine protection will likely persist for at least 20 years [33]. As such, we consider three possibilities, namely 20-year, 30-year, and lifelong protection.

Cervical cancer screening
We assume that vaccination does not affect screening behavior. The Cervical Screening Programme (CSP) in Hong Kong recommends women aged between 25 and 65 years to follow the 1-, 1-, 3-yearly cycle of cervical screening (i.e., screening annually for their first 2 years of screening and then triennially if their screening results remain negative) [27]. Based on the screening uptake data from the Behavioral Risk Factor Surveillance System surveys [27] and published literature [34, 35], we assume that screening uptake increased linearly from 40% in 1980 to 70% in 2004 when CSP was launched and remained at 70% thereafter. We assume that the sensitivity of cervical cytology at the threshold of atypical squamous cells of undetermined significance in detecting CIN2/3 and cervical cancer are 80% and 100%, respectively [36] (see Additional file 1 for details).

CBA and CEA
In the CBA, we used the human capital approach to monetize health and life-year loss into productivity

loss based on average personal income [37] (see Additional file 1 for details). In the CEA, we set the willingness-to-pay threshold for the incremental cost-effectiveness ratio (defined as the additional cost per each quality-adjusted life-year gained when comparing two interventions) at one local gross domestic product (GDP) per capita which is the lowest threshold used in cost-effectiveness studies of vaccination programs for Hong Kong [38]. The average GDP per capita in Hong Kong during 2012–2016 was US\$40,099 [39]. To assess the long-term impact of HPV vaccination, we estimated the changes in costs and health across the lifetimes of all female cohorts over a time horizon of 100 years. For example, at year 99, the incoming cohort will incur costs and benefits over its lifetime. The costs of screening and treatments were based on (1) charges for private patients in public hospitals, which account for over 90% of inpatient care in Hong Kong [40], and (2) expert opinions among local oncologists and gynecologists. Health utility parameters were based on overseas studies due to the lack of local data [41, 42]. Following the WHO guidelines, we discounted cost and health utility for women regardless of their ages after year 1 at 3% per annum [43]; the first age that discounting began was age 10 years. All cost figures were denominated in US dollars.

Cost of vaccination

We set the vaccine cost in the status quo scenario at US\$284 based on the price list in the FPAHK (which is a non-profit organization) [14] and the two-dose regime as recommended for individuals aged 9–14 years in Hong Kong [27]. Instead of explicitly modeling vaccine dose schedules and costs for routine HPV vaccination, we considered the cost required to fully vaccinate one girl (which includes the procurement, logistical, and administrative costs) as the outcome of our CBA and CEA. With this approach, we performed a head-to-head comparison between the CBA and CEA threshold vaccine cost, which was defined as the highest cost of vaccination at which the routine HPV vaccination program is cost-beneficial (i.e., the net monetary benefit is positive) and cost-effective (i.e., the incremental cost-effectiveness ratio is below the willingness-to-pay threshold), respectively. We denoted the CBA and CEA threshold vaccine cost by TVC_{CBA} and TVC_{CEA}, respectively.

Probabilistic sensitivity analysis

For each vaccination uptake and protection scenario, we considered 10,000 probabilistic sensitivity analysis scenarios which comprise all combinations of (i) 100 sets of transmission and natural history parameters randomly generated from their posterior distributions obtained from model parameterization (Additional file 1: Table S2); and (ii) 100 sets of vaccine efficacy, screening, cost,

and health utility parameters randomly generated from their plausible ranges shown in Additional file 1: Tables S3–S5 [4, 41, 42].

Results
Transmissibility and duration of natural immunity
The fitted model was largely congruent with the epidemiologic data used for model parameterization (Fig. 1). The baseline probability of transmission per partnership was 0.75 (95% credible interval 0.50–0.96), 0.88 (0.60–0.98), 0.93 (0.80–0.99), and 0.61 (0.50–0.71) for HPV-16, HPV-18, HPV-OV, and HPV-NV, respectively (Fig. 2a). The mean duration of natural immunity was 16 (3–83), 17 (4–75), and 0.7 (0.5–1.7) years for HPV-16, HPV-18, and HPV-OV, respectively (Fig. 2b). The inferred ephemeralness of natural immunity for HPV-OV was consistent with its multi-type nature (i.e., clearance of one type of HPV-OV will unlikely prevent infection by other types of HPV-OV). As individuals reach age 21 (16–24), their susceptibility and infectiousness began to fall gradually until they reached age 24 (21–27) (Fig. 2c). The total decrease in susceptibility and infectiousness over this period was 53% (47%–59%).

Assortativity of sexual mixing
Sexual mixing was highly assortative by both age (ε_A = 0.77 (0.29 – 0.99); σ_g = 2.1 (0.2 – 0.49)) and sexual activity level (ε_S = 0.98 (0.89 – 0.99)) (Fig. 2d, e). The inferred level of age assortativity in sexual mixing was comparable with that empirically observed in sexual surveys from the UK [44] and Australia [17]. In our fitted model, 74% (43%–97%) and 84% (60%–99%) of adult heterosexual partnerships had less than 5 and 10 years of age difference between the two partners, respectively.

Epidemiologic impact of routine female adolescent HPV vaccination
The prevalence of HPV-16, HPV-18, and HPV-OV decrease monotonically over time and reached a steady state 50–60 years after routine female vaccination began (Fig. 3a). This agrees with intuition because, in order for the routine vaccination program to confer maximal population-level benefit, all sexually active women in the population must have had the opportunity to receive the vaccine at age 12. Unsurprisingly, the prevalence of HPV-NV was constant over time because the nonavalent vaccine provides no protection against these HR-HPV types. Vaccine-type HR-HPV prevalence decreased with vaccine uptake as the latter increased from 10% to 90% with weak decreasing marginal return (Fig. 3b). Vaccine-type HR-HPV would have been eliminated if vaccine protection lasted for more than 30 years and routine vaccine uptake was higher than 90%. This result is consistent with the recent review of herd immunity threshold for HPV

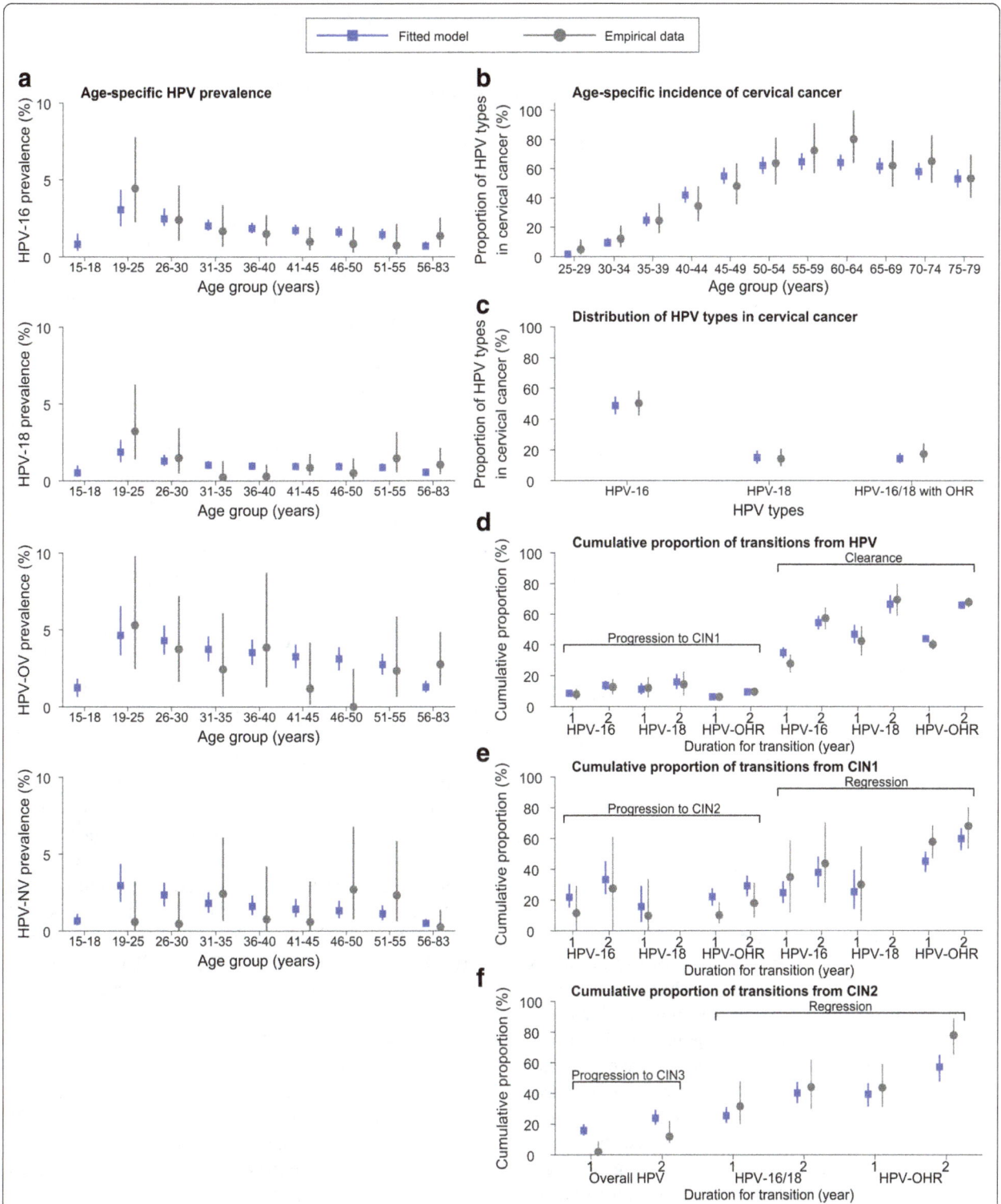

Fig. 1 Comparison of the empirical data and the fitted model. **a** Age-specific HPV prevalence. **b** Age-specific incidence of cervical cancer. **c** Distribution of HPV types in cervical cancer lesions. **d–f** Cumulative proportions of disease progression and clearance within 2 years for HPV infections without lesions, CIN1 and CIN2. Error bars indicate the 95% credible intervals for the fitted model and 95% confidence intervals for the data

vaccination [6, 45]. The decrease in age-standardized incidence of cervical cancer during the first 20 years is not caused by vaccination but instead attributed to increased screening uptake in Hong Kong since CSP was launched in 2004 (Fig. 3c; see Additional file 1 for details of cervical screening in Hong Kong). Because HPV infections take at

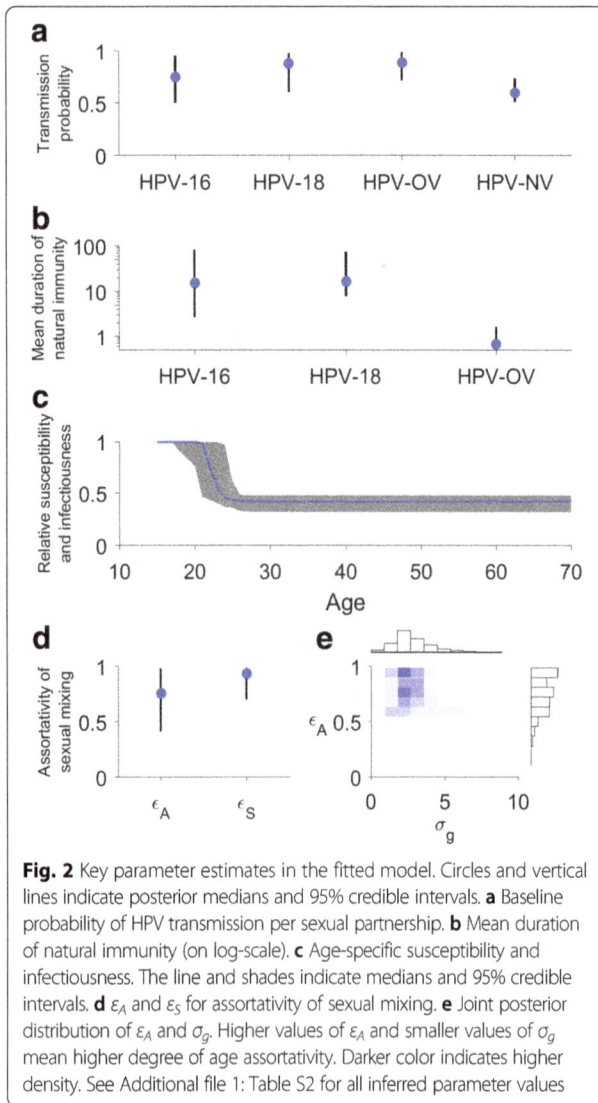

Fig. 2 Key parameter estimates in the fitted model. Circles and vertical lines indicate posterior medians and 95% credible intervals. **a** Baseline probability of HPV transmission per sexual partnership. **b** Mean duration of natural immunity (on log-scale). **c** Age-specific susceptibility and infectiousness. The line and shades indicate medians and 95% credible intervals. **d** ε_A and ε_S for assortativity of sexual mixing. **e** Joint posterior distribution of ε_A and σ_g. Higher values of ε_A and smaller values of σ_g mean higher degree of age assortativity. Darker color indicates higher density. See Additional file 1: Table S2 for all inferred parameter values

decreased (Fig. 4a). As vaccine uptake increased, TVC_{CBA} decreased but TVC_{CEA} increased with $TVC_{CBA} > TVC_{CEA}$ across all scenarios considered: TVC_{CBA} was lower than TVC_{CEA} by approximately 13%, 30%, and 36% when vaccine uptake was 25%, 50%, and 75%, respectively (Fig. 4a). When the vaccine provided only 20 years of protection and vaccine uptake was 75% (i.e., the scenario under which TVC_{CBA} was the lowest), the total cost for fully vaccinating one girl would need to be less than US$444 ($373–506) and $689 ($646–734) for routine HPV vaccination to be cost-beneficial and cost-effective, respectively. Compared to this scenario, TVC_{CBA} (TVC_{CEA}) increased by 2.3% (3.9%) if vaccine protection duration increased to 30 years or longer. If vaccine uptake decreased from 75% to 50%, TVC_{CBA} increased by 6.6% whereas TVC_{CEA} decreased by 2.3%. For TVC_{CBA} and TVC_{CEA} to be similar, the willingness-to-pay threshold would need to be approximately US$30,000 for vaccine uptake at 25% and US$20,000 for vaccine uptake at 75% (Fig. 4b).

Discussion

Main conclusions and their implications

We have evaluated the cost-benefit and cost-effectiveness of routine female adolescent nonavalent HPV vaccination for reducing cervical cancer burden in Hong Kong. Our results suggest that, at a vaccine uptake of between 25% and 75%, routine vaccination for 12-year-old girls (i.e., regardless of their sexual activity characteristics) as part of a centrally funded program represents good value for money if the cost of fully vaccinating one girl is no greater than US$444 ($373–506) and $689 ($646–734), respectively. The current market price of fully vaccinating one girl at age 12 at the FPAHK (as of November 2017) is $284, and the tender prices for bulk purchases in Italy, Norway, South Africa, and Spain were 66–77% lower than market prices [46]. Thus, we believe that the tender price of a centrally procured HPV vaccine in Hong Kong is likely to be well below the lower limit of our most conservative TVC estimate ($373) and thus provide the basis for a routine female adolescent HPV vaccination program that is both cost-beneficial and cost-effective.

Furthermore, because of the lack of local data, our analysis did not examine many of the benefits of HPV vaccination such as protection against anogenital warts, recurrent respiratory papillomatoses, or vulvar, vaginal, penile, anal, and oropharyngeal cancers. The value of protection against these non-cervical cancers has been estimated to be almost as great as the value of protecting against cervical cancers in some scenarios [47]. Further, our CBA is based on human capital calculations, valuing health in terms of a woman's productive capacity, and does not capture the additional value that people put on averting suffering due to disease. If these considerations

least 20 years to progress into malignancy in most cases of cervical cancer, the differential impact of vaccine uptake between status quo and routine vaccination on cervical cancer incidence would not be apparent until 20 years after routine vaccination had begun. Population-level benefit of routine vaccination on cancer incidence reached steady state 70–80 years after routine vaccination began. Compared to status quo opportunistic vaccination, routine vaccination with 25%, 50%, and 75% uptake further reduced the age-standardized cervical cancer incidence in year 100 by 21%, 57%, and 85%, respectively, with lifelong vaccine-induced protection, and by 19%, 51%, and 78%, respectively, with 20-year protection.

Comparative threshold vaccine costs (TVC) between CBA and CEA

As expected, the TVC decreased (i.e., became economically more stringent) as the duration of vaccine protection

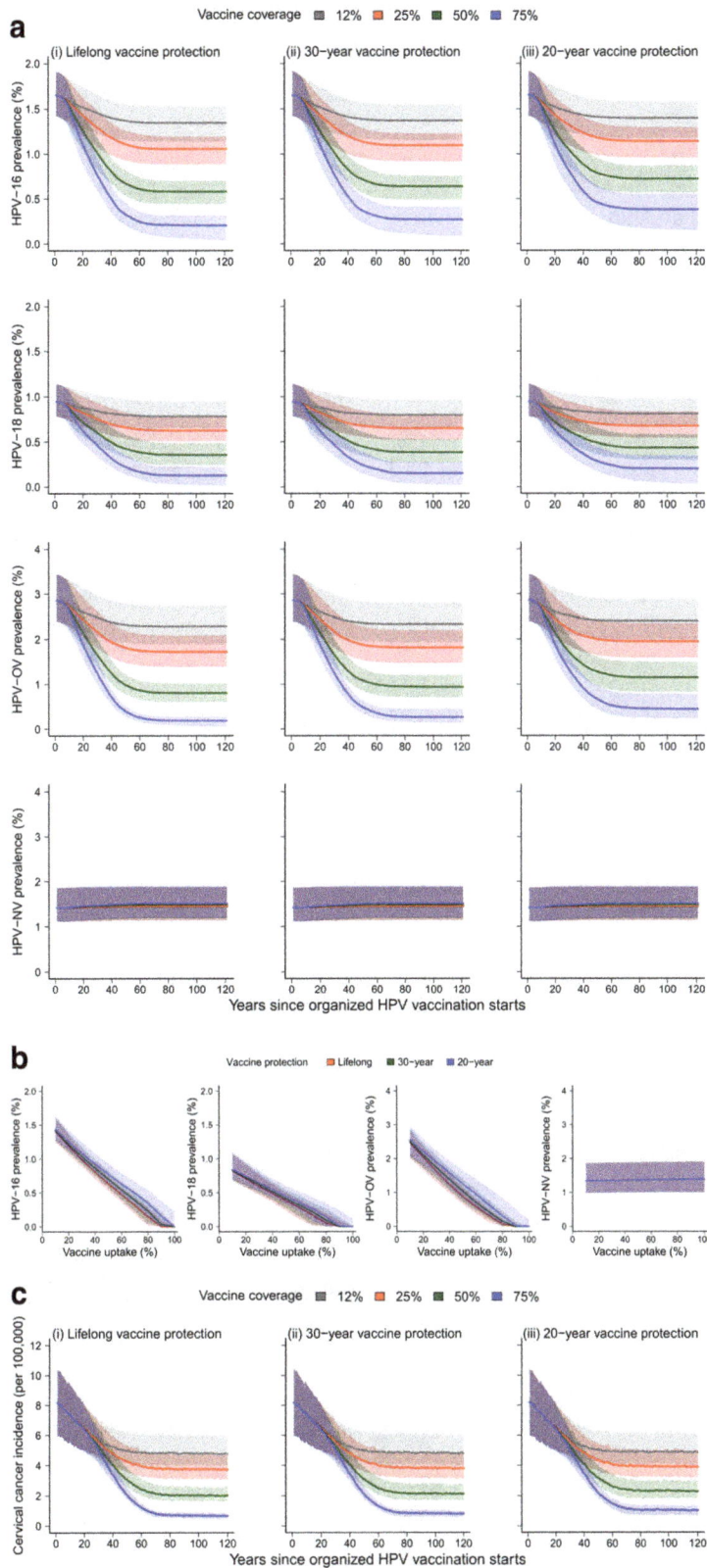

Fig. 3 (See legend on next page.)

(See figure on previous page.)
Fig. 3 Epidemiologic impact of routine female adolescent HPV vaccination. The curves and shades indicate the medians and 95% central ranges of the outcomes across all 100 probabilistic sensitivity analysis scenarios on natural history parameters, respectively. **a** Age-standardized HPV prevalence over time. **b** Age-standardized HPV prevalence after 100 years of routine vaccination as a function of vaccine uptake. **c** Age-standardized incidence of cervical cancer over time

are taken into account, then the TVC for the CBA is likely to be even greater than that for the CEA. Therefore, it is almost certain that centrally funded routine HPV vaccination for 12-year-old girls will be both cost-beneficial and cost-effective in Hong Kong.

To our knowledge, our study is the first to compare the CBA and CEA implications of HPV vaccination. For Hong Kong, the CBA threshold vaccine cost is always lower (i.e., economically more stringent) than its CEA counterpart, i.e., $TVC_{CBA}/TVC_{CEA} < 1$. The generalizability of this finding to other populations hinges on two other factors. The first factor is that CBAs in Hong Kong consider only changes in economic productivity (and not individual willingness-to-pay to avoid premature death as in the US or UK). Intuitively, TVC_{CBA}/TVC_{CEA} increases with the ratio of average personal income to willingness-to-pay threshold. The second factor is the age distribution of cervical cancer in relation to retirement age and life expectancy. HPV vaccination will be (1) more cost-beneficial if the gap between the average age of cervical cancer cases and retirement age increases; and (2) more cost-effective if the gap between the average age of cervical cancer and life expectancy increases. Consider an illustrative comparison among Hong Kong, the US (with one GDP per capita as the willingness-to-pay threshold, i.e., approximately $58,000), and the UK (with £20,000–30,000 as the willingness-to-pay threshold). The ratio of average personal income to willingness-to-pay threshold is approximately 0.5 for Hong Kong, 0.72 for the US, and > 0.7 for the UK. On the other hand, the median age of cervical

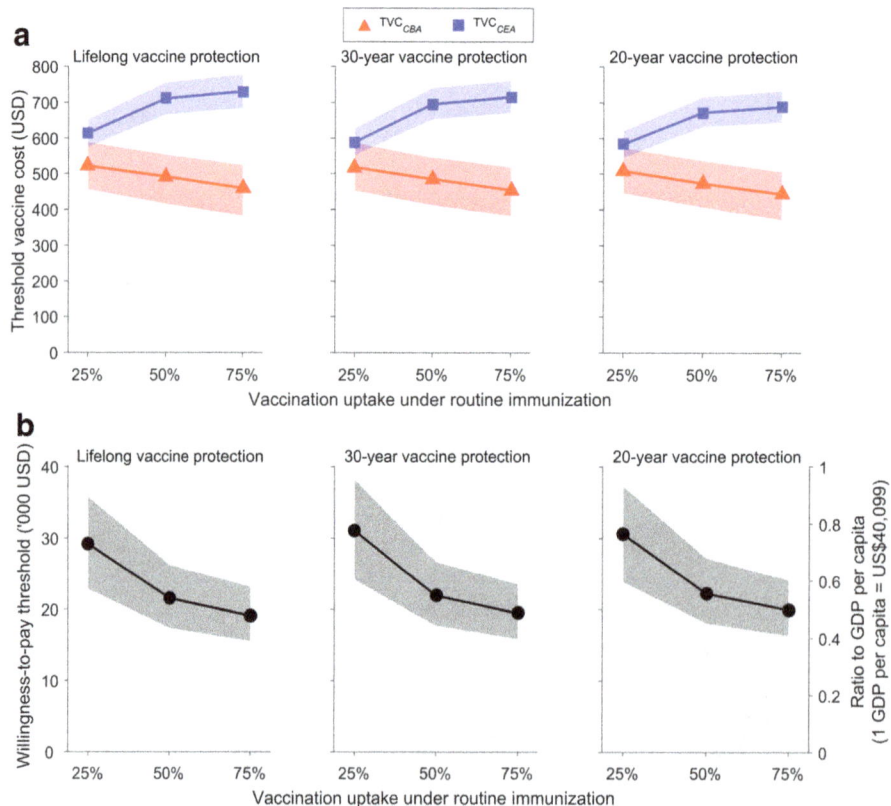

Fig. 4 Comparative threshold vaccine cost between cost-benefit analysis and cost-effectiveness analysis. The curves and shades indicate the medians and 95% central ranges of the outcomes, respectively, across all 10,000 probabilistic sensitivity analysis combinations of natural history and health economic parameter values. The outcomes at 25%, 50%, and 75% vaccine uptake are used to estimate the outcomes at other vaccine uptake levels using linear interpolation. **a** Threshold vaccine cost, i.e., the maximum cost for vaccination at which routine vaccination of girls at age 12 is cost-beneficial (TVC_{CBA}) and cost-effective (TVC_{CEA}) compared to status quo vaccine uptake (12%) at the current market price (US$284 for the two-dose schedule). **b** The willingness-to-pay threshold at which $TVC_{CBA} = TVC_{CEA}$. The GDP per capita in Hong Kong is US$40,099

cancer diagnosis is 45 in the UK, 49 in the US, and 52 in Hong Kong, whereas the female life expectancy is 82, 79, and 87, respectively. The retirement age in these populations are similar. Applying the rationale above, the difference between TVC_{CBA} and TVC_{CEA} is likely to be significantly smaller for the US and UK compared to Hong Kong, and thus CBA and CEA will likely result in similar conclusions on the health economics of HPV vaccination in the US and UK.

Comparison to other studies

A recently published review of cost-effectiveness studies of HPV vaccination [48], together with a more updated literature search, generated seven CEAs of nonavalent HPV vaccination in high-income countries [10, 49–54] and two for low- and middle-income countries [55, 56]. Most of these studies focused on switching from the use of either the bivalent or quadrivalent vaccines to nonavalent vaccine in existing vaccination programs [10, 49, 50, 52–54], while one study examined providing additional nonavalent vaccines to females who have already received three doses of quadrivalent vaccine [51]. Thus, they all differed from our study, which focused on comparing a scenario of an organized program using nonavalent vaccination at high coverage to an existing opportunistic program also using nonavalent vaccination.

Despite the different model scenarios, some results from previous studies can be compared with ours. We estimate that the female-only organized HPV vaccination with 75% vaccine uptake and lifelong vaccine protection would reduce cervical cancer incidence by 85% compared to 12% opportunistic vaccine uptake. In the CEAs for high-income countries, the additional reduction in cervical cancer for routine vaccination compared to no vaccination (which is the most similar scenario to the opportunistic vaccination scenario in our study) ranged between 70% and 92%, depending on vaccine uptake of females and males [10, 49, 50, 52, 54].

Although not explicitly stated, the TVC of nonavalent HPV vaccines for routine vaccination compared to no vaccination can be estimated from two previous studies where sufficient detail about the overall cost of vaccination is reported [52, 53]. In the Canadian CEA [53], the derived TVC for vaccination of 12-year-old females with a three-dose nonavalent vaccine schedule (as considered in the study) compared to no vaccination was estimated to be US$798. The estimation was based on a willingness-to-pay threshold of US$38,000 (CAD$40,000) per QALY gained, with a healthcare payer perspective, 80% female vaccination coverage, and 20-year duration of vaccine-induced protection. In another CEA for vaccinating both sexes in the US with a three-dose nonavalent vaccine schedule [52], the estimated TVC was US$959, using a willingness-to-pay threshold of US$50,000, a societal

perspective, lifelong vaccine protection, and vaccine uptake of 46% and 29% among females and males aged 13–17 years, respectively. Given current opportunistic vaccine uptake of 12% [26] and assuming that the nonavalent vaccine is used for both organized and opportunistic vaccination, our study estimates that the TVC for organized female vaccination is US$689 at a willingness-to-pay threshold of US$40,099 per QALY gain, societal perspective, two-dose regimen, 75% vaccine coverage, and 20-year duration of vaccine-induced protection. The slightly lower TVC in our study is probably because (1) we did not consider non-cervical diseases in our study; (2) the opportunistic program that we considered already generates some herd protection so less benefit is expected from an organized program; and (3) we assumed only 20-year duration of vaccine protection.

Strengths and limitations of the study

Our study has several other important limitations. First, we assumed that the duration and transmissibility of HPV infection are the same for males and females. While some evidence from other settings suggests that this is not generally true [9], Hong Kong does not have the necessary data (e.g., HPV prevalence or seroprevalence among males) for us to account for such heterogeneity. Second, we have not considered potential changes to cervical cancer screening (cytology is the most common primary screening method) and coverage after routine HPV vaccination begins. Depending on vaccine uptake, screening guidelines may be updated accordingly to optimize the cost-effectiveness and/or cost-benefit of screening [57]. Moreover, the use of primary HPV testing for cervical cancer screening will likely improve the positive predictive value of screening when the uptake of HPV vaccination is high [49]. Third, for model parsimony, we have assumed that assortativity in sexual mixing is the same for both sexes, which may not be accurate. Fourth, the health utility parameters in this study are based on studies from other settings that may not accurately reflect the situation in Hong Kong. Fifth, because there is no evidence on the societal willingness-to-pay threshold for cervical cancer in Hong Kong, we used one GDP per capita, which is the lowest willingness-to-pay threshold used by all the vaccination CEA studies in Hong Kong reviewed in Wong et al. [38]. The TVC from a CEA would be lower if the willingness-to-pay threshold is lower than that assumed here. Sixth, our CBA relies on valuing avoided morbidity and mortality using human capital calculations. The CBA threshold vaccine cost might be different if other methods are used (e.g., friction cost method [58] or approaches based on value of statistical life years [59]). Finally, the validity of the inferred parameters is limited by the data available for model parameterization and the associated assumptions imposed for fitting the model to these data. For example, transitions between CIN grades are based on data with 2-year follow-up periods and assumed to be Markovian, which might be inaccurate (e.g., we assume that a lesion is equally likely to clear regardless of how long it has persisted within the same CIN1 or CIN2 grade).

A major strength of our study is that, as we evaluate the health economics of HPV vaccination, we simultaneously characterize sexual mixing in Hong Kong by fitting the transmission model to epidemiological data [60]. The resulting parameter estimates suggest that sexual mixing in Hong Kong is, as would be anticipated, highly assortative by both age and sexual activity level. The level of age assortativity inferred in our study is comparable to that reported in sexual surveys from the UK and Australia, which lends support to the validity of our estimates. Given the substantial costs of sexual surveys and the difficulty of eliciting truthful responses on sexual behaviors, inference of sexual mixing parameters from epidemiologic data of sexually transmitted diseases (including HPV, chlamydia, etc.) is a potentially fruitful but underused methodology for understanding sexual behaviors in the population. Our study provides a first step in this direction.

The Greater Bay Area (GBA) Initiative in the 13th 5-year plan (2016–2020) of China aims to link the cities of Hong Kong, Macau, Guangzhou, Shenzhen, Zhuhai, Foshan, Zhongshan, Dongguan, Huizhou, Jiangmen, and Zhaoqing into an integrated economic, business, and technology hub that constitutes an area of 56,000 km^2, a combined population of 68 million, and an economy of $1.51 trillion. Given the low uptake of HPV vaccination and cervical cancer screening and the high burden of cervical cancer in these cities, prevention of cervical cancer will likely be a top-priority public health issue in the GBA Initiative. Over the next decade, demographics, sexual mixing, and disease transmission in these heterogeneous cities will be substantially impacted by the massive increase in short- and long-term human mobility and interaction brought about by the GBA Initiative. A recent study showed that interstate migration has a strong impact on the population-level benefit of HPV vaccination in the US because of herd immunity and the long duration between HPV infection and resultant cervical cancer [61]. As such, the GBA cities will need to coordinate their evaluations and policies to maximize the benefit of their HPV vaccination programs. Our study for Hong Kong provides a robust basis for the development of such a cooperative framework.

Conclusions

Routine HPV vaccination of 12-year-old females is highly likely to be cost-beneficial and cost-effective in Hong Kong. Inference of sexual mixing parameters from epidemiologic data of prevalent sexually transmitted diseases (i.e., HPV, chlamydia, etc.) is a potentially fruitful but largely untapped methodology for understanding sexual behaviors in the population.

Abbreviations

CBA: cost-benefit analysis; CEA: cost-effectiveness analysis; CIN: cervical intraepithelial neoplasia; CSP: cervical screening programme; FPAHK: The Family Planning Association of Hong Kong; GBA: Greater Bay Area; GDP: gross domestic product; HPV: human papillomavirus; HPV-NV: HPV non-vaccine HR-HPV; HPV-OV: HPV other vaccine types; HR-HPV: high-risk HPV; TVC: threshold vaccine cost

Acknowledgements

We thank Hextan YS Ngan, Karen KL Chan, Victor HF Lee, and Pauline PS Woo for their valuable discussion in the cost evaluation on cervical screening and cervical cancer treatment in Hong Kong. The computations were performed using research computing facilities offered by Information Technology Services, the University of Hong Kong. This work formed part of the dissertation requirement for HCWC's doctoral studies at the University of Hong Kong.

Funding

This study was supported by a commissioned grant from the Health and Medical Research Fund from the Government of the Hong Kong Special Administrative Region (HKS-15-E04 and HKS-17-E12) and Award Number U54GM088558 from the National Institute of General Medical Sciences. The content is solely the responsibility of the authors and does not necessarily represent the official views of the National Institute of General Medical Sciences or the National Institutes of Health. HCWC received financial support from the Graduate School, University of Hong Kong.

Authors' contributions

GML and JTW conceived the study design. HCWC performed the literature search, model simulation, data analysis, and figure preparation. HCWC, MJ, GML, KLT, and JTW were substantilly involved in data interpretation. HCWC, MJ, GML, and JTW wrote the manuscript. All authors approved the final reversion. HCWC and JTW contributed equally to this research.

Competing interests

The authors declare that they have no competing interests.

Author details

[1]WHO Collaborating Centre for Infectious Disease Epidemiology and Control, School of Public Health, Li Ka Shing Faculty of Medicine, The University of Hong Kong, 1/F North Wing, Patrick Manson Building, 7 Sassoon Road, Pok Fu Lam, Hong Kong. [2]Department of Systems Engineering and Engineering Management, City University of Hong Kong, Kowloon Tong, Hong Kong. [3]Department of Clinical Oncology, Li Ka Shing Faculty of Medicine, The University of Hong Kong, Pok Fu Lam, Hong Kong. [4]Modelling and Economics Unit, Public Health England, London, UK. [5]Department of Infectious Disease Epidemiology, London School of Hygiene and Tropical Medicine, London, UK.

References

1. Pink J, Parker B, Petrou S. Cost effectiveness of HPV vaccination: a systematic review of modelling approaches. Pharmacoeconomics. 2016;34(9):847–61.
2. Bloom DE. Valuing vaccines: deficiencies and remedies. Vaccine. 2015; 33(Suppl 2):B29–33.

3. Brisson M, Edmunds WJ. Impact of model, methodological, and parameter uncertainty in the economic analysis of vaccination programs. Med Decis Mak. 2006;26(5):434–46.

4. Joura EA, Giuliano AR, Iversen O-E, Bouchard C, Mao C, Mehlsen J, Moreira ED Jr, Ngan Y, Petersen LK, Lazcano-Ponce E, et al. A 9-valent HPV vaccine against infection and intraepithelial neoplasia in women. N Engl J Med. 2015;372(8):711–23.

5. Chen W, Zheng R, Baade PD, Zhang S, Zeng H, Bray F, Jemal A, Yu XQ, He J. Cancer statistics in China, 2015. CA Cancer J Clin. 2016;66(2):115–32.

6. Drolet M, Benard E, Boily M-C, Ali H, Baandrup L, Bauer H, Beddows S, Brisson J, Brotherton JML, Cummings T, et al. Population-level impact and herd effects following human papillomavirus vaccination programmes: a systematic review and meta-analysis. Lancet Infect Dis. 2015;15(5):565–80.

7. Korostil IA, Peters GW, Cornebise J, Regan DG. Adaptive Markov chain Monte Carlo forward simulation for statistical analysis in epidemic modelling of human papillomavirus. Stat Med. 2013;32(11):1917–53.

8. Korostil IA, Peters GW, Law MG, Regan DG. Herd immunity effect of the HPV vaccination program in Australia under different assumptions regarding natural immunity against re-infection. Vaccine. 2013;31(15):1931–6.

9. Beachler DC, Jenkins G, Safaeian M, Kreimer AR, Wentzensen N. Natural acquired immunity against subsequent genital human papillomavirus infection: a systematic review and meta-analysis. J Infect Dis. 2016;213(9):1444–54.

10. Boiron L, Joura E, Largeron N, Prager B, Uhart M. Estimating the cost-effectiveness profile of a universal vaccination programme with a nine-valent HPV vaccine in Austria. BMC Infect Dis. 2016;16:153.

11. Kim JJ, Goldie SJ. Health and economic implications of HPV vaccination in the United States. N Engl J Med. 2008;259(8):821–32.

12. The Hong Kong College of Obstetricians and Gynaecologists. Guidelines on the Management of Abnormal Cervical Cytology. Hong Kong: The Hong Kong College of Obstetricians and Gynaecologists; 2008.

13. Van de Velde N, Brisson M, Boily M-C. Modeling human papillomavirus vaccine effectiveness: quantifying the impact of parameter uncertainty. Am J Epidemiol. 2007;165(7):762–75.

14. The Family Planning Association of Hong Kong. https://www.famplan.org.hk/. Accessed 20 Mar 2018.

15. Walker R, Nickson C, Lew J-B, Smith M, Canfell K. A revision of sexual mixing matrices in models of sexually transmitted infection. Stat Med. 2012;31(27):3419–32.

16. Mercer CH, Copas AJ, Sonnenberg P, Johnson AM, McManus S, Erens B, Cassell JA. Who has sex with whom? Characteristics of heterosexual partnerships reported in a national probability survey and implications for STI risk. Int J Epidemiol. 2009;38(1):206–14.

17. Badcock PB, Smith AMA, Richters J, Rissel C, de Visser RO, Simpson JM, Grulich AE. Characteristics of heterosexual regular relationships among a representative sample of adults: the second Australian study of health and relationships. Sex Health. 2014;11(5):427–38.

18. Mosher WD, Chandra A, Jones J. Sexual behavior and selected health measures: men and women 15-44 years of age, United States, 2002. Adv Data. 2005;(362):1–55.

19. The Family Planning Association of Hong Kong. Youth Sexuality Study 2011. Hong Kong: The Family Planning Association of Hong Kong; 2014. https://www.famplan.org.hk/en/products/detail/P83.

20. Chan PKS, Ho WCS, Wong MCS, Chang AR, Chor JSY, Yu M-Y. Epidemiologic risk profile of infection with different groups of human papillomaviruses. J Med Virol. 2009;81:1635–44.

21. Liu SS, Chan KYK, Leung RCY, Chan KKL, Tam KF, Luk MHM, Lo SST, Fong DYT, Cheung ANY, Lin ZQ, et al. Prevalence and risk factors of human papillomavirus (HPV) infection in southern Chinese women - a population-based study. PLoS One. 2011;6(5):e19244.

22. Hong Kong Cancer Registry. http://www3.ha.org.hk/cancereg/. Accessed 3 Mar 2016.

23. Chan PKS, Ho WCS, Yu M-Y, Pong W-M, Chan ACL, Chan AKC, Cheung T-H, Wong MCS, To K-F, Ng H-K. Distribution of human papillomavirus types in cervical cancers in Hong Kong: current situation and changes over the last decades. Int J Cancer. 2009;125(7):1671–7.

24. Insinga RP, Perez G, Wheeler CM, Koutsky LA, Garland SM, Leodolter S, Joura EA, Ferris DG, Steben M, Hernandez-Avila M, et al. Incident cervical HPV infections in young women: transition probabilities for CIN and infection clearance. Cancer Epidemiol Biomarker Prev. 2011;20(2):287–96.

25. Moscicki A-B, Ma Y, Wibbelsman C, Darragh TM, Powers A, Farhat S, Shiboski S. Rate of and risks for regression of cervical intraepithelial neoplasia 2 in adolescents and young women. Obstet Gynecol. 2010;116:1373–80.

26. The Family Planning Association of Hong Kong Youth Sexuality Study 2016. https://www.famplan.org.hk/en/media-centre/press-releases/detail/fpahk-report-on-youth-sexuality-study. Accessed 4 Dec 2017.

27. Cervical Screening Programme, Department of Health. https://www.cervicalscreening.gov.hk/eindex.php. Accessed 6 Jan 2016.

28. Choi HCW, Leung GM, Woo PPS, Jit M, Wu JT. Acceptability and uptake of female adolescent HPV vaccination in Hong Kong: a survey of mothers and adolescents. Vaccine. 2013;32(1):78–84.

29. Public Health England. Vaccine Uptake Guidance and the Latest Coverage Data. https://www.gov.uk/government/collections/vaccine-uptake. Accessed 28 Jun 2016.

30. National HPV Vaccination Program Register. http://www.hpvregister.org.au/Default.aspx. Accessed 28 Jun 2016.

31. Malagon T, Drolet M, Boily M-C, Franco EL, Jit M, Brisson J, Brisson M. Cross-protective efficacy of two human papillomavirus vaccines: a systematic review and meta-analysis. Lancet Infect Dis. 2012;12(10):781–9.

32. Ferris DG, Samakoses R, Block SL, Lazcano-Ponce E, Restrepo JA, Mehlsen J, Chatterjee A, Iversen O-E, Joshi A, Chu J-L, et al. 4-valent human papillomavirus (4vHPV) vaccine in preadolescents and adolescents after 10 years. Pediatrics. 2017;140(6):e20163947.

33. Fraser C, Tomassini JE, Xi L, Golm G, Watson M, Giuliano AR, Barr E, Ault KA. Modeling the long-term antibody response of a human papillomavirus (HPV) virus-like particle (VLP) type 16 prophylactic vaccine. Vaccine. 2007;25:4324–33.

34. Leung GM, Woo PPS, Cowling BJ, Tsang CSH, Cheung ANY, Ngan HYS, Galbraith K, Lam T-H. Who receives, benefits from and is harmed by cervical and breast cancer screening among Hong Kong Chinese? J Public Health. 2008;30(3):282–92.

35. Wu JT. Cervical cancer prevention through cytologic and human papillomavirus DNA screening in Hong Kong Chinese women. Hong Kong Med J. 2011;17(Suppl 3):S20–4.

36. Kim JJ, Wright TC, Goldie SJ. Cost-effectiveness of alternative triage strategies for atypical squamous cells of undetermined significance. JAMA. 2002;287(18):2382–90.

37. Hutton G, Rehfuess E. Guidelines for Conducting Cost-Benefit Analysis of Household Energy and Health Interventions. Geneva: WHO Press; 2006.

38. Wong CKH, Liao Q, Guo VYW, Xin Y, Lam CLK. Cost-effectiveness analysis of vaccinations and decision makings on vaccination programmes in Hong Kong: a systematic review. Vaccine. 2017;35(24):3153–61.

39. Census and Statistics Department. Table 30: Gross domestic product (GDP), implicit price deflator of GDP and per capita GDP. https://www.censtatd.gov.hk/hkstat/sub/sp250.jsp?subjectID=250&tableID=030&ID=0&productType=8. Accessed 3 Feb 2017.

40. Census and Statistics Department. 2011 Population Census. https://www.census2011.gov.hk/en/index.html. Accessed 5 Oct 2012.

41. Insinga RP, Glass AG, Myers ER, Rush BB. Abnormal outcomes following cervical cancer screening: event duration and health utility loss. Med Decis Mak. 2007;27(4):414–22.

42. Gold MR, Franks P, McCoy KI, Fryback DG. Toward consistency in cost-utility analyses: using national measures to create condition-specific values. Med Care. 1998;36(6):778–92.

43. World Health Organization. Making choices in health: WHO guide to cost-effectiveness analysis. In: Tan-Torres Edejer T, Baltussen RMPM, Adam T, Hutubessy R, Acharya A, Evans DB, Murray CJL, editors. . Geneva: WHO; 2003.

44. Prah P, Copas AJ, Mercer CH, Nardone A, Johnson AM. Patterns of sexual mixing with respect to social, health and sexual characteristics among heterosexual couples in England: analyses of probability sample survey data. Epidemiol Infect. 2015;173(7):1500–10.

45. Brisson M, Benard E, Drolet M, Bogaards JA, Baussano I, Vanska S, Jit M, Boily MC, Smith MA, Berkhof J, et al. Population-level impact, herd immunity, and elimination after human papillomavirus vaccination: a systematic review and meta-analysis of predictions from transmission-dynamic models. Lancet Public Health. 2016;1(1):e8–e17.

46. Herlihy N, Hutubessy R, Jit M. Current global pricing for HPV vacc brings the greatest econ benefits to rich countries. Health Aff. 2015;35(2):227–34.

47. Jit M, Chapman R, Hughes O, Choi YH. Comparing bivalent and quadrivalent human papillomavirus vaccines: economic evaluation based on transmission model. Br Med J. 2011;343:d5775.

48. Ng SS, Hutubessy R, Chaiyakunapruk N. Systematic review of cost-effectiveness studies of human papillomavirus (HPV) vaccination: 9-valent vaccine, gender-neutral and multiple age cohort vaccination. Vaccine. 2018; 36(19):2529–44.

49. Simms KT, Laprise J-F, Smith MA, Lew J-B, Caruana M, Brisson M, Canfell K. Cost-effectiveness of the next generation nonavalent human papillomavirus vaccine in the context of primary human papillomavirus screening in Australia: a comparative modelling analysis. Lancet Public Health. 2016;1(2):e66–75.

50. Brisson M, Laprise J-F, Chesson HW, Drolet M, Malagon T, Boily M-C, Markowitz LE. Health and economic impact of switching from a 4-valent to a 9-valent HPV vaccination program in the United States. J Natl Cancer Inst. 2016;108(1):djv282.

51. Chesson HW, Laprise J-F, Brisson M, Markowitz LE. Impact and cost-effectiveness of 3 doses of 9-valent human papillomavirus (HPV) vaccine among US females previously vaccinated with 4-valent HPV vaccine. J Infect Dis. 2016;213(11):1694–700.

52. Chesson HW, Markowitz LE, Hariri S, Ekwueme DU, Saraiya M. The impact and cost-effectiveness of nonavalent HPV vaccination in the United States: estimates from a simplified transmission model. Hum Vaccin Immunother. 2016;12(6):1363–72.

53. Drolet M, Laprise J-F, Boily M-C, Franco EL, Brisson M. Potential cost-effectiveness of the nonavalent human papillomavirus (HPV) vaccine. Int J Cancer. 2014;134(9):2264–8.

54. Largeron N, Petry KU, Jacob J, Bianic F, Anger D, Uhart M. An estimate of the public health impact and cost-effectiveness of universal vaccination with a 9-valent HPV vaccine in Germany. Expert Rev Pharmacoecon Outcomes Res. 2016;17(1):85–98.

55. Kiatpongsan S, Kim JJ. Costs and cost-effectiveness of 9-valent human papillomavirus (HPV) vaccination in two east African countries. PLoS One. 2014;9(9):e106836.

56. Mo X, Tobe RG, Wang L, Liu X, Wu B, Luo H, Nagata C, Mori R, Nakayama T. Cost-effectiveness analysis of different types of human papillomavirus vaccination combined with a cervical cancer screening program in mainland China. BMC Infect Dis. 2017;17:502.

57. Beer H, Hibbitts S, Brophy S, Rahman MA, Waller J, Paranjothy S. Does the HPV vaccination programme have implications for cervical screening programmes in the UK? Vaccine. 2014;32(16):1828–33.

58. Koopmanschap MA, Rutten FF, van Ineveld BM, van Roijen L. The friction cost method for measuring indirect costs of disease. J Health Econ. 1995; 14(2):171–89.

59. Laxminarayan R, Jamison DT, Krupnick AJ, Norheim OF. Valuing vaccines using value of statistical life measures. Vaccine. 2014;32(39):5065–70.

60. Mercer CH, Tanton C, Prah P, Erens B, Sonnenberg P, Clifton S, Macdowall W, Lewis R, Field N, Datta J, et al. Changes in sexual attitudes and lifestyles in Britain through the life course and over time: findings from the National Surveys of sexual attitudes and lifestyles (Natsal). Lancet. 2013;382(9907): 1781–94.

61. Durham DP, Ndeffo-Mbah ML, Skrip LA, Jones FK, Bauch CT, Galvani AP. National- and state-level impact and cost-effectiveness of nonavalent HPV vaccination in the United States. Proc Natl Acad Sci U S A. 2016;113(18): 5107–12.

9

Adult height and risk of 50 diseases: a combined epidemiological and genetic analysis

Florence Y. Lai[1,2], Mintu Nath[1,2], Stephen E. Hamby[1,2], John R. Thompson[1,3], Christopher P. Nelson[1,2] and Nilesh J. Samani[1,2*]

Abstract

Background: Adult height is associated with risk of several diseases, but the breadth of such associations and whether these associations are primary or due to confounding are unclear. We examined the association of adult height with 50 diseases spanning multiple body systems using both epidemiological and genetic approaches, the latter to identify un-confounded associations and possible underlying mechanisms.

Methods: We examined the associations for adult height (using logistic regression adjusted for potential confounders) and genetically determined height (using a two-sample Mendelian randomisation approach with height-associated genetic variants as instrumental variables) in 417,434 individuals of white ethnic background participating in the UK Biobank. We undertook pathway analysis of height-associated genes to identify biological processes that could link height and specific diseases.

Results: Height was associated with 32 diseases and genetically determined height associated with 12 diseases. Of these, 11 diseases showed a concordant association in both analyses, with taller height associated with reduced risks of coronary artery disease (odds ratio per standard deviation (SD) increase in height $OR_{epi} = 0.80$, 95% CI 0.78–0.81; OR per SD increase in genetically determined height $OR_{gen} = 0.86$, 95% CI 0.82–0.90), hypertension ($OR_{epi} = 0.83$, 95% CI 0.82–0.84; $OR_{gen} = 0.88$, 95% CI 0.85–0.91), gastro-oesophageal reflux disease ($OR_{epi} = 0.85$, 95% CI 0.84–0.86; $OR_{gen} = 0.94$, 95% CI 0.92–0.97), diaphragmatic hernia ($OR_{epi} = 0.81$, 95% CI 0.79–0.82; $OR_{gen} = 0.91$, 95% CI 0.88–0.94), but increased risks of atrial fibrillation ($OR_{epi} = 1.42$, 95% CI 1.38–1.45; $OR_{gen} = 1.33$, 95% CI 1.26–1.40), venous thromboembolism ($OR_{epi} = 1.18$, 95% CI 1.16–1.21; $OR_{gen} = 1.15$, 95% CI 1.11–1.19), intervertebral disc disorder ($OR_{epi} = 1.15$, 95% CI 1.13–1.18; $OR_{gen} = 1.14$, 95% CI 1.09–1.20), hip fracture ($OR_{epi} = 1.19$, 95% CI 1.12–1.26; $OR_{gen} = 1.27$, 95% CI 1.17–1.39), vasculitis ($OR_{epi} = 1.15$, 95% CI 1.11–1.19; $OR_{gen} = 1.20$, 95% CI 1.14–1.28), cancer overall ($OR_{epi} = 1.09$, 95% CI 1.08–1.11; $OR_{gen} = 1.06$, 95% CI 1.04–1.08) and breast cancer ($OR_{epi} = 1.08$, 95% CI 1.06–1.10; $OR_{gen} = 1.07$, 95% CI 1.03–1.11). Pathway analysis showed multiple height-associated pathways associating with individual diseases.

Conclusions: Adult height is associated with risk of a range of diseases. We confirmed previously reported height associations for coronary artery disease, atrial fibrillation, venous thromboembolism, intervertebral disc disorder, hip fracture and cancer and identified potential novel associations for gastro-oesophageal reflux disease, diaphragmatic hernia and vasculitis. Multiple biological mechanisms affecting height may affect the risks of these diseases.

Keywords: Adult height, Genetically determined height, Mendelian randomisation, Instrumental variables, Disease risk

* Correspondence: njs@le.ac.uk
[1]Department of Cardiovascular Sciences, University of Leicester, Leicester, UK
[2]NIHR Leicester Biomedical Research Centre, Glenfield Hospital, Leicester, UK
Full list of author information is available at the end of the article

Background

Epidemiological studies have associated higher adult height with lower risk of mortality from coronary artery disease (CAD) and respiratory diseases [1–7] and increased risk of atrial fibrillation (AF) [8, 9], venous thromboembolism (VTE) [9–11], cancer and cancer in specific sites [1, 7, 12–16]. Although such studies have typically adjusted for age, sex and some socio-economic and behavioral risk factors, the observed associations may still be due to unmeasured confounding. Height itself is determined by genetics and early-life factors, such as nutrient availability, socio-economic circumstances and diseases [17–19], and some of these can themselves impact on risk of some diseases in later life. Precise reason(s) for the association of adult height with risk of these diseases are not known. In particular, it is unclear whether the associations are primary (due to shared biological pathways affecting both adult height and risk of diseases) and not due to confounding.

Genetic approaches (Mendelian randomisation) that use genetic variants as instrumental variables have been used to test for causal relationships between exposure and disease outcomes [20]. Genotypes are generated at conception with alleles randomly passed on from each parent and are independent of environmental and life style factors that can confound epidemiological analysis. Also, they cannot be altered by disease and therefore remove the possibility of reverse causality. Several recent studies have used a Mendelian randomisation approach to assess the relationship of height with selected diseases, including CAD [21, 22], stroke [22], VTE [23] and cancers [16, 24–28].

A recent genome-wide association studies (GWAS) meta-analysis involving 253,288 individuals of European ancestry by the GIANT consortium identified 697 height-associated variants which explain ~ 20% of the heritability of adult height [29]. Here, using this set of genetic variants and the breadth and scale of the UK Biobank [30], we comprehensively evaluated the associations of adult height with 50 diseases in multiple body systems in the same population using both traditional epidemiological and genetic approaches. We additionally undertook pathway analysis of the height-associated genes to explore potential biological processes underlying the associations.

Methods

Study design and setting

Details of the design of the UK Biobank have been reported elsewhere [30]. Briefly, the UK Biobank is a population-based longitudinal study that recruited ~ 500,000 participants aged 40–69 years during 2006–2010 from throughout the United Kingdom (UK). Participants were recruited by inviting just over 9 million individuals from central NHS registration databases in the appropriate age group and living within around 20–25 miles of 22 recruitment centres established in England, Scotland and Wales with an eventual participation rate of around 5%. Detailed data on sociodemographic, health status, family history and life style were collected via questionnaires. Standing height was measured by the Seca 202 device, and other physical measurements such as weight and blood pressure were measured at the assessment centres and biological samples were taken for further analysis.

The UK Biobank data have been linked to Hospital Episode Statistics (HES), as well as national death registries and cancer registries. HES data covers admissions to NHS hospitals in the UK between April 1997 and March 2015, with the Scottish data dating back as early as 1981. HES uses International Classification of Diseases ICD 9 and 10 to record diagnosis information, and OPCS-4 (Office of Population, Censuses and Surveys: Classification of Interventions and Procedures, version 4) to code operative procedures. Death registries include all deaths in the UK up to mid-2015, with both primary and contributory causes of death coded in ICD-10. Cancer registries cover registrations across the UK from 1970s to 2014 with diagnoses (coded in ICD9 and 10) acquired from a variety of sources including NHS and private hospitals, cancer screening programmes, cancer centres, hospices and nursing homes, general practices as well as HES, death certificates and Cancer Waiting Time (CWT) data.

The UK Biobank performed genome-wide genotyping using the Affymetrix UK BiLEVE Axiom array on first 50,000 participants as part of the BiLEVE study [31] and subsequently using the Affymetrix UK Biobank Axiom® array for the remaining cohort. The two arrays are very similar with over 95% overlap content. Details on genotyping, quality control and imputation methodology have been described elsewhere [32]. The assayed genotype data from both stages have been jointly imputed providing genome-wide genotypes on over 70 million SNPs for each subject.

Study participants

We included 459,324 UK Biobank participants with genotype data who self-reported as having a white ethnic background. We excluded 985 participants with missing height and 22 participants whose height was > 4 standard deviation (SD) away from the mean (< 131.6 and > 205.6 cm). On the basis of the genetic data, we further excluded subjects because of uncertain gender ($n = 354$), genotype data quality (high missingness, QC failure, etc.) ($n = 7025$) and relatedness (kinship coefficient > 0.088) ($n = 33,504$). Altogether, we investigated 417,434 unrelated individuals of white ethnic background with valid height measures and genotype data.

Disease definition

We examined 50 diseases covering six broad categories:

(i) Cardiovascular diseases—coronary artery disease (CAD), hypertension, peripheral vascular disease (PVD), heart failure (HF), atrial fibrillation (AF), venous thromboembolism (VTE), aortic valve stenosis (AS) and stroke

(ii) Musculoskeletal diseases—osteoarthritis, osteoporosis, gout, sciatica, and intervertebral disc disorder (IDD), and hip fracture

(iii) digestive diseases—liver cirrhosis, peptic ulcer, gastro-oesophageal reflux disease (GORD), irritable bowel syndrome (IBS), inflammatory bowel disease (IBD), gallstone, appendicitis, diaphragmatic hernia and inguinal hernia

(iv) Psychiatric and neurological diseases—anxiety disorder, depression, bipolar disorder, multiple sclerosis (MS), epilepsy, dementia and Parkinson's disease

(v) Other non-neoplastic diseases—chronic obstructive pulmonary disease (COPD), asthma, diabetes, hyperthyroidism, hypothyroidism, glaucoma, cataract and vasculitis

(vi) Cancer including cancer overall and 11 specific sites—lung, colorectum, prostate, female breast, uterus, ovary, kidney, bladder, melanoma, non-Hodgkin lymphoma and leukemia

We defined cases using both self-reported and registry data and included both prevalent and incident cases. Case definition and the proportion of cases that were self-reported are shown in Additional file 1: Table S1. All diseases have a minimum of 1000 cases from 417,434 subjects in this study, providing 80% power to detect a relative 15% difference in disease risk (i.e. an odds ratio of at least 1.15 or 0.85) per one SD change in height at $\alpha = 0.001$.

Statistical analysis

Epidemiological analysis

We used logistic regression to estimate the association of height with risk of diseases, adjusted for age, sex, obesity (BMI ≥ 30 kg/m^2), socio-economic status (based on quintiles of Townsend Deprivation Index [33] (an area-based measure of material deprivation calculated from census household data with a higher index indicating more deprived), smoking status (ever smoker, exposed to environmental tobacco smoke, none), physical activity and for individual diseases, other relevant factors, which included, where appropriate, waist-hip-ratio (WHR), systolic blood pressure (SBP), use of insulin, presence of hay fever/eczema and family history of relevant diseases, and for female diseases, parity, nulliparous, ever use of contraceptive pills and ever on hormone

replacement therapy. Further details of the adjustments are given in the legend to Fig. 1.

Genetic analysis

We used a two-sample Mendelian randomisation (MR) approach to assess the association of genetically determined height with various diseases. Summary statistics for effect size of the height-associated SNPs were extracted from Wood et al. [29]. Of the 697 height-associated SNPs, 8 were unavailable in the genotype data imputed from the Haplotype Reference Consortium panel. Of the 691 variants serving as instrumental variables, 146 were genotyped and 545 were imputed with excellent imputation quality (mean 0.99 and the lowest 0.84). Effects of these height-associated SNPs on the risk of diseases were estimated with the UK Biobank data under an additive model adjusting for age, sex, array type (BiLEVE or main study) and five principal components. We calculated the ratio estimate for each height-associated variant [20] and then combined the estimates across all variants using meta-analysis [34]. For each height-associated variant, we extracted β_1 (the effect size of the association between the variant and height) from published table [29], estimated β_2 (the effect size of the association between the variant and the disease) under an additive mode of inheritance and computed β_3 (the putative association between height and risk of disease mediated through that variant) using the equation

$\beta_3 = \frac{\beta_2}{\beta_1}$ and its standard error $s_3 = \sqrt{\frac{1}{\beta_1^2 s_2^2}}$, where s_2 is the standard error of β_2.

Estimates of β_3 across all the height-associated SNPs were then pooled using inverse-variance-weighted fixed-effect meta-analysis to obtain the overall association of genetically determined height on the risk of the disease [34]. In cases of high heterogeneity ($I^2 > 40\%$), we conducted a random-effects meta-analysis. The estimated β_3 reflect the logarithm of the odds ratio of developing the disease per one SD increase in genetically determined height. We adjusted the p values for testing 50 diseases using Bonferroni correction in both epidemiological and genetic analyses.

Sensitivity analysis

The MR analysis assumes a linear relationship between height and risk of diseases. It relies on certain assumptions on the selected SNPs as instruments [20]: they are (1) associated with height, (2) not associated with confounding factors and (3) associated with the diseases only through their effect on height. We assessed the potential impact of violation of these assumptions using MR-Egger regression [35] and median-based methods [36] as sensitivity analysis. Standard MR analysis is equivalent to performing a weighted regression of the effect sizes of variant-disease associations (β_2) against the effect sizes of variant-height associations (β_1) with no

A *Cardiovascular diseases*

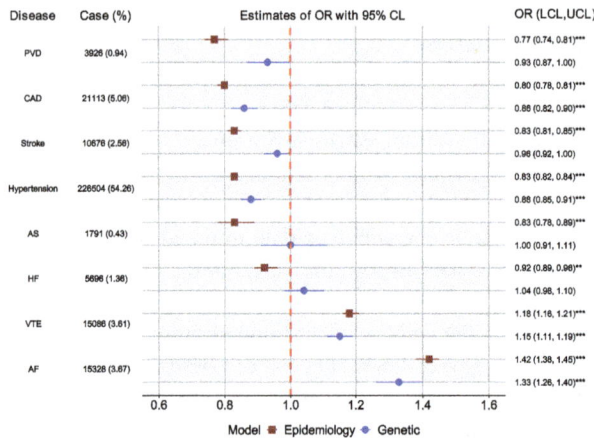

Disease	Case (%)	Estimates of OR with 95% CI	OR (LCL,UCL)
PVD	3926 (0.94)		0.77 (0.74, 0.81)***
			0.93 (0.87, 1.00)
CAD	21113 (5.06)		0.80 (0.78, 0.81)***
			0.86 (0.82, 0.90)***
Stroke	10676 (2.56)		0.83 (0.81, 0.85)***
			0.96 (0.92, 1.00)
Hypertension	226504 (54.26)		0.83 (0.82, 0.84)***
			0.88 (0.85, 0.91)***
AS	1791 (0.43)		0.83 (0.78, 0.89)***
			1.00 (0.91, 1.11)
HF	5696 (1.36)		0.92 (0.89, 0.96)**
			1.04 (0.98, 1.10)
VTE	15086 (3.61)		1.18 (1.16, 1.21)***
			1.15 (1.11, 1.19)***
AF	15328 (3.67)		1.42 (1.38, 1.45)***
			1.33 (1.26, 1.40)***

Model ■ Epidemiology ● Genetic

B *Musculoskeletal diseases*

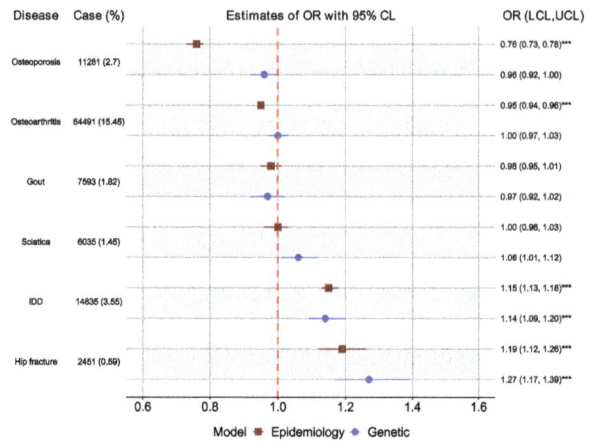

Disease	Case (%)	Estimates of OR with 95% CI	OR (LCL,UCL)
Osteoporosis	11281 (2.7)		0.76 (0.73, 0.78)***
			0.96 (0.92, 1.00)
Osteoarthritis	64491 (15.46)		0.95 (0.94, 0.96)***
			1.00 (0.97, 1.03)
Gout	7593 (1.82)		0.98 (0.95, 1.01)
			0.97 (0.92, 1.02)
Sciatica	6035 (1.45)		1.00 (0.96, 1.03)
			1.06 (1.01, 1.12)
IDD	14835 (3.55)		1.15 (1.13, 1.18)***
			1.14 (1.09, 1.20)***
Hip fracture	2451 (0.59)		1.19 (1.12, 1.26)***
			1.27 (1.17, 1.39)***

Model ■ Epidemiology ● Genetic

C *Digestive diseases*

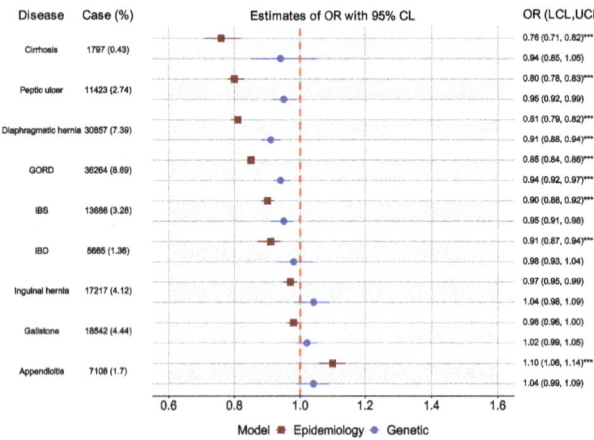

Disease	Case (%)	Estimates of OR with 95% CI	OR (LCL,UCL)
Cirrhosis	1797 (0.43)		0.76 (0.71, 0.82)***
			0.94 (0.85, 1.05)
Peptic ulcer	11423 (2.74)		0.80 (0.78, 0.83)***
			0.95 (0.92, 0.99)
Diaphragmatic hernia	30857 (7.39)		0.81 (0.79, 0.82)***
			0.91 (0.88, 0.94)***
GORD	36264 (8.69)		0.85 (0.84, 0.86)***
			0.94 (0.92, 0.97)***
IBS	13686 (3.28)		0.90 (0.88, 0.92)***
			0.95 (0.91, 0.98)
IBD	5665 (1.36)		0.91 (0.87, 0.94)***
			0.98 (0.93, 1.04)
Inguinal hernia	17217 (4.12)		0.97 (0.95, 0.99)
			1.04 (0.98, 1.09)
Gallstone	18542 (4.44)		0.98 (0.96, 1.00)
			1.02 (0.99, 1.05)
Appendicitis	7108 (1.7)		1.10 (1.06, 1.14)***
			1.04 (0.99, 1.09)

Model ■ Epidemiology ● Genetic

D *Psychiatric and neurological diseases*

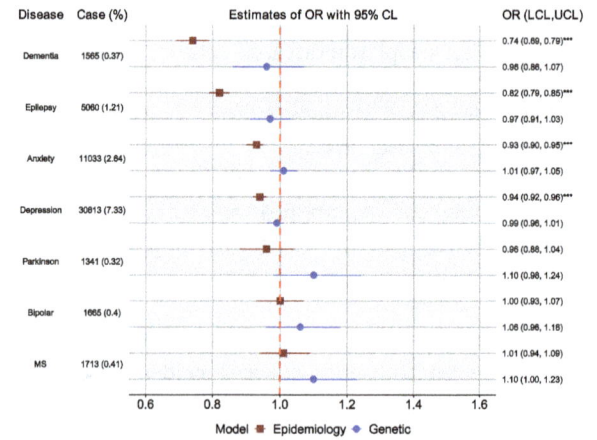

Disease	Case (%)	Estimates of OR with 95% CI	OR (LCL,UCL)
Dementia	1565 (0.37)		0.74 (0.69, 0.79)***
			0.96 (0.86, 1.07)
Epilepsy	5060 (1.21)		0.82 (0.79, 0.85)***
			0.97 (0.91, 1.03)
Anxiety	11033 (2.64)		0.93 (0.90, 0.95)***
			1.01 (0.97, 1.05)
Depression	30813 (7.33)		0.94 (0.92, 0.96)***
			0.99 (0.96, 1.01)
Parkinson	1341 (0.32)		0.96 (0.88, 1.04)
			1.10 (0.98, 1.24)
Bipolar	1665 (0.4)		1.00 (0.93, 1.07)
			1.06 (0.96, 1.16)
MS	1713 (0.41)		1.01 (0.94, 1.09)
			1.10 (1.00, 1.23)

Model ■ Epidemiology ● Genetic

E *Other non-neoplastic diseases*

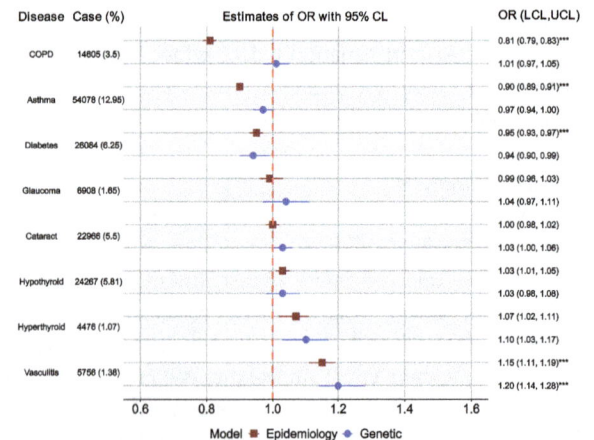

Disease	Case (%)	Estimates of OR with 95% CI	OR (LCL,UCL)
COPD	14605 (3.5)		0.81 (0.79, 0.83)***
			1.01 (0.97, 1.05)
Asthma	54078 (12.95)		0.90 (0.89, 0.91)***
			0.97 (0.94, 1.00)
Diabetes	26084 (6.25)		0.95 (0.93, 0.97)***
			0.94 (0.90, 0.99)
Glaucoma	6908 (1.65)		0.99 (0.96, 1.03)
			1.04 (0.97, 1.11)
Cataract	22966 (5.5)		1.00 (0.98, 1.02)
			1.03 (1.00, 1.06)
Hypothyroid	24267 (5.81)		1.03 (1.01, 1.05)
			1.03 (0.98, 1.08)
Hyperthyroid	4476 (1.07)		1.07 (1.02, 1.11)
			1.10 (1.03, 1.17)
Vasculitis	5758 (1.38)		1.15 (1.11, 1.19)***
			1.20 (1.14, 1.28)***

Model ■ Epidemiology ● Genetic

F *Cancer*

Disease	Case (%)	Estimates of OR with 95% CI	OR (LCL,UCL)
Cancer	66818 (16.01)		1.09 (1.08, 1.11)***
			1.06 (1.04, 1.08)***
Lung cancer	2232 (0.53)		0.93 (0.87, 0.99)
			1.15 (1.05, 1.26)
Prostate cancer	7462 (3.68)		1.03 (1.00, 1.05)
			0.99 (0.94, 1.04)
Bladder cancer	1651 (0.4)		1.03 (0.96, 1.10)
			1.06 (0.97, 1.20)
Uterine cancer	1870 (0.83)		1.03 (0.98, 1.08)
			1.01 (0.92, 1.12)
Ovarian cancer	1388 (0.62)		1.05 (0.99, 1.11)
			1.05 (0.94, 1.18)
Colorectal cancer	5052 (1.21)		1.07 (1.03, 1.11)
			1.11 (1.05, 1.18)*
Breast cancer	13396 (5.95)		1.08 (1.06, 1.10)***
			1.07 (1.03, 1.11)*
Leukaemia	1183 (0.28)		1.10 (1.01, 1.20)
			1.08 (0.96, 1.23)
Kidney cancer	1292 (0.31)		1.17 (1.08, 1.27)**
			1.09 (0.97, 1.23)
Non-Hodgkin lymphoma	1997 (0.48)		1.19 (1.12, 1.27)***
			1.13 (1.02, 1.24)
Melanoma	4835 (1.16)		1.21 (1.16, 1.26)***
			1.08 (1.02, 1.15)

Model ■ Epidemiology ● Genetic

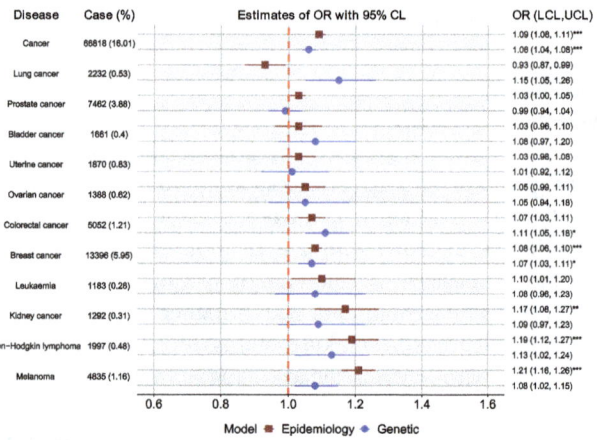

Fig. 1 (See legend on next page.)

Fig. 1 Epidemiological and genetic associations of height with diseases. Legend: Odds ratio (OR) and 95% confidence intervals per one standard deviation (SD) increase in height based on observed (epidemiology model) and genetically determined height (genetic model) are shown for **a** cardiovascular diseases (coronary artery disease (CAD), peripheral vascular disease (PVD), stroke, hypertension, aortic valve stenosis (AS), heart failure (HF), venous thromboembolism (VTE) and atrial fibrillation (AF)), **b** musculoskeletal diseases (osteoporosis, osteoarthritis, gout, sciatica, intervertebral disc disorder (IDD) and hip fracture), **c** digestive disorders (liver cirrhosis, peptic ulcer, diaphragmatic hernia, inguinal hernia, gastro-oesophageal reflux disease (GORD), irritable bowel syndrome (IBS), inflammatory bowel disease (IBD), gallstones and appendicitis), **d** psychiatric and neurological disorders (dementia, epilepsy, anxiety disorder, depression, bipolar disorder, Parkinson's disease and multiple sclerosis (MS)), **e** other non-neoplastic diseases (chronic obstructive pulmonary disease (COPD), asthma, diabetes, glaucoma, cataract, hypothyroidism and hyperthyroidism and vasculitis), and **f** cancers and various sites. One SD is 9.2 cm; for men and women specific diseases, 1-SD corresponds to 6.8 cm and 6.2 cm, respectively. All epidemiological models were adjusted for age, sex, obesity (BMI ≥ 30), socio-economic status (Townsend deprivation index in highest quintile), Smoking status (ever smoker, exposed to environmental tobacco smoke, none), physical activity (vigorous exercise at least once a week or more) and other relevant disease-specific risk factors as described below: models for CAD—waist-hip-ratio, systolic blood pressure, use of insulin and family history of heart diseases; models for AF, VTE, PVD and heart failure—systolic blood pressure, use of insulin and family history of heart diseases; model for hypertension—use of insulin and family history of hypertension; model for stroke—waist-hip-ratio, systolic blood pressure, use of insulin and family history of stroke; model for COPD—family history of COPD; model for asthma—presence of hay fever or eczema; model for dementia—family history of dementia; depression—family history of depression; Parkinson's disease—family history of Parkinson's disease; model of glaucoma—systolic blood pressure and use of insulin; model for diabetes—waist-hip-ratio, systolic blood pressure and family history of diabetes; model of cataract—use of insulin; model for cancer overall—family history of lung/breast/prostate/bowel cancer; model for cancer of the breast—nulliparous, ever use of contraceptive pills, ever on hormone replacement therapy and family history of breast cancer; models for lung, prostate and colorectal cancers—family history of respective cancers. *p < 0.05, **p < 0.01, ***p < 0.001 after Bonferroni correction for 50 tests

intercept term, but MR-Egger conducts such regression with an unconstrained intercept. The estimated intercept in the MR-Egger regression [35] can be interpreted as an estimate of the average pleiotropic effects across the genetic variants. A non-zero intercept is indicative of directional pleiotropy, that is, the pleiotropic effects do not cancel out resulting in a biased MR estimate. We also conducted three median-based methods [36]: (1) simple median method which takes the median β_3 estimate assuming all variants carry equal weight, (2) weighted median method which gives more weight to variants with more precise estimates and (3) penalised weighted median method which down-weights the contribution of heterogeneous variants. MR-Egger regression can give consistent estimates even when 100% of variants are invalid but requires the variants to satisfy a weaker assumption (the InSIDE assumption), whilst the weighted median methods can give consistent estimates as long as at least 50% of the weight comes from variants without pleiotropic effects. Additionally, we examined the association of genetically determined height with risk factors and repeated the genetic analysis excluding SNPs that showed a nominal association ($p < 0.05$) with suggested confounding factors. We restricted these sensitivity analyses to diseases showing evidence of association in primary genetic analysis (Bonferroni adjusted $p < 0.05$).

In this study, we defined cases using both self-reported and registry (hospital episodes, cancer and death registries) information. To assess any impact of including self-reported data, we repeated the epidemiological and genetic analyses defining cases based on registry data only. Furthermore, we defined cases including both prevalent and incident cases and have assumed that there were little changes in exposure of risk factors over time in the epidemiological analysis. To assess any

impact of this assumption, we repeated the epidemiological analysis defining cases based on incidence only.

Genetic score for height
We calculated a genetic score for height to evaluate the effect of inheriting number of height-increasing alleles on risk of diseases. For each variant, we computed a score based on the posterior probabilities for the height-increasing allele, which is then multiplied by the effect size for height estimated by Wood et al. [29]. The genetic score is the sum of these weighted values across all 691 height-associated variants. We used regression analysis to assess the proportion of variance of height that can be explained by the genetic score. We divided the study subjects into quartiles based on their genetic scores with quartile 1 (Q1) carrying the least number of height-increasing alleles and Q4 carrying the most number of height-increasing alleles. We then used the Cochran-Armitage trend test to assess the presence of diseases across quartiles, and logistic regression to estimate the ORs for the quartiles.

Pathway analysis
To identify possible shared biologic processes between height and diseases, we identified pathways represented by the 691 height-associated SNPs using the Ingenuity Pathway Analysis Software (analysis performed on September 19, 2017). This analysis requires the assignment of each height-associated SNP to a specific gene. We selected the genes identified by Wood et al. [29] through their extensive bioinformatics analysis of each locus. From the pathways identified, we selected those that contained at least five genes from among the height-related genes and tested the association of height and risk of diseases through the specific pathway by combining disease-specific β_3 estimates for all height variants in the pathway using

Table 1 Baseline characteristics of participants in the UK Biobank by quartiles of adult height

Characteristic	Height (cm)				Overall
	Quartile 1	Quartile 2	Quartile 3	Quartile 4	
Height (cm)—female	132–< 158	158–< 163	163–< 167	167–199	132–199
Height (cm)—male	132–< 171	171–< 176	176–< 180	180–205	132–205
N	87,358	117,771	97,416	114,889	417,434
Age	58.8 (7.5)	57.5 (7.8)	56.4 (7.9)	54.9 (8.1)	56.8 (8.0)
Sex—female	52.8%	55.7%	55.7%	51.6%	54.0%
Body mass index (BMI)	28.1 (4.9)	27.6 (4.8)	27.2 (4.7)	26.8 (4.6)	27.4 (4.8)
Obese (BMI ≥ 30)	28.9%	25.4%	23.0%	20.4%	24.2%
Waist-hip-ratio (WHR)	0.88 (0.1)	0.87 (0.1)	0.87 (0.1)	0.87 (0.1)	0.87 (0.1)
Townsend deprivation index[a]	22.5%	18.1%	16.7%	16.1%	18.1%
Ever smoker	47.1%	46.2%	45.5%	45.5%	46.0%
Vigorous activity[b]	55.5%	58.8%	60.6%	63.0%	59.7%
Systolic BP (mmHg)	145.3 (21.3)	142.3 (20.8)	140.1 (20.5)	137.8 (19.5)	141.2 (20.7)
Diastolic BP (mmHg)	85.4 (11.3)	84.6 (11.3)	84.0 (11.3)	83.4 (11.2)	84.3 (11.3)
Female only					
Nulliparous	15.9%	17.3%	19.0%	22.7%	18.8%
Ever oral contraceptive	78.1%	81.3%	83.3%	84.9%	82.0%
Ever on hormone replacement therapy	45.0%	41.6%	38.1%	33.4%	39.3%

Data expressed as mean (SD) for continuous variables or as percentages for categorical variables; missing data—BMI ($n = 464$), WHR ($n = 162$), systolic BP ($n = 348$), diastolic BP ($n = 346$), Townsend deprivation index ($n = 489$), smoking status ($n = 1481$), physical activity ($n = 547$), nulliparous ($n = 143$), oral contraceptive ($n = 34$) and hormone replacement therapy ($n = 87$)

BP blood pressure

[a]Townsend deprivation index—highest quantile

[b]Vigorous activity—at least once a week for 10+ min

meta-analysis. The results were not adjusted for multiple testing as this analysis was exploratory.

Results

Of the 417,434 people included in the study, 54.0% were women, the mean age at recruitment was 56.8 years (range 38–73), and the mean height was 168.7 cm (SD 9.2). Taller people were younger, more likely to have a lower BMI, a lower WHR, and lower blood pressure (Table 1). They were also less likely to have ever smoked or be socio-economically deprived and more likely to be physically active. Taller women were more likely to be nulliparous and to have ever used the oral contraceptive pill and less likely to have ever been on hormone replacement therapy. Given that taller women were younger, this observation is likely to be confounded by age.

As expected, people carrying more height-increasing alleles are taller (Table 2). Regression analyses showed that the weighted genetic score explained 16.7 and 16.5% of variation of height for women and men, respectively. Individuals in the upper quartiles were marginally older, with similar sex composition across quartiles, and appeared to be associated with a slightly lower BMI, lower blood pressure and lower Townsend Deprivation Index, but not with smoking history, or

undertaking vigorous physical activity. Women with higher genetic score are more likely to be nulliparous and ever on hormone replacement therapy.

Association of height with diseases based on epidemiological and genetic analyses

The estimated odds ratio (OR) per one SD (9.2 cm) increase in height (epidemiological analysis) and genetically determined height (genetic analysis) are shown in Fig. 1. For men and women specific diseases, 1-SD of height corresponds to 6.8 and 6.2 cm respectively. Overall, 39 and 23 diseases showed evidence suggestive of epidemiological and genetic associations with height ($p < 0.05$), respectively. The height association remained for 32 and 12 diseases (11 in common) after adjusting for multiple testing.

Among cardiovascular diseases, we found inverse epidemiological associations of height with CAD, PVD, stroke, hypertension, AS and HF with an estimated OR between 0.77 (PVD) and 0.92 (HF) (Fig. 1a). With genetic analyses, we found strong evidence for inverse association for CAD (OR = 0.86, 95% CI 0.82–0.90, $p < 0.0001$) and hypertension (OR = 0.88, 95% CI 0.85–0.91, $p < 0.0001$). In contrast to these inverse associations, taller height was associated with increased risk of VTE and AF in both epidemiological (VTE: OR = 1.18, 95% CI

Table 2 Characteristics of participants in the UK Biobank by quartiles of weighted genetic score for height

Characteristic	Weighted genetic score for height[a]			
	Quartile 1	Quartile 2	Quartile 3	Quartile 4
N	90,170	107,870	109,390	110,004
Height (cm)—female	159.2 (5.7)	161.6 (5.6)	163.3 (5.7)	165.8 (6.0)
Height (cm)—male	172.1 (6.2)	174.7 (6.2)	176.6 (6.2)	179.3 (6.5)
Age	56.7 (8.0)	56.8 (8.0)	56.8 (8.0)	56.9 (7.9)
Sex—female	53.9%	54.0%	53.8%	54.2%
Body mass index (BMI)	27.6 (4.9)	27.5 (4.8)	27.3 (4.7)	27.2 (4.7)
Obese (BMI ≥ 30)	25.5%	24.5%	23.8%	23.1%
Waist-hip-ratio (WHR)	0.87 (0.09)	0.87 (0.09)	0.87 (0.09)	0.87 (0.09)
Townsend deprivation index[b]	19.5%	18.2%	17.8%	17.4%
Ever smoker	46.2%	46.2%	45.8%	45.9%
Vigorous activity[c]	59.4%	59.7%	60.1%	59.4%
Systolic BP (mmHg)	141.7 (20.9)	141.4 (20.7)	141.0 (20.6)	140.6 (20.5)
Diastolic BP (mmHg)	84.6 (11.3)	84.4 (11.3)	84.2 (11.2)	84.1 (11.3)
Female only				
Nulliparous	18.7%	18.4%	18.7%	19.5%
Ever contraceptive pill	81.9%	82.0%	82.2%	82.0%
Ever on hormone replacement therapy	38.8%	39.2%	39.4%	39.8%

Data expressed as mean (SD) for continuous variables or as percentages for categorical variables; missing data—BMI ($n = 464$), WHR ($n = 162$), systolic BP ($n = 348$), diastolic BP ($n = 346$), Townsend deprivation index ($n = 489$), smoking status ($n = 1481$), physical activity ($n = 547$), nulliparous ($n = 143$), oral contraceptive ($n = 34$) and hormone replacement therapy ($n = 87$)

BP blood pressure

[a]Quartile 1 of the genetic score carrying the least number and quartile 4 the most number of height-increasing alleles

[b]Townsend deprivation index—highest quantile

[c]Vigorous activity—at least once a week for 10+ min

1.16–1.21, $p < 0.0001$; AF: OR = 1.42, 95% CI 1.38–1.45, $p < 0.0001$) and genetic analyses (VTE: OR = 1.15, 95% CI 1.11–1.19, $p < 0.0001$; AF: OR = 1.33, 95% CI 1.26–1.40, $p < 0.0001$).

Among musculoskeletal diseases, taller stature was strongly associated with an increased risk of IDD (epidemiological OR = 1.15, 95% CI 1.13–1.18, $p < 0.0001$; genetic OR = 1.14, 95% CI 1.09–1.20, $p < 0.0001$) and hip fracture (epidemiological OR = 1.19, 95% CI 1.12–1.26, $p < 0.0001$; genetic OR = 1.27, 95% CI 1.17–1.39, $p < 0.0001$) (Fig. 1b). The observed inverse associations of height with osteoporosis (OR = 0.76, 95% CI 0.73–0.78, $p < 0.0001$) and osteoarthritis (OR = 0.95, 95% CI 0.94–0.96, $p < 0.0001$) in epidemiological analyses were attenuated in genetic analyses (osteoporosis: OR = 0.96, 95% CI 0.92–1.00; osteoarthritis: OR = 1.00, 95% CI 0.97–1.03).

Among digestive diseases (Fig. 1c), we found inverse epidemiological associations between height and risks of liver cirrhosis, peptic ulcer, diaphragmatic hernia, GORD, IBS and IBD, with an estimated OR ranging from 0.76 to 0.91. For genetic analyses, the inverse height association was observed for diaphragmatic hernia (OR = 0.91, 95% CI 0.88–0.94, $p < 0.0001$) and GORD (OR = 0.94, 95% CI 0.92–0.97, $p = 0.0001$) only. We also observed epidemiological association of height with appendicitis (OR = 1.10, 95% CI 1.06–

1.14, $p < 0.0001$), but the association was attenuated in genetic analysis (OR = 1.04, 95% CI 0.99–1.09).

Among psychiatric/ neurological diseases, we observed inverse epidemiological association for dementia, epilepsy, anxiety and depression; however, the corresponding genetic associations were much weakened (Fig. 1d). Similarly, the inverse associations observed for COPD, asthma and diabetes in epidemiological analysis were not found in genetic analysis (Fig. 1e). However, we observed taller height being associated with increased risks of vasculitis in both epidemiological (OR = 1.15, 95% CI 1.11–1.19, $p < 0.0001$) and genetic analyses (OR = 1.20, 95% CI 1.14–1.28, $p < 0.0001$).

Both epidemiological (OR = 1.09, 95% CI 1.08–1.11, $p < 0.0001$) and genetic analysis (OR = 1.06, 95% CI 1.04–1.08, $p < 0.0001$) showed evidence of a positive association of height with overall cancer (Fig. 1f). Of the 11 sites, height was associated with 8 and 5 sites at $p < 0.05$ (unadjusted) in epidemiological and genetic analyses, respectively. After adjusting for multiple testing, epidemiological association remained for four sites: female breast (OR = 1.08, 95% CI 1.06–1.10, $p < 0.0001$), kidney (OR = 1.17, 95% CI 1.08–1.27, $p = 0.0053$), non-Hodgkin lymphoma (OR = 1.19, 95% CI 1.12–1.27, $p < 0.0001$) and melanoma (OR = 1.21, 95% CI 1.16–1.26, $p < 0.0001$), and genetic association

Table 3 Association between genetically determined height and risks of diseases based on inverse-variance-based, MR-Egger and median-based approaches

Disease	Inverse-variance-based method	p value intercept (MR-Egger)	MR-Egger	p value intercept (robust MR-Egger)	Robust MR-Egger	Simple median	Weighted median	Penalised weighted median
CAD	0.86 (0.82–0.90)	0.163	0.93 (0.84–1.03)	0.500	0.89 (0.80–1.00)	0.87 (0.83–0.92)	0.88 (0.83–0.93)	0.88 (0.83–0.93)
Hypertension	0.88 (0.85–0.91)	0.224	0.92 (0.86–0.99)	0.138	0.96 (0.88–1.04)	0.90 (0.88–0.93)	0.91 (0.88–0.93)	0.91 (0.88–0.93)
AF	1.33 (1.26–1.40)	0.444	1.39 (1.24–1.56)	0.436	1.40 (1.23–1.60)	1.36 (1.28–1.44)	1.34 (1.26–1.42)	1.34 (1.26–1.43)
VTE	1.15 (1.11–1.19)	0.147	1.23 (1.11–1.36)	0.434	1.18 (1.06–1.32)	1.14 (1.08–1.21)	1.18 (1.11–1.24)	1.16 (1.10–1.23)
GORD	0.94 (0.92–0.97)	0.595	0.93 (0.87–1.00)	0.695	0.94 (0.86–1.02)	0.96 (0.92–1.00)	0.95 (0.91–0.99)	0.96 (0.92–0.99)
Diaphragmatic hernia	0.91 (0.88–0.94)	0.516	0.88 (0.81–0.96)	0.813	0.91 (0.83–1.00)	0.94 (0.90–0.98)	0.93 (0.89–0.97)	0.93 (0.89–0.97)
IDD	1.14 (1.09–1.20)	0.041	1.29 (1.15–1.45)	0.198	1.22 (1.08–1.38)	1.14 (1.07–1.20)	1.13 (1.06–1.20)	1.12 (1.05–1.19)
Hip fracture	1.27 (1.17–1.39)	0.104	1.52 (1.20–1.92)	0.134	1.48 (1.17–1.87)	1.24 (1.08–1.42)	1.23 (1.07–1.42)	1.23 (1.07–1.41)
Vasculitis	1.20 (1.14–1.28)	0.139	1.33 (1.15–1.54)	0.240	1.32 (1.11–1.57)	1.21 (1.10–1.32)	1.22 (1.12–1.34)	1.22 (1.11–1.33)
Cancer overall	1.06 (1.04–1.08)	0.514	1.04 (0.99–1.10)	0.536	1.04 (0.99–1.09)	1.05 (1.02–1.09)	1.05 (1.02–1.08)	1.05 (1.02–1.08)
Colorectal cancer	1.11 (1.05–1.18)	0.234	1.02 (0.86–1.20)	0.173	0.99 (0.85–1.16)	1.10 (1.00–1.21)	1.06 (0.96–1.16)	1.04 (0.95–1.15)
Breast cancer	1.07 (1.03–1.11)	0.573	1.10 (0.98–1.23)	0.930	1.06 (0.94–1.19)	1.03 (0.97–1.10)	1.04 (0.98–1.11)	1.02 (0.96–1.09)

Association is expressed as odds ratios per 1 standard deviation increase in genetically determined height and its 95% confidence interval

CAD coronary artery disease, AF atrial fibrillation, VTE venous thromboembolism, GORD gastro-oesophageal reflux disease, IDD intervertebral disc disorder

The intercept term in MR-Egger regression can be interpreted as an estimate of the average pleiotropic effect across the genetic variants, with a non-zero intercept indicative of directional pleiotropy. MR-Egger uses standard regression in the analysis, whilst robust MR-Egger uses robust regression that down-weights the influence of outliers. The median-based method calculates a median of the causal estimates across all SNPs. The simple method calculates the simple unweighted median, the weighted method calculates the median using the inverse-variance weights, and the penalised method calculates the median down-weighting heterogeneous variants

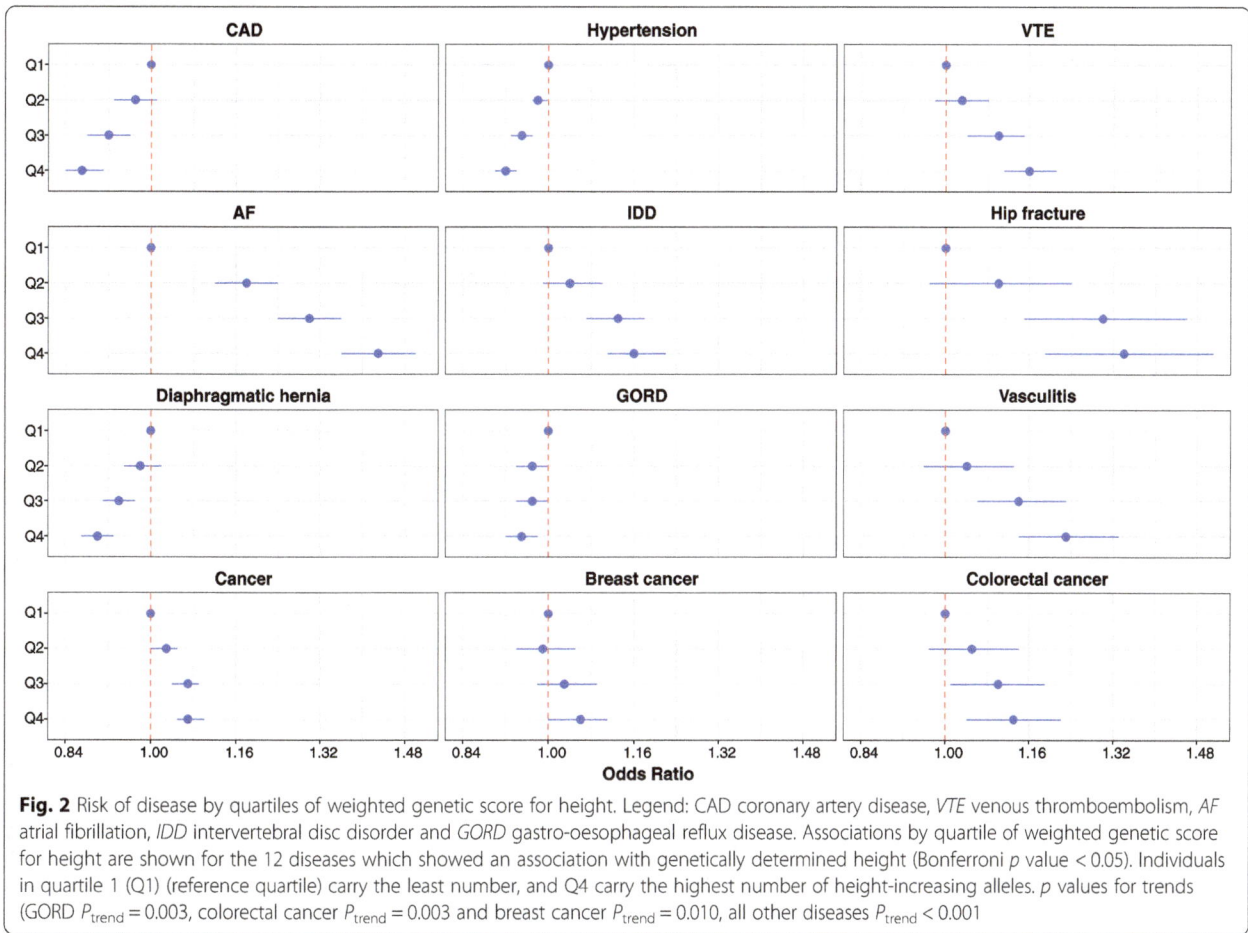

Fig. 2 Risk of disease by quartiles of weighted genetic score for height. Legend: CAD coronary artery disease, *VTE* venous thromboembolism, *AF* atrial fibrillation, *IDD* intervertebral disc disorder and *GORD* gastro-oesophageal reflux disease. Associations by quartile of weighted genetic score for height are shown for the 12 diseases which showed an association with genetically determined height (Bonferroni p value < 0.05). Individuals in quartile 1 (Q1) (reference quartile) carry the least number, and Q4 carry the highest number of height-increasing alleles. p values for trends (GORD $P_{trend} = 0.003$, colorectal cancer $P_{trend} = 0.003$ and breast cancer $P_{trend} = 0.010$, all other diseases $P_{trend} < 0.001$)

remained for two sites: breast (OR = 1.07, 95% CI 1.03–1.11, $p = 0.0366$) and colorectum (OR = 1.11, 95% CI 1.05–1.18, $p = 0.0307$).

Sensitivity analysis

For the 12 diseases showing an association with genetically determined height, the intercept tests from the MR-Egger regression revealed little evidence for pleiotropy (Table 3). The associations revealed by MR-Egger regression and median-based methods were broadly similar to the primary genetic analyses for the nine non-neoplastic diseases. For cancer overall, the OR estimates from MR-Egger and weighted median methods remained similar to the primary genetic analysis. For breast cancer and colorectal cancer, the sensitivity analysis appears to suggest a weaker or null genetic association.

We found that genetically determined height was associated with obesity, blood pressure, Townsend Deprivation Index and nulliparity (Additional file 2: Table S2). We repeated the genetic analyses excluding SNPs that were associated with these factors. This showed little impact on the estimates of the genetic associations, apart from the

anticipated effect when excluding SBP-associated SNPs, which weakened the genetic association for hypertension. (Additional file 2: Table S3).

The estimates for using registry-based cases only were similar to that for using both self-reported and registry-based cases (Additional file 2: Table S4). This suggests little impact on using self-reported data. In addition, we repeated the epidemiological analysis excluding prevalent cases at baseline. There were no significant changes in the estimates, except for IDD in which the association appeared to have become much weakened (Additional file 2: Table S5). The confidence intervals for the estimates as expected became wider due to reduced statistical power.

Genetic score of height and odds ratios of diseases

For the 12 diseases associated with genetically determined height, all exhibited a trend ($p < 0.05$) in either increasing or decreasing risk with carriage of more height-raising alleles (Fig. 2), and the directions were compatible with the findings from the primary genetic analysis. Compared with subjects in Q1, those in Q4 had a decreased risk of CAD (OR = 0.87, 95% CI 0.84–0.91, $p < 0.001$),

Table 4 Top pathways showing the association of height with diseases

Disease	Pathway	Height-associated genes in the pathway	Number of genes	Odds ratio	p value	Rank of height pathway#
Coronary artery diseases (CAD)	Caveolar-mediated endocytosis signalling	FLNB, COPA, COPB1, INSR, ITGB8, HLA-C	6	0.50	< 0.001	189
CAD	Production of nitric oxide and reactive oxygen species in macrophages	FGFR2, PIK3R3, PIK3C2A, RHOD, PIK3R1, NFKBIA, MAP2K4, FRS2, GRB2, CREBBP, FGFR4, PRKCZ, MAP3K3	13	0.65	< 0.001	159
CAD	Dendritic cell maturation	FGFR2, COL10A1, PIK3R3, PIK3C2A, PIK3R1, NFKBIA, CREB5, MAP2K4, FRS2, GRB2, HLA-C, CREBBP, TAB1, COL11A2, FGFR4	15	0.66	< 0.001	106
CAD	NGF signalling	FGFR2, PIK3R3, PIK3C2A, RAF1, PIK3R1, TP53, CREB5, MAP2K4, FRS2, GRB2, CREBBP, FGFR4, PRKCZ, MAP3K3	14	0.67	< 0.001	45
CAD	Germ cell-sertoli cell junction signalling	FGFR2, PIK3R3, PIK3C2A, CTNNB1, RHOD, TGFB2, FER, PIK3R1, MAP2K4, FRS2, GRB2, FGFR4, MAP3K3	13	0.69	< 0.001	135
Hypertension	Hepatic cholestasis	MAP2K4, TGFB2, RXRA, INSR, SLCO1C1, FGFR4, PRKCZ, NFKBIA, ESR1, ADCY9	10	0.58	< 0.001	186
Hypertension	RAR activation	PML, PIK3R3, NCOA1, TGFB2, SMAD6, NSD1, BMP2, PIK3R1, SMAD7, RDH14, MAP2K4, SMAD3, RXRA, CREBBP, IGFBP3, PRKCZ, ADCY9	17	0.75	< 0.001	59
Hypertension	IL-1 signalling	GNAS, MAP2K4, GNA12, TAB1, NFKBIA, ADCY9	6	0.57	< 0.001	200
Hypertension	TGF-β signalling	SMAD7, MAP2K4, SMAD3, RAF1, TGFB2, GRB2, SMAD6, CREBBP, TAB1, BMP2, RUNX2	11	0.75	0.001	64
Hypertension	Dopamine-DARPP32 feedback in cAMP signalling	GNAS, ITPR3, CREB5, PRKG1, PRKG2, ITPR1, KCNJ15, KCNJ12, CREBBP, KCNJ16, PRKCZ, ADCY9	12	0.74	0.001	150
Atrial fibrillation	ERK5 signalling	CREB5, GNA12, CREBBP, PRKCZ, MAP3K3, MEF2C, FOXO3	7	1.83	< 0.001	154
Atrial fibrillation	Wnt/β-catenin signalling	LRP5, SOX8, CTNNB1, WNT5A, SOX5, TGFB2, TP53, AXIN2, TLE3, SFRP4, SOX9, CREBBP, TAB1, WNT4	14	1.68	< 0.001	107
Atrial fibrillation	Androgen signalling	GNAS, NCOA1, POLR2A, SMAD3, GNA12, CREBBP, PRKCZ	7	2.14	0.001	197
Atrial fibrillation	Role of Oct4 in mammalian embryonic stem cell pluripotency	REST, FAM208A, RB1, WWP2, TP53, CCNF	6	1.90	0.004	146
Atrial fibrillation	Growth hormone signalling	FGFR2, SOCS5, PIK3R3, PIK3C2A, SOCS2, PIK3R1, IGF2, IGF1R, FRS2, GHR, GRB2, IGFBP3, FGFR4, PRKCZ	14	1.39	0.006	9
Venous thromboembolism (VTE)	Synaptic long-term depression	IGF1R, GNAS, ITPR3, RAF1, PRKG1, GNA12, PRKG2, ITPR1, PRKCZ	9	1.75	< 0.001	192
VTE	Glioma signalling	FGFR2, MTOR, PIK3R3, PIK3C2A, RBL2, RAF1, PIK3R1, TP53, IGF2, IGF1R, FRS2, GRB2, RBL1, CDK6, FGFR4,	17	1.59	< 0.001	5

Table 4 Top pathways showing the association of height with diseases (*Continued*)

Disease	Pathway	Height-associated genes in the pathway	Number of genes	Odds ratio	p value	Rank of height pathway#
		RB1, PRKCZ				
VTE	Role of tissue factor in cancer	FGFR2, MTOR, PIK3R3, PIK3C2A, FRS2, GNA12, GRB2, PIK3R1, FGFR4, TP53	10	1.69	< 0.001	155
VTE	Molecular mechanisms of cancer	FGFR2, LRP5, PIK3C2A, PTCH1, WNT5A, RHOD, ARHGEF12, GNA12, SMAD6, BMP2, PIK3R1, MAX, NFKBIA, TP53, CCND3, SMAD7, FRS2, SMAD3, GRB2, BMP6, CREBBP, RBL1, CDK6, FGFR4, PRKCZ, PIK3R3, IHH, CTNNB1, RAF1, TGFB2, GNAS, MAP2K4, TAB1, WNT4, RB1, ADCY9	36	1.37	< 0.001	1
VTE	Role of NFAT in regulation of the immune response	FGFR2, NFATC4, PIK3R3, PIK3C2A, RAF1, GNA12, PIK3R1, NFATC1, NFKBIA, MEF2C, NFATC3, GNAS, ITPR3, FRS2, GRB2, ITPR1, FGFR4, ZAP70	18	1.51	< 0.001	41
Intervertebral disc disorder (IDD)	Protein kinase A signalling	FLNB, AKAP13, PTCH1, HIST1H1E, NFKBIA, PDE11A, SMAD3, ITPR1, PDE3A, CREBBP, PTPDC1, PRKCZ, NFATC4, PTPN14, IHH, CTNNB1, RAF1, TGFB2, NFATC1, ANAPC10, NFATC3, GNAS, ITPR3, CREB5, PTPRG, CDC16, ADCY9, PDE1A	28	1.31	0.005	42
IDD	Wnt/β-catenin signalling	LRP5, SOX8, CTNNB1, WNT5A, SOX5, TGFB2, TP53, AXIN2, TLE3, SFRP4, SOX9, CREBBP, TAB1, WNT4	14	1.49	0.009	107
IDD	PI3K signalling in B lymphocytes	NFATC3, NFATC4, ITPR3, RAF1, PLEKHA1, ITPR1, PIK3R1, NFATC1, PRKCZ, NFKBIA, FOXO3	11	1.80	0.022	132
IDD	VDR/RXR activation	LRP5, NCOA1, TGFB2, RXRA, IGFBP3, PRKCZ, RUNX2	7	1.52	0.023	174
IDD	Factors promoting cardiogenesis in vertebrates	LRP5, CTNNB1, TGFB2, BMP6, BMP2, PRKCZ, MEF2C	7	1.95	0.027	187
Hip fracture	Actin cytoskeleton signalling	FGFR2, PIK3R3, PIK3C2A, SLC9A1, RAF1, ARHGEF12, GNA12, FGF18, PIK3R1, FN1, FRS2, GRB2, FGFR4, SSH2	14	3.46	< 0.001	166
Hip fracture	SAPK/JNK signalling	FGFR2, PIK3R3, PIK3C2A, GNA12, PIK3R1, NFATC1, TP53, NFATC3, MAP2K4, FRS2, GRB2, TAB1, FGFR4, MAP3K3	14	2.56	< 0.001	20
Hip fracture	NRF2-mediated oxidative stress response	FGFR2, FKBP5, PIK3R3, PIK3C2A, MAP2K4, FRS2, RAF1, GRB2, CREBBP, PIK3R1, FGFR4, PRKCZ	12	3.18	0.002	176
Hip fracture	Glucocorticoid receptor signalling	FGFR2, NFATC4, PIK3R3, NCOA1, PIK3C2A, POLR2A, RAF1, TGFB2, PIK3R1, NFATC1, NFKBIA, NFATC3, FKBP5, MAP2K4, FRS2, SMAD3, GRB2, CREBBP, TAB1, FGFR4, ESR1, FOXO3, PRKAB2	23	2.18	0.002	43
Hip fracture	Signalling by rho family GTPases	FGFR2, PIK3R3, PIK3C2A, SLC9A1, RHOD, RAF1, ARHGEF12, GNA12, PIK3R1, GNAS, MAP2K4, FRS2, GRB2, CDC42EP3, FGFR4, PRKCZ	16	2.31	0.003	141
Diaphragmatic hernia	ERK5 signalling	CREB5, GNA12, CREBBP, PRKCZ, MAP3K3, MEF2C, FOXO3	7	0.78	0.013	154
Diaphragmatic hernia	Protein kinase A signalling	FLNB, AKAP13, PTCH1, HIST1H1E, NFKBIA, PDE11A,	28	0.85	0.015	42

Table 4 Top pathways showing the association of height with diseases (Continued)

Disease	Pathway	Height-associated genes in the pathway	Number of genes	Odds ratio	p value	Rank of height pathway#
Diaphragmatic hernia	Androgen signalling	SMAD3, ITPR1, PDE3A, CREBBP, PTPDC1, PRKCZ, NFATC4, PTPN14, IHH, CTNNB1, RAF1, TGFB2, NFATC1, ANAPC10, NFATC3, GNAS, ITPR3, CREB5, PTPRG, CDC16, ADCY9, PDE1A	7	0.77	0.015	197
Diaphragmatic hernia	GPCR-mediated integration of enteroendocrine signalling exemplified by an L cell	GNAS, NCOA1, POLR2A, SMAD3, GNA12, CREBBP, PRKCZ	5	0.63	0.018	201
Diaphragmatic hernia	SUMOylation pathway	SENP3, RFC1, PML, CTBP2, MAP2K4, RHOD, SENP6, SP3, CREBBP, NFKBIA, TP53	11	0.77	0.025	77
Gastro-oesophageal reflux disease (GORD)	Virus entry via endocytic pathways	FGFR2, FLNB, PIK3R3, PIK3C2A, FRS2, GRB2, ITGB8, HLA-C, PIK3R1, FGFR4, PRKCZ	11	0.69	0.013	90
GORD	HER-2 signalling in breast cancer	FGFR2, PIK3R3, PIK3C2A, FRS2, GRB2, ITGB8, CDK6, PIK3R1, FGFR4, PRKCZ, TP53	11	0.81	0.015	69
GORD	Role of Oct4 in mammalian embryonic stem cell pluripotency	REST, FAM208A, RB1, WWP2, TP53, CCNF	6	0.71	0.018	146
GORD	mTOR signalling	RPS27L, FGFR2, MTOR, PIK3R3, PIK3C2A, RHOD, INSR, PIK3R1, FRS2, GRB2, EIF3H, MLST8, FGFR4, PRKCZ, PRKAB2	15	0.81	0.020	115
GORD	eNOS signalling	FGFR2, LPAR1, PIK3R3, SLC7A1, PIK3C2A, PRKG1, PIK3R1, GNAS, ITPR3, FRS2, GRB2, ITPR1, CCNA2, FGFR4, PRKCZ, ESR1, ADCY9, PRKAB2	18	0.83	0.024	18
Vasculitis	Glioma signalling	FGFR2, MTOR, PIK3R3, PIK3C2A, RBL2, RAF1, PIK3R1, TP53, IGF2, IGF1R, FRS2, GRB2, RBL1, CDK6, FGFR4, RB1, PRKCZ	17	1.82	< 0.001	5
Vasculitis	Molecular mechanisms of cancer	FGFR2, LRP5, PIK3C2A, PTCH1, WNT5A, RHOD, ARHGEF12, GNA12, SMAD6, BMP2, PIK3R1, MAX, NFKBIA, TP53, CCND3, SMAD7, FRS2, SMAD3, GRB2, BMP6, CREBBP, RBL1, CDK6, FGFR4, PRKCZ, PIK3R3, IHH, CTNNB1, RAF1, TGFB2, GNAS, MAP2K4, TAB1, WNT4, RB1, ADCY9	36	1.52	0.002	1
Vasculitis	Growth hormone signalling	FGFR2, SOCS5, PIK3R3, PIK3C2A, SOCS2, PIK3R1, IGF2, IGF1R, FRS2, GHR, GRB2, IGFBP3, FGFR4, PRKCZ	14	1.71	0.004	9
Vasculitis	Chronic myeloid leukemia signalling	FGFR2, PIK3R3, PIK3C2A, RBL2, RAF1, TGFB2, PIK3R1, TP53, CTBP2, FRS2, SMAD3, GRB2, RBL1, CDK6, FGFR4, RB1	16	1.70	0.006	7
Vasculitis	Synaptic long-term depression	IGF1R, GNAS, ITPR3, RAF1, PRKG1, GNA12, PRKG2, ITPR1, PRKCZ	9	1.66	0.006	192
Cancer overall	Adipogenesis pathway	FGFR2, NFATC4, WNT5A, BMP2, CLOCK, TP53, KLF3, EZH2, ARNTL, CTBP2, SMAD3, SOX9, FGFR4	13	1.34	< 0.001	85
Cancer overall	Molecular mechanisms of cancer	FGFR2, LRP5, PIK3C2A, PTCH1, WNT5A, RHOD, ARHGEF12, GNA12, SMAD6, BMP2, PIK3R1, MAX, NFKBIA, TP53, CCND3, SMAD7, FRS2, SMAD3, GRB2, BMP6, CREBBP, RBL1, CDK6, FGFR4, PRKCZ, PIK3R3, IHH, CTNNB1, RAF1, TGFB2, GNAS, MAP2K4, TAB1, WNT4, RB1, ADCY9	36	1.14	0.002	1
Cancer overall	CTLA4 signalling in cytotoxic T	FGFR2, PIK3R3, PIK3C2A, FRS2, GRB2, HLA-C, PIK3R1, FGFR4,	9	1.25	0.006	148

Table 4 Top pathways showing the association of height with diseases (Continued)

Disease	Pathway	Height-associated genes in the pathway	Number of genes	Odds ratio	p value	Rank of height pathway#
	lymphocytes	ZAP70				
Cancer overall	Systemic lupus erythematosus signalling	FGFR2, NFATC4, MTOR, PIK3R3, PIK3C2A, SNRPE, PIK3R1, NFATC1, NFATC3, FRS2, GRB2, HLA-C, FGFR4	13	1.21	0.006	182
Cancer overall	Sphingosine-1-phosphate signalling	S1PR2, FGFR2, PIK3R3, PIK3C2A, FRS2, RHOD, GNA12, GRB2, PIK3R1, FGFR4, ADCY9	11	1.20	0.008	122
Breast cancer	Hypoxia signalling in the cardiovascular system	CREB5, UBE2Z, CREBBP, NFKBIA, TP53	5	0.36	< 0.001	202
Breast cancer	PCP pathway	WNT5A, MAP2K4, ROR2, WNT4, DAAM1	5	2.06	0.038	198
Colorectal cancer	SAPK/JNK signalling	FGFR2, PIK3R3, PIK3C2A, GNA12, PIK3R1, NFATC1, TP53, NFATC3, MAP2K4, FRS2, GRB2, TAB1, FGFR4, MAP3K3	14	2.32	< 0.001	20
Colorectal cancer	Signalling by rho family GTPases	FGFR2, PIK3R3, PIK3C2A, SLC9A1, RHOD, RAF1, ARHGEF12, GNA12, PIK3R1, GNAS, MAP2K4, FRS2, GRB2, CDC42EP3, FGFR4, PRKCZ	16	2.27	< 0.001	141
Colorectal cancer	Small cell lung cancer signalling	FGFR2, PIK3R3, PIK3C2A, PIK3R1, MAX, NFKBIA, TP53, FRS2, GRB2, RXRA, CDK6, FGFR4, RB1	13	2.45	< 0.001	17
Colorectal cancer	Sphingosine-1-phosphate signalling	S1PR2, FGFR2, PIK3R3, PIK3C2A, FRS2, RHOD, GNA12, GRB2, PIK3R1, FGFR4, ADCY9	11	2.47	< 0.001	122
Colorectal cancer	Xenobiotic metabolism signalling	FGFR2, PIK3R3, NCOA1, SMOX, PIK3C2A, RAF1, PIK3R1, MAP2K4, FRS2, GRB2, RXRA, CREBBP, FGFR4, PRKCZ, MAP3K3	15	2.16	< 0.001	185

\# Rank indicates the rank of the height pathway as shown in Additional file 1: Table S6; Odds ratio and p value indicate the association of the height and the risks of diseases through the pathways

Abbreviations: *cAMP* cyclic adenosine monophosphate, *CLTA4* cytotoxic T-lymphocyte-associated protein 4, *DARPP32* dopamine- and cAMP-regulated phosphoprotein Mr 32 kDa, *eNOS* endothelial nitric oxide synthesis, *ERK5* extracellular signal regulated kinase 5, *GPCR* G protein-coupled receptor, *GTP* guanosine-5'-triphosphate, *HER-2* human epidermal growth factor 2, *JNK* Jun amino terminal kinase, *IL* interlukin, *mTOR* mammalian target of rapamycin, *NFAT* nuclear factor of activated T cells, *NGF* nerve growth factor, *NRF2* nuclear factor erythroid 2–related factor 2, *Oct4* octamer-binding transcription factor 4, *PCP* planar cell polarity, *PI3K* phosphoinositide-3-kinase, *RAR* retinoic acid receptor, *RXR* retinoid X receptor, *SAPK* stress-activated protein kinase, *TGF-β* transforming growth factor beta, *Wnt* wingless-related integration site, *VDR* vitamin D receptor hypertension (OR = 0.92, 95% CI 0.90–0.94, $p < 0.001$), GORD (OR = 0.95, 95% CI 0.92–0.98, $p = 0.002$) and diaphragmatic hernia (OR = 0.90, 95% CI 0.87–0.93, $p < 0.001$). In contrast, there were increased risks of AF (OR = 1.43, 95% CI 1.36–1.50, $p < 0.001$), VTE (OR = 1.16, 95% CI 1.11–1.21, $p < 0.001$), IDD (OR = 1.16, 95% CI 1.11–1.21, $p < 0.001$), hip fracture (OR = 1.34, 95% CI 1.19–1.51, $p < 0.001$), vasculitis (OR = 1.23, 95% CI 1.14–1.33, $p < 0.001$) and cancer (OR = 1.07, 95% CI 1.05–1.10, $p < 0.001$) along with two specific sites female breast (OR = 1.06, 95% CI 1.004–1.11, $p = 0.035$) and colorectum (OR = 1.13, 95% CI 1.04–1.22, $p = 0.004$) for subjects in Q4 compared with Q1.

Biological pathways

We identified 202 Ingenuity pathways which included five or more genes from amongst the 691 height-related variants (Additional file 1: Table S6). Table 4 shows the top five pathways associated with each disease. There was little overlap in the pathways showing the strongest association with individual diseases. Furthermore, no individual pathway explains the majority of the association with any disease.

Discussion

Our combined epidemiological and genetic analysis showed that adult height is associated with risk of many diseases affecting multiple body systems. We observed a concordance between the epidemiological and genetic analyses for 11 diseases suggesting a primary association between height and risk of these diseases. For colorectal cancer, the genetic analyses suggested a strong association with height but the epidemiological association was slightly weaker. For some diseases (e.g. HF, COPD), we observed an epidemiological association but a much weaker or null genetic association suggesting that the epidemiological associations, despite adjustment for potential confounders, likely remain subject to residual confounding.

We used a large number of genetic variants as instruments in our analysis. It is plausible that some of these variants have effects on disease development that are not linked/mediated through their effects on height (pleiotropy). However, among diseases that showed an association with genetically determined height, we observed trends between carrying more height-raising alleles and disease risk (Fig. 2), evidencing a dose response relationship that supports the role of height, or shared biological mechanisms related to both height and the development of disease.

Our analysis does not exclude the possibility that height itself induces behaviour or reflects circumstances that impact on disease risk. For example, genetically determined height appeared to be associated with a lower Townsend Deprivation Index suggesting the potential impact of genetically determined traits on socio-economic outcomes,

which could subsequently impact on disease (Additional file 2: Table S2). However, excluding height-related variants that also associated with Townsend Deprivation Index did not attenuate the observed associations (Additional file 2: Table S3). In the sensitivity analysis, the weighted penalised median produced a weakened association compared with the primary genetic analysis for breast and colorectal cancer, suggesting the possibility of non-homogeneity of the casual effect across variants. Whilst this may lead to incorrect estimate and affect the interpretation of the results, this may not lead to inappropriate inferences [37]. For most diseases in this study, the MR-Egger and weighted median analysis provided consistent estimates with the standard genetic analysis, together with the intercept tests of MR-Egger, supporting the validity of the selected genetic instruments (Table 3).

Turning to individual sets of diseases, the concordant inverse associations between height and risks of CAD in both epidemiological and genetic analyses, together with the absence of any attenuation of the genetic association from exclusion of lipid-related variants [21], suggests a primary impact of shorter height on the vasculature that predisposes to atherosclerotic disease. Our estimate of OR of 0.86 per 1-SD (9.2 cm) increase in genetically determined height agrees with previous reports [21, 22] which showed an estimated equivalent OR of 0.83–0.86. Shorter people have smaller caliber vessels which could cause symptomatic disease despite similar plaque burden [38, 39]. Height also affects pulsatile arterial haemodynamics with increased augmentation of central systolic pressure in shorter people [40] that could influence disease risk in multiple vascular beds.

Our study found evidence of a possible primary association between taller height and risk for AF. Increased atrial size has been recognised as a risk factor of AF [41]. Given the association between body size and left atrial size [42], it is plausible that the height-AF association may be mediated through atrial size. Previous epidemiological studies have reported a positive association between height and VTE [9–11], and our study supports a genetic role of height. One recent study showed an OR = 1.34 per 10 cm increase in genetically determined height [23], which appeared to be strong than our estimate of OR = 1.15 per 9.2 cm increase in genetically determined height, but this study used the genetic risk score (GRS) as the single instrumental variable as opposed to using the variants that comprise the GRS as the instrumental variables in our study and this may lead to the difference in the effect estimates [35]. Taller height is associated with an increased risk of VTE. It is possible that greater venous surface area in taller people increases the risk of VTE.

Extending previous epidemiological studies [43, 44], we found a positive relationship between height and risk of IDD. Whilst the mechanisms remain to be identified, one possible mechanism may be through facet tropism (asymmetry in left and right facet joint angles of lumbar spine) [45]. In addition, our result agrees with a recent meta-analysis of prospective cohort studies which concluded a positive association between height and risk of hip fracture [46]. It is plausible that the association might be mediated with hip axis length, given that height is positively associated with hip axis length [47], which has been reported as a risk factor of hip fracture [48]. Our study also found evidence for a negative association between height and risks of diaphragmatic hernia and GORD. Given that hiatal hernia is the most common type of diaphragmatic hernia, and that it plays an important role in the pathogenesis of GORD [49], it is not surprising height has the same directional impact to the risk of developing these two diseases. Whilst the mechanisms remain unclear, a prior hypothesis is that shorter people have greater intra-abdominal pressure, which increases the risk of developing hiatal hernia and subsequent reflux symptoms [50]. Our study also found strong evidence for a positive association between adult height and vasculitis. This suggests a possible link between height and some aspects of immune function although this requires further investigation. To our knowledge, this is the first analysis performed to evaluate the association of height with risks of diaphragmatic hernia, GORD and vasculitis.

Consistent with previous epidemiological reports [1, 7, 12–15], we found that taller height was associated with a higher overall risk of cancer. One recent study [27] using the UK Biobank showed an OR of 1.10 (95% CI 1.07–1.13) per 1-SD increase in genetically determined height, which appeared to be slightly stronger than our estimate (OR = 1.06, 95% CI 1.04–1.08 per 1-SD in genetically determined height), but one should note the difference in the study designs. Ong et al. [27] excluded self-reported cancer cases, used 2059 genetic variants as instrumental variables and conducted the analysis using the SNP-height and SNP-cancer effects all derived within the UK Biobank. Overlapping subjects in a two-sample MR is known to induce bias [51], and our estimate is potentially more accurate. Nonetheless, these studies strongly suggested that the positive association of height and cancer is primary (not due to confounding), potentially reflecting multiple shared mechanisms influencing cellular growth (Table 4). There were concordant trends towards higher risk with both observed and genetically determined height for various site-specific cancers (Fig. 1f). The diversity of the types of cancers associated with height and their magnitude of associations suggested that there may be different biological mechanisms by which height affects the risks. We observed concordant epidemiological and genetic evidence for breast cancer. Our genetic estimate of OR = 1.07 per 6.2 cm

increase (equivalent to OR = 1.12 per 10 cm increase) is similar to previous reports of OR = 1.19 and 1.22 per 10 cm increase in genetically determined height [16, 24]. Our study also agrees with previous studies showing evidence of genetically determined height with risk of colorectal cancer [26], and little evidence with prostate cancer [16, 25]. It is interesting to note that for lung cancer, the genetic and epidemiological associations were in opposite directions, although both associations were not found statistically significant after adjustment for multiple testing suggesting that the observed associations could be due to chance. It is also possible that the epidemiological finding here for lung cancer remains subject to confounding. Our genetic estimate of OR = 1.15 per 9.2 cm increase is consistent with previous report of OR = 1.10 per 10 cm increase in genetically determined height [16]. Previous epidemiological report in women population suggested possible effect modification by smoking status for smoking-related cancers [14], but our epidemiological analysis did not show evidence of difference in height-lung cancer risks between ever and never smokers (interaction of height with smoking status $p = 0.723$).

Our pathway analysis showed that there were different height-associated pathways influencing risks of individual diseases (Table 4). Several of these pathways have been linked to diseases or disease risk in their respective categories, although in many cases, the relationship between the pathways and the disease risks are not very well understood. Nitric oxide signalling has a known relationship to CAD risk [52], and Wnt signalling has been linked to AF [53]. We also found a link between Wnt signalling and IDD, but its role with the disease remains to be investigated. In addition, we observed a link of glioma signalling with VTE and the role of tissue factor in cancer. Several studies suggested possible link of VTE with malignant glioma [54, 55] and other forms of cancer [56]. In this study, we also noted an association of Sphingosine-1-phosphate (S1P) signalling with both the 'cancer overall' and colorectal cancer disease categories. S1P is known to have a role in tumorigenesis and tumor growth [57] and has been linked with multiple cancer types and has an association with intestinal inflammation and tumorigenesis [58]. The role of Rho GTPases in the development of colorectal cancer has been reported [59], and this is consistent with our finding of the link of 'signalling by Rho family GTPases' pathway with colorectal cancer.

Limitations of study

Whilst the scale and breadth of the UK Biobank and the ability to examine and directly compare both epidemiological and genetic associations in the same population are particular strengths of our analysis, some limitations need to be highlighted. Although large, the UK Biobank may not be representative of the UK population. There is a skew towards individuals in higher socio-economic groups [30]. Despite a low response rate, the fact that the associations reported in this paper largely agree with other studies, is reassuring. We included both prevalent and incident cases in the primary epidemiological analysis and assumed the exposure of risk factors recorded at baseline remained constant. Our sensitivity analysis revealed generally little impact of the current design as opposed to a prospective design which includes incident cases only. Our design allowed consistent case definition for both genetic and epidemiological analyses and enabled maximum statistical power for detection of association. Finally, there were a small minority of non-White participants in the UK Biobank. We restricted our analysis to individuals of a White ethnic background, and it remains to be shown whether the height-related associations apply to other ethnic groups.

Conclusion

Adult height is associated with risks of diseases in multiple body systems. Our study, using both epidemiological and genetic approaches, not only confirmed previously reported height associations for CAD, AF, VTE, IDD, hip fracture and cancer, but also identified potential novel associations for GORD, diaphragmatic hernia and vasculitis. It suggests complex relationship between adult height and risk of diseases and shared biological mechanisms underpinning many of the observed height-disease associations.

Abbreviations
AF: Atrial fibrillation; AS: Aortic valve stenosis; BMI: Body mass index; CAD: Coronary artery disease; CI: Confidence interval; COPD: Chronic obstructive pulmonary disease; GORD: Gastro-oesophageal reflux disease; GRS: Genetic risk score; GWAS: Genome-wide association studies; HES: Hospital Episode Statistics; HF: Heart failure; IBD: Inflammatory bowel disease; IBS: Irritable bowel syndrome; ICD: International Classification of Diseases; IDD: Intervertebral disc disorder; MR: Mendelian Randomization; MS: Multiple sclerosis; PVD: Peripheral vascular disease; OR: Odds ratio; SBP: Systolic blood pressure; SNP: Single nucleotide polymorphisms; SD: Standard deviation; VTE: Venous thromboembolism; WHR: Waist-hip-ratio

Acknowledgements
This study uses the data from the UK Biobank. We are grateful to the UK Biobank for access to their data.

Funding
FYL and SEH are funded by the National Institute for Health Research Leicester Biomedical Research Centre. CPN and NJS are funded by the British Heart Foundation. The funders had no role in study design, data collection and analysis, decision to publish or preparation of the manuscript.

Authors' contributions
FYL, CPN and NJS conceived and designed the study. FYL, MN and SEH performed the analysis under the guidance from CPN, JRT and NJS. FYL and NJS wrote the first draft of the manuscript. All authors reviewed and approved the final manuscript.

Competing interests
The authors declare that they have no competing interests.

Author details
[1]Department of Cardiovascular Sciences, University of Leicester, Leicester, UK. [2]NIHR Leicester Biomedical Research Centre, Glenfield Hospital, Leicester, UK. [3]Department of Health Sciences, University of Leicester, Leicester, UK.

References
1. Davey Smith G, Hart C, Upton M, Hole D, Gillis C, Watt G, et al. Height and risk of death among men and women: aetiological implications of associations with cardiorespiratory disease and cancer mortality. J Epidemiol Community Health. 2000;54:97–103.
2. Jousilahti P, Tuomilehto J, Vartiainen E, Eriksson J, Puska P. Relation of adult height to cause-specific and total mortality: a prospective follow-up study of 31,199 middle-aged men and women in Finland. Am J Epidemiol. 2000; 151:1112–20.
3. Strandberg TE. Inverse relation between height and cardiovascular mortality in men during 30-year follow-up. Am J Cardiol. 1997;80:349–50.
4. McCarron P, Okasha M, McEwen J, Smith GD. Height in young adulthood and risk of death from cardiorespiratory disease: a prospective study of male former students of Glasgow University, Scotland. Am J Epidemiol. 2002;155:683–7.
5. Paajanen TA, Oksala NK, Kuukasjärvi P, Karhunen PJ. Short stature is associated with coronary heart disease: a systematic review of the literature and a meta-analysis. Eur Heart J. 2010;31:1802–9.
6. Lee CM, Barzi F, Woodward M, Batty GD, Giles GG, Wong JW, Asia Pacific Cohort Studies Collaboration, et al. Adult height and the risks of cardiovascular disease and major causes of death in the Asia-Pacific region: 21,000 deaths in 510,000 men and women. Int J Epidemiol. 2009;38:1060–71.
7. Emerging Risk Factors Collaboration. Adult height and the risk of cause-specific death and vascular morbidity in 1 million people: individual participant meta-analysis. Int J Epidemiol. 2012;41:1419–33.
8. Rosenberg MA, Patton KK, Sotoodehnia N, Karas MG, Kizer JR, Zimetbaum PJ, et al. The impact of height on the risk of atrial fibrillation: the Cardiovascular Health Study. Eur Heart J. 2012;33:2709–17.
9. Schmidt M, Bøtker HE, Pedersen L, Sørensen HT. Adult height and risk of ischemic heart disease, atrial fibrillation, stroke, venous thromboembolism, and premature death: a population based 36-year follow-up study. Eur J Epidemiol. 2014;29:111–8.
10. Braekkan SK, Borch KH, Mathiesen EB, Njølstad I, Wilsgaard T, Hansen JB. Body height and risk of venous thromboembolism: the Tromsø Study. Am J Epidemiol. 2010;171:1109–15.
11. Flinterman LE, van Hylckama Vlieg A, Rosendaal FR, Cannegieter SC. Body height, mobility, and risk of first and recurrent venous thrombosis. J Thromb Haemost. 2015;13:548–54.
12. Batty GD, Shipley MJ, Langenberg C, Marmot MG, Davey Smith G. Adult height in relation to mortality from 14 cancer sites in men in London (UK): evidence from the original Whitehall study. Ann Oncol. 2006;17:157–66.
13. Wirén S, Häggström C, Ulmer H, Manjer J, Bjørge T, Nagel G, et al. Pooled cohort study on height and risk of cancer and cancer death. Cancer Causes Control. 2014;25:151–9.
14. Green J, Cairns BJ, Casabonne D, Wright FL, Reeves G, Beral V, Million Women Study collaborators. Height and cancer incidence in the Million Women Study: prospective cohort, and meta-analysis of prospective studies of height and total cancer risk. Lancet Oncol. 2011;12:785–94.
15. Kabat GC, Kim MY, Hollenbeck AR, Rohan TE. Attained height, sex, and risk of cancer at different anatomic sites in the NIH-AARP diet and health study. Cancer Causes Control. 2014;25:1697–706.

16. Khankari NK, Shu XO, Wen W, Kraft P, Lindström S, Peters U, et al. Association between adult height and risk of colorectal, lung, and prostate cancer: results from meta-analyses of prospective studies and Mendelian randomization analyses. PLoS Med. 2016;13:e1002118. https://doi.org/10.1371/journal.pmed.1002118.

17. Webb E, Kuh D, Peasey A, Pajak A, Malyutina S, Kubinova R, et al. Childhood socioeconomic circumstances and adult height and leg length in central and eastern Europe. J Epidemiol Community Health. 2008;62:351–7.

18. Gunnell D. Can adult anthropometry be used as a 'biomarker' for prenatal and childhood exposures? Int J Epidemiol. 2002;31:390–4.

19. Bozzoli C, Deaton A, Quintana-Domeque C. Adult height and childhood disease. Demography. 2009;46:647–69.

20. Lawlor DA, Harbord RM, Sterne JAC, Timpson N, Davey Smith G. Mendelian randomization: using genes as instruments for making causal inferences in epidemiology. Stat Med. 2008;27:1133–63.

21. Nelson CP, Hamby SE, Saleheen D, Hopewell JC, Zeng L, Assimes TL, et al. Genetically-determined height and coronary artery disease. N Engl J Med. 2015;372:1608–18.

22. Nüesch E, Dale C, Palmer TM, White J, Keating BJ, van Iperen EP, et al. Adult height, coronary heart disease and stroke: a multi-locus Mendelian randomization meta-analysis. Int J Epidemiol. 2016;45:1927–37.

23. Roetker NS, Armasu SM, Pankow JS, Lutsey PL, Tang W, Rosenberg MA, et al. Taller height as a risk factor for venous thromboembolism: a Mendelian randomization meta-analysis. J Thromb Haemost. 2017;15:1334–43.

24. Zhang B, Shu XO, Delahanty RJ, Zeng C, Michailidou K, Bolla MK, et al. Height and breast cancer risk: evidence from prospective studies and Mendelian randomization. J Natl Cancer Inst. 2015;107(11). https://doi.org/10.1093/jnci/djv219.

25. Davies NM, Gaunt TR, Lewis SJ, Holly J, Donovan JL, Hamdy FC, et al. The effects of height and BMI on prostate cancer incidence and mortality: a Mendelian randomization study in 20,848 cases and 20,214 controls from the PRACTICAL consortium. Cancer Causes Control. 2015;26:1603–16.

26. Thrift AP, Gong J, Peters U, Chang-Claude J, Rudolph A, Slattery ML, et al. Mendelian randomization study of height and risk of colorectal cancer. Int J Epidemiol. 2015;44:662–72.

27. Ong JS, An J, Law MH, Whiteman DC, Neale RE, Gharahkhani P, et al. Height and overall cancer risk and mortality: evidence from a Mendelian randomisation study on 310,000 UK Biobank participants. Br J Cancer. 2018;118:1262–7.

28. Dixon-Suen SC, Nagle CM, Thrift AP, Pharoah PDP, Ewing A, Pearce CL, et al. Adult height is associated with increased risk of ovarian cancer: a Mendelian randomisation study. Br J Cancer. 2018;118:1123–9.

29. Wood AR, Esko T, Yang J, Vedantam S, Pers TH, Gustafsson S, et al. Defining the role of common variation in the genomic and biological architecture of adult human height. Nat Genet. 2014;46:1173–86.

30. Sudlow C, Gallacher J, Allen N, Beral V, Burton P, Danesh J, et al. UK biobank: an open access resource for identifying the causes of a wide range of complex diseases of middle and old age. PLoS Med. 2015;12(3):e1001779. https://doi.org/10.1371/journal.pmed.1001779.

31. Wain LV, Shrine N, Miller S, Jackson VE, Ntalla I, Soler Artigas M, et al. Novel insights into the genetics of smoking behaviour, lung function, and chronic obstructive pulmonary disease (UK BiLEVE): a genetic association study in UK Biobank. Lancet Respir Med. 2015;3:769–81.

32. Bycroft C, Freeman C, Petkova D, Band G, Elliott LT, Sharp K, et al. Genome-wide genetic data on ~500,000 UK Biobank participants. bioRxiv. 2017. https://doi.org/10.1101/166298.

33. Townsend P, Phillimore P, Beattie A. Health and deprivation: inequality and the north. London: Croom Helm; 1988.

34. Burgess S, Dudbridge F, Thompson SG. Combining information on multiple instrumental variables in Mendelian randomization: comparison of allele score and summarized data methods. Stat Med. 2016;35:1880–906.

35. Bowden J, Davey Smith G, Burgess S. Mendelian randomization with invalid instruments: effect estimation and bias detection through Egger regression. Int J Epidemiol. 2015;44:512–25.

36. Bowden J, Davey Smith G, Haycock PC, Burgess S. Consistent estimation in Mendelian randomization with some invalid instruments using a weighted median estimator. Genet Epidemiol. 2016;40:304–14.

37. Burgess S, Thompson SG. Interpreting findings from Mendelian randomization using the MR-Egger method. Eur J Epidemiol. 2017;32:377–89.

38. Lemos PA, Ribeiro EE, Perin MA, Kajita LJ, de Magalhães MA, Falcão JL, et al. Angiographic segment size in patients referred for coronary intervention is influenced by constitutional, anatomical, and clinical features. Int J Card Imaging. 2007;23:1–7.

39. O'Connor NJ, Morton JR, Birkmeyer JD, Olmstead EM, O'Connor GT. Effect of coronary artery diameter in patients undergoing coronary bypass surgery. Circulation. 1996;93:652–5.

40. Smulyan H, Marchais SJ, Pannier B, Guerin AP, Safar ME, London GM. Influence of body height on pulsatile arterial hemodynamic data. J Am Coll Cardiol. 1998;31:1103–9.

41. Abhayaratna WP, Seward JB, Appleton CP, Douglas PS, Oh JK, Tajik AJ, et al. Left atrial size: physiologic determinants and clinical applications. J Am Coll Cardiol. 2006;47:2357–63.

42. Rosengren A, Hauptman PJ, Lappas G, Olsson L, Wilhelmsen L, Swedberg K. Big men and atrial fibrillation: effects of body size and weight gain on risk of atrial fibrillation in men. Eur Heart J. 2009;30:1113–20.

43. Heliövaara M. Body height, obesity, and risk of herniated lumbar intervertebral disc. Spine. 1987;12:469–72.

44. Kelsey JL. An epidemiological study of acute herniated lumbar intervertebral discs. Rheumatol Rehabil. 1975;14:144–59.

45. Karacan I, Aydin T, Sahin Z, Cidem M, Koyuncu H, Aktas I, et al. Facet angles in lumbar disc herniation: their relation to anthropometric features. Spine. 2004;29:1132–6.

46. Xiao Z, Ren D, Feng W, Chen Y, Kan W, Xing D. Height and risk of hip fracture: a meta-analysis of prospective cohort studies. Biomed Res Int. 2016;2016:2480693.

47. Greendale GA, Young JT, Huang MH, Bucur A, Wang Y, Seeman T. Hip axis length in mid-life Japanese and Caucasian U.S. residents: no evidence for an ethnic difference. Osteoporos Int. 2003;14:320–5.

48. Frisoli A Jr, Paula AP, Pinheiro M, Szejnfeld VL, Delmonte Piovezan R, Takata E, et al. Hip axis length as an independent risk factor for hip fracture independently of femoral bone mineral density in Caucasian elderly Brazilian women. Bone. 2005;37:871–5.

49. Hyun JJ, Bak YT. Clinical significance of hiatal hernia. Gut Liver. 2011;5:267–77.

50. Thrift AP, Risch HA, Onstad L, Shaheen NJ, Casson AG, Bernstein L, et al. Risk of esophageal adenocarcinoma decreases with height, based on consortium analysis and confirmed by Mendelian randomization. Clin Gastroenterol Hepatol. 2014;12:1667–76.e1.

51. Burgess S, Davies NM, Thompson SG. Bias due to participant overlap in two-sample Mendelian randomization. Genet Epidemiol. 2016;40:597–608.

52. Förstermann U, Xia N, Li H. Roles of vascular oxidative stress and nitric oxide in the pathogenesis of atherosclerosis. Circ Res. 2017;120:713–35.

53. Dawson K, Aflaki M, Nattel S. Role of the Wnt-Frizzled system in cardiac pathophysiology: a rapidly developing, poorly understood area with enormous potential. J Physiol. 2013;591:1409–32.

54. Marras LC, Geerts WH, Perry JR. The risk of venous thromboembolism is increased throughout the course of malignant glioma. Cancer. 2000;89(3):640–6.

55. Thaler J, Ay C, Kaider A, Reitter EM, Haselböck J, Mannhalter C, et al. Biomarkers predictive of venous thromboembolism in patients with newly diagnosed high-grade gliomas. Neuro-Oncology. 2014;16:1645–51.

56. Horsted F, West J, Grainge MJ. Risk of venous thromboembolism in patients with cancer: a systematic review and meta-analysis. PLoS Med. 2012;9(7):e1001275.

57. Pyne NJ, Pyne S. Sphingosine 1-phosphate and cancer. Nat Rev Cancer. 2010;10:489–503.

58. Nagahashi M, Hait NC, Maceyka M, Avni D, Takabe K, Milstien S, Spiegel S. Sphingosine-1-phosphate in chronic intestinal inflammation and cancer. Adv Biol Regul. 2014;54:112–20.

59. Leve F, Morgado-Díaz JA. Rho GTPase signaling in the development of colorectal cancer. J Cell Biochem. 2012;113:2549–59.

10

Poor reporting of multivariable prediction model studies: towards a targeted implementation strategy of the TRIPOD statement

Pauline Heus[1,2]* (iD), Johanna A. A. G. Damen[1,2], Romin Pajouheshnia[2], Rob J. P. M. Scholten[1,2], Johannes B. Reitsma[1,2], Gary S. Collins[3], Douglas G. Altman[3], Karel G. M. Moons[1,2] and Lotty Hooft[1,2]

Abstract

Background: As complete reporting is essential to judge the validity and applicability of multivariable prediction models, a guideline for the Transparent Reporting of a multivariable prediction model for Individual Prognosis Or Diagnosis (TRIPOD) was introduced. We assessed the completeness of reporting of prediction model studies published just before the introduction of the TRIPOD statement, to refine and tailor its implementation strategy.

Methods: Within each of 37 clinical domains, 10 journals with the highest journal impact factor were selected. A PubMed search was performed to identify prediction model studies published before the launch of TRIPOD in these journals (May 2014). Eligible publications reported on the development or external validation of a multivariable prediction model (either diagnostic or prognostic) or on the incremental value of adding a predictor to an existing model.

Results: We included 146 publications (84% prognostic), from which we assessed 170 models: 73 (43%) on model development, 43 (25%) on external validation, 33 (19%) on incremental value, and 21 (12%) on combined development and external validation of the same model. Overall, publications adhered to a median of 44% (25th–75th percentile 35–52%) of TRIPOD items, with 44% (35–53%) for prognostic and 41% (34–48%) for diagnostic models. TRIPOD items that were completely reported for less than 25% of the models concerned abstract (2%), title (5%), blinding of predictor assessment (6%), comparison of development and validation data (11%), model updating (14%), model performance (14%), model specification (17%), characteristics of participants (21%), model performance measures (methods) (21%), and model-building procedures (24%). Most often reported were TRIPOD items regarding overall interpretation (96%), source of data (95%), and risk groups (90%).

Conclusions: More than half of the items considered essential for transparent reporting were not fully addressed in publications of multivariable prediction model studies. Essential information for using a model in individual risk prediction, i.e. model specifications and model performance, was incomplete for more than 80% of the models. Items that require improved reporting are title, abstract, and model-building procedures, as they are crucial for identification and external validation of prediction models.

Keywords: TRIPOD, Reporting guideline, Prediction model, Risk score, Prediction rule, Risk assessment, Prognosis, Diagnosis, Development, Validation, Incremental value

* Correspondence: p.heus@umcutrecht.nl
[1]Cochrane Netherlands, University Medical Center Utrecht, Utrecht University, Utrecht, The Netherlands
[2]Julius Center for Health Sciences and Primary Care, University Medical Center Utrecht, Utrecht University, Utrecht, The Netherlands
Full list of author information is available at the end of the article

Background

Multivariable prediction models (risk scores or prediction rules) estimate an individual's probability or risk that a specific disease or condition is present (diagnostic models) or that a specific event will occur in the future (prognostic models) based on multiple characteristics or pieces of information for that individual [1]. Such models are increasingly used by healthcare providers to support clinical decision making or to inform patients or relatives. Studies about prediction models may address the development of a new model, validation of an existing, previously developed model in other individuals (with or without adjusting or updating the model to the validation setting), or a combination of these two types [2–5]. Some prediction model studies evaluate the addition of a single predictor to an existing model (incremental value) [4].

In addition to appropriate design, conduct, and analysis, reporting of prediction model studies should be complete and accurate. Complete reporting of research facilitates study replication, assessment of the study validity (risk of bias), interpretation of the results, and judgment of applicability of the study results (e.g. the prediction model itself) to other individuals or settings. Clinicians and other stakeholders can only use previously developed and validated prediction models when all relevant information is available for calculating predicted risks at an individual level. High-quality information about prediction model studies is therefore essential.

Previous systematic reviews showed that within different clinical domains the quality of reporting of prediction models is suboptimal [6–11]. To improve the reporting of studies of prediction models, a guideline for the Transparent Reporting of a multivariable prediction model for Individual Prognosis Or Diagnosis (TRIPOD) was launched in January 2015 in more than 10 medical journals [12, 13]. The TRIPOD statement is a checklist of 22 items considered essential for informative reporting of prediction model studies. Both diagnostic and prognostic prediction model studies are covered by the TRIPOD statement, and the checklist can be used for all types of prediction model studies (development, external validation, and incremental value) within all clinical domains.

In this comprehensive literature review, we assessed the completeness of reporting of prediction model studies that were published just before the introduction of the TRIPOD statement. Our results provide key clues to further refine and tailor the implementation strategy of the TRIPOD statement.

Methods

Identification of prediction model studies

To cover a wide range of clinical domains, we started with 37 subject categories (2012 Journal Citation Reports®) [14] from which we selected the 10 journals with the highest journal impact factor (Additional file 1). After deduplication, 341 unique journals remained. We performed a search in PubMed to identify prediction model studies published in these journals before the launch of TRIPOD (May 2014), using a validated search filter for identifying prognostic and diagnostic prediction studies (Additional file 2) [15].

Eligible publications described the development or external validation of a multivariable prediction model (either diagnostic or prognostic) or evaluated the incremental value of adding a predictor to an existing model [1–5, 16]. We excluded so-called prognostic factor or predictor finding studies, as well as studies evaluating the impact of the use of a prediction model on management or patient outcomes [3, 7, 17]. We excluded prediction model studies using non-regression techniques (e.g. classification trees, neural networks, and machine learning) or pharmacokinetic models. Titles and abstracts of the retrieved publications were screened by one of two authors (JAAGD or PH). After reading the full text report, they judged whether to include or exclude a potentially eligible publication. Any doubts regarding definitive eligibility were discussed, if necessary, with a third author. If we were not able to retrieve the full text of a publication via our institutions, it was excluded.

Data extraction

For each included publication we recorded the journal impact factor (2012 Journal Citation Reports®) [14], clinical domain, and whether the purpose of prediction was diagnostic or prognostic. Furthermore, we classified publications into four types of prediction model studies: development, external validation, incremental value, or combination of development and external validation of the same model. A publication could be categorised as more than one type of prediction model study. For example, if a publication reported on both development and external validation, but of different models, it was classified as development as well as external validation. If a publication included multiple prediction model studies of the same type, e.g. if two models were developed, we extracted data for only one model. If there was no primary model, we used the model that was studied in the largest sample. Information about study design, sample size, number of predictors in the final model, and predicted outcome was extracted for all included prediction models.

To judge the completeness of the reporting, we transformed items of the TRIPOD statement (Box 1) into a data extraction form, which was piloted extensively to ensure consistent extraction of the data. The TRIPOD statement consists of 22 main items, 10 of which are divided in two (items 3, 4, 6, 7, 14, 15, and 19), three (items 5 and 13), or five (item 10) subitems [12, 13]. For TRIPOD items (main or subitems, hereafter just called

---

Box 1 Items of the TRIPOD statement

Title and abstract

1. **Title (D; V)**: Identify the study as developing and/or validating a multivariable prediction model, the target population, and the outcome to be predicted

2. **Abstract (D; V)**: Provide a summary of objectives, study design, setting, participants, sample size, predictors, outcome, statistical analysis, results, and conclusions

Introduction

3. **Background and objectives**:

   a. **(D; V)** Explain the medical context (including whether diagnostic or prognostic) and rationale for developing or validating the multivariable prediction model, including references to existing models

   b. **(D; V)** Specify the objectives, including whether the study describes the development or validation of the model or both

Methods

4. **Source of data**:

   a. **(D; V)** Describe the study design or source of data (e.g. randomised trial, cohort, or registry data), separately for the development and validation data sets, if applicable

   b. **(D; V)** Specify the key study dates, including start of accrual, end of accrual, and, if applicable, end of follow-up

5. **Participants**:

   a. **(D; V)** Specify key elements of the study setting (e.g. primary care, secondary care, general population) including number and location of centres

   b. **(D; V)** Describe eligibility criteria for participants

   c. **(D; V)** Give details of treatments received, if relevant

6. **Outcome**:

   a. **(D; V)** Clearly define the outcome that is predicted by the prediction model, including how and when assessed

   b. **(D; V)** Report any actions to blind assessment of the outcome to be predicted

7. **Predictors**:

   a. **(D; V)** Clearly define all predictors used in developing or validating the multivariable prediction model, including how and when they were measured

   b. **(D; V)** Report any actions to blind assessment of predictors for the outcome and other predictors

8. **Sample size (D; V)**: Explain how the study size was arrived at

9. **Missing data (D; V)**: Describe how missing data were handled (e.g. complete-case analysis, single imputation, multiple imputation) with details of any imputation method

10. **Statistical analysis methods**:

    a. **(D)** Describe how predictors were handled in the analyses

    b. **(D)** Specify type of model, all model-building procedures (including any predictor selection), and method for internal validation

    c. **(V)** For validation, describe how the predictions were calculated

    d. **(D; V)** Specify all measures used to assess model performance and, if relevant, to compare multiple models

    e. **(V)** Describe any model updating (e.g. recalibration) arising from the validation, if done

11. **Risk groups (D; V)**: Provide details on how risk groups were created, if done

12. **Development vs. validation (V)**: For validation, identify any differences from the development data in setting, eligibility criteria, outcome, and predictors

Results

13. **Participants**:

    a. **(D; V)** Describe the flow of participants through the study, including the number of participants with and without the outcome and, if applicable, a summary of the follow-up time. A diagram may be helpful

    b. **(D; V)** Describe the characteristics of the participants (basic demographics, clinical features, available predictors), including the number of participants with missing data for predictors and outcome

    c. **(V)** For validation, show a comparison with the development data of the distribution of important variables (demographics, predictors, and outcome)

(Continued)

14. **Model development**:

    a. **(D)** Specify the number of participants and outcome events in each analysis

    b. **(D)** If done, report the unadjusted association between each candidate predictor and outcome

15. **Model specification**:

    a. **(D)** Present the full prediction model to allow predictions for individuals (i.e. all regression coefficients, and model intercept or baseline survival at a given time point)

    b. **(D)** Explain how to the use the prediction model

16. **Model performance (D;V)**: Report performance measures (with confidence intervals [CIs]) for the prediction model

17. **Model updating (V)**: If done, report the results from any model updating (i.e. model specification, model performance)

Discussion

18. **Limitations (D;V)**: Discuss any limitations of the study (such as non-representative sample, few events per predictor, missing data)

19. **Interpretation**:

    a. **(V)** For validation, discuss the results with reference to performance in the development data and any other validation data

    b. **(D;V)** Give an overall interpretation of the results, considering objectives, limitations, results from similar studies, and other relevant evidence

20. **Implications (D;V)**: Discuss the potential clinical use of the model and implications for future research

Other information

21. **Supplementary information (D;V)**: Provide information about the availability of supplementary resources, such as study protocol, Web calculator, and data sets

22. **Funding (D;V)**: Give the source of funding and the role of the funders for the present study

D;V item relevant to both development and external validation, *D* item only relevant to development, *V* item only relevant to external validation

---

items) containing multiple reporting elements, we extracted information regarding each of these elements. For example, for item 4b, 'Specify the key study dates, including start of accrual, end of accrual, and, if applicable, end of follow-up', we used three data extraction elements to record information regarding (1) the start of accrual, (2) end of accrual, and (3) end of follow-up. The data extraction form including all data extraction elements can be found on the website of the TRIPOD statement (www.tripod-statement.org/).

For each data extraction element we judged whether the requested information was available in the publication. If a publication reported both the development and external validation of the same prediction model, we extracted data on the reporting of either separately, and subsequently combined the extracted information for each data extraction element.

Three authors extracted data (JAAGD, PH, RP). If the authors disagreed or were unsure about the reporting of a data extraction element, it was discussed in consensus meetings with the other co-authors.

Analyses

Based on the extracted data elements, we first determined whether the reporting of each TRIPOD item was complete (completeness is defined in the following subsection). We then calculated overall scores for completeness of reporting per model, per publication, and per item of the TRIPOD statement (across models).

Completeness of reporting of each TRIPOD item

The reporting of a TRIPOD item was judged to be complete if the requested information for all elements of that particular TRIPOD item was present. For elements belonging to TRIPOD items 4b, 5a, 6a, and 7a, we considered a reference to information in another article acceptable. If an element was not applicable to a specific model (e.g. follow-up might be not relevant in a diagnostic prediction model study) (item 4b), or blinding was a non-issue (e.g. if the predicted outcome was for example overall mortality) (items 6b and 7b), this element was regarded as being reported.

Overall completeness of reporting per model

To calculate the overall completeness of reporting for each included model, we divided the number of completely reported TRIPOD items by the total number of TRIPOD items for that model. The total number of TRIPOD items varies per type of prediction model study, as six of the TRIPOD items only apply to development of a prediction model (10a, 10b, 14a, 14b, 15a, and 15b) and six only to external validation (10c, 10e, 12, 13c, 17, and 19a). This resulted in a total number of 31 TRIPOD items for the reporting of either development or external validation of a prediction model, 37 for the combined reporting of development and external validation of the same prediction model, and 36 for reporting incremental value.

Five items of the TRIPOD statement include an 'if done' or 'if applicable' statement (items 5c, 10e, 11, 14b, and 17). If we considered such an item not applicable for a particular study, it was excluded when calculating the completeness of reporting (in both the numerator and denominator). Furthermore, item 21 of the TRIPOD statement was excluded from all calculations, as it refers to whether supplementary material was provided.

Overall completeness of reporting per publication

The overall reporting per publication equals the reporting per model (see previous subsection) for publications classified as development, external validation, incremental value, or combined development and external validation of the same model. For publications classified as more than one type of prediction model study, e.g. development of a model and external validation of a different model, we combined the reporting of the different prediction model types within that publication. Reporting was considered complete when the reporting of the different types of prediction model studies was complete, except for TRIPOD items 3a and 18–20, for which complete reporting for either type was considered sufficient.

We used linear regression to investigate possible relationships between completeness of reporting per publication as dependent variable, and sample size, journal impact factor, number of predictors in the final model, and prospective study design (as dichotomous variable, yes/no) as independent variables.

Overall completeness of reporting per item of the TRIPOD statement

We assessed the overall completeness of reporting of individual items of the TRIPOD statement by dividing the number of models with complete reporting of a particular TRIPOD item by the total number of models in which that item was applicable.

Results

We included a total of 146 publications (Fig. 1). Most publications (122 [84%]) reported prognostic models. From the 146 publications we scored the reporting of 170 prediction models: 73 (43%) concerned model development, 43 (25%) external validation of an existing model, 33 (19%) incremental value of adding a predictor

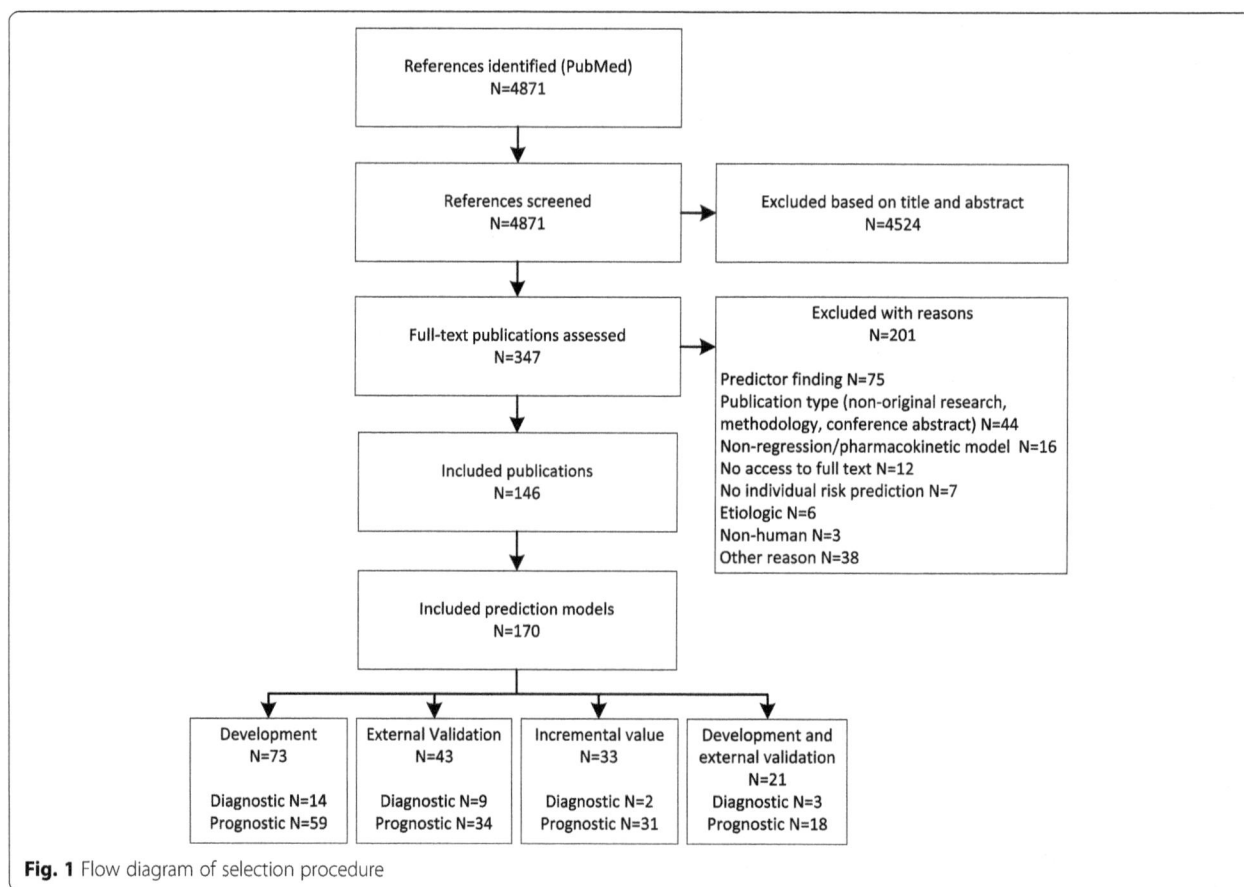

Fig. 1 Flow diagram of selection procedure

to a model, and 21 (12%) a combination of development and external validation of the same model.

The three clinical domains with the most publications of prediction models were critical care medicine (18 [11%]), obstetrics and gynaecology (15 [9%]), and gastroenterology and hepatology (12 [7%]). The median journal impact factor of the publications was 5.3 (25th–75th percentile [P_{25}–P_{75}] 4.0–7.1). The median sample size of the populations in which a model was studied was 450 (P_{25}–P_{75} 200–2005). In the final models a median of 5 (P_{25}–P_{75} 3–8) predictors were included, and in 23 models (16%) all-cause mortality was the predicted outcome.

Completeness of reporting per publication

Overall, publications adhered to between 16 and 81% of the items of the TRIPOD statement with a median of 44% (P_{25}–P_{75} 35–52%) (Fig. 2). The reporting quality for prognostic and diagnostic prediction models was comparable, with a median adherence of 44% (P_{25}–P_{75} 35–53%) and 41% (P_{25}–P_{75} 34–48%), respectively. The most complete reporting was seen for the combined reporting of development and external validation of the same model (47%; P_{25}–P_{75} 35–54%), followed by the reporting of model development (43%; P_{25}–P_{75} 35–53%), external validation (43%; P_{25}–P_{75} 37–54%), and incremental value (38%; P_{25}–P_{75} 33–49%). No associations were found

between completeness of reporting and sample size, journal impact factor, number of predictors in the final model, and prospective study design (data not shown).

Reporting of individual TRIPOD items

Six TRIPOD items were reported in 75% or more of the 170 models, and 10 items in less than 25% (Table 1).

Completeness of reporting of individual TRIPOD items is presented in Fig. 3 and Additional file 3 over all 170 models, and per type of prediction model study. The most notable findings for each section of the TRIPOD statement (title and abstract, introduction, methods, results, discussion, and other information) are described below.

Title and abstract (items 1 and 2)

According to the TRIPOD statement, an informative title contains (synonyms for) the term *risk prediction model*, the *type of prediction model* study (i.e. development, external validation, incremental value, or combination), the *target population*, and *outcome to be predicted*. Eight of the 170 models (5%) addressed all four elements. The description of the type of prediction model study was the least reported element (12%). Complete reporting of abstracts required information for 12 elements. Three of the models (2%) fulfilled all the requirements.

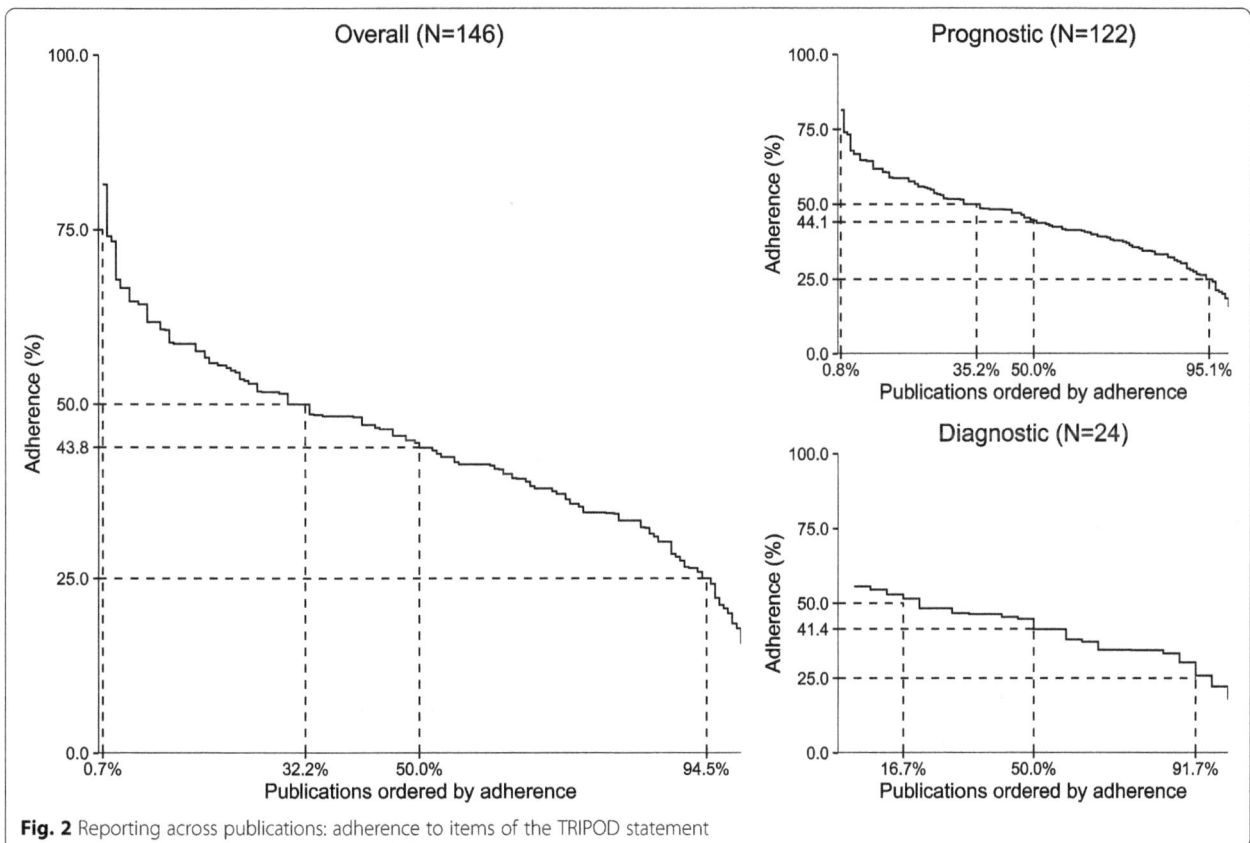

Fig. 2 Reporting across publications: adherence to items of the TRIPOD statement

Table 1 Completeness of reporting of individual TRIPOD items ($n = 170$ models)

Complete reporting for > 75% of the models		Complete reporting for < 25% of the models	
TRIPOD items	%	TRIPOD items	%
19b Give an overall interpretation of the results, considering objectives, limitations, results from similar studies, and other relevant evidence	96	10b Specify type of model, all model-building procedures (including any predictor selection), and method for internal validation	24
4a Describe the study design or source of data (e.g. randomised trial, cohort, or registry data), separately for the development and validation data sets, if applicable	95	10d Specify all measures used to assess model performance and, if relevant, to compare multiple models	21
11 Provide details on how risk groups were created, if done	90	13b Describe the characteristics of the participants (basic demographics, clinical features, available predictors), including the number of participants with missing data for predictors and outcome	21
18 Discuss any limitations of the study (such as non-representative sample, few events per predictor, missing data)	88	15a Present the full prediction model to allow predictions for individuals (i.e. all regression coefficients, and model intercept or baseline survival at a given time point)	17
3a Explain the medical context (including whether diagnostic or prognostic) and rationale for developing or validating the multivariable prediction model, including references to existing models	81	16 Report performance measures (with confidence intervals [CIs]) for the prediction model	14
5b Describe eligibility criteria for participants	79	17 If done, report the results from any model updating (i.e. model specification, model performance)	14
		12 For validation, identify any differences from the development data in setting, eligibility criteria, outcome, and predictors	11
		7b Report any actions to blind assessment of predictors for the outcome and other predictors	6
		1 Identify the study as developing and/or validating a multivariable prediction model, the target population, and the outcome to be predicted	5
		2 Provide a summary of objectives, study design, setting, participants, sample size, predictors, outcome, statistical analysis, results, and conclusions	2

Introduction (item 3)

For 81% of the models complete information about background and rationale was provided (item 3a), and in 63% reporting of study objectives (item 3b), including a specification of the type of prediction model study, was considered complete.

Methods (items 4–12)

Source of data (item 4a; 95% reported) and eligibility criteria (item 5b; 79%) were among the best reported items for all four types of prediction model studies. Actions to blind assessment of (non-objective) outcomes (item 6b; 28%) and predictors (item 7b; 7%) were less well reported. Detailed predictor definitions (item 7a) were provided for 25% of the models. Also, information about how missing data were handled (item 9) was incomplete for the majority of models (reported in 39%). Most aspects of statistical analysis were inadequately reported as well. How predictors were handled (item 10a) was described in 29% of the models. Model-building procedures (item 10b) were specified in 24% overall, and were particularly poorly represented in

incremental value reports (3%). Few studies (21%) described both discrimination and calibration as measures of model performance (item 10d).

Results (items 13–17)

Characteristics of participants (item 13b, complete reporting in 21%) were often reported without information regarding missing data for predictors and outcome. Two (5%) of the external validations presented demographics, distribution of predictors, and outcomes alongside those of the original development study (item 13c), and in combined reports of development and external validation this was done in 43%. The final model was presented in full (item 15a) in 17% of the models. For many models the intercept (or the cumulative baseline hazard, or baseline survival, for at least one time point in the case of survival models) was not provided. A small number of models provided information on both discrimination and calibration when reporting model performance (item 16; 14%). Discrimination was more frequently reported (79%) than calibration (29%).

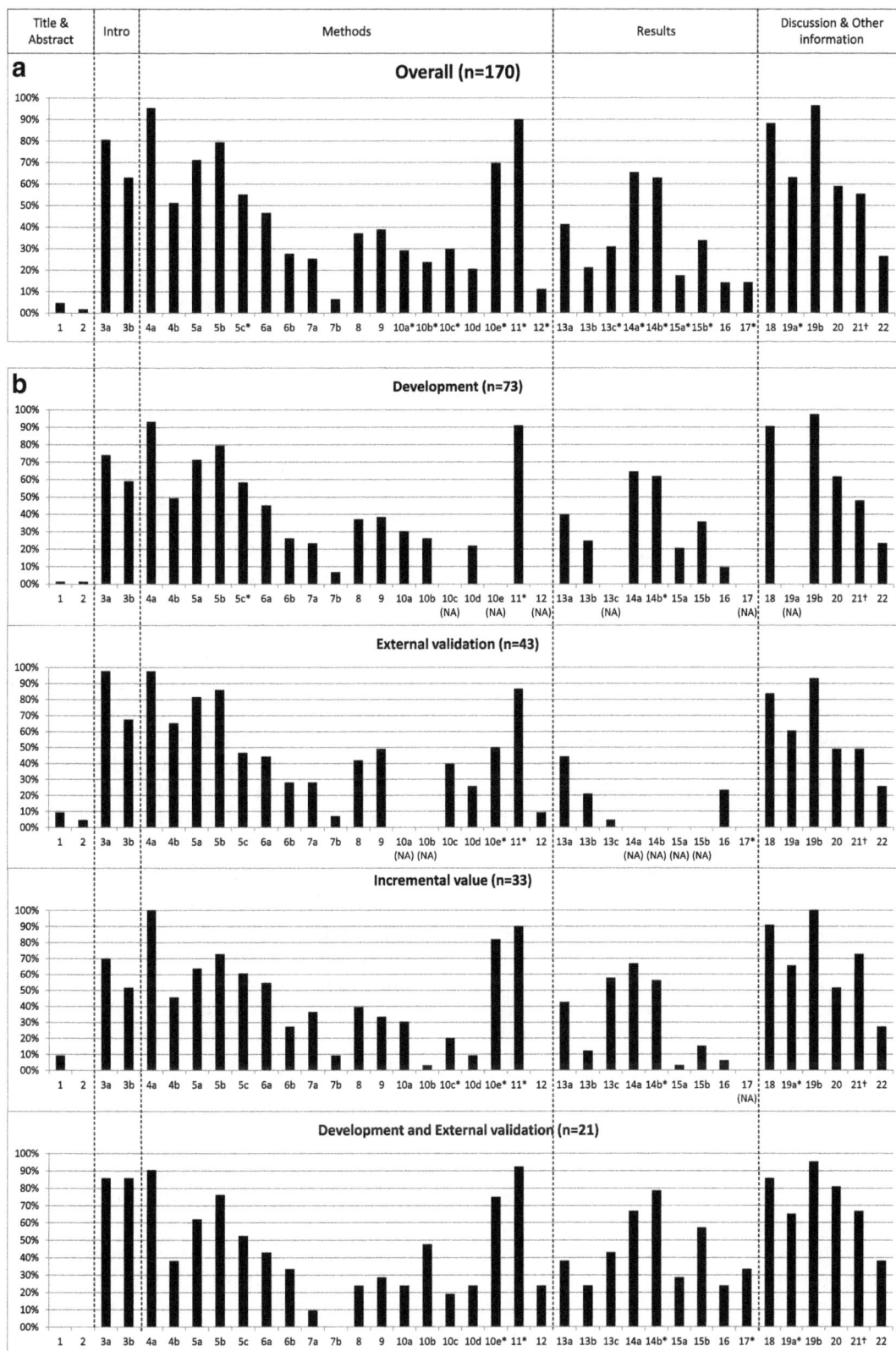

Fig. 3 (See legend on next page.)

Discussion (items 18–20)

An overall interpretation of the results (item 19b) was given for almost all included models of all types of prediction model studies (97%). The potential for clinical use and implications for future research (item 20) were discussed in 59% of the models.

Other information (items 21 and 22)

Information about the availability of supplementary resources (item 21) was provided in 55% of the models. Complete information regarding funding (item 22) was reported in 27%.

Discussion

Complete and accurate reporting of prediction model studies is required to critically appraise, externally validate, evaluate the impact of, and eventually use prediction models in clinical practice. Our study shows that, regardless of the type of prediction model study and whether diagnostic or prognostic, more than half of the items deemed essential to report in prediction model publications according to the TRIPOD statement were not completely reported.

Highly problematic TRIPOD items in terms of reporting were items regarding title and abstract. These items, for which complete reporting requires information on multiple elements, were adequately reported for less than 10% of the models. In addition, details of study methods, especially blinding of outcome and predictor assessments, were provided for only a minority of reported models. Furthermore, information on follow-up, predictor definitions, model-building procedures, and handling of missing data were often lacking. Notable findings regarding the reporting of study results were that in more than 70% of the included models the final model was not presented in enough detail to make predictions for new patients, and that the reporting of model performance was often incomplete. Items of the TRIPOD statement that were generally well reported addressed the source of data and eligibility criteria, risk groups (if applicable), study limitations, and overall interpretation of results.

Comparison with other studies

Our main finding of inadequate reporting in the majority of publications within 37 clinical domains is comparable to the findings of systematic reviews of prediction model studies performed in general medicine or specific clinical domains [6–11]. Inadequate reporting is considered to be a form of research waste [18, 19]. Therefore, for many study types, reporting guidelines were published in the last 20 years, such as the Consolidated Standards of Reporting Trials (CONSORT) statement in 1996 (updates in 2001 and 2010), the Standards for Reporting of Diagnostic Accuracy (STARD) statement in 2003 (update in 2015), and Reporting recommendations for tumour marker prognostic studies (REMARK) in 2005 [20–24]. Completeness of reporting before the introduction of these reporting guidelines was similar to our result of 44% adherence. Moher and colleagues (2001) evaluated 97 reports of randomised trials before the introduction of CONSORT and found adequate reporting for just over half of the items (58%) [25]. In a systematic review of 16 studies evaluating the adherence to STARD, overall, 51% of items were adequately reported [26]. For six included studies with quantitative data before publication of STARD, a range of 44–61% adherence was reported. An assessment of the reporting of prognostic studies of tumour markers was done shortly after the introduction of REMARK [27, 28]. Ten (out of 20) items were evaluated, and, overall, articles adhered to 53% of these.

Strengths and limitations of this study

With this literature review we cover a broad literature base by including three major types of prediction model studies, both prognostic and diagnostic, across 37 clinical domains. Despite the use of a validated search strategy, we may have missed publications on prediction models. It is likely that the completeness of reporting of prediction models in these studies would have been worse. Furthermore, we selected studies from high impact journals. Therefore, our results on the completeness of reporting might be an optimistic representation of the reporting of prediction model studies in general.

In accordance with the TRIPOD statement, we included prediction models based on regression modelling approaches [13]. Although most TRIPOD items would apply, transparent reporting of prediction models using non-regression modelling techniques may require additional details, especially regarding model-building procedures, and specific guidance might be desirable.

We were strict in scoring adherence by requiring complete information on all elements of a TRIPOD item; e.g. complete reporting of model performance required the provision of both discrimination and calibration measures. This is in line with the nature of TRIPOD as having essential items needed to appraise and utilise a prediction model. However, authors might have good reasons not to provide specific details regarding an item. For example, if they believe that their model should not be validated or used in clinical practice, they may have decided not to present the coefficients of the full model. In the current study we would have scored TRIPOD item 15a as 'incompletely reported'. Although strict scoring potentially leads to poorer adherence results, it is needed for reasons of consistency.

We used two different denominators in our analyses, the number of publications ($n = 146$) and the number of models ($n = 170$), which implies that in the 'model' analysis a number of publications were included multiple times. It is likely that results from the same publication, although based on the reporting of different models, are correlated. Given the descriptive nature of our analysis, we did not adjust for such a possible correlation.

We present results from studies that were published 4 years ago; nevertheless, we expect these findings to still be applicable and relevant to current publications of prediction models. From evaluations of other reporting guidelines, like CONSORT and STARD, we know that it takes time to demonstrate the impact of a reporting guideline on completeness of reporting, and changes over several years might be small [25, 26, 28–33]. In our opinion, therefore, it is too early for a before-after comparison at this moment, and the focus should first be on optimal implementation of TRIPOD.

Implications for practice and areas for future research

Inadequate reporting impedes the use of all available evidence regarding a prediction model. First, as title and abstract were among the least well-reported items, identifying publications of prediction model studies might be challenging. In addition, we found the reporting of model development often insufficiently detailed, which makes external validation almost impossible. As a consequence, a new model might be developed, rather than making use of an existing model. Also, without model specifications it is impossible to use the model in clinical practice. Finally, inadequate reporting hinders critical

appraisal and, thereby, the possibility of methodological investigation of sources of variation and bias in prediction model studies.

Experiences from other research areas indicate that the improvement in reporting after the introduction of a guideline is often slow and might be subtle [25, 26, 28–33]. Improving the completeness of reporting of prediction models is probably even more challenging, as it is a relatively young, less well-known research field, with methodology still in development and not yet strongly embedded in education. Moreover, the multivariable nature of prediction model studies and their focus on absolute probabilities rather than on comparative measures require the reporting of many details on methods and results. In addition, practical issues, like word limits or journal requirements, could act as barriers for complete reporting.

The introduction of the TRIPOD statement was the first step in improving the reporting of prediction model studies. However, more activities should be undertaken to enhance the implementation of the TRIPOD statement. Active implementation involves a collaborative effort of developers of a reporting guideline and other stakeholders within the academic community, like journal editors and educational institutions. Apart from raising awareness and providing training, possible post-publication activities that are recommended are encouraging guideline endorsement, asking for feedback, and evaluating the impact of the reporting guideline [34].

By highlighting the flaws in the reporting of prediction model studies, our results enable a targeted implementation strategy for the TRIPOD statement. Possible future activities are the development of educational materials and training regarding specific aspects of the reporting of prediction model studies. The examples of both adequate and suboptimal reporting within our data set can be used in the training of different stakeholders. An initiative that already has been started by the TRIPOD Group is the development of specific guidance on informative reporting of prediction model studies in abstracts [35]. Furthermore, as TRIPOD is periodically being reappraised and will be updated if necessary, our study will provide useful input for modifications of specific TRIPOD items, related to content, phrasing, or more detailed explanation [12]. Finally, our study will serve as a baseline measurement for future studies evaluating the impact of the introduction of the TRIPOD statement.

Conclusions

Prediction models are poorly reported: more than half of the items that are considered essential for transparent reporting of a prediction model were not or were inadequately reported, especially with regard to details of the title, abstract, blinding, model-building procedures, the final model, and model performance. The results of this study can be used to further develop and refine the implementation and increase the impact of the TRIPOD statement.

Abbreviations

CONSORT: CONsolidated Standards Of Reporting Trials; REMARK: REporting recommendations for tumour MARKer prognostic studies; STARD: STAndards for Reporting of Diagnostic accuracy; TRIPOD: Transparent Reporting of a multivariable prediction model for Individual Prognosis Or Diagnosis

Acknowledgements

We thank René Spijker for performing the search for this comprehensive literature survey and Daan Michels for his assistance with data extraction.

Funding

GSC was supported by the National Institute for Health Research (NIHR) Biomedical Research Centre, Oxford. KGMM received a grant from the Netherlands Organisation for Scientific Research (ZONMW 918.10.615 and 91208004). None of the funding sources had a role in the design, conduct, analyses, or reporting of the study, or in the decision to submit the manuscript for publication.

Authors' contributions

All authors contributed to the design of the study. Article selection was done by JAAGD and PH. Data were extracted by JAAGD, PH, and RP, and the other authors were involved in consensus meetings regarding data extraction. PH analysed the data. JAAGD, JBR, KGMM, LH, and RJPMS assisted in interpreting the data. PH wrote the first draft of the manuscript, which was revised by all authors. All authors approved the final version of the submitted manuscript.

Competing interests

JBR, GSC, DGA, and KGMM are members of the TRIPOD Group. All authors declare that they have no competing interests.

Author details

[1]Cochrane Netherlands, University Medical Center Utrecht, Utrecht University, Utrecht, The Netherlands. [2]Julius Center for Health Sciences and Primary Care, University Medical Center Utrecht, Utrecht University, Utrecht, The Netherlands. [3]Centre for Statistics in Medicine, NDORMS, Botnar Research Centre, University of Oxford, Oxford, UK.

References

1. Steyerberg EW, Moons KG, van der Windt DA, Hayden JA, Perel P, Schroter S, et al. Prognosis Research Strategy (PROGRESS) 3: prognostic model research. PLoS Med. 2013;10(2):e1001381.

2. Altman DG, Vergouwe Y, Royston P, Moons KG. Prognosis and prognostic research: validating a prognostic model. BMJ. 2009;338:b605.

3. Moons KG, Kengne AP, Grobbee DE, Royston P, Vergouwe Y, Altman DG, et al. Risk prediction models: II. External validation, model updating, and impact assessment. Heart. 2012;98(9):691–8.

4. Moons KG, Kengne AP, Woodward M, Royston P, Vergouwe Y, Altman DG, et al. Risk prediction models: I. Development, internal validation, and assessing the incremental value of a new (bio)marker. Heart. 2012;98(9):683–90.

5. Royston P, Moons KG, Altman DG, Vergouwe Y. Prognosis and prognostic research: developing a prognostic model. BMJ. 2009;338:b604.

6. Collins GS, Mallett S, Omar O, Yu LM. Developing risk prediction models for type 2 diabetes: a systematic review of methodology and reporting. BMC Med. 2011;9:103.

7. Bouwmeester W, Zuithoff NP, Mallett S, Geerlings MI, Vergouwe Y, Steyerberg EW, et al. Reporting and methods in clinical prediction research: a systematic review. PLoS Med. 2012;9(5):1–12.

8. Collins GS, Omar O, Shanyinde M, Yu LM. A systematic review finds prediction models for chronic kidney disease were poorly reported and often developed using inappropriate methods. J Clin Epidemiol. 2013;66(3):268–77.

9. Collins GS, de Groot JA, Dutton S, Omar O, Shanyinde M, Tajar A, et al. External validation of multivariable prediction models: a systematic review of methodological conduct and reporting. BMC Med Res Methodol. 2014;14:40.

10. Damen JA, Hooft L, Schuit E, Debray TP, Collins GS, Tzoulaki I, et al. Prediction models for cardiovascular disease risk in the general population: systematic review. BMJ. 2016;353:i2416.

11. Wen Z, Guo Y, Xu B, Xiao K, Peng T, Peng M. Developing risk prediction models for postoperative pancreatic fistula: a systematic review of methodology and reporting quality. Indian J Surg. 2016;78(2):136–43.

12. Collins GS, Reitsma JB, Altman DG, Moons KG. Transparent Reporting of a multivariable prediction model for Individual Prognosis or Diagnosis (TRIPOD): the TRIPOD statement. Ann Intern Med. 2015;162(1):55–63.

13. Moons KG, Altman DG, Reitsma JB, Ioannidis JP, Macaskill P, Steyerberg EW, et al. Transparent Reporting of a multivariable prediction model for Individual Prognosis or Diagnosis (TRIPOD): explanation and elaboration. Ann Intern Med. 2015;162(1):W1–73.

14. 2012 Journal Citation Reports® In: Science edition.Philadelphia: Clarivate Analytics; 2017.

15. Ingui BJ, Rogers MA. Searching for clinical prediction rules in MEDLINE. J Am Med Inform Assoc. 2001;8(4):391–7.

16. Moons KG, Royston P, Vergouwe Y, Grobbee DE, Altman DG. Prognosis and prognostic research: what, why, and how? BMJ. 2009;338:b375.

17. Riley RD, Hayden JA, Steyerberg EW, Moons KG, Abrams K, Kyzas PA, et al. Prognosis Research Strategy (PROGRESS) 2: prognostic factor research. PLoS Med. 2013;10(2):e1001380.

18. Chalmers I, Glasziou P. Avoidable waste in the production and reporting of research evidence. Lancet. 2009;374(9683):86–9.

19. Glasziou P, Altman DG, Bossuyt P, Boutron I, Clarke M, Julious S, et al. Reducing waste from incomplete or unusable reports of biomedical research. Lancet. 2014;383(9913):267–76.

20. Moher D, Hopewell S, Schulz KF, Montori V, Gotzsche PC, Devereaux PJ, et al. CONSORT 2010 explanation and elaboration: updated guidelines for reporting parallel group randomised trials. BMJ. 2010;340:c869.

21. Schulz KF, Altman DG, Moher D. CONSORT 2010 statement: updated guidelines for reporting parallel group randomized trials. Ann Intern Med. 2010;152(11):726–32.

22. Bossuyt PM, Reitsma JB, Bruns DE, Gatsonis CA, Glasziou PP, Irwig L, et al. STARD 2015: an updated list of essential items for reporting diagnostic accuracy studies. BMJ. 2015;351:h5527.

23. Cohen JF, Korevaar DA, Altman DG, Bruns DE, Gatsonis CA, Hooft L, et al. STARD 2015 guidelines for reporting diagnostic accuracy studies: explanation and elaboration. BMJ Open. 2016;6(11):e012799.

24. McShane LM, Altman DG, Sauerbrei W, Taube SE, Gion M, Clark GM. REporting recommendations for tumour MARKer prognostic studies (REMARK). Br J Cancer. 2005;93(4):387–91.

25. Moher D, Jones A, Lepage L. Use of the CONSORT statement and quality of reports of randomized trials: a comparative before-and-after evaluation. JAMA. 2001;285(15):1992–5.

26. Korevaar DA, van Enst WA, Spijker R, Bossuyt PM, Hooft L. Reporting quality of diagnostic accuracy studies: a systematic review and meta-analysis of investigations on adherence to STARD. Evid Based Med. 2014;19(2):47–54.

27. Mallett S, Timmer A, Sauerbrei W, Altman DG. Reporting of prognostic studies of tumour markers: a review of published articles in relation to REMARK guidelines. Br J Cancer. 2010;102(1):173–80.
28. Sekula P, Mallett S, Altman DG, Sauerbrei W. Did the reporting of prognostic studies of tumour markers improve since the introduction of REMARK guideline? A comparison of reporting in published articles. PLoS One. 2017; 12(6):e0178531.
29. Hopewell S, Dutton S, Yu LM, Chan AW, Altman DG. The quality of reports of randomised trials in 2000 and 2006: comparative study of articles indexed in PubMed. BMJ. 2010;340:c723.
30. Korevaar DA, Wang J, van Enst WA, Leeflang MM, Hooft L, Smidt N, et al. Reporting diagnostic accuracy studies: some improvements after 10 years of STARD. Radiology. 2015;274(3):781–9.
31. Smidt N, Rutjes AW, van der Windt DA, Ostelo RW, Bossuyt PM, Reitsma JB, et al. The quality of diagnostic accuracy studies since the STARD statement: has it improved? Neurology. 2006;67(5):792–7.
32. Turner L, Shamseer L, Altman DG, Weeks L, Peters J, Kober T, et al. Consolidated Standards of Reporting Trials (CONSORT) and the completeness of reporting of randomised controlled trials (RCTs) published in medical journals. Cochrane Database Syst Rev. 2012;11:Mr000030.
33. Chan AW, Altman DG. Epidemiology and reporting of randomised trials published in PubMed journals. Lancet. 2005;365(9465):1159–62.
34. Moher D, Schulz KF, Simera I, Altman DG. Guidance for developers of health research reporting guidelines. PLoS Med. 2010;7(2):e1000217.
35. Heus P, Hooft L, Reitsma JB, Scholten RJPM, Altman DG, Collins GS, et al. Reporting of clinical prediction model studies in journal and conference abstracts: TRIPOD for Abstracts. In: 24th Cochrane Colloquium; 2016 23–27 Oct: 2016. Seoul: Wiley; 2016.

11

Is telephone health coaching a useful population health strategy for supporting older people with multimorbidity? An evaluation of reach, effectiveness and cost-effectiveness using a 'trial within a cohort'

Maria Panagioti[1], David Reeves[1], Rachel Meacock[2], Beth Parkinson[2], Karina Lovell[3], Mark Hann[1], Kelly Howells[1], Amy Blakemore[3], Lisa Riste[1], Peter Coventry[4], Thomas Blakeman[5], Mark Sidaway[6] and Peter Bower[1]*

Abstract

Background: Innovative ways of delivering care are needed to improve outcomes for older people with multimorbidity. Health coaching involves 'a regular series of phone calls between patient and health professional to provide support and encouragement to promote healthy behaviours'. This intervention is promising, but evidence is insufficient to support a wider role in multimorbidity care. We evaluated health coaching in older people with multimorbidity.

Methods: We used the innovative 'Trials within Cohorts' design. A cohort was recruited, and a trial was conducted using a 'patient-centred' consent model. A randomly selected group within the cohort were offered the intervention and were analysed as the intervention group whether they accepted the offer or not.
The intervention sought to improve the skills of patients with multimorbidity to deal with a range of long-term conditions, through health coaching, social prescribing and low-intensity support for low mood.

Results: We recruited 4377 older people, and 1306 met the eligibility criteria (two or more long-term conditions and moderate 'patient activation'). We selected 504 for health coaching, and 41% consented. More than 80% of consenters received the defined 'dose' of 4+ sessions.
In an intention-to-treat analysis, those selected for health coaching did not improve on any outcome (patient activation, quality of life, depression or self-care) compared to usual care.
We examined health care utilisation using hospital administrative and self-report data. Patients selected for health coaching demonstrated lower levels of emergency care use, but an increase in the use of planned services and higher overall costs, as well as a quality-adjusted life year (QALY) gain. The incremental cost per QALY was £8049, with a 70–79% probability of being cost-effective at conventional levels of willingness to pay.

Conclusions: Health coaching did not lead to significant benefits on the primary measures of patient-reported outcome. This is likely related to relatively low levels of uptake amongst those selected for the intervention. Demonstrating effectiveness in this design is challenging, as it estimates the effect of being selected for treatment, regardless of whether treatment is adopted. We argue that the treatment effect estimated is appropriate for health coaching, a proactive model relevant to many patients in the community, not just those seeking care.

(Continued on next page)

* Correspondence: peter.bower@manchester.ac.uk
[1]NIHR School for Primary Care Research, Centre for Primary Care, Manchester Academic Health Science Centre, University of Manchester, Williamson Building, Oxford Road, Manchester M13 9PL, UK
Full list of author information is available at the end of the article

(Continued from previous page)

Trial registration: International Standard Randomised Controlled Trial Number (ISRCTN12286422).

Keywords: multimorbidity, older adults, health coaching, depression

Background

Multimorbidity, defined as 'the co-existence of two or more chronic conditions, where one is not necessarily more central than the others' [1], is highly prevalent [2]. Patients with multimorbidity are a major focus of health systems, but they face barriers to accessing high-quality care [3–5], and they incur high costs [6]. Recently, clinical guidelines for multimorbidity have highlighted the need for innovative models of care [7]. Successful self-management will be crucial for improving the health outcomes of patients with multimorbidity, but the current evidence for effectively managing multimorbidity is weak. A recent Cochrane review reported only 18 trials [8], with some evidence for interventions targeted at risk factors such as depression or specific functional difficulties. The review concluded that there is an urgent need for interventions that can help patients with multimorbidity to better self-manage their conditions to prevent exacerbations and avoid expensive care utilisation [9].

For self-management to be cost-effective at a population level, interventions must be delivered to a significant proportion of the population in need, not just those motivated to participate. This is described as 'reach' [10]. Evidence of reach is often lacking in trials of self-management, because only a proportion of those meeting the eligibility criteria actually participate [11]. Evidence of reach can be particularly problematic amongst people with multimorbidity because they are often excluded from trials [12]. This study aimed to evaluate the impact of an intervention that can be used with a large number of patients, using a trial design that can better assess the likely population benefit of the intervention.

The 'trial within a cohort' as a test of intervention 'reach'

In a conventional trial, participants receive information, then provide consent to participate and are randomised. Critically, patients are told about the different treatments available, but only half are randomised to each. Patients with preferences for one treatment may be less likely to take part [13].

The 'Trials within Cohorts' (TWiCs) design more closely mimics the way treatment decisions are made in routine care [14]. A cohort of participants are recruited and followed up systematically. Under the form of TWiCs used here, all eligible participants in the cohort are identified, and a sample is *selected at random*. Patients selected for the intervention are contacted and offered the treatment, which they can either decide to receive — and provide informed consent — or decline. Whether or not a patient consents to treatment, for the purposes of this design, they remain part of the intervention arm. All those eligible but not selected are not contacted for participation and become controls.

The TWiCs design has two potential advantages. It more closely mimics the process of treatment decision-making in routine care, as patients are offered a treatment (which they can decline) rather than being offered two treatments, then allocated at chance. The design also provides a different (and in some contexts more useful) estimate of the effects of the *offer of treatment* amongst all those who are eligible, rather than amongst a subset who agree to receive the treatment. As such, it may have greater relevance for treatments designed to have broad 'reach' amongst the wider population. Examples would include diabetes prevention programmes [15] and self-management programmes for older people with long-term conditions [16, 17].

Health coaching as a population health intervention

Self-management is critical for patients with long-term conditions. A model that has received significant attention is health coaching, defined as 'a regular series of phone calls between patient and health professional...to provide support and encouragement to the patient, and promote healthy behaviours such as treatment control, healthy diet, physical activity and mobility, rehabilitation, and good mental health' [18].

Various types of health coaching exist that differ in content, delivery (face to face, remote), and personnel. An important issue is whom is targeted for health coaching. It can be provided for patients predicted to be high users of services or following events such as hospital discharge [19]. Although the rationale for such targeting is clear, many patients identified as high users of care revert to lower patterns over time without intervention [20]. There may be an argument for broader strategies targeting the wider population of patients who are currently well but whose current self-management is not optimal. These patients can be described as being less 'activated'. Patient activation is defined as how well a patient understands his/her own role in personal health care, reflecting knowledge, skills and confidence [21, 22]. Activation may be a method of targeting coaching to maximise benefit. Another important factor may be depression, which is associated with poor outcomes in multimorbidity and may be important in self-management [23]. Treatment burden is an additional factor of relevance in this patient population. It is defined as 'the impact of the "work of being a patient" on functioning and well-being' [24, 25] and occurs when the tasks of managing multiple conditions become a detriment to health and well-being.

An increasing number of systematic reviews have been published on the effectiveness of health coaching. Most suggest significant, modest short-term benefits, and some also support longer term gains [26–33]. However, it is difficult to generalise these findings to care for people with multimorbidity, as many trials are focussed on people with only one long-term condition [28, 32]. Further research is indicated to examine the impact of health coaching, assessing reach and the cost-effectiveness of this intervention amongst patients with multimorbidity.

Methods
Study design and participants
The study was embedded in a wider integrated care programme to improve care for older people with long-term conditions in North West England. The CLASSIC study is a longitudinal cohort study evaluating this integrated care programme. Embedded within CLASSIC, the Proactive Telephone Coaching and Tailored Support (PROTECTS) trial used the TWiCs design to assess the cost-effectiveness of health coaching for patients with multimorbidity. PROTECTS is reported as per Consolidated Standards of Reporting Trials (CONSORT) guidelines (see Additional file 1: CONSORT checklist). The trial protocol is also included as an additional file (Additional file 2).

The integrated care programme was delivered to patients over the age of 65 with at least one long-term condition, and we recruited these patients to the CLASSIC cohort [34]. FARSITE is a software package (http://nweh.co.uk/products/farsite) that enables centralised searching of general practitioner (GP) records. FARSITE was used to generate a list of eligible patients in each practice, and the results were provided to general practices to allow them to remove any patients meeting the exclusion criteria (patients in palliative care or with reduced capacity to consent) prior to asking them for consent. A total of 12,989 patients were eligible between November 2014 and February 2015. If they did not respond, they were sent a reminder 3 weeks later. Participants were offered an incentive of a £10 voucher. At baseline, 4377 people (34.2%) returned a questionnaire. We did not have access to data on non-respondents.

For inclusion in PROTECTS, patients had to have 2 or more self-reported long-term conditions from a list of 15 [35], and must have been assessed as needing some

assistance with self-management, defined via scores on the Patient Activation Measure (PAM) [36]. The PAM allows activation to be categorised into four levels. Level 1 includes passive recipients of care, level 2 includes those who lack the basic knowledge and confidence to self-manage, level 3 is those who have the basic knowledge but lack the confidence and skills to engage in self-management and level 4 is those who have the knowledge, confidence and skills and may only require support during times of stress [36]. We included patients in PROTECTS whose scores placed them in level 2 or 3 of activation, because these patients showed some evidence of self-management which could be improved by health coaching.

Randomisation and masking
As noted earlier, patients eligible for the trial are identified from the cohort and randomly selected for treatment. We piloted these procedures in 50 patients to test the rate of uptake of the new treatment. After assessment of eligibility, we selected patients to be offered health coaching at random, using appropriate central randomisation through a clinical trials unit to ensure concealment of allocation. In this pragmatic evaluation, we did not blind either patients or providers.

Procedures
The intervention was health coaching, as defined earlier. The content of the health coaching was based on three core mechanisms:

1. *Telephone health coaching* involved support and encouragement to the patient to promote healthy behaviours around diet, exercise, smoking and alcohol, through provision of information and motivation for long-term conditions. The core health coaching materials include telephone and associated patient tracking and management software, and health coaching scripts for lifestyle support.
2. *Social prescribing* involved links to resources in the wider community through the community and voluntary sector [37, 38]. Access to local resources was provided through either PLANS (http://www.plansforyourhealth.org/, a self-assessment tool for users to assess their health and social needs, with links to relevant community resources and local support) or the Ways to Wellbeing site (on-line resources and information, no longer available in the form used in the trial).
3. *Low-intensity support for low mood* included assessment of common mental health problems, simple lifestyle advice and behavioural techniques to manage mood, and use of appropriate risk assessment protocols [39, 40].

Six monthly phone calls to participants were planned. The receipt of four out of the six planned calls was considered a complete 'dose' of the intervention.

The PROTECTS intervention was delivered by a 'health advisor' (a National Health Service (NHS) Agenda for Change Band 4 worker) with skills in information technology and communication, as well as experience in working with the general public. Advisors already had experience with coaching for diabetes and use of social prescribing. The health advisor attended 3 days of training specific to working with low mood. They were given a manual which outlined the key elements of the low-intensity intervention used (behavioural activation, cognitive restructuring, problem solving). They also received monthly group clinical supervision which focussed on working with low mood. The health advisor were further supported by a specialist nurse manager and received additional advice on mental health and social prescribing (i.e. referral to relevant community resources) from the research team. Patients routinely had continuity in their coach for the duration of their treatment. There were no formal links with primary care as part of the intervention. The health coaching was delivered via telephone from a central NHS facility. Proactive, monthly calls of around 20 min were made for a period of 6 months, with the option for additional calls to deal with complex patients or issues of risk. Health coaching staff were trained to customize calls to the individual patient. Provision of support for low mood and social prescribing were made where appropriate.

The design meant that the comparator for patients meeting the eligibility criteria who were not selected for the intervention was usual NHS care. We collected details of that care for the economic evaluation.

Outcomes

PROTECTS was nested within the CLASSIC cohort, which used a wide range of measures, varying at different time points. A pre-specified subgroup of primary outcomes were used in PROTECTS. All outcomes were collected via postal survey at four time points across the study: at baseline, then at 6, 12 and 20 months. The protocol was registered and updated in a registry (ISRCTN 12286422).

The primary outcome measures were:

- *Self-management.* The PAM is a self-report measure of patient knowledge, skills and confidence in self-management for long-term conditions [22, 36, 41]. We used the short 13-item version. The score is categorised into four levels for eligibility determination, although we used the continuous score in the analyses.

- *Quality of life.* The World Health Organization Quality of Life brief measure (WHOQOL-BREF) is a 26-item measure of global quality of life (QOL), which has been validated in a large international population with physical and mental long-term conditions. QOL is measured across four domains: physical, psychological, social and environmental, as well as a single-item scale for QOL [42]. We used the physical domain score as the most relevant in relation to the PROTECTS intervention.

Secondary outcome measures were:

- *Depression.* The Mental Health Inventory (MHI-5) is a 5-item scale which measures general mental health [43]. This measure is well validated for identifying depression symptoms, with a higher score indicating better mental health [44, 45]. The recommended cutoff score of 60 was used to indicate the presence of 'probable depression' [45], although we used the continuous score in the analyses.
- *Self-care.* The Summary of Diabetes Self-Care Activities (SDSCA) is a 7-item measure assessing the number of days per week respondents engage in healthy and unhealthy behaviours (i.e. eating fruits and vegetables, eating red meat, undertaking exercise, drinking alcohol and smoking) [46].

Power and statistical analysis

At the time of study development, there were no bespoke methods for powering this TWiCs design, and we used conventional methods [47]. We powered the study to have 80% power (alpha 5%) to detect a standardised effect size of 0.25 on any continuous outcome measure. Allowing for 25% attrition amongst participants — and assuming that outcome measures at baseline correlate 0.5 with their respective follow-ups — 504 patients were indicated, with 252 randomised to treatment. The CLASSIC cohort included 1306 patients eligible for PROTECTS, and we randomly selected 252 to be offered the intervention. The uptake rate was lower than anticipated, and we therefore offered the intervention to a further 252 patients. This resulted in a final intervention group of 504 of which 207 consented to the intervention, with the remaining 802 as controls. However, under the TWiCs framework, all 504 patients offered treatment remain in the treatment group in analysis, including those who declined. In consequence, the eventual effect size detectable at 80% power was 0.39 amongst the subsample consenting to treatment.

The analysis followed intention-to-treat principles and a pre-specified analysis plan. In summary, we report the trial and analysis according to updated CONSORT standards and utilising the extension for pragmatic trials

[48]. The main hypothesis test of the intervention was that the overall effect of the intervention is zero. The primary analysis used complete cases only. Condition group was used as a binary variable. All outcomes were treated as though continuous and normally distributed (in all cases both skewness and kurtosis were < =1.0) and analysed using linear multiple regression. Baseline values of outcomes and a set of pre-specified covariates considered prognostic of outcome were included in all analyses: gender, age (categorised as 65–69, 0–79, 80–98), health literacy [49], social support [50], patient activation, depression and quality of life (physical health domain). Robust estimates of variance were used accounting for the clustering of patients within practices.

We ran two sensitivity analyses. The first repeated the primary analyses using multiple imputation to include cases with missing baseline or follow-up data. Missing data values were imputed using chained-equation multiple imputation and scores on all available outcome measures and patient demographics at baseline and follow-up. Twenty multiple imputation sets were used to ensure stability of results. The second sensitivity analysis assessed the robustness of the primary analysis results to removal of the pre-specified covariates from the model (not including the outcome at baseline).

Health coaching in the trial was delivered by an existing service managing other patients outside the trial, rather than a bespoke service. This, combined with the time taken to administer and analyse the cohort and randomly select the groups, meant that no patient was offered treatment until 6 months after the baseline assessment for the CLASSIC cohort, and for some the offer was not made until month 12 or later. This caused variations in the duration of time before start of the treatment (range 259 to 513 days after baseline assessment). Length of follow-up from end of treatment to 20 months follow-up was similarly variable. Thus, the trial is considered to have run over 20 months, with patients receiving treatment at any time after the initial 6 months. As these implementation delays were not anticipated, the pre-specified analysis plan stated that the primary analysis would assess the change in outcomes between baseline and 20 months follow-up.

The design provides an estimate of the mean effect in people offered treatment. Compared to a pragmatic trial, which provides an estimate of the mean effect in people agreeing to treatment, the effect is 'diluted' by the proportion of patients in the treatment arm who do not consent to treatment. An estimate of the treatment effect in those patients consenting to treatment was derived through application of a complier average causal effect (CACE) analysis [51, 52]. The CACE estimator was obtained by dividing the mean effect estimate by the proportion giving consent [51]. The CACE estimate is typically larger, but the power to detect an effect is not greater, since the variance of the estimate increases proportionately [53].

Cost-effectiveness analysis

The primary outcome measure for the economic evaluation was the EuroQOL 5-Dimension 5-Level (EQ-5D-5L) [54], a generic measure of health-related QOL covering five domains (mobility, self-care, usual activities, pain/discomfort, anxiety/depression). This new version was developed due to concerns over the lack of sensitivity to change of the original scale, and consists of five severity levels for each domain. Published English general population preference weightings were used to convert responses to a single utility index [55].

The perspective of the economic analysis was that of the English NHS. Individual patient-level health care resource utilisation over the trial period was collected from two sources. The number of GP contacts in the previous 6 months was collected from self-report data at 6-monthly intervals. Hospital utilisation was extracted from linked administrative patient records provided by the NHS, divided into emergency admissions (short stays ≤5, long stays > 5 days), elective admissions, elective day cases, outpatient attendances and accident and emergency (A&E) department attendances.

The economic analysis assessed the incremental cost-effectiveness of the offer of health coaching compared with usual care from the perspective of the NHS. EQ-5D-5L data were combined with in-hospital mortality information from the secondary care utilisation data, applying a utility value of 0 upon death. Quality-adjusted life years (QALYs) were calculated using the area under the curve method assuming linear extrapolation of utility between time points. QALYs in the second year of the trial were discounted at an annual rate of 3.5% as specified by NICE [56].

Intervention costs were estimated combining the cost of training and supervision, written materials and delivery of the health coaching sessions. The intervention was offered to all participants selected, although only 189 received at least one call. Only patients receiving at least one call were assigned treatment costs, and the intervention costs were therefore estimated based on these 189 participants.

Patient-level resource utilisation data were combined with relevant unit cost data for the price year 2014–2015 to calculate total costs. Unit costs not available for this price year were inflated to 2014/2015 prices using the consumer price index [57]. Costs occurring in the second year were discounted at a rate of 3.5% [56]. Unit cost figures were sourced from the Personal Social

Services Research Unit's unit costs of Health and Social Care 2015 and national NHS Reference Costs [58, 59].

Follow-up questionnaire completion dates were missing in a small number of cases ($n = 2$). In these instances, dates were imputed using the mean length of time between baseline and follow-up for the sample for the purpose of QALY and cost calculations. Missing information on age and gender were sourced from the linked hospital administrative data, where available (gender $n = 6$, age $n = 35$). For the remaining individuals with missing age ($n = 30$) or missing baseline EQ-5D-5L ($n = 29$), mean imputation was used to ensure independence from treatment allocation [60].

For missing EQ-5D-5L and resource use data, we used multiple imputation by chained equations (ICE) to generate 50 imputed datasets assuming the data were missing at random. The independent variables specified in the imputation models were age, gender, treatment arm and baseline EQ-5D-5L. To account for non-normality, predictive mean matching was used which forces imputations to only take values observed in the original dataset. Multiple imputation (MI) was conducted using Stata's ICE package, and analysis using Stata's MI package.

The incremental cost-effectiveness ratio (ICER) was calculated, adjusting for age, gender, and baseline EQ-5D-5L index score [61]. To assess uncertainty surrounding the estimates and to account for the typically skewed nature of cost data, incremental costs and QALYs were bootstrapped using pairwise bootstrapping with replacement using 10,000 replications. Cost-effectiveness planes plot these 10,000 bootstrap replications of the ICER estimates to illustrate the uncertainty around the point estimate of the ICER in probabilistic terms. Finally, cost-effectiveness acceptability curves (CEACs) were plotted to graphically represent the probability of the intervention being cost-effective across a range of cost-effectiveness thresholds.

The primary economic analysis was based on a comparison on the full sample with MI. A sensitivity analysis was performed using only the complete case sample for which there were no missing data. We also took advantage of the implementation delays to perform a further sensitivity analysis separating the trial period into two parts: baseline to 6 months follow-up, where no treatment had yet been received; and 6 months to 20 months follow-up, where we expect any treatment effects to occur. Stata version 14 was used in the analysis.

Results

Recruitment, retention and baseline characteristics

In total, 12,989 patients were identified as eligible for the cohort, and at baseline 4377 (33.6%) participated. Of those, 1306 were eligible for PROTECTS. Of the 1306, 504 were randomly selected to the intervention, and the remaining 802 eligible participants acted as controls. The flow of participants is shown in Fig. 1. The baseline characteristics of participants are presented in Table 1.

Treatment uptake and adherence

Signed consent to health coaching amongst those eligible was received from 207/504 (41%) of those selected, although only 189 actually received calls (38%). The baseline characteristics of consenters and non-consenters are reported in Additional file 3: Table A. A multivariate logistic regression exploring baseline factors associated with consent found that only younger age (odds ratio (OR) = 1.08, 95% confidence interval (CI) = 1.03–1.14) and higher education (OR = 4.07, 95% CI = 2.08–7.94) predicted consent to health coaching.

Among those who consented, 167/189 (85%) received 4+ calls (the predefined 'dose'). Assessment of call content showed that diet and exercise were the most common areas dealt with (in 70% and 57% of patients respectively), whereas 25% of patients received social prescribing and around 23% received support for low mood.

Outcomes

Table 2 shows the patient-reported outcomes for patients selected for the offer of health coaching and those not selected. The adjusted mean differences were small for all of the primary and secondary outcome measures and did not reach statistical significance ($p > 0.05$). The non-significance of all group differences was confirmed in both sensitivity analyses.

Using CACE analysis, the estimated treatment effects on participants who took up the intervention were higher, but with correspondingly wider non-significant confidence intervals (Table 2).

Economic analysis

Complete data necessary for the economic analysis were available for 45% of the sample (584/1306).

Table 3 shows EQ-5D-5L utility scores at each time point and the total QALY gain over 18 months for the complete case sample. Patients selected for the offer of health coaching reported slightly lower EQ-5D-5L scores at baseline. This steadily fell at each time point for the usual care group (0.664 at 18 months follow-up), whilst remaining stable for the health coaching group (0.691). The mean unadjusted QALYs for usual care were 1.105, and 1.124 for health coaching over the study period.

The resources required to deliver the health coaching intervention are presented in Additional file 3: Table B. The average cost per individual receiving the full course of health coaching (6 calls) was £148.27. In addition to

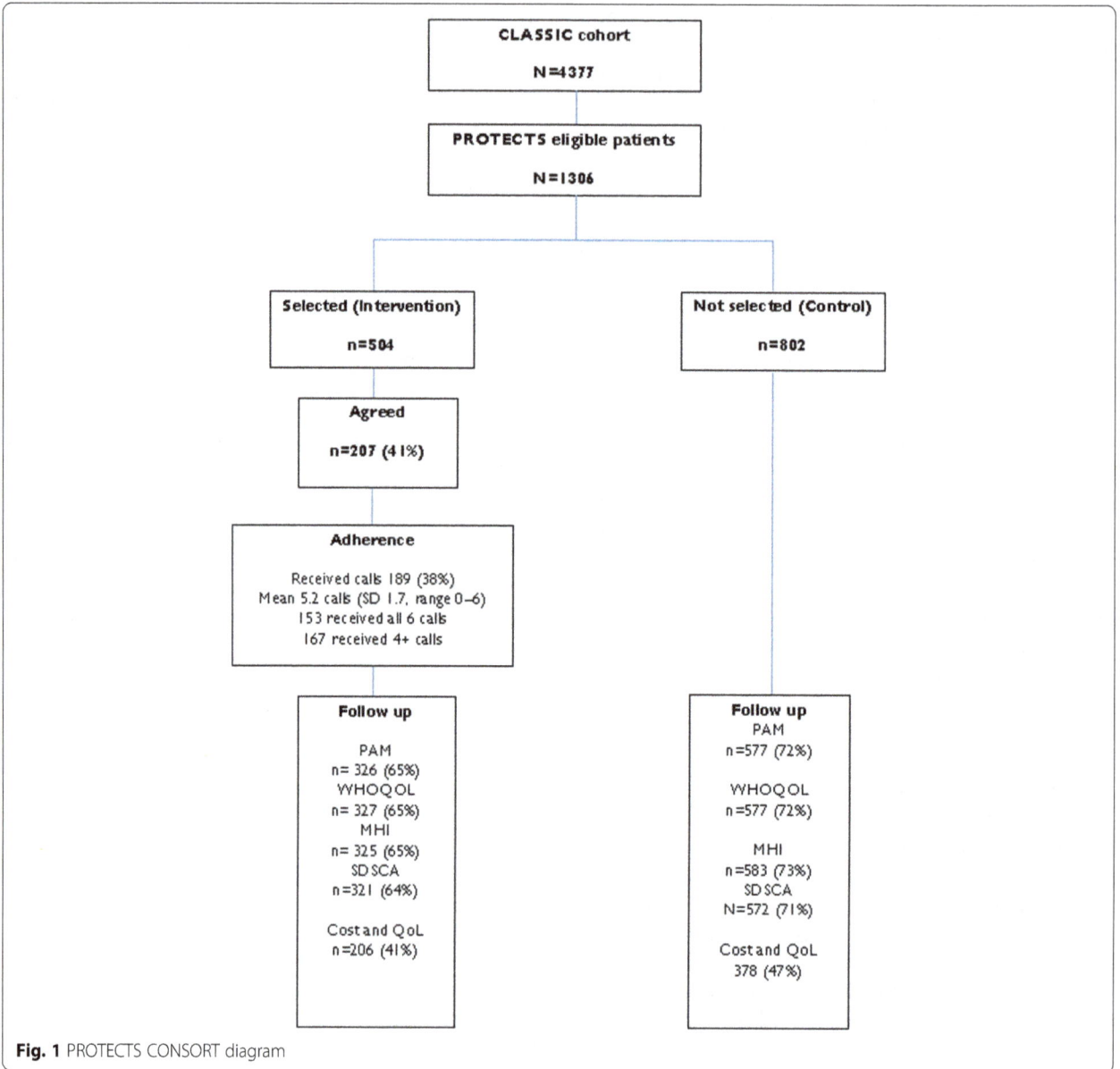

Fig. 1 PROTECTS CONSORT diagram

the direct costs, the analysis also considered the wider NHS resource utilisation. Table 4 reports the average utilisation by resource category for the complete case sample. Overall, there was a pattern of greater use of emergency care amongst the control group, whilst the group offered health coaching used more planned services.

Table 5 presents the average costs of the resource utilisation of the complete case sample. The list of unit costs and resources is available in Additional file 3: Table C. The most costly category was outpatient appointments, followed by elective admissions and GP appointments. These are all planned care services, the costs of which were higher in the health coaching group. Conversely, the costs of emergency admissions (short and long stays), day cases, and A&E attendances were higher in usual care. Overall, mean costs were higher in health coaching (£4000.88) than usual care (£3424.16). The average intervention costs in health coaching were £79. 29. This is lower than the £148.27 estimated for a course of health coaching because not all individuals took up or completed the health coaching.

Cost-effectiveness analysis: full sample with imputation

Table 6 presents the adjusted estimates of the effects of the offer of health coaching on the incremental costs and QALYs compared to usual care in the full sample with imputed data, controlling for age, gender and baseline utility.

Table 1 Baseline characteristics of participants

Characteristics	Not selected (n = 802)	Selected (n = 504)	Total (n = 1306)
Mean (SD) age	74.2 (6.4)	75.4 (6.8)	74.7 (6.6)
Age in categories:			
65–69 years	216 (26.9)	115 (22.8)	331 (25.3)
70–79 years	385 (48.0)	230 (45.6)	615 (47.1)
80–98 years	155 (19.3)	140 (27.8)	295 (22.6)
Sex (%):			
Female	441 (55.0)	270 (53.6)	711 (54.4)
Male	357 (44.5)	232 (46.0)	589 (45.1)
Health literacy:			
Never	536 (66.8)	322 (63.9)	858 (65.7)
Rarely	100 (12.5)	57 (11.3)	157 (12.0)
Sometimes	87 (10.9)	63 (12.5)	150 (11.5)
Often/always	59 (7.4)	44 (8.7)	103 (7.9)
Living status (%):			
Live with partner or others	509 (63.5)	315 (62.5)	824 (63.1)
Live alone	288 (35.9)	188 (37.3)	476 (36.5)
Education (%):			
No qualifications	352 (43.9)	221 (43.9)	573 (43.9)
School level qualifications	68 (8.5)	56 (11.1)	124 (9.5)
College degree or higher	349 (43.5)	191 (37.9)	540 (41.4)
Mean (SD) chronic conditions	6.8 (2.6)	6.8 (2.5)	6.8 (2.6)
Mean (SD) index of multiple deprivation	31.0 (18.8)	33.0 (18.6)	31.8 (18.7)
Employment (%):			
Retired or not economically active	748 (93.3)	472 (93.7)	1220 (93.4)
Working or other	39 (4.7)	23 (4.6)	62 (4.8)
Ethnicity (%):			
White	786 (98.0)	489 (97.0)	1275 (97.6)
Non-white	11 (1.37)	12 (2.4)	23 (1.8)
Mean (SD) GP visits in past 6 months	3.1 (2.0)	3.0 (1.9)	3.1 (1.9)
Mean (SD) patient activation	57.8 (6.0)	57.6 (5.6)	57.8 (5.9)
Mean (SD) quality of life (physical health)	55.3 (19.8)	54.0 (18.8)	54.8 (19.4)
Mean (SD) depressive symptoms	65.3 (21.3)	65.3 (21.8)	65.3 (21.3)
Possible depression diagnosis (%):			
Depression	371 (46.3)	227 (45.0)	598 (45.8)
No depression	426 (53.1)	265 (52.9)	691 (52.9)
Mean (SD) self-care activities	3.8 (0.9)	3.8 (0.9)	3.8 (0.9)

The offer of health coaching is associated with a mean incremental total cost increase of £150.58 (95% CI £–470.611, £711.776) and a mean incremental QALY gain of 0.019 (95% CI –0.006, 0.043).

Whilst there are no statistically significant differences in either costs or QALYs, the point estimate of the ICER is £8049.96 per QALY. This would represent a cost-effective intervention at the standard cost-per-QALY threshold of £20,000–30,000. However, it is important to consider the uncertainty surrounding this estimate. The cost-effectiveness plane plots the 10,000 bootstrap replications of incremental cost and QALY estimates (Fig. 2). The replications are clustered in the north-east quadrant in Fig. 2 (positive health gain and increased cost). Health coaching resulted in an incremental QALY gain in 94% of bootstrap replications and was higher cost in 69% of replications.

Table 2 Intention-to-treat analyses of primary and secondary outcomes, using complete cases

	Intervention group (eligible patients selected for treatment)		Control group (eligible patients not selected for treatment)		Comparison		CACE estimates (estimated points change in those consenting to treatment)
	N	Mean (SD)	N	Mean (SD)	Adjusted difference in means[a] (95% CI)	p value	Adjusted difference in means[a] (95% CI)
Primary outcomes							
Patient Activation Measure (PAM)	326	62.88 (14.39)	577	61.92 (13.24)	1.44 (−0.46 to 3.33)	0.133	3.69 (−1.17 to 8.53)
WHO Quality of Life —- physical health (WHOQOL)	327	55.74 (19.15)	577	55.41 (18.72)	1.62 (−0.32 to 3.56)	0.099	4.15 (−0.82 to 9.12)
Secondary outcomes							
Depression (Mental Health Inventory, MHI-5)	325	75.74 (16.40)	583	74.29 (17.26)	1.00 (−1.25 to 3.26)	0.373	2.56 (−3.20 to 8.36)
Self-care (SDSCA)	321	3.49 (1.09)	572	3.54 (1.10)	−0.04 (−0.19 to 0.11)	0.58	−0.10 (−0.49 to 0.28)

[a]Adjusted for covariates gender, age, health literacy, social support, patient activation, depression and quality of life

The CEAC (Fig. 3) demonstrates how the probability that health coaching is cost-effective increases with the decision-maker's willingness to pay. At the lower bound threshold of £20,000 per QALY, there is a 70% probability of health coaching being cost-effective. This rises to 79% at the upper bound of £30,000. Compared with usual care, health coaching is likely to be cost-effective in 50% or more cases if decision-makers are willing to pay £8180 or more for a QALY.

The results of the cost-effectiveness analyses were similar when a complete case analysis was undertaken (see Additional file 4). The post hoc sensitivity analysis analysing costs and outcomes separately in the first 6 months post baseline (when no health coaching was received) confirmed that the period in which participants actually received treatment was driving outcomes, as the effects were restricted to the period in which health coaching was delivered (see Figures C to F in Additional file 4).

Table 3 HRQOL outcomes (EQ-5D-5L) amongst the complete case sample

	Usual care (n = 378)				Health coaching (n = 206)			
	Mean	SD	Min	Max	Mean	SD	Min	Max
Baseline	0.708	0.23	−0.18	1	0.696	0.236	−0.102	1
6 months	0.691	0.247	−0.185	1	0.709	0.228	0.018	1
12 months	0.685	0.254	−0.246	1	0.694	0.237	0	1
18 months	0.664	0.264	−0.18	1	0.691	0.26	0	1
QALYs	1.105	0.374	−0.29	1.723	1.124	0.355	0.055	1.683

Discussion
Principal outcomes
We evaluated the role of health coaching in the care of multimorbidity. We showed reasonable levels of intervention uptake amongst older patients with multimorbidity who were not actively seeking help with self-management. A large proportion of those who accepted the referral to health coaching received a defined 'dose'. Assistance with diet and exercise were the most common interventions within health coaching, although support for low mood and social prescribing were also present for a significant minority.

Analysis of health outcomes demonstrated no significant benefit associated with health coaching. However, the economic analysis suggested that health coaching resulted in an incremental increase in both costs and QALYs. When a QALY was valued at £20,000, there was a 70% probability that health coaching was cost-effective. The economic analysis suggested that health coaching led to higher utilisation of planned services and lower use of emergency hospital services than usual care.

Strengths and limitations
In addition to its large size and focus on multimorbidity, this trial employed the novel 'Trials within Cohorts' design. This design provides evidence of 'reach' because it assesses uptake amongst people not actively seeking treatment. A major criticism of conventional trials is that they show effectiveness of an innovation in a very selected group of patients, which then fails to 'scale' because of issues such as low rates of acceptability amongst the wider population, and differences between those who take part in trials and those eligible for the intervention [11].

Table 4 Resource utilisation amongst the complete case sample

Type of service	Baseline to 6 months	
	Usual care ($n = 378$)	Health coaching ($n = 206$)
	Mean (95% CI)	Mean (95% CI)
Secondary care contacts		
Emergency short stay	0.063 (0.039—0.088)	0.058 (0.026–0.091)
Emergency long stay	0.026 (0.009–0.044)	0.024 (0.003–0.045)
Day case	0.172 (0.104–0.240)	0.112 (0.059–0.165)
Elective admission	0.024 (0.008–0.039)	0.029 (0.002–0.056)
Outpatient	4.992 (4.162–5.823)	6.553 (4.977–8.130)
A&E attendance	0.156 (0.110–0.203)	0.131 (0.083–0.179)
GP appointments	3.111 (2.791–3.431)	3.039 (2.641–3.437)
	6 months to 12 months	
Secondary care contacts	Mean (95% CI)	Mean (95% CI)
Emergency short stay	0.050 (0.027–0.074)	0.039 (0.006–0.072)
Emergency long stay	0.040 (0.010–0.069)	0.019 (0.000–0.038)
Day case	0.127 (0.069–0.185)	0.053 (0.017–0.090)
Elective admission	0.029 (0.009–0.049)	0.029 (0.002–0.056)
Outpatient	4.595 (3.650–5.540)	6.403 (5.126–7.680)
A&E attendance	0.159 (0.108–0.209)	0.097 (0.041–0.153)
GP appointments	2.783 (2.527–3.039)	3.058 (2.696–3.421)
	12 months to 18 months	
Secondary care contacts	Mean (95% CI)	Mean (95% CI)
Emergency short stay	0.132 (0.091–0.174)	0.068 (0.028–0.108)
Emergency long stay	0.045 (0.022–0.068)	0.034 (0.009–0.059)
Day case	0.196 (0.107–0.284)	0.180 (0.105–0.254)
Elective admission	0.040 (0.020–0.059)	0.063 (0.027–0.099)
Outpatient	7.185 (6.064–8.307)	9.893 (8.570–11.217)
A&E attendance	0.275 (0.207–0.343)	0.170 (0.112–0.228)
GP appointments	2.865 (2.599–3.131)	2.922 (2.543–3.302)

Table 5 Resource use costs amongst the complete case sample

Type of service	Usual care ($n = 378$)	Health coaching ($n = 206$)
	Mean (£) 95% CI	Mean (£) 95% CI
Secondary care costs		
Emergency short stay	146.87 (112.25–181.48)	98.95 (64.27–133.63)
Emergency long stay	313.76 (190.97–436.54)	219.08 (101.92–336.24)
Day case	343.61 (212.29–474.93)	238.36 (166.87–309.86)
Elective admission	310.71 (203.04–418.38)	405.96 (201.93–609.99)
Outpatient appointment	1851.42 (1605.13–2097.70)	2521.95 (2139.57–2904.32)
A&E attendance	76.66 (62.69–90.63)	51.79 (39.33–64.24)
Mean total costs of secondary care contacts	3043.02 (2626.02–3460.03)	3536.09 (2979.87–4092.31)
GP appointments	381.14 (350.96–411.32)	392.50 (351.72–433.28)
Health coaching costs	–	79.29 (69.59–88.99)
Mean total cost	3424.16 (2999.98–3848.34)	4007.88 (3444.57–4571.18)

Table 6 Cost-effectiveness analysis: full sample with imputation

Health coaching ($n = 504$) over usual care ($n = 802$)	Mean	Bootstrapped standard error	Bootstrapped 95% CI	
Incremental cost (£)	150.583	316.941	−470.611	771.776
Incremental QALYs	0.019	0.012	−0.006	0.043
ICER	£8049.96			

However, this trial also has important limitations, some of which are directly associated with the TWiCs design. A conventional pragmatic trial assesses intervention effects on those consenting to treatment, with an assumption that there will be non-adherence amongst consenters which will reduce any intervention effect (as these are included in any intention-to-treat analysis). The current design estimates the mean effect of selection for treatment, and again all patients selected for treatment must remain in that group in the intention-to-treat analysis. The proportion of selected patients who do not take up the intervention in a 'trial within a cohort' will likely always be larger than the proportion of consenting patients who do not comply with treatment in a conventional pragmatic trial. In consequence, the inclusion in the PRO-TECTS treatment group of 59% of participants selected for the intervention who did not take it up — including 10% who were uncontactable — greatly diluted the overall treatment effect compared to controls, and resulted in a detectable standardised effect (amongst those consenting to treatment) of 0.39, rather than the 0.25 initially powered for. We have since published specific methods for estimating sample sizes for this type of design [47].

Our ability to detect an effect is likely to have been further reduced by the use of data collected at fixed time intervals, as start of treatment varied greatly relative to the collection of baseline measures — with correspondingly wide variation between end of treatment and 20 months follow-up. The logistics of the research and capacity within the service meant that no participant was offered the intervention prior to the 6 months follow-up. Changes in health or behaviours over this period may have an impact on the effectiveness of an intervention, possibly reducing differences between groups. Nevertheless, delays in accessing treatment are common in routine service delivery. Another 'trial within a cohort' (the Depression in South Yorkshire (DEPSY) trial) achieved a somewhat higher consent rate of 51%, but with 19% of those selected uncontactable [62]. DEPSY experienced a much higher attrition rate in the treatment arm, 32% compared to 13% of controls, and we found some evidence for differential attrition. These and other TWiCs design-related issues are considered in a related publication [47].

The trial cannot answer the question of whether health coaching is effective and cost-effective for multimorbidity in the longer term. The health coaching intervention consisted of three mechanisms, but the design does not allow us to estimate their distinct contribution. Nearly half of the patients reported symptoms of depression, and although support for low mood was provided frequently, it may have to be a more significant aspect of interventions in patients with multimorbidity [63]. The economic analysis was based on 45% of patients who

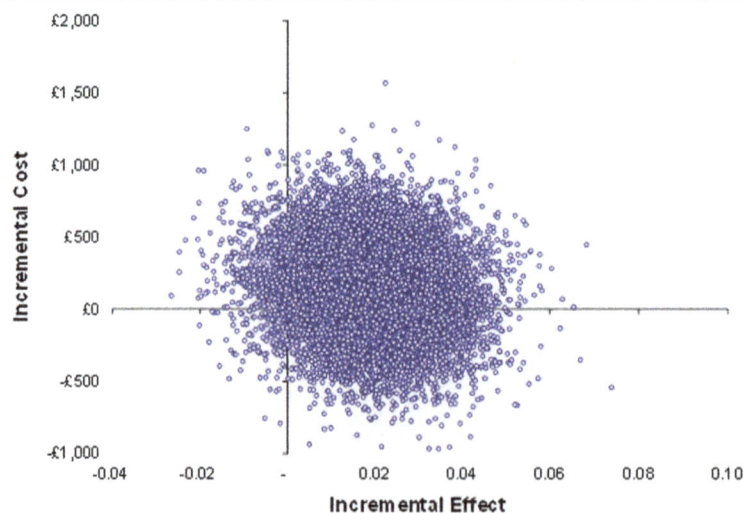

Fig. 2 Cost-effectiveness plane: full sample with imputed data

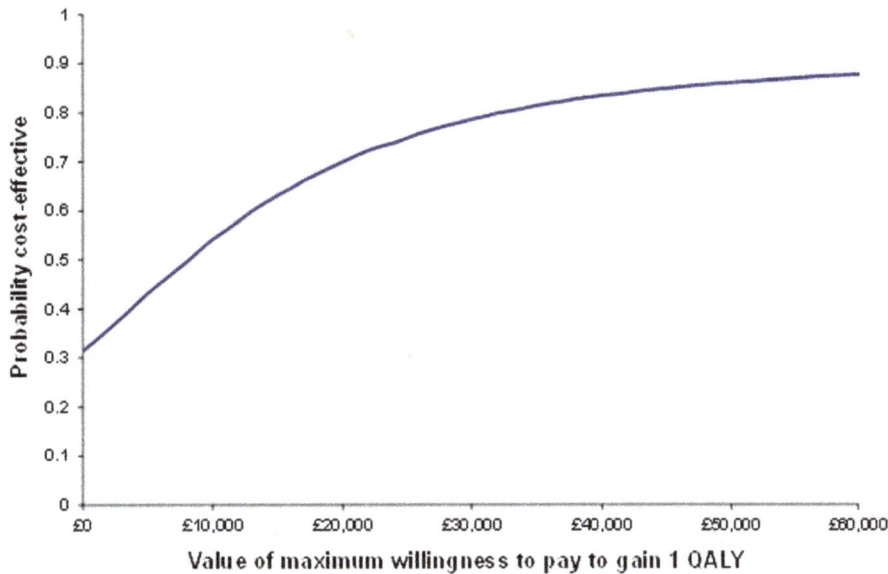

Fig. 3 Cost-effectiveness acceptability curve: full sample with imputed data

returned complete data, which may limit the general conclusions. Although multiple imputation was used to impute missing data values, this cannot fully adjust for unmeasured factors that may affect both outcomes and questionnaire completion; hence, the cost-effectiveness findings may be subject to residual confounding. However, a sensitivity analysis comparing cost-effectiveness in the 6 months prior to the intervention — in which time the majority of attrition occurred — with cost-effectiveness under the intervention found the effects restricted to the latter period.

Finally, this trial was conducted amongst patients with multimorbidity in one area in the UK primarily composed of white patients. Ethnic minority groups report poorer experience of care [64], and we do not know whether the effectiveness, reach and cost-effectiveness of health coaching are different in ethnic minority groups with multimorbidity. Although we have described this as a population health approach, we did restrict to certain groups depending on baseline activation, so 'reach' was somewhat limited by design. The response rate of patients to the initial cohort recruitment was in line with previous studies in this area [65, 66], but is potentially another source of bias, and with very limited demographic data on non-responders to the initial cohort, we were unable to assess overall representativeness. Although patient inclusion in the cohort was based on data within clinical records, patients self-reported types of long-term conditions, and these were not validated against clinical diagnosis.

Interpretation of the results in the context of the wider literature

It was felt that this design was a relevant test of health coaching as a population health strategy, reaching out to patients assessed as in need, but who may not necessarily be seeking self-management support. There will naturally be interest in the effects on those patients who engaged. Although per-protocol analyses can be used, such an approach is vulnerable to bias. Some published trials have assessed the effects through propensity matching of the subset who engaged [67]. The CACE analysis is the preferred model for assessment of effects in those who receive the intervention, as under certain, though usually reasonable, assumptions it provides an unbiased estimate of effect.

Further development of the intervention may have to consider different approaches to targeting, or more choice around the exact nature of the intervention to better align with patient preferences. Qualitative research conducted alongside the trial will be published in the full study report and may provide insights into these issues [68]. The group entering the trial did report significant numbers of conditions, and it is possible that they were too ill to benefit from the intervention. As noted earlier, existing treatment burden may be high in these patients, and although the coaching is designed to support self-management, it is possible that adding more self-management may exacerbate issues in treatment burden [69]. Our model of using activation to target the intervention is in line with the suggested uses of the measure [21] and reflects previous health coaching studies which have suggested the importance of avoiding patients who are too ill or too well to benefit [70]. There is good evidence that activation predicts many outcomes, but the evidence that activation can predict differential benefit from interventions is not as strong [34].

The pattern of health utilisation shown in the different groups is of interest. Many interventions for older people target those who demonstrate high levels of health care utilisation, on the basis that this is where reductions are most likely to be made. Nevertheless, it can be difficult to reduce utilisation in such patients in a comparative study [19], as patients identified on the basis of high use may demonstrate regression to the mean, may not be particularly amenable to intervention and may be present in small numbers in the population [20]. One of the largest trials of health coaching undertaken used a risk prediction score for inclusion in the trial, but it failed to demonstrate overall benefits in terms of admission rates [67]. The approach taken in PROTECTS was different, as patients were identified on the basis of showing capacity for improvement in activation. Such patients are prevalent, and the results suggested that the intervention might reduce emergency use of care. However, the positive impacts of such change were ameliorated by increases in elective use and overall increases in costs. Another very large trial of health coaching which showed reductions in costs had an additional focus on 'preference sensitive' shared decision-making rather than self-management alone [70].

As noted earlier, the recent Cochrane review reported only limited evidence for patients with multimorbidity [8], although there was a suggestion that interventions targeted at risk factors such as depression or specific functional difficulties might be more effective. Whilst our intervention had a depression component, it was not the primary focus as in other interventions in multimorbidity [63], and it is possible that the broad focus on self-management behaviour change is less impactful than a specific focus on a single area such as depression, especially in the context of an intervention of limited duration. Alternatively, our focus on depression may have paid insufficient attention to other psychosocial issues that might be present in these patients, such as anxiety or functional disorders. It is equally possible that for patients with fairly high levels of multimorbidity, the dose of the coaching was simply insufficient [67]. A longer treatment might have increased effectiveness, although with restricted resources, increasing the length of treatment will clearly restrict 'reach'.

Conclusions

Patients with multimorbidity are a major part of the workload of health systems, and findings from large evaluations of new models of care for this patient group are directly relevant to clinicians and policy decision-makers. The interpretation of the results will depend on the relative weight placed by decision-makers on clinical and economic outcomes. To readers focussed on clinical

outcomes, the trial demonstrated that health coaching led to no changes in activation or quality of life. However, the economic analyses showed that the intervention was likely to represent a cost-effective use of resources at conventional levels of willingness to pay. The economic analysis examines the effect of health coaching using a generic measure of health-related quality of life, which may detect broader impacts of the intervention not captured by the primary trial outcomes. It also considers the trade-off between differences in costs and effects associated with the intervention.

Decision-makers may not be convinced of the benefits of health coaching in the absence of evidence of clinical improvement. However, resource utilisation patterns highlighted interesting results which warrant further investigation. Individuals offered health coaching had higher utilisation of planned services and lower use of emergency hospital services. Health coaching may have had a positive impact by increasing individuals' wider engagement in the health service. Due to the limited follow-up period of the trial, we are not able to assess whether such increased engagement with planned services is maintained.

Health coaching in patients with multimorbidity did not lead to significant benefits on the primary measures of patient-reported outcome. The optimal role of this model of care within integrated care systems for patients with multiple long-term conditions remains unclear.

Abbreviations
CACE: Complier Average Causal Effect; CEACs: Cost-effectiveness acceptability curves; CLASSIC: Comprehensive Longitudinal Assessment of Salford's Integrated Care; ICER: Incremental cost-effectiveness ratio; MHI-5: Mental Health Inventory; NHS: National Health Service; NICE: National Institute of Health and Clinical Excellence; PAM: Patient Activation Measure; PROTECTS: Proactive Telephone Coaching and Tailored Support; QALYs: Quality-adjusted life years; QOL: Quality of life; SDSCA: Summary of Self-Care Activities; TwiCs: 'trial within a cohort'; WHOQoL-BREF: World Health Organization Quality of Life brief measure

Acknowledgements
We thank North West E Health and the National Institute for Health Research (NIHR) Clinical Research Network: Greater Manchester for assistance with the recruitment of the CLASSIC cohort, as well as staff at the participating practices. We thank the health advisors and their managers for their assistance in delivering the intervention. For assistance with the CLASSIC study, we thank 'Salford Together' — a partnership of Salford City Council, NHS Salford Clinical Commissioning Group, Salford Royal NHS Foundation Trust, Greater Manchester Mental Health NHS Foundation Trust and Salford Primary Care Together.

Funding

Funding was provided by the UK NIHR (grant 12/130/33). This paper represents independent research funded by the NIHR, project 12/130/33. Views and opinions are those of the authors and do not necessarily reflect those of the NHS, NIHR, NIHR Evaluation, Trials and Studies Coordinating Centre (NETSCC), Health Services and Delivery Research (HS&DR) or Department of Health.

Authors' contributions

PB, DR, KL, PC and TB were involved in the acquisition of funding and design of the trial. LR, KH, AB, LR and MS were involved in the administration of the study and recruitment of the patients. The statistical analysis was conducted by MP, MH and DR, with the economic analysis conducted by BP and RM. MP and PB drafted the manuscript, and all authors provided comments and approved the final manuscript.

Competing interests

The authors declare that they have no competing interests.

Author details

[1]NIHR School for Primary Care Research, Centre for Primary Care, Manchester Academic Health Science Centre, University of Manchester, Williamson Building, Oxford Road, Manchester M13 9PL, UK. [2]Manchester Centre for Health Economics, Division of Population Health, Health Services Research & Primary Care, Manchester Academic Health Science Centre, University of Manchester, Manchester M13 9PL, UK. [3]School of Nursing, Midwifery & Social Work, University of Manchester, Manchester M13 9PL, UK. [4]Mental Health and Addiction Research Group, Department of Health Sciences and Hull York Medical School, University of York, York YO10 5DD, UK. [5]NIHR Collaboration for Leadership in Applied Health Research and Care – Greater Manchester and Manchester Academic Health Science Centre, University of Manchester, Manchester M13 9PL, UK. [6]Salford Royal NHS Foundation Trust, Stott Lane, Salford M6 8HD, UK.

References

1. Boyd CM, Fortin M. Future of multimorbidity research: how should understanding of multimorbidity inform health system design? Public Health Rev. 2010;32(2):451–74.
2. Salisbury C. Multimorbidity: redesigning health care for people who use it. Lancet. 2012;380(9836):7–9.
3. Sinnott C, McHugh S, Browne J, Bradley C. GPs' perspectives on the management of patients with multimorbidity: systematic review and synthesis of qualitative research. BMJ Open. 2014;3(9):e003610.
4. Coventry P, Fisher L, Kenning C, Bee P, Bower P. Capacity, responsibility, and motivation: a critical qualitative evaluation of patient and practitioner views about barriers to self-management in people with multimorbidity. BMC Health Serv Res. 2014;14:536.
5. Paddison C, Roland M. Better management of patients with multimorbidity. BMJ. 2013;346:f2510.
6. Yoon J, Zulman D, Scott J, Mciejewski M. Costs associated with multimorbidity among VA patients. Med Care. 2014;52:S31–6.
7. Farmer C, Fenu E, O'Flynn N, Guthrie B. Clinical assessment and management of multimorbidity: summary of NICE guidance. BMJ. 2016;354: i4843.
8. Smith SM, Wallace E, O'Dowd T, Fortin M. Interventions for improving outcomes in patients with multimorbidity in primary care and community settings. Cochrane Database Syst Rev. 2016;3 https://doi.org/10.1002/14651858.CD006560.pub3.
9. Bodenheimer T, Lorig K, Holman H, Grumbach K. Patient self-management of chronic disease in primary care. JAMA. 2002;288(19):2469–75.
10. Glasgow R, McKay H, Piette J, Reynolds K. The RE-AIM framework for evaluating interventions: what can it tell us about approaches to chronic disease management? Patient Educ Couns. 2001;44:119–27.
11. Treweek S, Dryden R, McCowan C, Harrow A, Thompson AM. Do participants in adjuvant breast cancer trials reflect the breast cancer patient population? Eur J Cancer. 2015;51(8):907–14.
12. Kenning C, Coventry P, Bower P. Self-management interventions in patients with long-term conditions: a structured review of the role of multimorbidity in patient inclusion, assessment and outcome. J Comorb. 2014;4(1):37–45.
13. King M, Nazareth I, Lampe F, Bower P, Chandler M, Morou M, Sibbald B, Lai R: Conceptual framework and systematic review of the effects of participants' and professionals' preferences in randomised controlled trials. Health Technol Assess 2005, 9(35):1-186.
14. Relton C, Torgerson D, O'Cathain A, Nicholl J. Rethinking pragmatic randomised controlled trials: introducing the 'cohort multiple randomised controlled trial' design. BMJ. 2013;340:c1066.
15. Aziz Z, Absetz P, Oldroyd J, Pronk N, Oldenburg B. A systematic review of real-world diabetes prevention programs: learnings from the last 15 years. Implement Sci. 2015;10:172.
16. Lorig KR, Sobel D, Ritter P, Laurent D, Hobbs M. Effect of a self-management program on patients with chronic disease. Eff Clin Pract. 2001;4(6):256–62.
17. Kennedy A, Reeves D, Bower P, Lee V, Middleton E, Richardson G, Gardner C, Gately C, Rogers A. The effectiveness and cost effectiveness of a national lay led self care support programme for patients with long-term conditions: a pragmatic randomised controlled trial. J Epidemiol Community Health. 2007;61:254–61.
18. McLean S, Protti D, Sheikh A. Telehealthcare for long term conditions. BMJ. 2011;342:d120.
19. Steventon A, Tunkel S, Blunt I, Bardsley M. Effects of telephone health coaching (Birmingham OwnHealth) on hospital use and associated costs: cohort study with matched controls. BMJ. 2013;347:f4585.
20. Roland M, Abel G. Reducing emergency admissions: are we on the right track? BMJ. 2012;345:e6017.
21. Hibbard J, Gilburt H. Supporting people to manage their health: an introduction to patient activation. London: The King's Fund; 2014.
22. Hibbard J, Stockard E, Mahoney E, Tusler M. Development of the Patient Activation Measure (PAM): conceptualizing and measuring activation in patients and consumers. Health Serv Res. 2004;39:1005–26.
23. Katon WJ, Lin EHB, Von Korff M, Ciechanowski P, Ludman EJ, Young B, Peterson D, Rutter CM, McGregor M, McCulloch D. Collaborative care for patients with depression and chronic illnesses. N Engl J Med. 2010;363(27): 2611–20.
24. Eton D, de Oliveira D, Egginton J, Ridgeway J, Odell L, May C, Montori V. Building a measurement framework of burden of treatment in complex patients with chronic conditions: a qualitative study. Patient Relat Outcome Meas. 2012;3:39–49.
25. May C, Montori V, Mair F. We need minimally disruptive medicine. BMJ. 2009;339(aug11_2):b2803.
26. Dejonghe LAL, Becker J, Froboese I, Schaller A. Long-term effectiveness of health coaching in rehabilitation and prevention: a systematic review. Patient Educ Couns. 2017;100(9):1643–53.
27. Oliveira JS, Sherrington C, Amorim AB, Dario AB, Tiedemann A. What is the effect of health coaching on physical activity participation in people aged 60 years and over? A systematic review of randomised controlled trials. Br J Sports Med. 2017;51(19):1425–32.
28. Boehmer KR, Barakat S, Ahn S, Prokop LJ, Erwin PJ, Murad MH. Health coaching interventions for persons with chronic conditions: a systematic review and meta-analysis protocol. Syst Rev. 2016;5(1):146.
29. Hill B, Richardson B, Skouteris H. Do we know how to design effective health coaching interventions: a systematic review of the state of the literature. Am J Health Promot. 2015;29(5):e158–68.
30. Wolever RQ, Simmons LA, Sforzo GA, Dill D, Kaye M, Bechard EM, Southard ME, Kennedy M, Vosloo J, Yang N. A systematic review of the literature on health and wellness coaching: defining a key behavioral intervention in healthcare. Global Adv Health Med. 2013;2(4):38–57.
31. Ammentorp J, Uhrenfeldt L, Angel F, Ehrensvard M, Carlsen EB, Kofoed PE. Can life coaching improve health outcomes? — A systematic review of intervention studies. BMC Health Serv Res. 2013;13:428.
32. Barakat S, Boehmer K, Abdelrahim M, Ahn S, Al-Khateeb AA, Villalobos NA, Prokop L, Erwin PJ, Fleming K, Serrano V, et al. Does health coaching grow capacity in cancer survivors? A systematic review. Popul Health Manag. 2018;21:63–81.
33. Kivela K, Elo S, Kyngas H, Kaariainen M. The effects of health coaching on adult patients with chronic diseases: a systematic review. Patient Educ Couns. 2014;97(2):147–57.
34. Blakemore A, Hann M, Howells K, Panagioti M, Sidaway M, Reeves D, Bower P. Patient activation in older people with long-term conditions and multimorbidity: correlates and change in a cohort study in the United Kingdom. BMC Health Serv Res. 2016;16(1):582.

35. Bayliss E, Ellis J, Steiner J. Seniors' self-reported multimorbidity captured biopsychosocial factors not incorporated in two other data-based morbidity measures. J Clin Epidemiol. 2009;62(5):550–7.

36. Hibbard J, Mahoney ER, Stockard J, Tusler M. Development and testing of a short form of the patient activation measure. Health Serv Res. 2005;40(6 Pt 1):1918–30.

37. Brandling J, House W. Social prescribing in general practice: adding meaning to medicine. Br J Gen Pract. 2014;59(563):454–6.

38. South J, Higgins T, Woodall J, White P. Can social prescribing provide the missing link? Prim Health Care Res Dev. 2008;9(4):310–8.

39. Lovell K, Bower P, Richards D, Barkham M, Sibbald B, Roberts C, Davies L, Rogers A, Gellatly J, Hennessey S. Developing guided self-help for depression using the Medical Research Council complex interventions framework: a description of the modelling phase and results of an exploratory randomised controlled trial. BMC Psychiatry. 2008;8(1):91.

40. Lovell K, Richards D. A recovery programme for depression. London: Rethink Mental Illness; 2007. https://www.rethink.org/resources/r/recovery-programme-for-depression-booklet-april-2012. Accessed 7 Feb 2017

41. Schmittdiel J, Mosen D, Glasgow R, Hibbard J, Remmers C, Bellows J. Patient assessment of chronic illness care (PACIC) and improved patient-centered outcomes for chronic conditions. J Gen Intern Med. 2011;23(1):77–80.

42. Skevington S, Lotfy M, O'Connell K. The World Health Organization's WHOQOL-BREF quality of life assessment: psychometric properties and results of the international field trial — a report from the WHOQOL group. Qual Life Res. 2013;13(2):299–310.

43. Berwick DM, Murphy JM, Goldman PA, Ware JE Jr, Barsky AJ, Weinstein MC. Performance of a five-item mental health screening test. Med Care. 1991; 29(2):169–76.

44. Yamazaki S, Fukuhara S, Green J. Usefulness of five-item and three-item Mental Health Inventories to screen for depressive symptoms in the general population of Japan. Health Qual Life Outcomes. 2005;3:48.

45. Kelly MJ, Dunstan FD, Lloyd K, Fone DL. Evaluating cutpoints for the MHI-5 and MCS using the GHQ-12: a comparison of five different methods. BMC Psychiatry. 2008;8:10.

46. Toobert DJ, Hampson SE, Glasgow RE. The summary of diabetes self-care activities measure: results from 7 studies and a revised scale. Diabetes Care. 2000;23(7):943–50.

47. Reeves D, Howells K, Sidaway M, Blakemore A, Hann M, Panagioti M, Bower P. The cohort multiple randomized controlled trial design was found to be highly susceptible to low statistical power and internal validity biases. J Clin Epidemiol. 2018;95:111–9.

48. Zwarenstein M, Treweek S, Gagnier J, Altman D, Tunis S, Haynes B, Xman A, Oher D, CONSORT and Pragmatic Trials in Healthcare (Practihc) groups. Improving the reporting of pragmatic trials: an extension of the CONSORT statement. BMJ. 2008;337(nov11_2):a2390.

49. Morris NS, MacLean CD, Chew LD, Littenberg B. The Single Item Literacy Screener: evaluation of a brief instrument to identify limited reading ability. BMC Fam Pract. 2006;7:21.

50. Mitchell PH, Powell L, Blumenthal J, Norten J, Ironson G, Pitula CR, Froelicher ES, Czajkowski S, Youngblood M, Huber M, et al. A short social support measure for patients recovering from myocardial infarction: the ENRICHD Social Support Inventory. J Cardiopulm Rehabil. 2003;23(6):398–403.

51. Dunn G, Emsley R, Liu H, Landau S, Green J, White I, Pickles A. Evaluation and validation of social and psychological markers in randomised trials of complex interventions in mental health. Health Technol Assess. 2015;19:1–116.

52. Dunn G, Maracy M, Dowrick C, Ayuso-Mateos J-L, Dalgard O, Page H, Lehtinen V, Casey P, Wilkinson C, Vazquez-Barquero J, et al. Estimating psychological treatment effects from a randomised controlled trial with both non-compliance and loss to follow up. Br J Psychiatry. 2003;183: 323 31.

53. Koop JC. On an identity for the variances of a ratio of two random variables. J R Stat Soc Ser B Methodol. 1964;26(3):484–6.

54. Herdman M, Gudex C, Lloyd A, Janssen M, Kind P, Parkin D, Bonsel G, Badia X. Development and preliminary testing of the new five-level version of EQ-5D (EQ-5D-5L). Qual Life Res. 2011;20(10):1727–36.

55. Devlin N, Shah K, Feng Y, Mulhern B, van Hout B. Valuing health-related quality of life: an EQ-5D-5L value set for England. London: Office of Health Economics; 2016. https://www.ohe.org/publications/valuing-health-related-quality-life-eq-5d-5l-value-set-england. Accessed 7 Feb 2017

56. NICE. Developing NICE guidelines: the manual. Process and methods guides. London: National Institute for Health and Care Excellence; 2014.

57. NICE. Guide to the methods of technology appraisal 2013. Manchester: National Institute for Health and Care Excellence; 2013.

58. Curtis L, Burns A. Unit Costs of Health & Social Care 2015. Canterbury: Personal Social Services Research Unit; 2015. http://www.pssru.ac.uk/project-pages/unit-costs/2015/. Accessed 7 Feb 2017

59. Department of Health. NHS reference costs 2014 to 2015. London: Department of Health; 2015. https://www.gov.uk/government/publications/nhs-reference-costs-2014-to-2015. Accessed 7 Feb 2017

60. Faria R, Gomes M, Epstein D, White I. A guide to handling missing data in cost-effectiveness analysis conducted within randomised controlled trials. Pharmacoeconomics. 2014;32:1157–70.

61. Manca A, Hawkins N, Sculpher M. Estimating mean QALYs in trial-based cost-effectiveness analysis: the importance of controlling for baseline utility. Health Econ. 2005;14:487–96.

62. Viksveen P, Relton C, Nicholl J. Benefits and challenges of using the cohort multiple randomised controlled trial design for testing an intervention for depression. Trials. 2017;18:308.

63. Coventry P, Lovell K, Dickens C, Bower P, Chew-Graham C, McElvenny D, Hann M, Cherrington A, Garrett C, Gibbons CJ, et al. Integrated primary care for patients with mental and physical multimorbidity: cluster randomised controlled trial of collaborative care for patients with depression comorbid with diabetes or cardiovascular disease. BMJ. 2015;350:h638.

64. Burt J, Lloyd C, Campbell J, Roland M, Abel G. Variations in GP-patient communication by ethnicity, age, and gender: evidence from a national primary care patient survey. Brit J Gen Pract. 2016;66(642):E47–52.

65. Kennedy A, Bower P, Reeves D, Blakeman T, Bowen R, Chew-Graham C, Eden M, Fullwood C, Gaffney H, Gardner C, et al. Implementation of self management support for long term conditions in routine primary care settings: cluster randomised controlled trial. BMJ. 2013;346:f2882.

66. Reeves D, Hann M, Rick J, Rowe K, Small N, Burt J, Roland M, Protheroe J, Blakeman T, Richardson G, et al. Care plans and care planning in the management of long-term conditions in the United Kingdom: a controlled prospective cohort study. Br J Gen Pract. 2014;64(626):568–75.

67. Härter M, Dirmaier J, Dwinger S, Kriston L, Herbarth L, Siegmund-Schultze E, Bermejo I, Matschinger H, Heider D, König H-H. Effectiveness of telephone-based health coaching for patients with chronic conditions: a randomised controlled trial. PLoS One. 2016;11(9):e0161269.

68. Bower P, Reeves D, Sutton M, Lovell K, Bakemore A, Hann M, Howells H, Meacock R, Munford L, Panagioti M, et al. Comprehensive Longitudinal Assessment of Salford Integrated Care (CLASSIC): a mixed methods study of the implementation and effectiveness of a new model of care for long-term conditions. Health Serv Deliv Res. 2018. (in press)

69. Lin E, Katon W, Rutter C, Simon G, Ludman E, Von KM, Young B, Oliver M, Ciechanowski P, Kinder L, et al. Effects of enhanced depression treatment on diabetes self-care. Ann Fam Med. 2006;4(1):46–53.

70. Wennberg D, Marr A, Lang L, O'Malley S, Bennett G. A randomized trial of a telephone care-management strategy. N Engl J Med. 2010;363(13):1245–55.

Global variation in bacterial strains that cause tuberculosis disease

Kirsten E Wiens[1], Lauren P Woyczynski[1], Jorge R Ledesma[1], Jennifer M Ross[1,2], Roberto Zenteno-Cuevas[3], Amador Goodridge[4], Irfan Ullah[5,6], Barun Mathema[7], Joel Fleury Djoba Siawaya[8,9], Molly H Biehl[1], Sarah E Ray[1], Natalia V Bhattacharjee[1], Nathaniel J Henry[1], Robert C Reiner Jr[1], Hmwe H Kyu[1], Christopher J L Murray[1] and Simon I Hay[1*]

Abstract

Background: The host, microbial, and environmental factors that contribute to variation in tuberculosis (TB) disease are incompletely understood. Accumulating evidence suggests that one driver of geographic variation in TB disease is the local ecology of mycobacterial genotypes or strains, and there is a need for a comprehensive and systematic synthesis of these data. The objectives of this study were to (1) map the global distribution of genotypes that cause TB disease and (2) examine whether any epidemiologically relevant clinical characteristics were associated with those genotypes.

Methods: We performed a systematic review of PubMed and Scopus to create a comprehensive dataset of human TB molecular epidemiology studies that used representative sampling techniques. The methods were developed according to the Preferred Reporting Items for Systematic Reviews and Meta-Analyses (PRISMA). We extracted and synthesized data from studies that reported prevalence of bacterial genotypes and from studies that reported clinical characteristics associated with those genotypes.

Results: The results of this study are twofold. First, we identified 206 studies for inclusion in the study, representing over 200,000 bacterial isolates collected over 27 years in 85 countries. We mapped the genotypes and found that, consistent with previously published maps, Euro-American lineage 4 and East Asian lineage 2 strains are widespread, and West African lineages 5 and 6 strains are geographically restricted. Second, 30 studies also reported transmission chains and 4 reported treatment failure associated with genotypes. We performed a meta-analysis and found substantial heterogeneity across studies. However, based on the data available, we found that lineage 2 strains may be associated with increased risk of transmission chains, while lineages 5 and 6 strains may be associated with reduced risk, compared with lineage 4 strains.

Conclusions: This study provides the most comprehensive systematic analysis of the evidence for diversity in bacterial strains that cause TB disease. The results show both geographic and epidemiological differences between strains, which could inform our understanding of the global burden of TB. Our findings also highlight the challenges of collecting the clinical data required to inform TB diagnosis and treatment. We urge future national TB programs and research efforts to prioritize and reinforce clinical data collection in study designs and results dissemination.

Keywords: Tuberculosis, *Mycobacterium tuberculosis*, Genotype, Genetic variation, Epidemiology, Molecular epidemiology

* Correspondence: sihay@uw.edu
[1]Institute for Health Metrics and Evaluation, University of Washington, 2301 5th Ave, Suite 600, Seattle, WA 98121, USA
Full list of author information is available at the end of the article

Background

Tuberculosis (TB) is found in every population of the world today and kills 1.1–1.6 million people globally each year [1]. There is also significant geographic variation in the prevalence, incidence, and mortality of TB [1]. The factors that contribute to individual and geographic variation in TB infection and disease are incompletely understood. An intact immune response is required to prevent infection and progression to active disease as conditions that weaken the immune system are strongly associated with TB, including HIV co-infection, type II diabetes mellitus, undernutrition, and immunosuppressive medications such as anti-tumor necrosis factor (TNF) therapy [2]. Environmental factors likely also play a role in infection and disease progression, including population density, indoor and outdoor air pollution, and health care quality and access [2]. However, these risk factors are insufficient to explain the current burden of TB [3].

An additional driver of variation may be human and bacterial genetic variation [4]. There are human genetic polymorphisms associated with susceptibility to latent TB infection and progression to active disease [5], as well as polymorphisms in the *Mycobacterium tuberculosis* complex (MTBC) associated with the ability to cause disease [6] and with transmissibility [7]. The host-pathogen relationship in TB is sympatric [8], i.e., the host and pathogen tend to share a common ancestral geographic origin [8]. When patients are infected with an allopatric strain or a strain that originates from a different geographic origin than the patient, they may be at risk for greater pulmonary impairment [9]. Similarly, there is evidence for associations between human leukocyte antigen (HLA) type and susceptibility to TB disease caused by particular MTBC strains [10, 11]. However, there is considerable variation in studies that test for associations between MTBC genotypes and clinical characteristics [12, 13].

A better understanding of MTBC molecular epidemiology could improve our ability to treat and control TB. Genetic data are already being used by epidemiologists as tools for outbreak investigations to identify sources of mycobacterial infection [14] and as tools in surveillance to identify the strains most likely to spread rapidly through new human populations [3]. Additionally, understanding the risk factors associated with MTBC genetic data could help direct the development of biomarker-based diagnostic tests to identify patients early that are infected with strains associated with higher risk of treatment failure, relapse, drug resistance, or death [15]. Finally, there is accumulating evidence for variation in the immune response to distinct MTBC strains [16–21]. Therefore, understanding the global variation in MTBC strains will be important as new vaccines, biomarkers, and host-directed therapies are developed [13].

The objective of this study was to systematically synthesize all available information on MTBC genotypes in order to (1) map the global distribution of genotypes that cause TB disease and (2) determine whether any epidemiologically relevant clinical characteristics were associated with those genotypes. Previous systematic reviews that mapped MTBC genotype distribution focused on MTBC Beijing family strains and their association with drug resistance [22, 23]. We expanded on this previous work by considering data for all MTBC lineages, making this the most comprehensive synthesis of MTBC genotypes that has been conducted to date.

Methods

The methods for this systematic review, including literature search, inclusion criteria, and analysis, were developed according to the Preferred Reporting Items for Systematic Reviews and Meta-Analyses (PRISMA) [24, 25].

Information sources and search strategy

We identified studies by systematically searching PubMed and Scopus. The first search was run on June 8, 2017, and the final search was run on November 13, 2017. Articles identified in these searches were supplemented by six published studies in Papua New Guinea, India, Botswana, Nepal, Ethiopia, and Kenya, and two unpublished studies in Mexico and Panama, which we were directed to by manually checking the reference lists of studies and by reviewing the conference abstracts for the 48th Union World Conference on Lung Health. Complete details of search strings and dates searched are found in Additional file 1.

Eligibility criteria
Types of studies

In order to minimize sampling bias in the analysis, we restricted our analysis to human TB molecular epidemiology studies that used either probability sampling methods, such as random or cluster-based sampling, or that collected samples from all reported or all new TB cases in the study location and time period. For the majority of studies "all TB cases" included culture-positive TB cases only. For studies that used GeneXpert remnants for DNA collection, this included microscopy-positive TB cases. We excluded studies of sub-populations that may over- or underrepresent particular genotypes, such as studies restricted to hospital workers, prisoners, HIV-infected individuals, children, homeless individuals, immigrants, individuals living in slums, military personnel, individuals with drug-resistant strains, relapse or re-infection cases, or extrapulmonary TB cases. In addition, we excluded outbreak investigations, case studies, review articles, and studies not available in English or Spanish. When multiple studies used the same data, we included the study that provided the most detailed genotyping data and/or the most detailed corresponding clinical data. For the global mapping analysis, we excluded studies that only tested or reported data for one lineage. These latter studies were considered for the clinical characteristics analysis. We did not apply publication date restrictions.

Types of genotyping methods

We included studies that reported genotyping results by geographic location, year, and sampling method and that met the eligibility criteria described above. We considered genotypes determined by whole-genome sequencing (WGS), large sequence polymorphism (LSP) as determined by polymerase chain reaction (PCR), spacer oligonucleotide typing (spoligotyping), and multi-locus variable number of tandem repeats (VNTR) analysis (MLVA).

Types of clinical characteristics

In a secondary step, we screened all studies that met our initial inclusion criteria for studies that also reported clinical characteristics associated with genotypes, including transmission chains, progression to active TB, treatment failure, duration of symptoms, relapse or retreatment, severity of pulmonary lesions, and extrapulmonary TB. For further analysis, we focused on the characteristics with clear case definitions and sufficient data available for meta-analysis, which included treatment failure and transmission chains. Treatment failure was defined as a TB case that had a positive sputum culture and/or smear at 5–8 months following the start of TB treatment. Transmission chains were inferred by genetic clusters, which were defined as two or more identical genotype patterns identified in the same study location and time period [26]. Genetic clustering appears not to be a perfect measure of transmission chains since it can be impacted by various factors including social mixing, immigration, age structure, and underlying TB incidence [27, 28]. However, we decided that it was an important measure to include because (1) it has been an important tool for TB surveillance [29–31] and (2) it currently has sufficient published data available for global analysis.

Data collection process and data items
Study screening and selection

Articles were reviewed for eligibility first by screening the titles and abstracts and then by reviewing the full texts in an unblinded standardized manner. One reviewer screened the titles and abstracts, and the selected articles were divided between three reviewers to screen and extract using a standardized data extraction form. When there was uncertainty about the eligibility, reviewers arrived at a decision by consensus.

Genotype data extraction

Information that was extracted from each study included (1) page number and table or figure the data was extracted from, (2) underlying study design [cohort or cross-sectional], (3) sampling approach [all cases, all new cases, cluster-based sample, or random sample], (4) geographic region and year(s) the sample represented, (5) genotyping method [spoligotyping, MLVA typing, PCR, or WGS], and (6) total count of each genotype identified in the sample. Additional file 2 contains the screening sheet detailing all studies reviewed, reason(s) for exclusion, and a log of any follow-up. Additional file 3 contains all raw genotyping data extracted and corresponding study meta-data. The original extraction sheet is available upon request.

Clinical characteristic data extraction

All studies that reported transmission chains or genetic clustering as defined above were included in a second extraction sheet. The following additional data were extracted in this sheet: (1) the total count of each genotype, (2) total count of each genotype that was part of a genetic cluster, and (3) potential confounders, when available (including the proportion of HIV co-infection and drug resistance in the sample, the mean age of the participants, and the proportion of participants that were male, had previously been diagnosed with TB, had extrapulmonary TB, or were immigrants). Additional file 4 contains raw genetic clustering data extracted and corresponding study meta-data.

Synthesis and analysis
Classification system for genotypes

In this study, we defined "strains" based on the seven phylogenetic lineages identified by S. Gagneaux and colleagues [32]. We included data on animal lineage strains isolated from human TB cases, which included *Mycobacterium bovis*, *Mycobacterium pinnipedii*, *Mycobacterium caprae*, *Mycobacterium origys*, and *Mycobacterium microti* strains. Some studies reported "other," "unknown," "undefined," "unclear," or "uncommon" genotypes, which we labeled as "unknown lineages." For each study, we extracted data at the most detailed genotype level available. When spoligotype octal codes were provided, we determined phylogenetic lineage using the central Bayesian network (CBN) method implemented in Run TB-Lineage [33, 34]. When spoligotype clade or family was provided, we used SITVIT Web and Run TB-Lineage to determine phylogenetic lineage [35]. When MLVA family was provided, we determined phylogenetic lineage using MIRU-VNTR*plus* [36, 37]. For Ethiopian MLVA families, we assigned strains to lineage 4 or lineage 7 using genetic relatedness based on published phylogenies [38, 39]. We implemented this method directly in the extraction sheet using Excel formulas. Additional file 1: Table S1 illustrates the online tools used in this method and Additional file 1: Table S2 and Additional file 5 detail how individual genotypes were related based on this method.

Data quality checks

We performed several data quality checks using code written in R software (version 3.3.3) to check for duplicate extractions and for discrepancies between the screening and extraction sheets. We checked that all extracted studies were included in the screening sheet, and vice versa, using PubMed ID or a unique study identifier. We checked for duplicate extractions by looking for any studies that (1) had duplicate PubMed ID or unique study identifiers, (2) had the same country and start year, or (3) had the same country and sample size. Each potentially duplicated or missed study was checked manually, and the decision to include or exclude was recorded.

Proportion of estimated TB cases represented in each country

We determined the proportion of estimated TB cases that were represented in each country for which we had data using estimates from the Global Burden of Disease Study 2016 [40]. We downloaded estimates of the total number of TB cases prevalent in each country and year across all ages and sexes from https://vizhub.healthdata.org/gbd-compare/ (accessed on July 29, 2018). We matched these country-year estimates to each study based on the country the study was conducted in and the year that corresponded to the mid-point of its sampling period. We divided the sample size of each study by the estimated prevalent TB cases in the corresponding country and year to get the proportion represented in each study. We then summed the proportions represented in all studies within each country to get final estimates of the proportion of TB cases represented per country.

Map of the global distribution of genotypes

We determined the proportion of each phylogenetic lineage present in each country for which we had data. If multiple studies were available in a country, we summed the strain counts across all studies and years to get the final proportions and sample sizes.

Meta-analysis of genetic clustering association with genotypes

We performed a random effects (RE) meta-analysis of the relative risk (RR) of genetic clustering associated with genotypes using the Reliability Method (RELM) method in the R software package "metafor" (version 3.3.3) [41]. We excluded studies that identified fewer than two isolates of the lineages under analysis. We examined inconsistency across studies using the I^2 test that

measures the percentage of total variation across studies due to heterogeneity [42]. We performed a subgroup analysis of genetic clustering within the regions West Asia, East Asia, Europe and the Americas, and Africa.

Results

Study selection

We identified 206 studies for inclusion in the study, representing over 200,000 bacterial isolates collected over 27 years in 85 countries. Of these studies, 30 also reported transmission chains and 4 reported treatment failure associated with genotypes. Figure 1 shows the PRISMA flow diagram detailing the study selection process. Additional file 1: Figure S1 shows a map of the numbers of studies per year that were included from each country.

Study variation

The 206 studies included 42 nationally representative samples and 164 samples representative of smaller geographic units. These included 34 studies that used a cluster or random sampling, 170 that collected samples from all reported or new TB cases in a given geographic location and time period, and 2 studies that used different sampling methods for different time periods. We illustrated how these study designs varied globally in Fig. 2. Sub-Saharan Africa was dominated by subnationally representative studies, while Caribbean Latin America was dominated by nationally representative studies (Fig. 2). In addition, we calculated the proportion of estimated prevalent TB cases that were represented in each country. Proportions ranged from 0.0012% in Nigeria to 5.4% in Greenland (Fig. 2). In general, the proportions were lower in countries where TB burden was highest (Fig. 2). The meta-data linked with each individual study is available in its raw format in Additional file 3.

Geographic variation in MTBC genotypes

We mapped the distribution of MTBC genotypes identified in our systematic review across all years and for all locations in each country for which we had data. A striking feature of the map was the widespread global distribution of Euro-American lineage 4 (Figs. 3 and 4). Lineage 4 was identified in every country where genotyping data was available for inclusion, and it was the majority lineage in 52 of the 85 countries (Additional file 1: Table S3). Our map also showed the fairly widespread distribution of East Asian lineage 2 (Figs. 3 and 4), which was identified in 67 of the 85 countries and was the majority lineage in 6 countries (Additional file 1: Table S3). In contrast, West African lineages 5 and 6 were identified in only 30 countries and were the majority lineages in zero countries (Additional file 1: Table S2). In addition, Indo-Oceanic lineage 1 and East African-Indian lineage 3 were identified

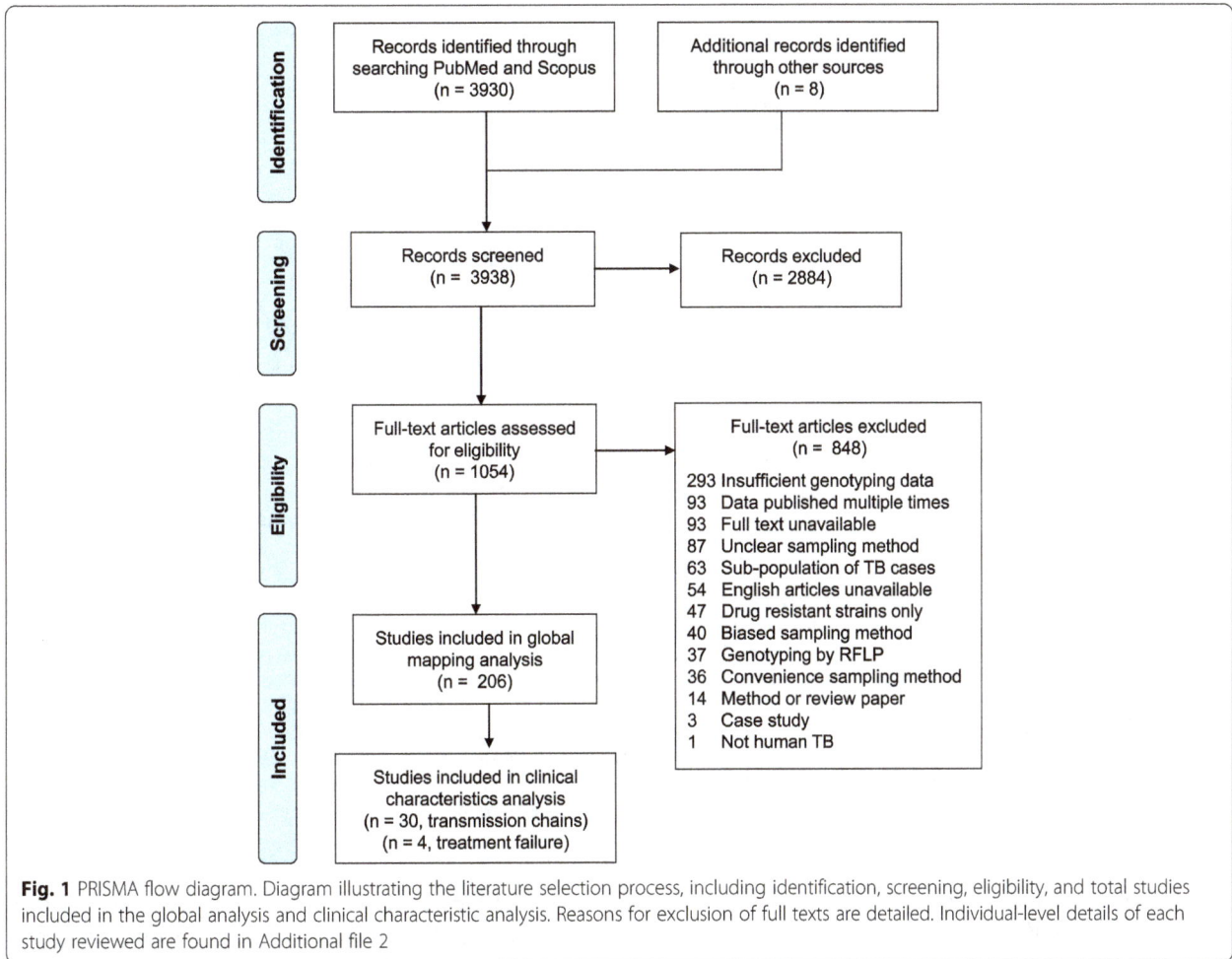

Fig. 1 PRISMA flow diagram. Diagram illustrating the literature selection process, including identification, screening, eligibility, and total studies included in the global analysis and clinical characteristic analysis. Reasons for exclusion of full texts are detailed. Individual-level details of each study reviewed are found in Additional file 2

in 64 and 59 countries, respectively, and each was the majority lineage in 2 countries (Additional file 1: Table S3).

The map also illustrated various regions of distinct mycobacterial distribution that may be independent of geopolitical country boundaries (Fig. 3 and Additional file 1: Figure S2). For example, Eastern Africa from Sudan to Mozambique was distinct from the rest of Africa in that it had a higher prevalence of lineages 1 and 3. Western Africa was distinct in that it had the highest prevalence of lineages 5 and 6, while Southern Africa had the highest prevalence of lineage 2 strains and Central Africa had the highest prevalence of lineage 4 strains. In addition, the Indian subcontinent and Australia had a similar genotype distribution, which was distinct from Russia and Eastern Asia. The UK was distinct from the rest of Europe in that it had a greater prevalence of lineages 1 and 3. Finally, Central America and northern South America had distinct genotype distributions from central and southern South America.

Temporal variation in MTBC genotypes
The results described above represent MTBC genotype distributions aggregated across all years from 1990 to 2017. In order to investigate the changes over time in genotype distribution, and to illustrate the time periods that more accurately represented the data in each country, we created maps of genotype distribution for three distinct time periods (Additional file 1: Figure S3). To synthesize these data, we plotted the total prevalence of each lineage in each time period by region (Fig. 5). Figure 5 should be used as a guide and interpreted with some caution as it represents data aggregated across diverse geographic locations. The plots showed that lineage 3 strains have increased in prevalence over time in the UK (Additional file 1: Figure S3A-C) and Europe (Fig. 5). In addition, the plots showed a decline in the prevalence of lineage 1 in West and Central Asia (Fig. 5 and Additional file 1: Figure S3B-C).

Clinical variation in MTBC genotypes
Transmission chains as measured by genetic clustering
We performed a random-effects meta-analysis [41] of the 30 studies that reported transmission chains or genetic clusters associated with MTBC genotypes. We defined genetic clusters as two or more identical genotype patterns

% of TB cases

○ 0.0012
○ 0.046
○ 5.4

● National: survey
○ National: all TB cases
● Sub–national: survey
○ Sub–national: all TB cases

Fig. 2 Variation in sampling methods of studies included in the systematic review. Variation in study design for the 206 studies that met the inclusion criteria for this systematic review. The proportion of studies in each country that collected a nationally representative sample versus a sample representative of a smaller geographic location are shown in purple and green, respectively. Light purple and green indicate the proportion of studies in each country that collected all reported or all new TB cases in a given location and time period. For the majority of studies, "all TB cases" represents culture-positive cases only; for studies that use GeneXpert remnants for DNA collection, this represents microscopy-positive cases. Dark purple and green indicate the proportion of studies in a given country that used a random or cluster-based survey sampling method to select a subset of cases. TB cases in each country were estimated by the Global Burden of Disease Study 2016 [40]. We calculated percent of all TB cases in each country using the total number of genotyped cases as the numerator and total estimated prevalent TB cases as the denominator. The radius of each pie is proportional to percent of total estimated TB cases that are represented across all studies in each country. Examples of percent of total estimated TB cases that correspond to pie sizes are shown in the legend in gray. The example pies show the minimum, mid-point, and maximum percent of estimated TB cases represented in this review

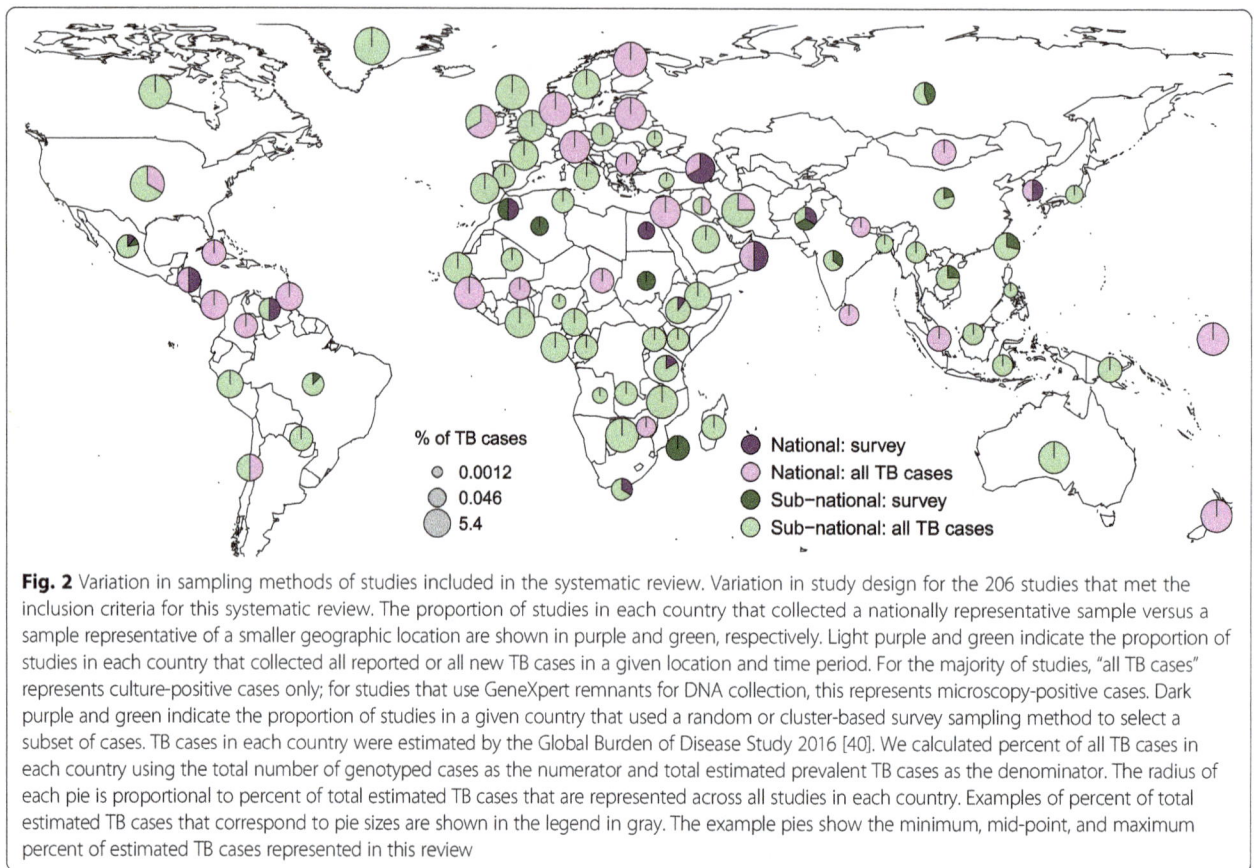

identified in the same study location and time period. We used lineage 4 as the reference group because lineage 4 strains were identified in each study included in the meta-analysis. The characteristics of each study included in the meta-analyses are shown in Additional file 1: Table S4. We analyzed transmission chain relative risk (RR) across all studies, as well as within subgroups of Africa, East Asia, West Asia, and Europe and the Americas.

The results of the meta-analyses are summarized in Table 1, and detailed forest plots are shown in Additional file 1: Figure S4. Lineage 1 strains overall were not associated with transmission chains (RR [95% CI] = 1.07 [0.83, 1.37]) (Table 1) but were associated with increased risk within East Asia (RR [95% CI] = 2.54 [1.02, 6.28]) (Additional file 1: Figure S4A). Lineage 2 Beijing strains were associated with increased risk of transmission chains overall (RR [95% CI] = 1.24 [1.07, 1.45]) (Table 1), and the risk was higher within East Asia (RR [95% CI] = 1.90 [1.14, 3.17]) (Additional file 1: Figure S4B). Lineage 3 strains were associated with reduced risk of transmission chains in Europe and the Americas (RR [95% CI] = 0.67 [0.50, 0.91]) (Additional file 1: Figure S4C). Lineages 5 and 6 strains were associated with reduced risk of transmission chains overall (RR [95% CI] = 0.61 [0.43, 0.86]) (Table 1, Additional file 1: Figure S4D), as were animal lineage strains (RR [95% CI] = 0.79 [0.64, 0.96]) (Table 1,

Additional file 1: Figure S4E). Unknown strains, which comprise orphans, undefined, and uncommon genotypes, were associated with reduced risk of transmission chains overall (RR [95% CI] = 0.56 [0.40, 0.79]) (Table 1, Additional file 1: Figure S4F).

RE meta-analysis of the RR of transmission chains associated with each MTBC lineage compared with MTBC lineage 4. Transmission chains in this analysis are defined as identification of two or more MTBC isolates with identical genetic patterns in the same study location and time period. "Cluster" indicates part of a transmission chain, and "unique" indicates not part of a transmission chain. Lineage 7 strains are grouped with "unknown" strains because there was insufficient data on these strains for meta-analysis. We performed the analysis across all studies that we identified in the systematic review, as well as within the regions West Asia, East Asia, Europe and the Americas, and Africa. RE meta-analysis was performed using the RELM method in R software package "metafor" (version 3.3.3) [41]. Forest plots for each analysis are shown in Additional file 1: Figure S4A-F.

These results should be interpreted with some caution as I^2 analysis showed significant heterogeneity across all studies (Table 1), as well as within most subgroups (Additional file 1: Figure S3), with a few exceptions. There was low heterogeneity between studies in the

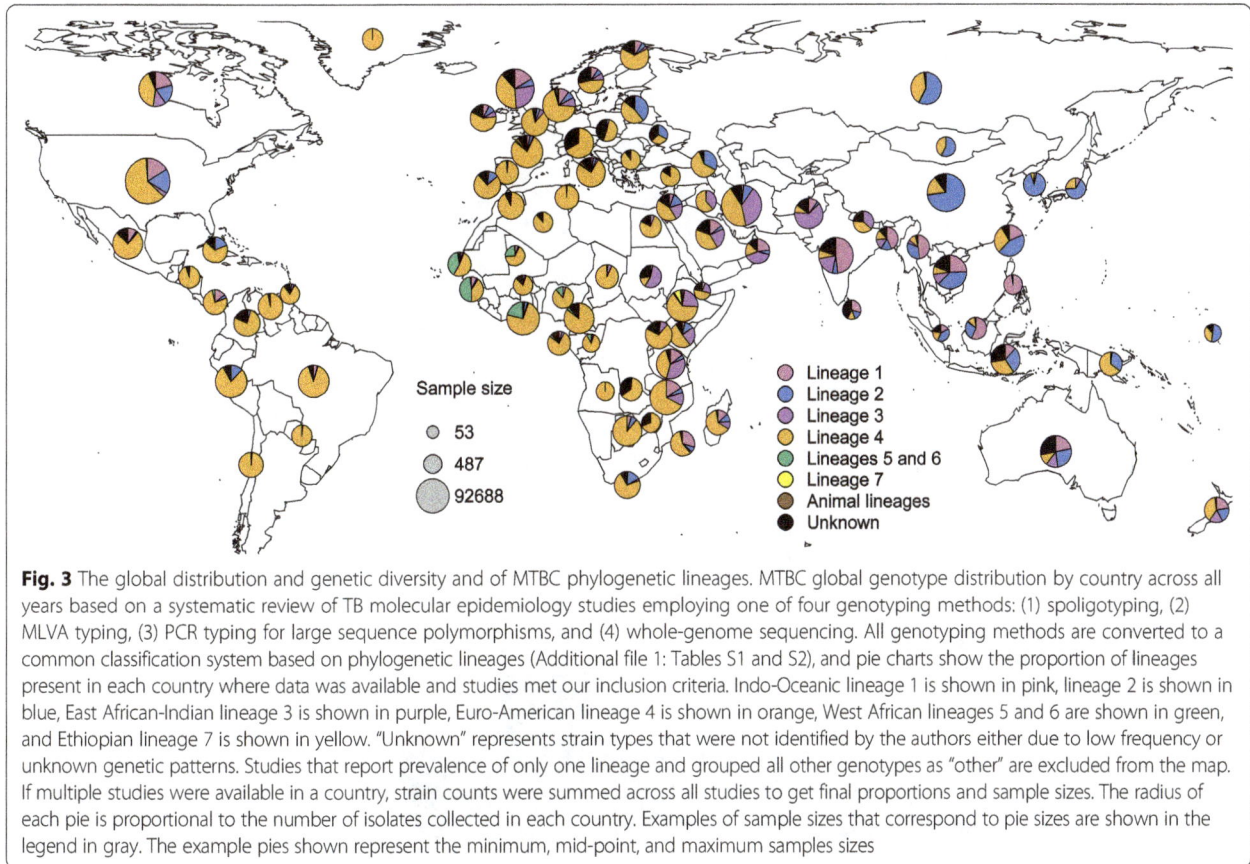

Fig. 3 The global distribution and genetic diversity and of MTBC phylogenetic lineages. MTBC global genotype distribution by country across all years based on a systematic review of TB molecular epidemiology studies employing one of four genotyping methods: (1) spoligotyping, (2) MLVA typing, (3) PCR typing for large sequence polymorphisms, and (4) whole-genome sequencing. All genotyping methods are converted to a common classification system based on phylogenetic lineages (Additional file 1: Tables S1 and S2), and pie charts show the proportion of lineages present in each country where data was available and studies met our inclusion criteria. Indo-Oceanic lineage 1 is shown in pink, lineage 2 is shown in blue, East African-Indian lineage 3 is shown in purple, Euro-American lineage 4 is shown in orange, West African lineages 5 and 6 are shown in green, and Ethiopian lineage 7 is shown in yellow. "Unknown" represents strain types that were not identified by the authors either due to low frequency or unknown genetic patterns. Studies that report prevalence of only one lineage and grouped all other genotypes as "other" are excluded from the map. If multiple studies were available in a country, strain counts were summed across all studies to get final proportions and sample sizes. The radius of each pie is proportional to the number of isolates collected in each country. Examples of sample sizes that correspond to pie sizes are shown in the legend in gray. The example pies shown represent the minimum, mid-point, and maximum samples sizes

animal strains analysis (Table 1, I^2 = 18%), as well as in the analysis of lineages 5 and 6 strains within Europe and the Americas (Additional file 1: Figure S3D, I^2 = 0.0%).

Treatment failure

Several studies identified in the systematic review showed that lineage 2 Beijing family strains were associated with treatment failure. Beijing strains were associated with treatment failure in Indonesia compared with all other genotypes after adjusting for drug resistance, non-adherence, age, diabetes mellitus, and severity of radiological lesions (relative risk [95% CI] = 1.94 [1.26, 3.0]) (Table 2) [43]. Beijing strains were also associated with treatment failure after adjusting for multi-drug resistance in India (odds ratio [95% CI] = 3.29 [1.29, 8.14]) (Table 2) [44]. However, Beijing strains were not associated with treatment failure after adjusting for multi-drug resistance in Vietnam (odds ratio [95% CI] = 0.7 [0.3, 2.0]) (Table 2) [45] and were not associated with treatment failure of drug-susceptible TB in South Africa (Table 2) [46]. Confounders that were not adjusted for in all these studies, such as HIV co-infection, diabetes mellitus, body mass index (BMI), cavitary TB, and quality of health care, may contribute to the variation in results (Table 2).

Summary of study design and findings for each study reported genotype associations with treatment failure. RR indicates relative risk, OR indicates odds ratio, and 95% CI indicates 95% confidence interval. The latter measures were taken directly from the studies and were not reanalyzed.

Discussion

To our knowledge, this study represents the most comprehensive dataset on MTBC lineages that has been created by systematically assembled genotyping data from studies that used representative sampling techniques. The data show geographic variation in MTBC genotypes, which is consistent with previously published studies that used convenience samples and much smaller datasets. We find some evidence for clinical variation between genotypes, though, we also show significant variation between studies, which highlights the need for additional data.

Global variation in bacterial strains that cause TB disease

The results presented in this study are consistent with previously published maps that showed that MTBC strains that evolved more recently in human history— lineage 2, lineage 3, and lineage 4 strains—tend to be more widely distributed around the world [22, 35, 47,

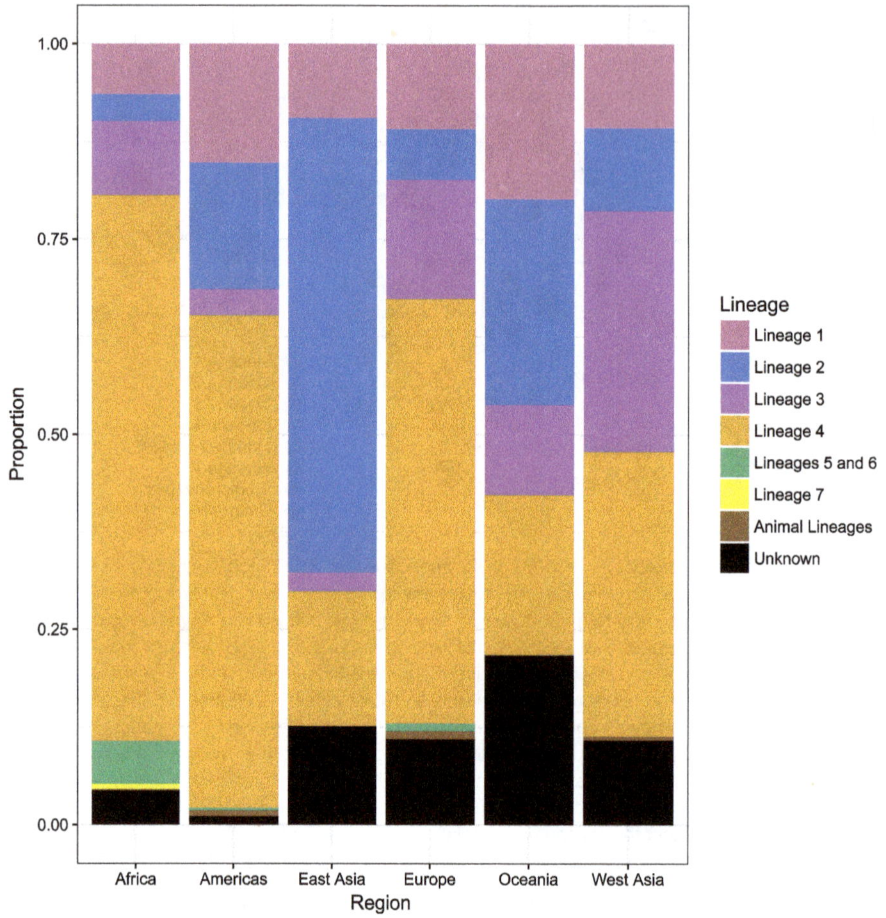

Fig. 4 Distribution of MTBC phylogenetic lineages by region. MTBC global genotype distribution by region corresponding to the data presented in Fig. 3. Lineage proportions broken down by countries within each region are shown in Additional file 1: Table S3 and Figure S2

48]. We also showed that lineage 1, lineage 2, and lineage 3 are more prevalent in Europe and in North and South America than shown in previously published maps [35, 47, 48]. Moreover, we show that lineage 3 strains may be increasing in prevalence in Europe, while lineage 1 strains may be decreasing in prevalence in West Asia. These patterns in genotype distribution likely reflect both historical and recent movement of strains with people from East Asia and the Indian subcontinent to Europe and the American continent. The dominance of lineage 4 globally, and in particular in South American countries, also supports the hypothesis that European colonialists aided in the dispersion of this lineage in the mid-sixteenth to nineteenth centuries [32, 48, 49]. If the first inhabitants of the American continent brought early forms of lineage 2 strains with them when they migrated from north-eastern Asia, these strains may have been eliminated with the arrival of strains from European colonialists.

Human migration is likely not the only determinant of MTBC genotype distribution. Lineages 5 and 6 are prevalent only in West Africa [35, 47, 48]. The reasons for this geographic restriction are largely unknown but may have to do with clinical characteristics of the patients infected with these strains. Patients infected with lineage 6 are more likely than patients infected with other strains to be older, HIV-infected, and severely malnourished [50]. In addition, we showed that lineages 5 and 6 strains may be less likely to cause transmission chains than lineage 4 strains and that these findings were more consistent in Europe and the Americas than in Africa, which may reflect biological differences and/or social mixing which prevents these strains from spreading through non-West African populations. We also found that lineage 3 strains were associated with reduced risk of transmission chains in Europe and the Americas, which is consistent with the findings from a household contact study in Montreal [51]. In contrast, we found that Beijing family strains may be more likely to cause transmission chains, which could reflect the ability of Beijing strains to spread quickly through human populations [46, 52, 53]. These findings are not consistent with previous work that showed no differences

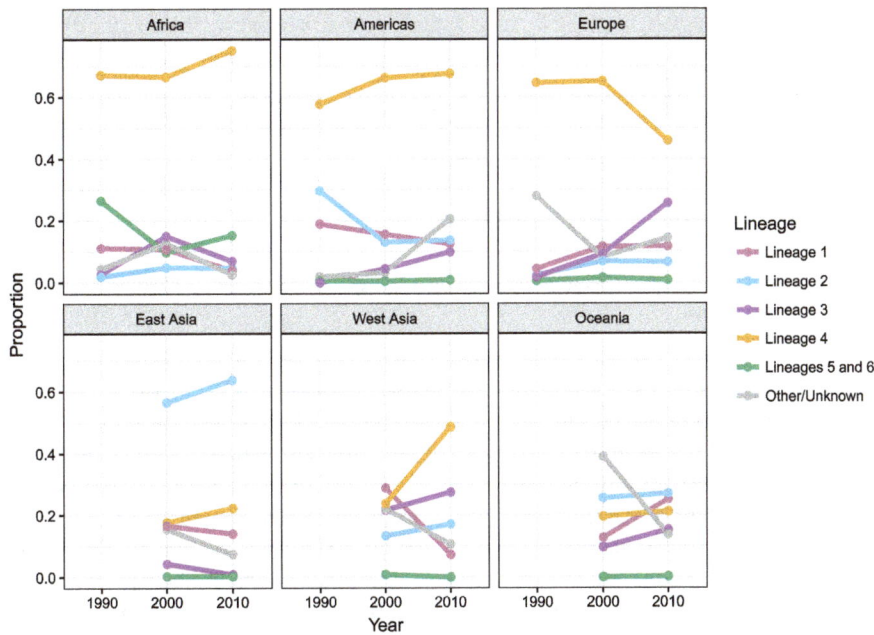

Fig. 5 Distribution of MTBC lineages over time by region. MTBC genotype distribution by region over time corresponding to results presented in Additional file 1: Figure S3. The year 1990 represents all studies from 1990 to 1999, the year 2000 represents all studies from 2000 to 2009, and the year 2010 represents all studies from 2010 to 2017. Indo-Oceanic lineage 1 is shown in pink, East Asian lineage 2 is shown in blue, East African-Indian lineage 3 is shown in purple, Euro-American lineage 4 is shown in orange, and West African lineages 5 and 6 are shown in green. Other/unknown strains are shown in gray and represent animal lineages, lineage 7, and strain types that were not identified by authors either due to low frequency or unknown genetic patterns. Strain counts and sample sizes were summed across all studies within the given regions and time periods to get proportions. There was no data from East Asia, West Asia, and Oceania in the 1990s, and therefore, these years are left blank

between lineages in transmission from household contacts [46, 54, 55]. Thus, further studies would be required to confirm our findings.

Several studies included in our analysis showed that treatment failure was associated with lineage 2 Beijing family strains [43, 44]. Beijing family strains are also associated with drug resistance [56], which has been reviewed previously [12, 22, 23]. Additionally, lineage 1 strains have been associated with more rapid response to treatment in drug-susceptible TB cases in the USA [57]. Thus, there is evidence for a relationship between bacterial genotype and treatment outcome, at least in certain populations or contexts. Future studies that carefully control for potential confounders that may impact

treatment failure are required to confirm these findings. This type of information could be particularly important to clinicians if it could inform the development of novel diagnostic tools that test for bacterial genotypes associated with poor response to treatment and development of drug resistance.

Variation between studies and implications for variation in MTBC genotypes

There was variation in the sampling methods and representativeness of the studies included in this systematic review. The majority of studies were representative of much smaller geographic locations than the national level, and despite the large number of bacterial isolates

Table 1 Summary of random effects (RE) meta-analyses of relative risk (RR) of transmission chains associated with MTBC lineages

Lineage number	Lineage name	RR	p value (RR)	CI, lower	CI, upper	Q	p value (Q)	I^2 (%)	Number of studies
4	Euro-American	1.00							
1	Indo-Oceanic	1.07	0.61	0.83	1.37	228.3	0.00	95.4	17
2	East Asian	1.24	0.01	1.07	1.45	220.6	0.00	97.8	20
3	East African-Indian	0.98	0.84	0.81	1.18	130.6	0.00	84.9	17
5, 6	West African	0.61	0.01	0.43	0.86	39.4	0.00	95.0	8
–	Animal	0.79	0.02	0.64	0.96	7.43	0.28	18.0	7
–	Unknown	0.56	0.00	0.40	0.79	70.5	0.00	92.0	12

Table 2 Summary of treatment failure studies

Source	Location	Years	No. of patients	Confounders adjusted for	Findings	RR/OR [95% CI]
Parwati et al. [43]	Indonesia	2000–2005	818	Drug resistance, non-adherence, age, diabetes mellitus, and severity of radiological lesions	Lineage 2 Beijing family were associated with treatment failure.	RR 1.94 [1.26, 3.0]
Chatterjee et al. [44]	India	2004–2007	646	Multi-drug resistance	Lineage 2 Beijing family were associated with treatment failure.	OR 3.29 [1.29, 8.14]
Buu et al. [45]	Vietnam	2003–2007	1106	Multi-drug resistance	Lineage 2 Beijing family were not associated with treatment failure.	OR 0.7 [0.3, 2.0]
van der Spuy et al. [46]	South Africa	1993–2004	1737	None (analysis included only drug-susceptible strains)	Lineage 2 Beijing family were not associated with treatment failure.	Not reported ($p > 0.05$)

included in this study, they represented only a small fraction of the total estimated TB cases. While the goal of this study was to summarize the MTBC genotyping data available, not to make nationally representative estimates, it is important to note that this variation was not distributed evenly throughout the world. There was less information available about MTBC genotype distribution in South America and Sub-Saharan Africa than in other regions, and the data in Central and Eastern Asia represented a smaller proportion of all estimated TB cases than elsewhere. Thus, the genetic diversity shown in the map in Fig. 3 for these regions is likely less representative of the underlying populations.

Another source of variation that may impact representativeness is whether studies were biased towards including either rural or urban populations. There is likely greater MTBC genetic diversity in patients from urban populations than patients from rural areas since urban areas experience higher rates of travel and migration. Most studies included in this analysis did not report the urban/rural composition of their sample, and the bias towards one or the other would likely vary depending on study location. For example, the majority of the studies included in our systematic review used samples collected from public hospitals or reference laboratories. Therefore, in countries such as India, where people in urban areas may be more likely to seek care from private health clinics [58], the urban population may be underrepresented and we may have underestimated genetic diversity. On the other hand, in countries such as Uganda, where the rural population has limited access to public health facilities [59], the rural population may be underrepresented and we may have overestimated genetic diversity. This highlights the importance of data from prevalence surveys that use active surveillance techniques to reach a broader subset of the population.

We also identified a significant amount of heterogeneity between studies in the meta-analysis of genetic clustering associated with genotypes. One source of this heterogeneity is likely methodological differences between the studies, such as genotyping method, sampling

method, and study duration, which have been shown to impact genetic clustering [27, 28]. For example, duration of sampling ranged from 2 months to 9 years, and genotyping methods ranged from the use of either spoligotyping or MLVA typing to the use of both methods (Additional file 1: Table S4). Studies that used shorter sampling durations may have missed transmission chains and underestimated clustering, while studies that used spoligotyping only may have overestimated clustering [60]. An additional source of heterogeneity may be confounders that impact genetic clustering and transmission, such as social mixing, immigration, age structure, comorbidities, and underlying TB incidence [27, 28]. These confounders likely also varied between these studies but were often not reported. For example, only 14 of the studies reported HIV prevalence (range 0 to 91%), only 6 reported proportion of immigrants (range 0 to 78%), and only 14 reported mean age of patients (range 25 to 50) included in the sample (Additional file 1: Table S4). If social mixing was high in each of the studies, this could have led us to overestimate the impact of genotype on transmission chains, while if migration was high, this could have led us to underestimate the presence of transmission chains.

Study limitations

A limitation of this study is that we grouped strains into seven lineages, which masks within-lineage variation. Distinct sub-lineages of the Beijing family are associated with differences in transmissibility in human populations [61, 62], and lineage 4 contains both geographically widespread and restricted sub-lineages [49]. However, we propose that this was the best method as it allowed us to (1) include a broad range of studies, including those that did not report sub-lineages, and (2) synthesize studies that used WGS- or PCR-based typing together with studies that used methods more common in resource-limited settings, such as spoligotyping and MLVA typing.

Another limitation is that we did not include data from WGS databases. A challenge of incorporating WGS data is identifying study meta-data, such as sampling methods and demographic characteristics of patients, linked with genomes. In addition, many of the WGS data available are poised for phylogeographic studies and for examining the presence of specific mutations [32, 49, 56], but are less representative of the populations they are isolated from. These data are often from outbreaks or studies of specific subpopulations, which we excluded in this analysis. As WGS data linked with meta-data become more available (through prevalence surveys [63] and endeavors such as ReSeqTB) including this data would be an important extension of our study. Our study supports these future studies by illustrating the importance of using genome sequences to determine phylogenetic lineages or sub-lineages. The dataset we have created could be used to fill geographic gaps in future WGS-based maps, particularly in regions where WGS technology is unavailable, and to verify results from convenience-based samples.

Conclusions

The evidence gathered in this systematic review support a role for bacterial genetic diversity in understanding global variation in TB disease. However, there are aspects of the studies that restrict our ability to confidently attribute clinical characteristics to genotypes. In order to address these conditions in the future, there will need to be a shift in the design of MTBC strain diversity studies such that data is collected in a way that is clinically and epidemiologically informative, wherever possible. We encourage future studies to carefully consider potential confounding variables in study design and analysis and to make all genotypes and study meta-data publicly available upon publication. We also encourage the analysis of less-studied strains from lineages 1 and 3 in order to increase comparability with the relative abundance of data on lineage 2 and lineage 4 strains. The evidence presented in this study demonstrate these types of data could potentially be used to create tools to inform the clinical diagnosis and treatment of TB and improve our understanding of the epidemiology of this disease.

Additional files

Additional file 1: Supplementary appendix. Document containing complete description of literature search strings and dates searched, as well as Tables S1-S4 and Figure S1-S4. (PDF 1440 kb)

Additional file 2: Literature screening sheet. Literature screening sheet including citation information for all literature included in the study. (XLSX 3109 kb)

Additional file 3: Raw genotype distribution data. Raw genotype distribution data extracted in the systematic review. (CSV 1975 kb)

Additional file 4: Raw genetic clustering data. Raw genetic clustering data extracted in the systematic review. (CSV 15 kb)

Additional file 5: Genotype classification system. Sheets containing MTBC genotype conversions for all genotyping methods included in this study. (XLSX 146 kb)

Abbreviations
CI: Confidence interval; LSP: Large sequence polymorphism; MIRU: Mycobacterial interspersed repetitive units; MLVA: Multi-locus variable number of tandem repeats analysis; MTBC: *Mycobacterium tuberculosis* complex; OR: Odds ratio; PCR: Polymerase chain reaction; PRISMA: Preferred Reporting Items for Systematic Reviews and Meta-Analyses; RE: Random effects; RFLP: Restriction fragment length polymorphism; RR: Relative risk; TB: Tuberculosis; VNTR: Variable number of tandem repeats; WGS: Whole-genome sequencing

Acknowledgements
We thank Diana Louden (University of Washington, Seattle, WA) for the assistance with the methods employed in the systematic review. We also thank Ian Pollock (Institute for Health Metrics and Evaluation, Seattle, WA) and Emilie Maddison (Institute for Health Metrics and Evaluation, Seattle, WA) for the assistance in organizing and indexing the literature collected in this study. We thank Brent Bell (Institute for Health Metrics and Evaluation, Seattle, WA) for the assistance with preparing the data for publication, and we thank Nicole Weaver (Institute for Health Metrics and Evaluation, Seattle, WA) and Laurie Marczak (Institute for Health Metrics and Evaluation, Seattle, WA) for the editorial assistance.

Funding
This work was primarily supported by grant OPP1132415 by the Bill & Melinda Gates Foundation. AG received support from the Sistema Nacional de Investigadores de Panamá (SNI), Network for Research and Training in Tropical Diseases, Central America (NeTropica) and Secretaría Nacional de Ciencia, Tecnología e Innovación (SENACYT). RZC received support from the CONACyT-Programa de desarrollo científico para atender problemas nacionales No. 213712. The funders had no role in the study design, collection, analysis, or interpretation of data, writing of the report, or the decision to submit the paper for publication.

Authors' contributions
KEW and SIH conceived and designed the study. KEW, LPW, and JRL extracted and cleaned the data and produced the tables and figures. RZC, AG, IU, BM, and JFDS provided data and guidance on methods development. KEW wrote the first draft. All authors provided intellectual inputs into the revisions of this study. All authors read and approved the final manuscript.

Competing interests
The authors declare that they have no competing interests.

Author details
[1]Institute for Health Metrics and Evaluation, University of Washington, 2301 5th Ave, Suite 600, Seattle, WA 98121, USA. [2]Departments of Global Health and Medicine, University of Washington, Seattle, WA, USA. [3]Public Health Institute, University of Veracruz, Veracruz, Mexico. [4]Tuberculosis Biomarker Research Unit, Instituto de Investigaciones Científicas y Servicios de Alta Tecnología (INDICASAT-AIP), City of Knowledge, Panama, Panama. [5]Gomal

Centre of Biochemistry and Biotechnology, Gomal University, Dera Ismail Khan, Khyber Pakhtunkhwa, Pakistan. [6]Programmatic Management of Drug-Resistant TB Unit, BSL-II TB Culture Laboratory, Mufti Mehmood Memorial Teaching Hospital, Dera Ismail Khan, Khyber Pakhtunkhwa, Pakistan. [7]Department of Epidemiology, Mailman School of Public Health, Columbia University, New York, NY, USA. [8]Unité de Recherche et de Diagnostics Spécialisés, Laboratoire National de Santé Publique, Libreville, Gabon. [9]Centre Hospitalier Universitaire Mère-Enfant Fondation Jeanne EBORI, Libreville, Gabon.

References

1. Kyu HH, Maddison ER, Henry NJ, Mumford JE, Barber R, Shields C, et al. The global burden of tuberculosis: results from the Global Burden of Disease (GBD) Study 2015. Lancet Infect Dis. 2018;18:261–84.

2. Getahun H, Matteelli A, Chaisson RE, Raviglione M. Latent *Mycobacterium tuberculosis* infection. https://doi.org/10.1056/NEJMra1405427. 2015. doi: https://doi.org/10.1056/NEJMra1405427.

3. Dye C. The population biology of tuberculosis. Princeton: Princeton University Press; 2015.

4. Comas I, Gagneux S. A role for systems epidemiology in tuberculosis research. Trends Microbiol. 2011;19:492–500.

5. Abel L, Fellay J, Haas DW, Schurr E, Srikrishna G, Urbanowski M, et al. Genetics of human susceptibility to active and latent tuberculosis: present knowledge and future perspectives. Lancet Infect Dis. 2017. https://doi.org/10.1016/S1473-3099(17)30623-0.

6. Orgeur M, Brosch R. Evolution of virulence in the *Mycobacterium tuberculosis* complex. Curr Opin Microbiol. 2018;41:68–75.

7. Nebenzahl-Guimaraes H, van Laarhoven A, Farhat MR, Koeken VACM, Mandemakers JJ, Zomer A, et al. Transmissible *Mycobacterium tuberculosis* strains share genetic markers and immune phenotypes. Am J Respir Crit Care Med. 2016;195:1519–27.

8. Fenner L, Egger M, Bodmer T, Furrer H, Ballif M, Battegay M, et al. HIV infection disrupts the sympatric host-pathogen relationship in human tuberculosis. PLoS Genet. 2013;9:e1003318.

9. Pasipanodya JG, Moonan PK, Vecino E, Miller TL, Fernandez M, Slocum P, et al. Allopatric tuberculosis host–pathogen relationships are associated with greater pulmonary impairment. Infect Genet Evol. 2013;16:433–40.

10. Toyo-oka L, Mahasirimongkol S, Yanai H, Mushiroda T, Wattanapokayakit S, Wichukchinda N, et al. Strain-based HLA association analysis identified HLA-DRB1*09:01 associated with modern strain tuberculosis. HLA. 2017; 90:149–56.

11. Salie M, van der Merwe L, Möller M, Daya M, Spuy VD, van der Spuy GD, et al. Associations between human leukocyte antigen class I variants and the *Mycobacterium tuberculosis* subtypes causing disease. J Infect Dis. 2014; 209:216–23.

12. Hanekom M, Gey van Pittius NC, McEvoy C, Victor TC, Van Helden PD, Warren RM. *Mycobacterium tuberculosis* Beijing genotype: a template for success. Tuberculosis. 2011;91:510–23.

13. Chae H, Shin SJ. Importance of differential identification of *Mycobacterium tuberculosis* strains for understanding differences in their prevalence, treatment efficacy, and vaccine development. J Microbiol Seoul Korea. 2018;56:300–11.

14. Gardy JL, Johnston JC, Sui SJH, Cook VJ, Shah L, Brodkin E, et al. Whole-genome sequencing and social-network analysis of a tuberculosis outbreak. N Engl J Med. 2011;364:730–9.

15. Köser CU, Ellington MJ, Cartwright EJP, Gillespie SH, Brown NM, Farrington M, et al. Routine use of microbial whole genome sequencing in diagnostic and public health microbiology. PLoS Pathog. 2012;8:e1002824.

16. Portevin D, Gagneux S, Comas I, Young D. Human macrophage responses to clinical isolates from the *Mycobacterium tuberculosis* complex discriminate between ancient and modern lineages. PLoS Pathog. 2011;7:e1001307.

17. Wiens KE, Ernst JD. The mechanism for type I interferon induction by *Mycobacterium tuberculosis* is bacterial strain-dependent. PLoS Pathog. 2016; 12. https://doi.org/10.1371/journal.ppat.1005809.

18. Shang S, Harton M, Tamayo MH, Shanley C, Palanisamy GS, Caraway M, et al. Increased Foxp3 expression in guinea pigs infected with W-Beijing strains of *M. tuberculosis*. Tuberc Edinb Scotl. 2011;91:378–85.

19. Manca C, Tsenova L, Freeman S, Barczak AK, Tovey M, Murray PJ, et al. Hypervirulent *M. tuberculosis* W/Beijing strains upregulate type I IFNs and increase expression of negative regulators of the Jak-Stat pathway. J Interf Cytokine Res. 2005;25:694–701.

20. Reiling N, Homolka S, Walter K, Brandenburg J, Niwinski L, Ernst M, et al. Clade-specific virulence patterns of *Mycobacterium tuberculosis* complex strains in human primary macrophages and aerogenically infected mice. MBio. 2013;4. https://doi.org/10.1128/mBio.00250-13.

21. Nahid P, Jarlsberg LG, Kato-Maeda M, Segal MR, Osmond DH, Gagneux S, et al. Interplay of strain and race/ethnicity in the innate immune response to *M. tuberculosis*. PLoS One. 2018;13:e0195392.

22. Glynn JR, Whiteley J, Bifani PJ, Kremer K, van Soolingen D. Worldwide occurrence of Beijing/W strains of *Mycobacterium tuberculosis*: a systematic review. Emerg Infect Dis. 2002;8:843–9.

23. Ramazanzadeh R, Sayhemiri K. Prevalence of Beijing family in *Mycobacterium tuberculosis* in world population: systematic review and meta-analysis. Int J Mycobacteriology. 2014;3:41–5.

24. Liberati A, Altman DG, Tetzlaff J, Mulrow C, Gøtzsche PC, Ioannidis JPA, et al. The PRISMA statement for reporting systematic reviews and meta-analyses of studies that evaluate health care interventions: explanation and elaboration. PLoS Med. 2009;6:e1000100.

25. Preferred reporting items for systematic reviews and meta-analyses: the PRISMA statement. http://journals.plos.org/plosmedicine/article?id=10.1371/journal.pmed.1000097. Accessed 30 Apr 2018.

26. Dheda K, Gumbo T, Maartens G, Dooley KE, McNerney R, Murray M, et al. The epidemiology, pathogenesis, transmission, diagnosis, and management of multidrug-resistant, extensively drug-resistant, and incurable tuberculosis. Lancet Respir Med. 2017;5:291–360.

27. Murray M, Alland D. Methodological problems in the molecular epidemiology of tuberculosis. Am J Epidemiol. 2002;155:565–71.

28. Kasaie P, Mathema B, Kelton WD, Azman AS, Pennington J, Dowdy DW. A novel tool improves existing estimates of recent tuberculosis transmission in settings of sparse data collection. PLoS One. 2015;10:e0144137.

29. Small PM, Hopewell PC, Singh SP, Paz A, Parsonnet J, Ruston DC, et al. The epidemiology of tuberculosis in San Francisco – a population-based study using conventional and molecular methods. N Engl J Med. 1994;330:1703–9.

30. van der SGD, Warren RM, Richardson M, Beyers N, Behr MA, van HPD. Use of genetic distance as a measure of ongoing transmission of *Mycobacterium tuberculosis*. J Clin Microbiol. 2003;41:5640–4.

31. Streicher EM, Sampson SL, Dheda K, Dolby T, Simpson JA, Victor TC, et al. Molecular epidemiological interpretation of the epidemic of extensively drug-resistant tuberculosis in South Africa. J Clin Microbiol. 2015;53:3650–3.

32. Comas I, Coscolla M, Luo T, Borrell S, Holt KE, Kato-Maeda M, et al. Out-of-Africa migration and Neolithic coexpansion of *Mycobacterium tuberculosis* with modern humans. Nat Genet. 2013;45:1176–82.

33. Shabbeer A, Cowan LS, Ozcaglar C, Rastogi N, Vandenberg SL, Yener B, et al. TB-Lineage: an online tool for classification and analysis of strains of *Mycobacterium tuberculosis* complex. Infect Genet Evol. 2012;12:789–97.

34. Aminian M, Shabbeer A, Bennett KP. A conformal Bayesian network for classification of *Mycobacterium tuberculosis* complex lineages. BMC Bioinformatics. 2010;11:S4.

35. Demay C, Liens B, Burguière T, Hill V, Couvin D, Millet J, et al. SITVITWEB – a publicly available international multimarker database for studying *Mycobacterium tuberculosis* genetic diversity and molecular epidemiology. Infect Genet Evol. 2012;12:755–66.

36. Allix-Béguec C, Harmsen D, Weniger T, Supply P, Niemann S. Evaluation and strategy for use of MIRU-VNTRplus, a multifunctional database for online analysis of genotyping data and phylogenetic identification of *Mycobacterium tuberculosis* complex isolates. J Clin Microbiol. 2008; 46:2692–9.

37. Weniger T, Krawczyk J, Supply P, Niemann S, Harmsen D. MIRU-VNTRplus: a web tool for polyphasic genotyping of *Mycobacterium tuberculosis* complex bacteria. Nucleic Acids Res. 2010;38(suppl_2):W326–31.

38. Yimer SA, Norheim G, Namouchi A, Zegeye ED, Kinander W, Tønjum T, et al. *Mycobacterium tuberculosis* lineage 7 strains are associated with prolonged patient delay in seeking treatment for pulmonary tuberculosis in Amhara region, Ethiopia. J Clin Microbiol. 2015;53:1301–9.

39. Tessema B, Beer J, Merker M, Emmrich F, Sack U, Rodloff AC, et al. Molecular epidemiology and transmission dynamics of *Mycobacterium tuberculosis* in Northwest Ethiopia: new phylogenetic lineages found in Northwest Ethiopia. BMC Infect Dis. 2013;13:131.

40. Institute for Health Metrics and Evaluation (IHME). GBD compare data visualization. Seattle: IHME, University of Washington; 2016. Available from http:// vizhub.healthdata.org/gbd-compare. Accessed 29 July 2018

41. Conducting meta-analyses in R with the metafor package | Viechtbauer |, editor. J Stat Softw. https://doi.org/10.18637/jss.v036.i03.

42. Quantifying heterogeneity in a meta-analysis - Higgins - 2002 - Statistics in Medicine - Wiley Online Library. https://onlinelibrary.wiley.com/doi/abs/10.1002/sim.1186. Accessed 23 Aug 2018

43. Parwati I, Alisjahbana B, Apriani L, Soetikno RD, Ottenhoff TH, van der Zanden AGM, et al. Mycobacterium tuberculosis Beijing genotype is an independent risk factor for tuberculosis treatment failure in Indonesia. J Infect Dis. 2010;201:553-7.

44. Chatterjee A, D'Souza D, Vira T, Bamne A, Ambe GT, Nicol MP, et al. Strains of Mycobacterium tuberculosis from Western Maharashtra, India, exhibit a high degree of diversity and strain-specific associations with drug resistance, cavitary disease, and treatment failure. J Clin Microbiol. 2010;48:3593-9.

45. Buu TN, Huyen MNT, van Soolingen D, Lan NTN, Quy HT, Tiemersma EW, et al. The Mycobacterium tuberculosis Beijing genotype does not affect tuberculosis treatment failure in Vietnam. Clin Infect Dis Off Publ Infect Dis Soc Am. 2010;51:879-86.

46. van der Spuy GD, Kremer K, Ndabambi SL, Beyers N, Dunbar R, Marais BJ, et al. Changing Mycobacterium tuberculosis population highlights clade-specific pathogenic characteristics. Tuberc Edinb Scotl. 2009;89:120-5.

47. Mathema B, Kurepina NE, Bifani PJ, Kreiswirth BN. Molecular epidemiology of tuberculosis: current insights. Clin Microbiol Rev. 2006;19:658-85.

48. Hershberg R, Lipatov M, Small PM, Sheffer H, Niemann S, Homolka S, et al. High functional diversity in Mycobacterium tuberculosis driven by genetic drift and human demography. PLoS Biol. 2008;6:e311.

49. Stucki D, Brites D, Jeljeli L, Coscolla M, Liu Q, Trauner A, et al. Mycobacterium tuberculosis lineage 4 comprises globally distributed and geographically restricted sublineages. Nat Genet. 2016;48:1535-43.

50. de Jong BC, Antonio M, Gagneux S. Mycobacterium africanum--review of an important cause of human tuberculosis in West Africa. PLoS Negl Trop Dis. 2010;4:e744.

51. Albanna AS, Reed MB, Kotar KV, Fallow A, McIntosh FA, Behr MA, et al. Reduced transmissibility of East African Indian strains of Mycobacterium tuberculosis. PLoS One. 2011;6:e25075.

52. Hu Y, Mathema B, Zhao Q, Zheng X, Li D, Jiang W, et al. Comparison of the socio-demographic and clinical features of pulmonary TB patients infected with sub-lineages within the W-Beijing and non-Beijing Mycobacterium tuberculosis. Tuberculosis. 2016;97(Supplement C):18-25.

53. Holt KE, McAdam P, Thai PVK, Thuong NTT, Ha DTM, Lan NN, et al. Frequent transmission of the Mycobacterium tuberculosis Beijing lineage and positive selection for the EsxW Beijing variant in Vietnam. Nat Genet. 2018;50:849-56.

54. de Jong BC, Hill PC, Aiken A, Awine T, Antonio M, Adetifa IM, et al. Progression to active tuberculosis, but not transmission, varies by M. tuberculosis lineage in the Gambia. J Infect Dis. 2008;198:1037-43.

55. Lalor MK, Anderson LF, Hamblion EL, Burkitt A, Davidson JA, Maguire H, et al. Recent household transmission of tuberculosis in England, 2010-2012: retrospective national cohort study combining epidemiological and molecular strain typing data. BMC Med. 2017;15:105.

56. Merker M, Blin C, Mona S, Duforet-Frebourg N, Lecher S, Willery E, et al. Evolutionary history and global spread of the Mycobacterium tuberculosis Beijing lineage. Nat Genet. 2015;47:242-9.

57. Click ES, Winston CA, Oeltmann JE, Moonan PK, Mac Kenzie WR. Association between Mycobacterium tuberculosis lineage and time to sputum culture conversion. Int J Tuberc Lung Dis. 2013;17:878-84.

58. Sengupta A, Nundy S. The private health sector in India. BMJ. 2005;331:1157-8.

59. Konde-Lule J, Gitta SN, Lindfors A, Okuonzi S, Onama VO, Forsberg BC. Private and public health care in rural areas of Uganda. BMC Int Health Hum Rights. 2010;10:29.

60. Comas I, Homolka S, Niemann S, Gagneux S. Genotyping of genetically monomorphic bacteria: DNA sequencing in Mycobacterium tuberculosis highlights the limitations of current methodologies. PLoS One. 2009;4:e7815.

61. Kato-Maeda M, Kim EY, Flores L, Jarlsberg LG, Osmond D, Hopewell PC. Differences among sublineages of the East-Asian lineage of Mycobacterium tuberculosis in genotypic clustering. Int J Tuberc Lung Dis Off J Int Union Tuberc Lung Dis. 2010;14:538-44.

62. DA L, Hanekom M, Mata D, van PNCG, van HPD, Warren RM, et al. Mycobacterium tuberculosis strains with the Beijing genotype demonstrate variability in virulence associated with transmission. Tuberculosis. 2010;90:319-25.

63. Zignol M, Cabibbe AM, Dean AS, Glaziou P, Alikhanova N, Ama C, et al. Genetic sequencing for surveillance of drug resistance in tuberculosis in highly endemic countries: a multi-country population-based surveillance study. Lancet Infect Dis. 2018;18:675-83.

13

A longitudinal, observational study of the features of transitional healthcare associated with better outcomes for young people with long-term conditions

A. Colver[1,2]* 🆔, H. McConachie[1], A. Le Couteur[1,3], G. Dovey-Pearce[2], K. D. Mann[1], J. E. McDonagh[4,5], M. S. Pearce[1], L. Vale[1], H. Merrick[1], J. R. Parr[3,6,7] and On behalf of the Transition Collaborative Group

Abstract

Background: Most evidence about what works in transitional care comes from small studies in single clinical specialties. We tested the hypothesis that exposures to nine recommended features of transitional healthcare were associated with better outcomes for young people with long-term conditions during transition from child-centred to adult-oriented health services.

Methods: This is a longitudinal, observational cohort study in UK secondary care including 374 young people, aged 14–18.9 years at recruitment, with type 1 diabetes ($n = 150$), cerebral palsy ($n = 106$) or autism spectrum disorder with an associated mental health problem ($n = 118$). All were pre-transfer and without significant learning disability. We approached all young people attending five paediatric diabetes centres, all young people with autism spectrum disorder attending four mental health centres, and randomly selected young people from two population-based cerebral palsy registers. Participants received four home research visits, 1 year apart and 274 participants (73%) completed follow-up. Outcome measures were Warwick Edinburgh Mental Wellbeing Scale, Mind the Gap Scale (satisfaction with services), Rotterdam Transition Profile (Participation) and Autonomy in Appointments.

Results: Exposure to recommended features was 61% for 'coordinated team', 53% for 'age-banded clinic', 48% for 'holistic life-skills training', 42% for 'promotion of health self-efficacy', 40% for 'meeting the adult team before transfer', 34% for 'appropriate parent involvement' and less than 30% for 'written transition plan', 'key worker' and 'transition manager for clinical team'.

Three features were strongly associated with improved outcomes. (1) 'Appropriate parent involvement', example association with Wellbeing ($b = 4.5$, 95% CI 2.0–7.0, $p = 0.001$); (2) 'Promotion of health self-efficacy', example association with Satisfaction with Services ($b = -0.5$, 95% CI -0.9 to -0.2, $p = 0.006$); (3) 'Meeting the adult team before transfer', example associations with Participation (arranging services and aids) (odds ratio 5.2, 95% CI 2.1–12.8, $p < 0.001$) and with Autonomy in Appointments (average 1.7 points higher, 95% CI 0.8–2.6, $p < 0.001$).

There was slightly less recruitment of participants from areas with greater socioeconomic deprivation, though not with respect to family composition.

(Continued on next page)

* Correspondence: allan.colver@ncl.ac.uk
[1]Institute of Health & Society, Sir James Spence Institute, Royal Victoria Infirmary, Newcastle University, Queen Victoria Road, Newcastle upon Tyne NE1 4LP, UK
[2]Northumbria Healthcare NHS Foundation Trust, North Tyneside General Hospital, Rake Lane, North Shields NE29 8NH, UK
Full list of author information is available at the end of the article

(Continued from previous page)

Conclusions: Three features of transitional care were associated with improved outcomes. Results are likely to be generalisable because participants had three very different conditions, attending services at many UK sites. Results are relevant for clinicians as well as for commissioners and managers of health services. The challenge of introducing these three features across child and adult healthcare services, and the effects of doing so, should be assessed.

Keywords: Transition, Adolescence, Health service delivery

Background

Young people with long-term conditions have a physical, mental or health impairment with the potential for a substantial and long-term adverse effect on their everyday lives [1]. Adolescence and young adulthood is a key developmental stage, extending into the mid-twenties, during which a young person experiences many developmental transitions such as leaving school, gaining training, employment or further education, forming romantic relationships and potentially leaving home. Simultaneously, the healthcare of young people with a long-term health condition 'transfers' from child to adult health services, with the expectation that young people take increasing responsibility for managing their health condition. Many young people with long-term health conditions have poor health and social outcomes following transition [2, 3]. The importance of healthcare transition and its challenges are recognised in the 2016 UK National Institute for Health and Clinical Excellence (NICE) Guideline 43 [4] and Quality Standard 140 [5]. 'Transition' is the purposeful, planned process that addresses the medical, psychosocial and educational/vocational needs of adolescents and young adults with long-term conditions as they move from child-centred to adult-oriented healthcare systems [6]. 'Transfer' is the formal event when the healthcare of a young person moves from children's services to adults' services.

The international research literature proposes service features that might promote better healthcare transition, both at national level [7, 8] and specialty level [9]. However, there is a lack of evidence about whether these 'proposed beneficial features' improve outcomes [10]. A systematic review [11] highlighted some evidence, mainly from diabetic services, and concluded that the most encouraging interventions were those oriented to patients (educational programmes and skills training), staffing (transition co-ordinators), and service delivery (young adult clinics or enhanced follow-up). The recent evidence overview, provided by NICE Guideline 43 [4], set out 9 overarching principles and 47 recommendations but recognised it could cite relatively little high-quality evidence to support them or to prioritise them.

Recommendations for particular service features should be supported by robust evidence that indicate improved outcomes across a range of conditions and settings before they are adopted into practice. With this challenge in mind, we designed our research to enable us to examine patient-level outcomes that would be applicable across a range of conditions. We focused on nine proposed beneficial features (PBFs, see Methods). The aim of this longitudinal, observational study was to test the hypothesis that exposure to these PBFs is associated with better outcomes for young people with long-term conditions, namely satisfaction with services, mental wellbeing, participation and autonomy in appointments.

Methods

The study methods and sample characteristics, described in detail elsewhere [12, 13], are summarised below.

Participants

The study recruited 374 young people from across England and Northern Ireland, on the basis of having one of three conditions – 150 young people with type 1 diabetes mellitus (exemplar of chronic health condition with national standards of care, recruited through five NHS Trusts); 118 young people with autism spectrum disorder (ASD) and additional mental health problems (exemplar of neurodevelopmental disorder, recruited through four NHS Trusts); and 106 young people with cerebral palsy (CP) (exemplar of complex physical disability, recruited through two regional population registers and one NHS Trust). Young people were aged 14 to 18.9 years at recruitment, did not have significant learning disability, and had not transferred to adult healthcare. For each young person, a parent or carer was also invited to participate.

Procedure

Recruitment was between June 2012 and October 2013. Local researchers visited the young people and parents, usually at home, took informed consent and administered independently completed questionnaires. Visits were arranged annually for 3 years. The local researchers attended joint training each year, and participated in group telephone discussions at around 3-month intervals to maintain consistency of approach. To maximise young person engagement and retention, outcome measures could be completed by post or electronically. At the baseline visit, the nature of the PBFs was discussed with the young person and a log-book was provided. Before each subsequent annual visit, the researcher consulted the young person's medical records to seek evidence of the PBFs having been provided (for example, inclusion of a member of the adult service at a paediatric appointment). Then, at the visit, the researcher and young person completed a summary sheet recording whether each PBF had been experienced or not in the previous year; the information gathered from medical notes acting as additional prompts for the discussion.

PBFs

Definition of the nine PBFs is provided in Box 1. 'Appropriate parent involvement' represents the perceptions of both the young person and parent being satisfied with level of parent involvement. These were chosen on the basis of being recommended in recent guidance

[4], identified as beneficial in a systematic review [11, 14], and following our own analysis of individual studies (Table two in Colver et al. [12]).

Outcome measures

We chose measures of satisfaction with services, mental wellbeing, participation and autonomy in appointments. They were chosen to be relevant across conditions and settings and correspond to measures subsequently proposed in international Delphi studies [15, 16]. In particular, we included a measure of mental wellbeing which captures what the young person feels about their life, as recommended by an International, Interdisciplinary Health Care Transition Research Consortium [15, 17]. The measure of participation reflects the importance that the International Classification of Functioning, Disability and Health [18] attaches to social as well as health outcomes.

Box 1 Definitions of Proposed Beneficial Features (PBFs)

Age-banded clinic. An intermediate clinic setting such as a young person's clinic or a young adult team. In child health services, it would mean that children less than approximately 12 years would not be at the clinic. In adult services, it would mean adults over 24 years of age would not be at the clinic.

Meet adult team before transfer. This could be in a joint clinic where child and adult healthcare professionals consult together, or an adult clinician might visit the child clinic to be introduced, or the young person might have been taken to the adult clinic by their key worker or child healthcare professional to meet the adult clinician(s).

Promotion of health self-efficacy. The young person is asked 'Have you received enough help to increase your confidence in managing your condition?'

Written transition plan. This should be created some time before transfer. It should include plans for wider aspects of transition, not just the arrangements for transfer to adult health services. The young person should have a copy of it and it should be reviewed at each appointment and updated as necessary.

Appropriate parent involvement in their child's care, but with changing responsibilities. Parent and young person are asked separately if they think the level of involvement is appropriate. Involvement concerns what happens in the clinic (parent being present or not and who does the talking). It is the perceptions of both the young person and parent being satisfied with the level of parent involvement.

Key worker. This is a single person known to the young person whom they can easily contact or go to if there were any problems of co-ordination or misunderstandings that needed to be sorted out. The role could cross into education and social services. Whilst a clinic may have a policy to 'appoint' a key worker, this needs to be negotiated with the young person who may report it to be someone else they feel most comfortable with.

Coordinated team. Some young people need to see a team of people; for example, those with diabetes may need to see doctor, nurse, dietician and psychologist. Those with cerebral palsy may need to see doctor, physiotherapist and orthopaedic surgeon. The members of these teams need to work and communicate well together, and demonstrate to the young person and family that this is happening. Coordination of appointments on the same day is one demonstration of such coordination.

Holistic life-skills training about education, gaining employment, finances, housing, social relationships, sexual health, substance use, mental health, etc. as well as health maintenance. The young person is asked whether they have had any formal life-skill training offered relevant to their long-term condition. The health service may not provide such training but, during consultations, staff should inquire about such matters and make referrals to other agencies as needed.

Transition manager for clinical team. This person may not be known to the young person, but should facilitate good working relationships between adult and child services, ensure appropriate materials are available (such as for health education or the transition plan), and will monitor that the young person has a suitable appointment in adult services and whether the appointment is kept.

Satisfaction with services was assessed using Mind the Gap [19]. This scale measures the difference or 'gap' between a young person's ideal service and the service they have received (thus higher scores indicate lower satisfaction). Service satisfaction is expressed as a total score, with subdomain scores for Management of the environment, Provider characteristics and Process issues.

Mental wellbeing was assessed using the Warwick Edinburgh Mental Wellbeing Scale [20]. This 14-item questionnaire collects responses to each item on a 5-point Likert scale ('none of the time' 1 to 'all of the time' 5). Higher scores (range 14–70) denote higher mental wellbeing.

Participation was measured by the Rotterdam Transition Profile [21]. This captures independence in participation across nine domains. Independence is categorised into three 'phases', phase 1 being the least independent (thus higher scores indicate higher participation). A further participation measure, not in the original protocol, was added on the advice of the Programme's External Advisory Board. This was Autonomy in Appointments, involving three questions about whether the young person makes their own appointments and asks and answers questions themselves (range 3–15) [22]. Higher scores indicate greater autonomy.

Other information
Baseline demographic information, including age, sex, index of multiple deprivation (IMD) [23] calculated from postcode in England, and the multiple deprivation measure [24] in Northern Ireland, and a number of socioeconomic indicators, including family composition, was collected for those who participated in the study.

'Date of transfer' was defined as the date of the last appointment with a paediatrician or adolescent psychiatrist. The young person's status at each visit was recorded as still in a children's service, transferred to dedicated adult service, transferred to General Practitioner in primary care, or lost to follow-up.

In order to maximise useable questionnaire data, the 'final visit' was defined as visit 4, or as visit 3 if visit 4 did not take place or questionnaire data were missing.

Our protocol [12] also proposed condition-specific outcomes and data relevant to economic analysis; these data will be or have been reported elsewhere [25, 26].

Data analysis and statistical methods
Age, Satisfaction with services (total and per domain), Mental wellbeing, and Autonomy in appointments were treated as continuous variables. Condition, site, sex, participation and exposure to PBFs were treated as categorical variables. Missing data were handled according to the suggested rules for each outcome measure. In the regression analyses, those with missing data for PBFs

(year-by-year and consolidated PBF indicator) were grouped together and included in the modelling.

Representativeness between young people who were retained to final visit and those lost to follow-up, by age, sex, condition, site and socioeconomic status, was assessed using t, Mann–Whitney and χ^2 tests as appropriate. The Kruskal–Wallis test was used to examine associations between outcome measures and condition. Comparisons of outcome measures between baseline and final visit were tested using Wilcoxon paired sign-rank and χ^2 tests.

Two approaches to analysis were undertaken to assess the association of PBFs with outcomes across the duration of follow-up. The first approach used the young person's experience of each PBF during the previous year (i.e. whether the PBF was present (yes) or absent (no) during that year) and tested this against each outcome at the end of that year. Hence, analyses were conducted 'year-by-year' and each was a cross-sectional analysis. The time between baseline (visit 1) and visit 2 was called 'Period' 1; similarly for periods 2 and 3.

The second approach used the young person's experience of each PBF throughout the 3 years of the study. This was a longitudinal analysis. It was not appropriate to model the exposure to PBFs by simple frequencies, as young people had varying numbers of contacts with clinicians; in some years, a young person experienced a PBF and the next year might not. Also there was variation in the times at which the PBFs were captured; although intended to be every year, appointments often fell 1 or 2 months either side for practical reasons. We therefore developed a consolidated indicator to estimate the extent to which each PBF was delivered over the duration of the study. The indicator was based on whether the PBF had been experienced or not in each follow-up period. It was defined to be 'optimal' or 'sub-optimal' for each PBF, based on the following criteria developed by consensus within the members of the research team:

- Group one optimal: for 'age-banded clinic', 'meet adult team before transfer', 'written transition plan', 'holistic life-skills training' and 'transition manager for clinical team'; evidence that the PBF was experienced or recorded in the 12 months before at least one of the research visits 2, 3 and 4 over the 3 years.
- Group two optimal: for 'key worker' and 'coordinated team'; the PBF should have been experienced in the 12 months before at least two of the research visits 2, 3 and 4 over the 3 years.
- Group three optimal: for 'promotion of health self-efficacy' and 'appropriate parent involvement'; the PBF should have been experienced in the 12 months before all research visits 2, 3 and 4 over the 3 years.

For both approaches, linear or logistic regression modelling was used, depending on the nature of the outcome variable, to test for association between each PBF individually or each consolidated PBF indicator and outcomes. All models were adjusted for age, sex, condition and potential for clustering by site.

Significant associations ($p < 0.05$) from these models were further adjusted for transfer status, time since transfer to final visit (if applicable) and time to first adult appointment (if applicable).

A significance threshold of $p \leq 0.01$ was used in final models to mitigate multiple testing (but associations at $p \leq 0.05$ are presented as supporting evidence). Data were analysed using STATA version 14.

Patient involvement

Throughout the 5 years of the Transition Research Programme, a young persons' advisory group (UP) met each month. All group members had long-term health conditions. The group provided advice on outcome measures, recruitment and data collection, and interpretation of findings. Details of UP's activities are on the Programme's website: http://research.ncl.ac.uk/transition/.

To support recruitment and retention during the study, all participants and referring clinicians received regular newsletters (approximately every 9 months) about the progress of the study. Feedback of the results at the end of the study to participants took place in two ways, (1) through displaying results of the research on the website, and (2) a summary of the results was included in the final newsletter sent to every participant who wanted to continue to receive information about the study.

Results

A total of 374 young people were recruited to the study (150 for diabetes, 106 for CP, 118 for ASD), mean age 16.2 years (standard deviation (SD) 1.3), along with 369 parents/carers. Demographic data are summarised in Additional file 1: Table S1. As previously reported [13], participants did not differ significantly from non-participants by age or sex. Overall, participants had significantly ($p < 0.001$) lower socioeconomic status scores (i.e. less deprived) than non-participants; however, the difference in overall IMD score on a continuous scale ranging from 0.5 to 87.8, was only 6.1. Further, the proportion of single parent families with dependent children in the UK Annual Families and Households Survey 2013 [27] was 25.1%, very similar to the proportion in our sample at 23.7% (Additional file 1: Table S1).

Attrition

A total of 304 (81.3%) young people remained in the study by visit 2, 259 (69.3%) by visit 3 and 274 (73%) by final visit (235 from visit 4 and 39 from visit 3, see Methods). Of these 274 young people, 58% were male and there were 112 with diabetes, 74 with CP and 88 with ASD. The mean time between baseline visit and final visit was 2.9 years (SD 0.4, range 1.8–3.9).

There were no significant differences between those remaining in the study and those not remaining with respect to sex ($p = 0.6$), age ($p = 0.6$), condition ($p = 0.6$), diabetes sites ($p = 0.4$) or ASD sites ($p = 0.6$). However, in Northern Ireland, those with CP lost to follow-up came from areas with, on average, greater socioeconomic deprivation ($p = 0.03$). Examining socioeconomic factors based on actual circumstances rather than area of residence, there was a significant reduction in the proportion of families with single parents (Additional file 1: Table S1).

Of the 100 participants not remaining in the study, one had died, 28 were lost to follow-up and 71 withdrew. Of those withdrawing, 22 said they were no longer interested, 19 had other commitments, 19 experienced personal issues such as major injuries or severe parental illness, and the remainder gave miscellaneous reasons.

The mean age at final visit was 19.1 years (SD 1.4, range 16.1–22.0). Of the 274 participants at final visit, 49 (18%) remained in child services and 225 (82%) had left child services. Very different proportions by condition transferred to primary care (General Practice) as compared to a dedicated adult service (Table 1).

Changes in outcomes during the study

The average changes in outcomes between baseline and final visits are shown in Additional file 1: Table S2. In summary, satisfaction with services decreased overall but remained stable for those with diabetes; mental wellbeing was steady overall but was always lower for those with ASD and associated mental health problems; participation increased overall but was always higher for those with diabetes; and autonomy in appointments increased overall but was again always higher for those with diabetes.

PBFs experienced over transition

Table 2 sets out the extent to which participants experienced optimal or suboptimal exposure to PBFs across

Table 1 Service attended by young people at final visit

Service	All	D	CP	ASD
	n (%)	n (%)	n (%)	n (%)
Remained in child services	49 (18)	19 (17)	10 (14)	20 (23)
Left child services:	225 (82)	93 (83)	64 (86)	68 (77)
To adult services	149	90	35	24
To primary care (General Practitioner)	76	3	29	44

D diabetes, *CP* cerebral palsy, *ASD* autism spectrum disorder

Table 2 Consolidated indicator of Proposed Beneficial Features at final visit, by condition group

Consolidated indicator of Proposed Beneficial Feature		n	%	n	%	n	%	n	%	p value
		All		D		CP		ASD		
Age-banded clinic	Optimal	145	53	109	97	16	22	20	23	< 0.001
	Sub-optimal	111	40	2	2	54	73	55	62	
	Missing	18	7	1	1	4	5	13	15	
Meet adult team before transfer	Optimal	111	40	73	65	16	22	22	25	< 0.001
	Sub-optimal	133	49	31	28	54	73	48	55	
	Missing	30	11	8	7	4	5	18	20	
Promotion of health self-efficacy	Optimal	116	42	76	68	18	24	22	25	< 0.001
	Sub-optimal	151	55	29	26	56	76	66	75	
	Missing	7	3	7	6	0	0	0	0	
Written transition plan	Optimal	48	17	32	29	11	15	5	6	< 0.001
	Sub-optimal	185	68	62	55	59	80	64	73	
	Missing	41	15	18	16	4	5	19	21	
Appropriate parent involvement										
Both young person and parent happy with parent involvement	Optimal	93	34	36	32	28	38	29	33	0.44
	Sub-optimal	141	51	55	49	33	45	53	60	
	Missing	38	14	21	19	12	16	5	6	
	Non-applicable	2	1	0	0	1	1	1	1	
Key worker	Optimal	79	29	56	50	3	4	20	23	< 0.001
	Sub-optimal	170	62	47	42	68	92	55	62	
	Missing	25	9	9	8	3	4	13	15	
Coordinated team	Optimal	167	61	104	93	25	34	38	43	< 0.001
	Sub-optimal	66	24	2	2	40	54	24	27	
	Missing	25	9	6	5	4	5	15	17	
	Non-applicable	16	6	0	0	5	7	11	13	
Holistic life-skills training	Optimal	132	48	74	66	18	24	40	45	< 0.001
	Sub-optimal	117	43	28	25	52	70	37	42	
	Missing	25	9	10	9	4	6	11	13	
Transition manager for clinical team	Optimal	60	22	27	24	14	19	19	21	0.95
	Sub-optimal	143	52	67	60	34	46	42	48	
	Missing	71	26	18	16	26	35	27	31	
Total n		274		112		74		88		

D diabetes, *CP* cerebral palsy, *ASD* autism spectrum disorder

the period of the study, using the consolidated indicator. Optimal exposure to features of transitional healthcare was 61% for 'coordinated team', 53% for 'age-banded clinic', 48% for 'holistic life-skills training', 42% for 'promotion of health self-efficacy', 40% for 'meeting the adult team before transfer', 34% for 'appropriate parent involvement', and less than 30% for 'written transition plan', 'key worker' and 'transition manager for clinical team'. Significantly more young people with diabetes experienced optimal exposure to PBFs compared to those with CP or ASD, particularly 'meeting the adult team before transfer' and 'promotion of health self-efficacy'.

PBFs as predictors of Mind the Gap scores
In the year-by-year analysis, there were significant positive associations ($p \leq 0.01$) during each period between 'appropriate parental involvement' and satisfaction with services (Mind the Gap) overall and in most domains of the instrument (Table 3). These were confirmed by significant associations of the consolidated PBF indicator with Mind the Gap at final visit.

The pattern of associations was similar for 'promotion of health self-efficacy' though the evidence for the association was not as strong (total Mind the Gap $p = 0.04$) for the influence of the consolidated PBF indicator.

Table 3 Associations of Proposed Beneficial Features (PBFs) with outcome measures

PBF	Period	PBFs by 'year-by-year' visits				Consolidated PBF indicator at final visit			
		Outcome	Coefficient or odds ratio[a]	95% confidence interval	p value	Outcome	Coefficient or odds ratio[a]	95% confidence interval	p value
Appropriate parent involvement	1	MTG: total	−0.48	−0.76 to −0.19	**0.001**	MTG: total	−0.67	−0.97 to −0.37	**<0.001**
	1	MTG: environment	−0.57	−0.92 to −0.21	**0.001**	MTG: environment	−0.71	−1.17 to −0.26	**0.006**
	1	MTG: provider	−0.52	−0.82 to −0.22	**0.001**	MTG: provider	−0.75	−0.99 to −0.52	**<0.001**
	1	RTP: domestic	[0.14a]	0.03 to 0.67	**0.01**	RTP: finances	[0.6a]	0.92 to 0.39	0.02
	1	RTP: healthcare	[0.35a]	0.17 to 0.72	**0.004**	WEMWBS	2.18	0.21 to 4.15	0.03
	1	RTP: services and aids	[0.42a]	0.18 to 0.97	0.04				
	2	MTG: total	−0.60	−1.00 to −0.21	**0.003**				
	2	MTG: environment	−0.65	−1.08 to −0.21	**0.004**				
	2	MTG: provider	−0.48	−0.90 to −0.06	0.03				
	2	MTG: process	−0.82	−1.32 to −0.31	**0.002**				
	2	WEMWBS	4.47	1.96 to 6.97	**0.001**				
	3	MTG: total	−0.87	0.45 to 1.29	**0.001**				
	3	MTG: environment	−0.91	−1.44 to −0.37	**<0.001**				
	3	MTG: provider	−0.95	−1.37 to −0.52	**<0.001**				
	3	MTG: process	−0.63	−1.18 to −0.07	0.03				
	3	WEMWBS	3.45	0.92 to 5.99	**0.008**				
Promotion of health self-efficacy	1	MTG: total	−0.51	−0.87 to −0.15	**0.006**	MTG: total	−0.32	−0.62 to −0.03	0.04
	1	MTG: environment	−0.63	−1.06 to −0.18	**0.005**	MTG: environment	−0.57	−1.03 to −0.11	0.02
	1	MTG: provider	−0.47	−0.85 to −0.09	0.02	MTG: process	−0.37	−0.70 to −0.04	0.03
	1	MTG: process	−0.46	−0.91 to −0.01	0.04				
	1	RTP: finances	[0.26a]	0.07 to 0.93	0.04				
	1	RTP: domestic	[0.04a]	0.01 to 0.21	**0.001**				
	2	MTG: total	−0.51	−0.91 to −0.11	**0.01**				
	2	MTG: provider	−0.49	−0.90 to −0.08	0.02				
	2	MTG: process	−0.70	−1.21 to −0.19	**0.007**				
	2	MTG: total	−0.60	−1.01 to −0.20	**0.004**				
	3	MTG: environment	−0.90	−1.40 to −0.40	**<0.001**				
	3	MTG: provider	−0.52	−0.95 to −0.11	**0.01**				

Table 3 Associations of Proposed Beneficial Features (PBFs) with outcome measures (*Continued*)

PBF	PBFs by 'year-by-year' visits					Consolidated PBF indicator at final visit			
	Period	Outcome	Coefficient or odds ratio[a]	95% confidence interval	p value	Outcome	Coefficient or odds ratio[a]	95% confidence interval	p value
Meet adult team before transfer	1	**RTP: domestic**	6.29[a]	1.60 to 24.80	**0.009**	**RTP: education/ employment**	2.33[a]	1.21 to 4.55	**0.01**
	1	**RTP: healthcare**	2.71[a]	1.24 to 5.90	**0.01**	RTP: finances	2.78[a]	1.10 to 7.14	0.03
	1	**RTP: services and aids**	5.15[a]	2.08 to 12.78	**< 0.001**	RTP: services and aids	2.50[a]	1.06 to 5.88	0.04
	1	RTP: transport	2.01[a]	1.06 to 3.79	0.03	Autonomy in appointments	1.60	0.32 to 2.87	0.02
	1	RTP: education/ employment	3.24[a]	1.09 to 9.65	0.04				
	1	**Autonomy in appointments**	1.69	0.80 to 2.58	**< 0.001**				
	2	RTP: finances	2.64[a]	0.92 to 6.62	0.02				
	2	RTP: transport	2.08[a]	1.11 to 3.90	0.02				
	2	Autonomy in appointments	1.00	0.01 to 2.0	0.05				
	3	**RTP: healthcare**	2.11[a]	1.03 to 4.34	**0.004**				
	3	**Autonomy in appointments**	1.46	0.34 to 2.59	**0.01**				
Key worker	1	RTP: leisure	[0.56[a]]	0.32 to 0.96	0.04				
	2	**MTG: provider**	− 0.66	− 1.04 to − 0.28	**0.001**				
	2	**MTG: process**	− 0.69	− 1.17 to − 0.21	**0.005**				
	3	RTP: education/employment	[0.40[a]]	0.20 to 0.95	0.02				
Holistic life-skills training	1	RTP: domestic	[0.19[a]]	0.04 to 0.93	0.04				
	1	RTP: services and aids	[0.34[a]]	0.12 to 0.94	0.04				
	2	MTG: provider	[0.43]	0.03 to 0.84	0.04				
	3	MTG: total	− 0.46	− 0.87 to − 0.05	0.03				
	3	**MTG: provider**	− 0.57	− 0.99 to − 0.14	**0.009**				
	3	**RTP: domestic**	2.47[a]	1.10 to 5.58	**0.003**				
	3	RTP: romantic relationships	[0.52[a]]	0.26 to 0.98	0.04				
Written transition plan	1	RTP: romantic relationships	[0.43[a]]	0.19 to 0.96	0.04				
	2	MTG: total	− 0.72	− 1.39 to − 0.04	0.04				
	2	**MTG: process**	− 1.19	− 1.39 to − 0.04	**0.007**				

Clinical and Translational Medicine

Table 3 Associations of Proposed Beneficial Features (PBFs) with outcome measures (*Continued*)

PBF	Period	Outcome	Coefficient or odds ratio[a]	95% confidence interval	p value	Outcome	Coefficient or odds ratio[a]	95% confidence interval	p value
						Consolidated PBF indicator at final visit			
Coordinated team	1	RTP: domestic	[0.19^a]	0.04 to 0.93	0.04	MTG: provider	−0.67	−1.25 to −0.09	0.03
	3	RTP: healthcare	[0.17^a]	0.04 to 0.82	0.03	RTP: education/employment	[0.31^a]	0.11 to 0.82	0.02
	3	RTP: services and aids	[0.22^a]	0.06 to 0.81	0.02	RTP: domestic	[0.41^a]	0.19 to 0.91	0.03
Transition manager for clinical team		No associations				RTP: domestic	2.63^a	1.16 to 5.88	0.02
						RTP: services and aids	[0.41^a]	0.20 to 0.86	0.02
						RTP: romantic relationships	[0.52^a]	0.31 to 0.89	0.02
Age-banded clinic	1	WEMWBS	3.08	0.18 to 5.98	0.04				
	1	**Autonomy in appointments**	1.44	0.48 to 2.4	**0.003**				
	2	RTP: education/employment	5.22^a	1.21 to 22.53	0.03				

Note 1 Coefficients and odds ratios 'year-by-year' and for the consolidated PBF indicator have sub-optimal PBF delivery as the reference group
Note 2 A larger Mind the Gap score means less satisfaction with services than a smaller score
MTG Mind the Gap, *RTP* Rotterdam Transition Profile, *WEMWBS* Warwick Edinburgh Mental Wellbeing Scale
[] negative association, i.e. satisfactory PBF was associated with worse outcome
^{a} indicates an odds ratio
Bold indicates $p \leq 0.01$

PBFs as predictors of wellbeing scores

'Appropriate parent involvement' was associated with wellbeing (Warwick Edinburgh Mental Wellbeing Scale) in the second and third periods of the year-by-year analysis, though at a lesser level of significance ($p = 0.03$) for the consolidated PBF indicator.

PBFs as predictors of the Rotterdam transition profile

'Meeting the adult team before transfer' was significantly associated ($p \leq 0.01$) with a number of domains of the Rotterdam Profile in all three periods of the year-by-year analysis and also the consolidated PBF indicator (Table 3).

A number of weaker year-by-year and consolidated PBF indicator associations with other domains of the Rotterdam Profile were seen, but they were not in the predicted direction.

PBFs as predictors of autonomy in appointments

There were significant associations ($p < 0.01$) of 'meeting the adult team before transfer' with 'autonomy in appointments' in periods 1 and 3 and with the consolidated PBF indicator ($p = 0.02$).

Thus, three PBFs of transitional healthcare had significant ($p \leq 0.01$) positive associations with better outcomes, namely 'appropriate parent involvement', 'promotion of health self-efficacy' and 'meeting the adult team before transfer'. The b-coefficients indicated changes of approximately 0.5 SDs with respect to the satisfaction with services scale (SD 1.5 in our population), wellbeing (SD 7.0 in our population) and autonomy in appointments (SD 3.0 in our population). The odds ratios indicated increased likelihoods of being in a more independent phase of transition. The other six PBFs had few statistically significant positive associations ($p \leq 0.01$, Table 3) with better outcomes in the year-by-year analysis, had a number of negative associations, and had no positive associations with the consolidated indicator of exposure to PBFs.

Discussion

Our study explored whether features of transitional healthcare, recommended in policy documents, were associated with positive outcomes. Three PBFs had significant positive associations with better outcomes, namely 'appropriate parent involvement', 'promotion of health self-efficacy', and 'meeting the adult team before transfer'. The b-coefficients indicated clinically significant changes of approximately 0.5 SDs with respect to the satisfaction with services scale, wellbeing and autonomy in appointments. The odds ratios indicated increased likelihoods of being in a more independent phase of transition.

The other six PBFs had few statistically significant positive associations with better outcomes in the year-by-year analysis, had a number of negative associations and had

no positive associations with the consolidated indicator of exposure to PBFs.

Two of the three key features which help ('appropriate parent involvement' and 'promotion of health self-efficacy') are not specific to transition; rather, they are features of developmentally appropriate healthcare for all young people. This finding reinforces the view that much of the essence of good transitional care is actually good developmentally appropriate healthcare [28, 29].

'Appropriate parent involvement' and 'promotion of health self-efficacy' were perceived to have been experienced satisfactorily by less than half of participants across transition across the three conditions. However, they were experienced by more young people with diabetes than by those with CP or ASD. For 'meeting the adult team before transfer', around two-thirds of young people with diabetes reported that they had met a member of the adult team but, for those with CP or ASD, it was less than a quarter. Thus, we found a different quality of experience of transitional healthcare for young people with a long-term illness (diabetes) compared to those with a long-term disability. These gaps in current practice need to be addressed through service development.

Strengths and weaknesses

Our study was hypothesis driven, with pre-planned outcome measures that were applicable over condition and setting. These measures examined young people's satisfaction with services, their wellbeing and participation, rather than focusing on process indicators such as attendance or loss to follow-up. There is a place for both outcomes and process indicators in transition evaluation. However, if service features do not improve the health or well-being of the young person, then it is hard to argue on clinical effectiveness grounds any basis for their adoption regardless of how process indicators may change. Our study has reported on wellbeing and participation which have rarely been used in this area, despite recommendations to do so [15, 17, 30]. Inclusion of a sample of young people with three contrasting conditions raises confidence in the generalisability of the findings to most young people with long-term health conditions. The retention rate of 73% to final visit was a considerable strength in this age group. Our data related to clinical practice for the three very different conditions, across several geographical locations. Unlike many previous studies [31–35], it was not an evaluation by a local team of their local intervention, which risks observer bias and limits generalisability of findings. Further, we collected data longitudinally over 3 years of transition. One limitation was lower average recruitment from a group with a special need for transitional care, namely those from areas of greater socioeconomic deprivation. However, the difference in overall IMD score on a continuous scale ranging from 0.5 to 87.8, was only 6.1; further, there was no difference in proportion of single parent families as compared to national norms. Regarding attrition, this was more marked by IMD score only for those with CP in Northern Ireland. There was, however, a reduction in the proportion of single parent families, which could be relevant to interpreting our finding that appropriate parent involvement in transition was significantly associated with better outcomes.

There was also lower than intended recruitment from the two disability groupings, so that analyses controlling for condition may have been underpowered. A further potential limitation was the accuracy of exposure to PBFs. The local researchers were trained together each year on this topic and then held the discussion each year with the young person, supplemented by the young person's notes and inspection of medical notes. The analysis by whether exposure to the consolidated PBF indicator had been 'optimal' was a more demanding interrogation of the data than the year-by-year analyses because it required there to be some degree of good practice throughout the 3 years, not just over 1 year. However, the decision rules (described in Methods) about what constitutes optimal exposure to each PBF were determined by the research team and have some subjectivity.

Strengths and weaknesses in relation to other studies

The three PBFs for which we found evidence of positive associations are supported by guidance and corroborating evidence discussed below. The link to current UK guidance (NICE) is also presented for each.

'Appropriate parent involvement'

The NICE [4] guideline 43 emphasised 'Appropriate parent involvement' throughout its report; it is an overarching principle in section "Background".1.1, and sections "Background".2.19–1.2.22 focusing on the involvement of parents. Heath and Farre's systematic review of studies of parents' perceptions of their role in Transition [36] concluded that *"Parents can be key facilitators of their child's healthcare Transition, supporting them to become experts in their own condition and care. However, to do so parents require clarification on their role and support from service providers"*. Akre's study [37] found parental satisfaction with their involvement was associated with easier transition from the young person's point of view. Allen's study of young people with diabetes emphasised the importance of parents during Transition [38]. A review of qualitative studies [39] and a subsequent study [40] identified the tension that young people experience between seeking autonomy and still needing their parents. Two further recent reports investigated the parent–young person dyad [41, 42] and reached similar conclusions to those of the current study, namely that the parent and young person

need to share care but that the change to adult autonomy is dynamic and will continuously change.

'Promotion of health self-efficacy'

In section "Background".2.17, NICE [4] recommended 'Promotion of health self-efficacy'. Sattoe and van Staa [43] found that *"continuing attention to self-management"* was associated with better health-related quality of life. There is conflicting evidence as to whether a structured approach, including motivational techniques, to increase health self-efficacy in diabetes influences glycaemic control [44, 45]. After liver transplant, higher perceived self-management competence was actually associated with poorer clinical outcomes [46]. Mackie [47] showed the benefit of a 1-hour nurse-led intervention to promote knowledge and confidence about one's condition, in this case congenital heart disease.

'Meeting the adult team before transfer'

In sections "Background".3.5 and 1.3.6, NICE [4] recommended 'Meeting the adult team before transfer'. Our definition of meeting the adult team before transfer included clinics where adult and paediatric clinicians consulted jointly. In other studies, such joint clinics have shown improvements in certain indicators in nephrology (transplant rejection) [34], urology (aspects of care) [33] and rheumatology (knowledge of one's condition) [48]. Crowley's review [11] found joint clinics were associated with improved outcomes in those with diabetes.

The remaining six PBFs, for which our study found little evidence of benefit, had been included because a number of small published studies suggested they might be associated with improved outcomes. 'Having a key worker' was recommended by NICE [4] (sections "Background".2.5–1.2.10 called for a 'Named Worker'). Sloper et al. [49] found strong evidence for introducing key workers. The difficulty with 'key worker' may be operational rather than the principle; staff changes, due to leaving post, restrictions in job plans, service restructuring, sickness or maternity leave, make it difficult to provide a consistent key worker for all young people with long-term conditions. Having access to *"holistic life-skills training"* was recommended by NICE (sections "Background".2.13–1.2.15). It was associated with greater satisfaction with service providers, and with more independent participation in domestic life in the third period of the year-by-year analysis, but not in the analysis by consolidated PBF indicators. Interpretation is difficult because few services provided this type of training. 'Having a written transition plan' was associated with greater satisfaction with services during the second study period but was otherwise negatively associated with many outcomes. NICE [4] (section "Background".3.4) recommended transition planning but did not specifically mention that it should be a written document. Data from our qualitative work [50] showed the potential for careful planning to mitigate some of the disruptive, disorienting consequences of transfer. However, there were conflicting views about a 'written' plan. Some professionals said such plans get forgotten or lost, and personal interaction was far more important. On the other hand, lack of a formal plan left many families disoriented and wondering whether services would have sufficient resources to provide for care after transfer. Having a 'transition manager for clinical team' had no associations in the year-by-year analysis and had largely negative associations with the consolidated PBF indicator. In pilot studies, some benefits of having such a manager were seen after liver transplant [32] and in rheumatology [51].

Which outcomes should be measured in transition studies? [52–54] There is a need to go beyond current Delphi studies, and crucially involve young people and their families in developing consensus. Our choice of outcomes was informed by the International Classification of Functioning [18] and by discussion with international transition researchers, and conformed with many of the recommendations of subsequent international surveys [15, 16]. Although carefully chosen and piloted, measures may not be ideal; for example, we found the domain Finances of the Rotterdam Transition Profile not to be sensitive to change by the end of the study, as most young people remained dependent in part on family financial support.

Conclusions

This study examined patient-level generic outcomes and provides new evidence about what may improve such outcomes. The findings are likely to be generalisable because participants had three very different conditions, attending services at many UK sites. Most previous studies have examined process indicators, which can be relevant to monitoring services but do not establish whether outcomes improve.

Three PBFs consistently associated with better outcomes were 'Appropriate parent involvement', 'Promotion of health self-efficacy' and 'Meeting the adult team before transfer'. Our findings are relevant to almost all physicians and surgeons as some of their patients are likely to be adolescents and/or young adults with long-term conditions. The findings are also relevant for commissioners and managers of both child and adult health services who should prioritise changes for which there is evidence of benefit. There may need to be different approaches to different conditions as current provision of the three features is better for those with long-term conditions such as diabetes than for those with disabling conditions such as CP or ASD.

The three features should be introduced or maintained to a high standard in both child and adult services and the challenge of doing so evaluated. Such change will also require staff training and organisational change across child and adult healthcare services.

Abbreviations

ASD: autism spectrum disorder; CP: cerebral palsy; IMD: Index of Multiple Deprivation; NICE: National Institute for Health and Clinical Excellence; PBF: proposed beneficial feature; SD: standard deviation

Acknowledgements

We acknowledge the support of the NIHR Clinical Research Network.
We thank the members of the Young Persons' Advisory Group (UP) for their work throughout the study. We thank the members of the External Advisory Board, which included PPI contributors, among them a parent with a son and daughter with long-term conditions, representatives of two patient organisations and members of the UP group.
We thank the research assistants: Kam Ameen-Ali, Sarah Balne, Shaunak Deshpande, Louise Foster, Charlotte George, Louisa Fear, Kate Hardenberg, Guio Garcia Jalon, Holly Roper, Tracy Scott, Catherine Sheppard, Louise Ting, and Hazel Windmill.
The Transition Collaborative Group consists of the authors of this paper and Caroline Bennett, Greg Maniatopoulos, Tim Rapley, Debbie Reape, Nichola Chater, Helena Gleeson, Amanda Billson, Anastasia Bem, Stuart Bennett, Stephen Bruce, Tim Cheetham, Diana Howlett, Zilla Huma, Mark Linden, Maria Lohan, Cara Maiden, Melanie Meek, Jenny Milne, Julie Owens, Jackie Parkes, Fiona Regan, and Nandu Thalange.

Funding

This article presents independent research funded by the National Institute for Health Research (NIHR) under the Programme Grants for Applied Research programme: RP-PG-0610-10112. The views expressed in this article are those of the authors and not necessarily those of the NHS, the NIHR or the Department of Health. The funder took no part in the collection, analysis or interpretation of the data, in the writing of the article nor in the decision to submit the article for publication.

Sponsor

The study sponsor, Northumbria Healthcare NHS Foundation Trust, had no role in the study design, in the collection, analysis and interpretation of data, in the writing of the report, nor in the decision to submit the article for publication. AFC had an honorary contract with Northumbria Healthcare, and GD-P was employed by Northumbria Healthcare.

Authors' contributions

AC, HMC, ALC, GD-P, MSP, JM, LV and JRP designed the study; KDM and MSP were principally responsible for analysis of the data and supervision of data collection; AC and HMC drafted the paper. All authors commented on and approved the paper's text. All authors had full access to all of the data (including statistical reports and tables) and take responsibility for the integrity of the data and the accuracy of the data analysis. The lead author (the manuscript's guarantor) affirms that the manuscript is an honest, accurate and transparent account of the study being reported, that no important aspects of the study have been omitted and that any discrepancies from the study as planned have been explained.

Competing interests

The authors declare that they have no competing interests.

Author details

[1]Institute of Health & Society, Sir James Spence Institute, Royal Victoria Infirmary, Newcastle University, Queen Victoria Road, Newcastle upon Tyne NE1 4LP, UK. [2]Northumbria Healthcare NHS Foundation Trust, North Tyneside General Hospital, Rake Lane, North Shields NE29 8NH, UK. [3]Northumberland, Tyne and Wear NHS Foundation Trust, St. Nicholas Hospital, Jubilee Road, Newcastle upon Tyne NE3 3XT, UK. [4]Centre for Musculoskeletal Research and Manchester Academic Health Science Centre, University of Manchester, Stopford Building, Oxford Rd, Manchester M13 9PT, UK. [5]NIHR Manchester Biomedical Research Centre, Manchester University NHS Foundation Trust, Manchester Royal Infirmary, Oxford Rd, Manchester M13 9WL, UK. [6]Institute of Neuroscience, Sir James Spence Institute, Newcastle University, Queen Victoria Road, Newcastle upon Tyne NE1 4LP, UK. [7]Great North Children's Hospital, Newcastle Upon Tyne Hospitals NHS Foundation Trust, Royal Victoria Infirmary, Queen Victoria Road, Newcastle upon Tyne NE1 4LP, UK.

References

1. UK Parliament. Disability Discrimination Act. London: The Stationery Office, 2005.
2. Stam H, Hartman EE, Deurloo JA, Groothoff J, Grootenhuis MA. Young adult patients with a history of pediatric disease: impact on course of life and transition into adulthood. J Adolesc Health. 2006;39(1):4–13.
3. Gorter J, Stewart D, Woodbury-Smith M, King G, Wright M, Nguyen T, et al. Pathways toward positive psychosocial outcomes and mental health for youth with disabilities: a knowledge synthesis of developmental trajectories. Can J Commun Ment Health. 2014;33(1):45–61.
4. National Institute for Health and Care Excellence (NICE). Transition from Children's to Adults' Services for Young People Using Health or Social Care Services, Guideline 43. London: National Institute for Health and Care Excellence (NICE); 2016.
5. National Institute for Health and Care Excellence (NICE). Transition from Children's to Adults' Services. Quality standard 140. London: National Institute for Health and Care Excellence (NICE); 2016.
6. Blum RW, Garell D, Hodgman CH, Jorissen TW, Okinow NA, Orr DP, et al. Transition from child-centered to adult health-care systems for adolescents with chronic conditions. A position paper of the Society for Adolescent Medicine. J Adolesc Health. 1993;14(7):570–6.
7. American Academy of Pediatrics, American Academy of Family Physicians, American College of Physicians, Transitions Clinical Report Authoring Group, Cooley WC, Sagerman PJ. Supporting the health care transition from adolescence to adulthood in the medical home. Pediatrics. 2011;128(1):182–200.
8. Mazur A, Dembinski L, Schrier L, Hadjipanayis A, Michaud PA. European Academy of Paediatric consensus statement on successful transition from paediatric to adult care for adolescents with chronic conditions. Acta Paediatr. 2017;106(8):1354–7.
9. Foster HE, Minden K, Clemente D, Leon L, McDonagh JE, Kamphuis S, et al. EULAR/PReS standards and recommendations for the transitional care of young people with juvenile-onset rheumatic diseases. Ann Rheum Dis. 2017;76(4):639–46.
10. Campbell FBK, Aldiss SK, O'Neill PM, Clowes M, McDonagh J, While A, Gibson F. Transition of care for adolescents from paediatric services to adult health services (Review). Cochrane Database Syst Rev. 2016;4:CD009794.
11. Crowley R, Wolfe I, Lock K, McKee M. Improving the transition between paediatric and adult healthcare: a systematic review. Arch Dis Child. 2011;96:548–53.
12. Colver AF, Merrick H, Deverill M, Le Couteur A, Parr J, Pearce MS, et al. Study protocol: longitudinal study of the transition of young people with complex health needs from child to adult health services. BMC Public Health. 2013; 13(1):675.
13. Merrick H, McConachie H, Le Couteur A, Mann K, Parr JR, Pearce MS, et al. Characteristics of young people with long term conditions close to transfer to adult health services. BMC Health Serv Res. 2015;15:435.
14. While A, Forbes A, Ullman R, Lewis S, Mathes L, Griffiths P. Good practices that address continuity during transition from child to adult care: synthesis of the evidence. Child Care Health Dev. 2004;30(5):439–52.
15. Fair C, Cuttance J, Sharma N, Maslow G, Wiener L, Betz C, et al. International and interdisciplinary identification of health care transition outcomes. JAMA Pediatr. 2016;170(3):205–11.
16. Suris JC, Akre C. Key elements for, and indicators of, a successful transition: an international Delphi study. J Adolesc Health. 2015;56(6):612–8.
17. Scal P. Improving health care transition services: just grow up, will you please. JAMA Pediatr. 2016;170(3):197–9.
18. World Health Organization. International Classification of Functioning, Disability and Health: Children and Youth Version. Geneva: ICF-CY; 2007.
19. Shaw KL, Southwood TR, McDonagh JE. Development and preliminary validation of the 'Mind the Gap' scale to assess satisfaction with transitional health care among adolescents with juvenile idiopathic arthritis. Child Care Health Dev. 2007;33(4):380–8.
20. Clarke A, Friede T, Putz R, Ashdown J, Martin S, Blake A, et al. Warwick-Edinburgh mental well-being scale (WEMWBS): validated for teenage school students in England and Scotland. A mixed methods assessment. BMC Public Health. 2011;11:487.
21. Donkervoort M, Wiegerink DJ, van Meeteren J, Stam HJ, Roebroeck ME. Transition to adulthood: validation of the Rotterdam transition profile for young adults with cerebral palsy and normal intelligence. Dev Med Child Neurol. 2009;51(1):53–62.
22. van Staa A, On Your Own Feet Research Group. Unraveling triadic communication in hospital consultations with adolescents with chronic conditions: the added value of mixed methods research. Patient Educ Couns. 2011;82:455–64.
23. Department for Communities and Local Government. English IMD 2010 Data. 2011; https://www.gov.uk/government/statistics/english-indices-of-deprivation-2015. Accessed June 2018.
24. Northern Ireland Statistics and Research Agency. Northern Ireland MDM 2010 Data. 2010; www.nisra.gov.uk/deprivation/nimdm_2010.htm. Accessed 22 Mar 2017.
25. Solanke F, Colver A, McConachie H. Transition Collaborative Group. Are the health needs of young people with cerebral palsy met during transition from child to adult health care? Child Care Health Dev. 2018; 44(3):355–63.
26. Gray S, Cheetham T, McConachie H, Mann KD, Parr JR, Pearce MS, et al. A longitudinal, observational study examining the relationships of patient satisfaction with services and mental well-being to their clinical course in young people with type 1 diabetes mellitus during transition from child to adult health services. Diabet Med. 2018; https://doi.org/10.1111/dme.13698.
27. Office for National Statistics. Families and Households Survey. 2013; https://www.ons.gov.uk/peoplepopulationandcommunity/birthsdeathsandmarriages/families/qmis/familiesandhouseholdsqmi. Accessed 15 Apr 2018.
28. Farre A, Wood V, McDonagh JE, Parr JR, Reape D, Rapley T, et al. Health professionals' and managers' definitions of developmentally appropriate healthcare for young people: conceptual dimensions and embedded controversies. Arch Dis Child. 2016;101(7):628–33.
29. Toolkit for introducing Developmentally Appropriate Healthcare. 2017; https://www.northumbria.nhs.uk/quality-and-safety/clinical-trials/for-healthcare-professionals/. Accessed 15 Dec 2017.
30. Le Roux E, Mellerio H, Guilmin-Crepon S, Gottot S, Jacquin P, Boulkedid R, et al. Methodology used in comparative studies assessing programmes of transition from paediatrics to adult care programmes: a systematic review. BMJ Open. 2017;7(1):e012338.
31. Fredericks EM, Magee JC, Eder SJ, Sevecke JR, Dore-Stites D, Shieck V, et al. Quality improvement targeting adherence during the transition from a pediatric to adult liver transplant clinic. J Clin Psychol Med Settings. 2015; 22(2–3):150–9.
32. Annunziato RA, Baisley MC, Arrato N, Barton C, Henderling F, Arnon R, et al. Strangers headed to a strange land? A pilot study of using a transition coordinator to improve transfer from pediatric to adult services. J Pediatr. 2013;163(6):1628–33.
33. Shalaby MS, Gibson A, Granitsiotis P, Conn G, Cascio S. Assessment of the introduction of an adolescent transition urology clinic using a validated questionnaire. J Pediatr Urol. 2015;11(2):89 e1–5.
34. Harden PN, Walsh G, Bandler N, Bradley S, Lonsdale D, Taylor J, et al. Bridging the gap: an integrated paediatric to adult clinical service for young adults with kidney failure. BMJ. 2012;344:e3718.
35. Huang JS, Terrones L, Tompane T, Dillon L, Pian M, Gottschalk M, et al. Preparing adolescents with chronic disease for transition to adult care: a technology program. Pediatrics. 2014;133(6):e1639–46.
36. Heath G, Farre A, Shaw K. Parenting a child with chronic illness as they transition into adulthood: a systematic review and thematic synthesis of parents' experiences. Patient Educ Couns. 2017;100(1):76–92.
37. Suris JC, Larbre JP, Hofer M, Hauschild M, Barrense-Dias Y, Berchtold A, et al. Transition from paediatric to adult care: what makes it easier for parents? Child Care Health Dev. 2017;43(1):152–5.
38. Allen D, Channon S, Lowes L, Atwell C, Lane C. Behind the scenes: the changing roles of parents in the transition from child to adult diabetes service. Diabet Med. 2011;28(8):994–1000.
39. Lugasi T, Achille M, Stevenson M. Patients' perspective on factors that facilitate transition from child-centered to adult-centered health care: a theory integrated metasummary of quantitative and qualitative studies. J Adolesc Health. 2011;48(5):429–40.
40. Pierce JS, Aroian K, Schifano E, Milkes A, Schwindt T, Gannon A, et al. Health care transition for young adults with type 1 diabetes: stakeholder engagement for defining optimal outcomes. J Pediatr Psychol. 2017;42(9):970–82.
41. Hanna KM, Dashiff CJ, Stump TE, Weaver MT. Parent-adolescent dyads: association of parental autonomy support and parent-adolescent shared diabetes care responsibility. Child Care Health Dev. 2013;39(5):695–702.
42. Nguyen T, Henderson D, Stewart D, Hlyva O, Punthakee Z, Gorter JW. You never transition alone! Exploring the experiences of youth with chronic health conditions, parents and healthcare providers on self-management. Child Care Health Dev. 2016;42(4):464–72.

43. Sattoe JN, Bal MI, Roelofs PD, Bal R, Miedema HS, van Staa A. Self-management interventions for young people with chronic conditions: a systematic overview. Patient Educ Couns. 2015;98(6):704–15.

44. Channon SJ, Huws-Thomas MV, Rollnick S, Hood K, Cannings-John RL, Rogers C, et al. A multicenter randomized controlled trial of motivational interviewing in teenagers with diabetes. Diabetes Care. 2007;30(6):1390–5.

45. Christie D, Thompson R, Sawtell M, Allen E, Cairns J, Smith F, et al. Structured, intensive education maximising engagement, motivation and long-term change for children and young people with diabetes: a cluster randomised controlled trial with integral process and economic evaluation - the CASCADE study. Health Technol Assess. 2014;18(20):1–202.

46. Annunziato RA, Bucuvalas JC, Yin W, Arnand R, Alonso EM, Mazariegos GV, et al. Self-management measurement and prediction of clinical outcomes in pediatric transplant. J Pediatr. 2018;193:128–33 e2.

47. Mackie AS, Islam S, Magill-Evans J, Rankin KN, Robert C, Schuh M, et al. Healthcare transition for youth with heart disease: a clinical trial. Heart. 2014; 100(14):1113–8.

48. Stringer E, Scott R, Mosher D, MacNeill I, Huber AM, Ramsey S, et al. Evaluation of a rheumatology transition clinic. Pediatr Rheumatol Online J. 2015;13:22.

49. Franklin A, Sloper T, Beecham J, Clarke S, Moran N. Models of Multi-agency Services for Transition to Adult Services for Disabled Young People and Those with Complex Health Needs: Impact and Costs. Progress Report. York: Social Policy Research Unit, University of York; 2009.

50. Colver A, Pearse R, Watson RM, Fay M, Rapley T, Mann KD, et al. How well do services for young people with long term conditions deliver features proposed to improve transition? BMC Health Serv Res. 2018;18(1):337.

51. Jensen PT, Karnes J, Jones K, Lehman A, Rennebohm R, Higgins GC, et al. Quantitative evaluation of a pediatric rheumatology transition program. Pediatr Rheumatol Online J. 2015;13:17.

52. Coyne B, Hallowell SC, Thompson M. Measurable outcomes after transfer from pediatric to adult providers in youth with chronic illness. J Adolesc Health. 2017;60(1):3–16.

53. Williamson PR, Altman DG, Blazeby JM, Clarke M, Devane D, Gargon E, et al. Developing core outcome sets for clinical trials: issues to consider. Trials. 2012;13:132.

54. Prior M, McManus M, White P, Davidson L. Measuring the "triple aim" in transition care: a systematic review. Pediatrics. 2014;134(6):e1648–61.

14

Chronic hepatitis B virus infection and risk of chronic kidney disease: a population-based prospective cohort study of 0.5 million Chinese adults

Jiahui Si[1†], Canqing Yu[1†], Yu Guo[2], Zheng Bian[2], Chenxi Qin[1], Ling Yang[3], Yiping Chen[3], Li Yin[4], Hui Li[5], Jian Lan[6], Junshi Chen[7], Zhengming Chen[3], Jun Lv[1,8*], Liming Li[1,2] and on behalf of the China Kadoorie Biobank Collaborative Group

Abstract

Background: Existing evidence remains inconclusive as to the association between chronic hepatitis B virus (HBV) infection and the risk of chronic kidney disease (CKD). We prospectively examined the association between chronic HBV infection and CKD risk, and the joint associations of HBV infection with established risk factors of several lifestyle factors and prevalent diseases on CKD risk.

Methods: Participants from the China Kadoorie Biobank were enrolled during 2004–2008 and followed up until 31 December 2015. After excluding participants with previously diagnosed CKD, cancer, heart disease, and stroke at baseline, the present study included 469,459 participants. Hepatitis B surface antigen (HBsAg) was qualitatively tested at baseline. Incident CKD cases were identified mainly through the health insurance system and disease and death registries.

Results: During a median follow-up of 9.1 years (4.2 million person-years), we documented 4555 incident cases of CKD. Cox regression yielded multivariable-adjusted hazard ratios (HRs) and 95% confidence intervals (CIs). Compared with HBsAg-negative participants, the multivariable-adjusted HR (95% CI) for CKD was 1.37 (1.18, 1.60) for HBsAg-positive participants. The association was stronger in men (HR = 1.77; 95% CI: 1.43, 2.20) than in women (HR = 1.10; 95% CI: 0.88, 1.36). HBsAg-positive participants, with or without hepatitis or cirrhosis, whether or not under treatment, all showed increased risk of developing CKD. We observed positive additive interactions of HBsAg positivity with smoking, physical inactivity, or diabetes on CKD risk. Compared with HBsAg-negative participants who were nonsmokers, more physically active, or did not have diabetes at baseline, the greatest CKD risk for HBsAg-positive participants was for those who were smokers (HR = 1.85; 95% CI: 1.44, 2.38), physically inactive (HR = 1.91; 95% CI: 1.52, 2.40), or diabetic (HR = 6.11; 95% CI: 4.47, 8.36).

Conclusions: In countries with a high endemicity of HBV infection, kidney damage associated with chronic HBV infection should be a non-negligible concern. Our findings also highlight the importance of health advice on quitting smoking, increasing physical activity, improving glucose control, and early screening for CKD in people with chronic HBV infection.

Keywords: Chronic hepatitis B virus infection, Chronic kidney disease, Prospective cohort study

* Correspondence: lvjun@bjmu.edu.cn
†Jiahui Si and Canqing Yu contributed equally to this work.
[1]Department of Epidemiology and Biostatistics, School of Public Health, Peking University Health Science Center, 38 Xueyuan Road, Beijing 100191, China
[8]Peking University Institute of Environmental Medicine, Beijing, China
Full list of author information is available at the end of the article

Background

Chronic kidney disease (CKD), which has important health and economic implications [1], had a prevalence of 10.8% in China in 2010 [2], as high as that in developed countries such as the USA (13.1%) and Norway (10.2%) [3, 4]. CKD is a general term for heterogeneous disorders and defined based on the presence of kidney damage or decreased kidney function for 3 months or more [5]. Several risk factors for CKD have been identified, including diabetes, hypertension, older age, tobacco smoking, obesity, cardiovascular diseases, and nephrotoxic drugs or toxins [5, 6]. However, possible effects of more adverse factors on the CKD risk remain to be clarified.

Hepatitis B virus (HBV) infection has been shown to have negative impacts on renal funtion [7–9]. A recently published systematic review showed that two prospective studies consistently linked HBV infection to increased risk of end-stage renal disease [10]. However, another two prospective studies examining the association between HBV infection and a broader CKD outcome showed mixed results [11, 12].

China is a higher-intermediate HBV endemicity country, with an estimated seroprevalence of hepatitis B surface antigen (HBsAg) of 5.49% [13]. If chronic HBV infection is causally related to CKD risk, this may partially explain the high burden of CKD and may guide prevention efforts in China. In the present study, we prospectively examined the association between chronic HBV infection and CKD risk in the China Kadoorie Biobank (CKB) study of 0.5 million adults. We additionally examined the joint associations of HBV infection with established risk factors of several lifestyle factors and prevalent diseases on CKD risk, applying both multiplicative and additive interaction analyses.

Methods

Study population

Detailed descriptions of the CKB have been given elsewhere [14, 15]. Briefly, a total of 512,891 participants aged 30–79 years were recruited in 2004–2008 from five urban and five rural regions in China. Eligible participants were invited to a community assessment center and completed an interviewer-administered electronic questionnaire, physical measurements, and blood spot tests for random blood glucose and HBsAg. A 10 ml non-fasting blood sample for each participant was also collected and shipped to the central blood repository for long-term storage. The study protocol was approved by the Ethics Review Committee of the Chinese Center for Disease Control and Prevention (Beijing, China) and the Oxford Tropical Research Ethics Committee, University of Oxford (UK). All participants provided written informed consent before taking part in the study.

In the present analysis, we excluded participants who reported having been diagnosed with CKD ($n = 7577$), heart disease ($n = 15,472$), stroke ($n = 8884$), or cancer ($n = 2577$) by a qualified doctor. We also excluded participants with missing data or an unclear result for HBsAg ($n = 11,136$) or missing data for body mass index (BMI; $n = 2$), plus one participant who was lost to follow-up shortly after baseline ($n = 1$). After these exclusions, 469,459 participants remained for the final analyses.

Assessment of exposure

At baseline, the whole venous blood of participants was qualitatively tested for HBsAg using on-site rapid test strips (ACON dipstick, USA) (negative, positive, or unclear). All participants also completed interviewer-administered laptop-based questionnaires and were asked if they had ever been diagnosed with chronic hepatitis (not limited to chronic viral hepatitis) or liver cirrhosis (yes or no) by a doctor. For those who reported a prior medical history of the disease, we further asked their age at the first diagnosis, and if they were still on treatment (not specifically anti-HBV treatment; yes or no).

Assessment of covariates

Covariate information was obtained from the baseline questionnaire, including socio-demographic status (age, sex, education, occupation, household income, and marital status), lifestyle behaviors (alcohol consumption, tobacco smoking, physical activity, and intake of red meat, fresh fruit, and fresh vegetables), personal medical history (hypertension, diabetes, and rheumatic arthritis) and women's menopause status. In the present analysis, we included in the current smoker category former smokers who had stopped smoking due to illness to avoid a misleadingly elevated risk. The daily level of physical activity was calculated by multiplying the metabolic equivalent tasks (METs) value for a particular type of physical activity by hours spent on that activity per day and summing the MET-hours for all activities.

Trained staff undertook baseline measurements of body weight, height, waist circumference, and blood pressure. BMI was calculated as weight in kilograms divided by the square of the height in meters. Prevalent hypertension was defined as measured systolic blood pressure ≥140 mmHg, measured diastolic blood pressure ≥90 mmHg, self-reported prior diagnosis of hypertension, or self-reported use of antihypertensive medication at baseline. Prevalent diabetes was defined as measured fasting blood glucose ≥7.0 mmol/l, measured random blood glucose ≥11.1 mmol/l, or self-reported prior diagnosis of diabetes at baseline.

Ascertainment of incident chronic kidney disease

Incident CKD cases were identified by linking local disease and death registries, linking the national health insurance (HI) system, and by active follow-up (i.e., visiting local communities or directly contacting participants). In particular, the electronic linkage with the HI claims database is one of the most important means of ascertaining CKD cases in the present study. The HI data are comprehensive and contain information on all diagnoses and treatments prescribed to patients who sought health care in a hospital. Successful linkage to the HI system was achieved for more than 96% of the CKB participants in 2015, which was similar across ten survey sites. Trained staff blinded to baseline information coded all diagnoses using the International Classification of Diseases, Tenth Revision (ICD-10). The outcome of the present analysis was CKD, including diabetes mellitus with renal complications (E10.2, E11.2, E12.2, E13.2, and E14.2), hypertensive renal disease (I12 and I13), glomerular disease (N03, N04, N05, and N07), renal tubulo-interstitial disease (N11, N12, N13, N14, and N15), and renal failure (N18 and N19).

Statistical analysis
Participants contributed person-time from baseline until the date of CKD diagnosis, death, loss to follow-up, or 31 December 2015, whichever came first. We used a multivariable Cox proportional hazards model to estimate the hazard ratio (HR) and 95% confidence interval (CI), with age as the underlying time scale, stratified by 5-year age groups and ten survey sites. The proportional hazards assumption for the Cox model was checked using Schoenfeld residuals, and no violation was found.

Multivariable models for association between chronic HBV infection and CKD risk were adjusted for age; sex (for whole cohort); level of education; marital status; alcohol consumption; smoking status; physical activity; frequencies of intake of red meat, fresh fruit, and fresh vegetables; menopausal status (for women only); BMI; prevalent diabetes; and prevalent hypertension. We further explored whether the association was mediated by the presence of chronic hepatitis or cirrhosis by adjusting for a composite variable of disease duration and treatment status at baseline.

In the sensitivity analyses, we excluded participants whose outcome occurred during the first 2 years of follow-up. We additionally adjusted for occupation, household income, waist circumference, systolic blood pressure, and prevalent rheumatic arthritis at baseline separately. We further included participants with medical histories of heart disease or stroke at baseline and additionally adjusted for these two variables. The risk estimates did not change materially (data not shown).

We examined whether the association of HBsAg status with CKD risk differed by demographics, lifestyles, and co-morbidities on both multiplicative and additive scales. Prespecified baseline subgroups included sex (men or

women), age at baseline (<50 or ≥50 years), residence (urban or rural), smoking status (daily smoker or not), alcohol consumption (daily drinker or not), level of physical activity (categorized using sex-specific tertile cutoffs, the lowest tertile or others), BMI (<24.0 or ≥24.0 kg/m^2), prevalent diabetes (presence or absence), and prevalent hypertension (presence or absence). We tested multiplicative interaction by using likelihood ratio test comparing models with and without a cross-product term. We assessed additive interaction by estimating the relative excess risk due to interaction (RERI) [16]. A RERI of 0 indicates no interaction on the additive scale and >0 indicates a synergistic interaction. We further decomposed the joint effect of two exposures, that is, comparing both exposures present to both absent, into three components: the proportions attributable to HBsAg positivity alone, to the prespecified baseline variable alone, and to their interaction [16, 17].

We used Stata version 14.2 (StataCorp, TX, USA) to analyze the data. Statistical significance was set at two-tailed $P < 0.05$.

Results
Of all 469,459 participants, 41.0% were men, and 56.4% resided in rural areas. HBsAg-positive participants were more likely to be men and urban residents, and report having prevalent chronic hepatitis or liver cirrhosis. Among participants with chronic hepatitis or liver cirrhosis, HBsAg-positive participants were more likely to be under treatment at baseline (Table 1).

During a median of 9.1 years (interquartile range 1.88 years; 4.2 million person-years) of follow-up, we documented 1762 incident CKD cases among men and 2793 among women. In the multivariable-adjusted model, HBsAg positivity was significantly associated with a higher risk of incident CKD (Table 2). In all eligible participants, compared with HBsAg-negative participants, the HRs (95% CIs) for CKD were 1.37 (1.18, 1.60) for HBsAg-positive participants. The association between HBsAg status and CKD risk was stronger in men (HR = 1.77; 95% CI: 1.43, 2.20) than in women (HR = 1.10; 95% CI: 0.88, 1.36) ($P = 0.007$ for interaction with sex). Further adjustment for the presence of chronic hepatitis or cirrhosis at baseline did not change the association materially.

We further examined the joint association of HBsAg status and presence of chronic hepatitis or cirrhosis and its treatment status with CKD risk (Table 3). Compared with HBsAg-negative participants without chronic hepatitis or cirrhosis, those who were HBsAg positive and had chronic hepatitis or cirrhosis under treatment at baseline had the greatest risk of developing CKD (HR = 4.74; 95% CI: 2.68, 8.36). The magnitude of risk was similar in men and women ($P = 0.061$ for interaction with sex). Male participants who were HBsAg positive but without chronic hepatitis or cirrhosis or not on

Table 1 Baseline characteristics according to HBsAg status at baseline for 469,459 participants

	HBsAg negative	HBsAg positive	p value
Number of participants	454,588	14,871	
Age (years)	51.1	48.6	<0.001
Men (%)	40.8	46.9	<0.001
Rural area (%)	56.7	48.7	<0.001
Married (%)	90.9	90.3	0.024
Middle school and higher (%)	49.5	47.4	<0.001
Daily smoker (%)			
Men	67.7	68.4	0.231
Women	2.6	2.9	0.104
Daily drinker (%)			
Men	20.9	20.2	0.165
Women	0.9	1.1	0.046
Physical activity (MET-h/day)	21.5	21.4	0.650
Weekly consumption*			
Red meat (day)	3.7	3.7	0.002
Fresh vegetables (day)	6.8	6.8	0.738
Fresh fruit (day)	2.5	2.5	0.014
Body mass index (kg/m^2)[†]	23.6	23.5	<0.001
Postmenopausal (%)	50.7	50.9	0.521
Prevalent diabetes (%)[†]	5.4	5.7	0.075
Prevalent hypertension (%)[†]	33.9	32.3	< 0.001
Prevalent rheumatic arthritis (%)	1.9	1.8	0.448
Prevalent chronic hepatitis or cirrhosis (%)	0.8	10.8	< 0.001
Medical history (years)[‡]	17.2	12.6	< 0.001
Under treatment at baseline (%)[‡]	10.4	19.1	< 0.001

All variables were adjusted for age, sex, and survey sites, as appropriate
HBsAg hepatitis virus B surface antigen, MET metabolic equivalent of task
*Weekly consumption of red meat, fresh vegetables, and fresh fruit was calculated by assigning participants to the midpoint of their consumption category
[†]Variables obtained or partly obtained by physical measurements. Other variables were obtained through the questionnaire
[‡]Among participants with prevalent chronic hepatitis or cirrhosis at baseline

Table 2 HRs (95% CIs) for incident chronic kidney disease according to HBsAg status among 469,459 participants

	HBsAg negative	HBsAg positive	p value
Whole cohort			
Number of cases	4381	174	
Cases/PY (1000)	1.07	1.33	
Age and sex adjusted	1.00	1.36 (1.17, 1.59)	<0.001
Multivariable adjusted*	1.00	1.37 (1.18, 1.60)	<0.001
+ Presence of hepatitis or cirrhosis[†]	1.00	1.33 (1.14, 1.55)	<0.001
Men			
Number of cases	1671	91	
Cases/PY (1000)	1.02	1.54	
Age adjusted	1.00	1.81 (1.46, 2.24)	<0.001
Multivariable adjusted*	1.00	1.77 (1.43, 2.20)	<0.001
+ Presence of hepatitis or cirrhosis[†]	1.00	1.72 (1.38, 2.14)	<0.001
Women			
Number of cases	2710	83	
Cases/PY (1000)	1.11	1.15	
Age adjusted	1.00	1.08 (0.86, 1.34)	0.517
Multivariable adjusted*	1.00	1.10 (0.88, 1.36)	0.414
+ Presence of hepatitis or cirrhosis[†]	1.00	1.06 (0.85, 1.33)	0.606

CI confidence interval, HBsAg hepatitis virus B surface antigen, HR hazard ratio, PY person-year
*Multivariable model was adjusted for: age (years); sex (men or women, for whole cohort); level of education (no formal school, primary school, middle school, high school, college, or university or higher); marital status (married, widowed, divorced or separated, or never married); alcohol consumption (less than weekly drinker, weekly drinker, daily drinker with an intake of <15, 15–29, 30–59, or ≥60 g/day); smoking status (nonsmoker, former smoker having quit smoking ≥5 or <5 years previously, or current daily smoker smoking <15, 15–24, or ≥25 cigarettes or equivalents per day); physical activity (MET-h/day); intake frequencies of red meat, fresh fruit, and fresh vegetables (daily, 4–6 days/week, 1–3 days/week, monthly, or rarely or never); body mass index (kg/m^2); menopausal status (premenopausal, perimenopausal, or postmenopausal; for women only); prevalent diabetes; and prevalent hypertension at baseline (presence or absence)
[†]A composite variable of disease status (absence or presence), duration (< 15 or ≥ 15 years), and treatment status at baseline (no or yes)

treatment also showed a moderate increase in the CKD risk. HBsAg-positive participants who had been diagnosed with chronic hepatitis or cirrhosis for ≥15 years had a slightly higher risk of developing CKD compared with those diagnosed for <15 years (see Additional file 1).

We examined the association between HBsAg status and CKD risk according to potential baseline risk factors. Notably, the effect of HBsAg positivity interacted with the effect of smoking, physical inactivity, or prevalent diabetes on CKD risk, on multiplicative and/or additive scales (Table 4). The positive association between HBsAg status and CKD risk was stronger in those who were smokers, less physically active, or diabetic. Compared

with HBsAg-negative participants who were non-smokers, more physically active, or did not have diabetes at baseline, HBsAg-positive participants had the greatest risk of developing CKD if they were smokers (HR = 1.85; 95% CI: 1.44, 2.38), physically inactive (HR = 1.91; 95% CI: 1.52, 2.40), or diabetic (HR = 6.11; 95% CI: 4.47, 8.36). We observed positive additive interactions of HBsAg positivity with smoking, physical inactivity, or diabetes on CKD risk, with all corresponding RERI > 0. The proportion of risk (%) in the doubly exposed group attributable to the interaction with HBsAg positivity was 66.3 (32.4, 100.3) for smoking, 79.1 (50.5, 107.7) for physical inactivity, and 48.0 (27.7, 68.3) for diabetes, respectively. No statistically significant interaction was observed

Table 3 HRs (95% CIs) for incident chronic kidney disease according to HBsAg status and presence of chronic hepatitis or cirrhosis and its treatment status at baseline for 469,459 participants

	HBsAg negative		HBsAg positive		
	Without hepatitis or cirrhosis	With hepatitis or cirrhosis	Without hepatitis or cirrhosis	With hepatitis or cirrhosis	
				Without treatment	With treatment
Whole cohort					
Number of cases	4339	42	143	19	12
Cases/PY (1000)	1.07	1.28	1.22	1.62	5.03
HR (95% CI)	1.00	0.99 (0.73, 1.35)	1.27 (1.08, 1.51)	1.57 (1.00, 2.46)	4.74 (2.68, 8.36)
p value	–	0.961	0.004	0.052	<0.001
Men					
Number of cases	1652	19	72	12	7
Cases/PY (1000)	1.02	0.99	1.41	1.86	4.26
HR (95% CI)	1.00	0.85 (0.54, 1.34)	1.63 (1.29, 2.07)	2.10 (1.19, 3.72)	4.64 (2.20, 9.80)
p value	–	0.484	<0.001	0.011	<0.001
Women					
Number of cases	2687	23	71	7	5
Cases/PY (1000)	1.11	1.69	1.08	1.32	6.71
HR (95% CI)	1.00	1.20 (0.79, 1.81)	1.03 (0.82, 1.31)	1.15 (0.55, 2.42)	5.25 (2.18, 12.66)
p value	–	0.390	0.775	0.712	<0.001

CI confidence interval, *HBsAg* hepatitis virus B surface antigen, *HR* hazard ratio, *PY* person-year

Multivariable model was adjusted for: age (years); sex (men or women, for whole cohort); level of education (no formal school, primary school, middle school, high school, college, or university or higher); marital status (married, widowed, divorced or separated, or never married); alcohol consumption (less than weekly drinker, weekly drinker, daily drinker with an intake of <15, 15–29, 30–59, or ≥60 g/day); smoking status (nonsmoker, former smoker having quit smoking ≥5 or <5 years previously, or current daily smoker smoking <15, 15–24, or ≥25 cigarettes or equivalents per day); physical activity (MET-h/day); intake frequencies of red meat, fresh fruit, and fresh vegetables (daily, 4–6 days/week, 1–3 days/week, monthly, rarely, or never); body mass index (kg/m^2); menopausal status (premenopausal, perimenopausal, or postmenopausal; for women only); prevalent diabetes; and prevalent hypertension at baseline (presence or absence)

for the following baseline factors on both multiplicative and additive scales: age, rural or urban residence, alcohol consumption, BMI, and prevalent hypertension (see Additional file 2).

Discussion

In this large prospective Chinese adult cohort, we found that chronic HBV infection was associated with a 37% increased risk of CKD. The association was stronger in men than in women. In addition, the joint effects of chronic HBV infection with smoking, physical inactivity, or prevalent diabetes on CKD risk were more than the addition of the risk associated with each of these factors.

To our knowledge, only two prospective studies have examined the association between HBV infection and CKD risk. In a study using claims data from the Taiwan National Health Insurance Research Database, 17,796 adults with untreated HBV infection and 71,184 matched controls were compared and showed an increased risk of CKD associated with chronic HBV infection (HR = 2.58; 95% CI: 1.95, 3.42) during a mean 6.5 years of follow-up [11]. However, in another study conducted for 4329 adults who received regular healthy check-ups in a Chinese hospital, occult HBV infection, defined as seropositive for antibodies to the HBV core

antigen, was not associated with CKD in the subsequent 5 years (odds ratio = 1.12; 95% CI: 0.65, 1.95) [12]. In the present study, we associated chronic HBV infection, characterized by HBsAg positivity, with a higher risk of incident CKD over a period of close to 10 years. The risk estimates of CKD did not change materially after adjusting for chronic hepatitis or cirrhosis at baseline, suggesting that these conditions might not be the causal intermediates from HBV infection to CKD. The presence of chronic hepatitis or cirrhosis and receiving treatment at baseline might be an indicator of long-term active virus replication with a higher risk of causing damage, and was associated with the greatest CKD risk in the present population. Also, we cannot rule out the possibility that some medications for chronic liver diseases are nephrotoxic. However, in the present study, HBsAg-positive participants, without hepatitis or cirrhosis or not on treatment at baseline, still showed an increased risk of developing CKD.

The pathogenesis of HBV-associated nephropathy remains unclear, and several mechanisms have been implicated. Steatosis, a typical feature of chronic HBV infection, could induce lipid peroxidation and increase plasma inflammatory biomarkers, leading to endothelial dysfunction and renal injury [18]. It is also suggested that

Table 4 HRs (95% CIs) for chronic kidney disease in relation to HBsAg status by potential baseline risk factors among 469,459 participants

Variable of interest	HBsAg	Number of cases	Cases/PY (1000)	Multiplicative interaction			Additive interaction			
				Stratum-specific HR (95% CI)	p_{Int-M}*	HR (95% CI) p_{Int-A}†	RERI	Attributable proportion, %		
								HBV infection	Variable of interest	Additive interaction
Daily smoking										
No	Negative	3166	1.09	1.00	0.030	1.00 0.030	0.56 (0.05, 1.07)	25.5 (−5.0, 56.1)	8.2 (−16.3, 32.6)	66.3 (32.4, 100.3)
No	Positive	108	1.20	1.20 (0.99, 1.45)		1.22 (1.00, 1.47)				
Yes	Negative	1215	1.03	1.00		1.07 (0.97, 1.18)				
Yes	Positive	66	1.59	1.83 (1.42, 2.34)		1.85 (1.44, 2.38)				
Physical inactivity‡										
No	Negative	2721	0.99	1.00	0.003	1.00 0.004	0.72 (0.23, 1.21)	15.9 (−10.6, 42.3)	5.0 (−18.4, 28.4)	79.1 (50.5, 107.7)
No	Positive	97	1.07	1.15 (0.94, 1.41)		1.14 (0.93, 1.40)				
Yes	Negative	1660	1.24	1.00		1.05 (0.97, 1.12)				
Yes	Positive	77	1.90	1.80 (1.43, 2.27)		1.91 (1.52, 2.40)				
Prevalent diabetes										
No	Negative	3519	0.91	1.00	0.068	1.00 0.012	2.45 (0.53, 4.38)	5.4 (0.7, 10.2)	46.6 (25.9, 67.2)	48.0 (27.7, 68.3)
No	Positive	134	1.07	1.28 (1.07, 1.52)		1.28 (1.08, 1.52)				
Yes	Negative	862	4.11	1.00		3.38 (3.13, 3.66)				
Yes	Positive	40	6.54	1.77 (1.28, 2.44)		6.11 (4.47, 8.36)				

CI confidence interval, *HBsAg* hepatitis virus B surface antigen, *HR* hazard ratio, *PY* person-year, *RERI* relative excess risk due to interaction

*p value for multiplicative interaction

†p value for additive interaction

‡Defined as <13.4 or <12.4 MET-h/day for men or women respectively

Multivariable model was adjusted for: age (years); sex (men or women, for whole cohort); level of education (no formal school, primary school, middle school, high school, college, or university or higher); marital status (married, widowed, divorced or separated, or never married); alcohol consumption (less than weekly drinker, weekly drinker, daily drinker with an intake of <15, 15–29, 30–59, or ≥60 g/day); intake frequencies of red meat, fresh fruit, and fresh vegetables (daily, 4–6 days/week, 1–3 days/week, monthly, rarely, or never); body mass index (kg/m²); menopausal status (premenopausal, perimenopausal, or postmenopausal; for women only); and prevalent hypertension at baseline (presence or absence). The variables of smoking status (nonsmoker, former smoker having quit smoking ≥5 or <5 years previously, or current daily smoker smoking <15, 15–24, or ≥25 cigarettes or equivalents per day), physical activity (MET-h/day), and prevalent diabetes were adjusted for in the multivariable model except for their own subgroup analysis

HBV carriers are more likely to have increased insulin resistance and a higher circulating level of transforming growth factor ß, contributing to the potentiation of apoptosis and renal fibrosis [19, 20]. It has been shown that men are more likely to develop steatosis [21] and have a lower HBV clearance than women [22]. It is consistent with our findings that the association between HBV infection and CKD is stronger in men than women.

Our in-depth analyses suggested important interactions of chronic HBV infection with tobacco smoking, physical inactivity, or diabetes on the CKD risk on both multiplicative and additive scales. The additive interaction is more relevant to public health measures than the multiplicative interaction. We found that about two-thirds of CKD cases among a population with chronic HBV infection who smoke tobacco would occur if both exposures were present but not if only one or the other was present. A similar additive interaction was found for HBV infection with physical inactivity or with diabetes on the CKD risk. These findings imply that the public health consequences of quitting smoking, increasing physical activity, and improving glucose control would be larger in participants with chronic HBV infection.

The synergistic effects of chronic HBV infection with individual lifestyle factors and conditions on CKD risk are biologically plausible, consistent with previous studies that the pathogenesis of HBV-associated nephropathy depends on interactions between viral, host, and environmental factors [23]. The adverse impact of chronic HBV infection on CKD might be exacerbated by smoking-induced renal atherosclerosis [24] and endothelial dysfunction [25], and attenuated by reduced oxidative stress and reduced inflammation with increasing physical activity [26]. Similarly, HBV infection and hyperglycemia-induced metabolic and hemodynamic pathways might be interwoven together in the pathogenesis of kidney injury [27, 28]. The mechanisms for their synergistic effects on CKD still warrant further elucidation.

To the best of our knowledge, the present study has been, by far, the largest prospective study examining the association between chronic HBV infection and CKD risk. For the first time, this study provides compelling evidence of the synergistic effects of chronic HBV infection with tobacco smoking, physical inactivity, or diabetes on CKD risk. Strengths of the study include its prospective design, large sample size, long follow-up period, the inclusion of a geographically spread Chinese population living in urban and rural areas, and careful adjustment for potential confounders.

This study acknowledges some limitations. We used an on-site HBsAg rapid test because it was feasible for a large-scale population study, but there was the possibility of misclassification. However, measurement errors in the prospective study may be nondifferential on subsequent disease status and may have attenuated our findings towards the null. Participants were excluded from the study based on self-reporting of a prediagnosed CKD at baseline. Underreporting of the subclinical or early stage of CKD might exist, leading to overestimation of CKD incidence during the follow-up. However, after excluding participants whose outcome occurred during the first 2 years of follow-up, the risk estimates remained largely unchanged. Also, the incident cases of CKD in this study were mainly identified using a linkage with the HI system. Some asymptomatic or mild cases might have been missed, resulting in nondifferential outcome misclassification and attenuation of the effect estimates. Lack of detailed information about viral load, antiviral treatment (especially the use of nephrotoxic drugs), or any biochemistry data indicating liver function precluded further analysis.

Conclusions

In this large prospective study, we found that participants with chronic HBV infection had an increased risk of CKD. HBV infection exhibited noticeable synergistic effects with smoking, less physical activity, or diabetes on the CKD risk. In countries with an intermediate and high endemicity of HBV infection, kidney damage associated with chronic HBV infection should be a non-negligible concern. Our study also highlights the importance of health advice on quitting smoking, increasing physical activity, improving glucose control, and early screening for the CKD in people with chronic HBV infection. More studies are warranted to confirm the results of this study and clarify the underlying mechanism of the association.

Abbreviations
BMI: Body mass index; CI: Confidence interval; CKB: China Kadoorie Biobank; CKD: Chronic kidney disease; HBsAg: Hepatitis B surface antigen; HBV: Hepatitis B virus; HI: Health insurance; HR: Hazard ratio; ICD-10: International Classification of Diseases, Tenth Revision; MET: Metabolic equivalent task; RERI: Relative excess risk due to interaction

Acknowledgments
The most important acknowledgment is to the participants in the study and the members of the survey teams in each of the ten regional centres, as well as to the project development and management teams based at Beijing, Oxford, and the ten regional centres.
The members of the steering committee and collaborative group are listed in the online-only supplementary appendix (see Additional file 3).

Funding
This work was supported by grants (81390540, 81390544, and 81390541; http://www.nsfc.gov.cn) from the National Natural Science Foundation of China and grants (2016YFC0900500, 2016YFC0900501, and 2016YFC0900504) from the National Key Research and Development Program of China. The CKB baseline survey and the first re-survey were supported by a grant from the Kadoorie Charitable Foundation in Hong Kong. The long-term follow-up is supported by grants from the UK Wellcome Trust (202922/Z/16/Z, 088158/Z/09/Z, and 104085/Z/14/Z; http://www.wellcome.ac.uk/) and the Chinese Ministry of Science and Technology (2011BAI09B01). The funders had no role in study design, data collection and analysis, decision to publish, or preparation of the manuscript.

Authors' contributions
JLv and LL conceived and designed the paper. LL, ZC, and JC, as members of the CKB steering committee, designed and supervised the conduct of the whole study, obtained funding, and together with YG, ZB, LYang, YC, LYin, HL, and JLan acquired the data. JS, CY, and CQ analyzed the data. JS and JLv drafted the manuscript. JLv, LL, CY, YG, ZB, CQ, LYang, YC, LYin, HL, JLan, JC, and ZC contributed to the interpretation of the results and critical revision of the manuscript for important intellectual content. All authors contributed to and approved the final manuscript. JLv is the study guarantor.

Competing interests
The authors declare that they have no competing interests.

Author details
[1]Department of Epidemiology and Biostatistics, School of Public Health, Peking University Health Science Center, 38 Xueyuan Road, Beijing 100191, China. [2]Chinese Academy of Medical Sciences, Beijing, China. [3]Clinical Trial Service Unit & Epidemiological Studies Unit (CTSU), Nuffield Department of Population Health, University of Oxford, Oxford, UK. [4]Hunan Center for Disease Control & Prevention, Changsha, Hunan, China. [5]Liuzhou Traditional Chinese Medical Hospital, Liuzhou, Guangxi, China. [6]Liuzhou Center for Disease Control & Prevention, Liuzhou, Guangxi, China. [7]China National Center for Food Safety Risk Assessment, Beijing, China. [8]Peking University Institute of Environmental Medicine, Beijing, China.

References
1. Nugent RA, Fathima SF, Feigl AB, Chyung D. The burden of chronic kidney disease on developing nations: a 21st century challenge in Global Health. Nephron Clin Pract. 2011;118(3):c269–77.
2. Zhang L, Wang F, Wang L, et al. Prevalence of chronic kidney disease in China: a cross-sectional survey. Lancet. 2012;379(9818):815–22.
3. Hallan SI, Coresh J, Astor BC, et al. International comparison of the

relationship of chronic kidney disease prevalence and ESRD risk. J Am Soc Nephrol JASN. 2006;17(8):2275–84.

4. Coresh J, Selvin E, Stevens LA, et al. Prevalence of chronic kidney disease in the United States. JAMA. 2007;298(17):2038–47.

5. Levey AS, Coresh J. Chronic kidney disease. Lancet. 2012;379(9811):165–80.

6. Drawz P, Rahman M. Chronic kidney disease. Ann Intern Med. 2015;162(11):1–16.

7. Johnson RJ, Couser WG. Hepatitis B infection and renal disease: clinical, immunopathogenetic and therapeutic considerations. Kidney Int. 1990;37(2):663–76.

8. Lai KN, Li PK, Lui SF, et al. Membranous nephropathy related to hepatitis B virus in adults. N Engl J Med. 1991;324(21):1457–63.

9. Amet S, Bronowicki J-P, Thabut D, et al. Prevalence of renal abnormalities in chronic HBV infection: the HARPE study. Liver Int. 2015;35(1):148–55.

10. Fabrizi F, Donato FM, Messa P. Association between hepatitis B virus and chronic kidney disease: a systematic review and meta-analysis. Ann Hepatol. 2017;16(1):21–47.

11. Chen YC, Su YC, Li CY, Hung SK. 13-year nationwide cohort study of chronic kidney disease risk among treatment-naïve patients with chronic hepatitis B in Taiwan. BMC Nephrol. 2015;16:110.

12. Kong XL, Ma XJ, Su H, Xu DM. Relationship between occult hepatitis B virus infection and chronic kidney disease in a Chinese population-based cohort. Chronic Dis Transl Med. 2016;2(1):55–60.

13. Schweitzer A, Horn J, Mikolajczyk RT, Krause G, Ott JJ. Estimations of worldwide prevalence of chronic hepatitis B virus infection: a systematic review of data published between 1965 and 2013. Lancet Lond Engl. 2015; 386(10003):1546–55.

14. Chen Z, Chen J, Collins R, et al. China Kadoorie biobank of 0.5 million people: survey methods, baseline characteristics and long-term follow-up. Int J Epidemiol. 2011;40(6):1652–66.

15. Chen Z, Lee L, Chen J, et al. Cohort profile: the Kadoorie study of chronic disease in China (KSCDC). Int J Epidemiol. 2005;34(6):1243–9.

16. VanderWeele TJ, Knol MJ. A tutorial on interaction. Epidemiol Methods. 2014;3(1):33–72.

17. VanderWeele TJ, Tchetgen Tchetgen EJ. Attributing effects to interactions. Epidemiol Camb Mass. 2014;25(5):711–22.

18. Chaabane NB, Loghmari H, Melki W, et al. Chronic viral hepatitis and kidney failure. Presse Med. 2008;37(4 Pt 2):665–78.

19. Ishizaka N, Ishizaka Y, Seki G, Nagai R, Yamakado M, Koike K. Association between hepatitis B/C viral infection, chronic kidney disease and insulin resistance in individuals undergoing general health screening. Hepatol Res Off J Jpn Soc Hepatol. 2008;38(8):775–83.

20. Deng CL, Song XW, Liang HJ, Feng C, Sheng YJ, Wang MY. Chronic hepatitis B serum promotes apoptotic damage in human renal tubular cells. World J Gastroenterol. 2006;12(11):1752–6.

21. Machado MV, Oliveira AG, Cortez-Pinto H. Hepatic steatosis in hepatitis B virus infected patients: meta-analysis of risk factors and comparison with hepatitis C infected patients. J Gastroenterol Hepatol. 2011;26(9):1361–7.

22. London WT, Drew JS. Sex differences in response to hepatitis B infection among patients receiving chronic dialysis treatment. Proc Natl Acad Sci U S A. 1977;74(6):2561–3.

23. Bhimma R, Coovadia HM. Hepatitis B virus-associated nephropathy. Am J Nephrol. 2004;24(2):198–211.

24. Barua RS, Sharma M, Dileepan KN. Cigarette smoke amplifies inflammatory response and atherosclerosis progression through activation of the H1R-TLR2/4-COX2 Axis. Front Immunol. 2015;6:572.

25. Li H, Horke S, Förstermann U. Oxidative stress in vascular disease and its pharmacological prevention. Trends Pharmacol Sci. 2013;34(6):313–9.

26. Samjoo IA, Safdar A, Hamadeh MJ, Raha S, Tarnopolsky MA. The effect of endurance exercise on both skeletal muscle and systemic oxidative stress in previously sedentary obese men. Nutr Diabetes. 2013;3(9):e88.

27. Satirapoj B. Nephropathy in diabetes. Adv Exp Med Biol. 2012;771:107–22.

28. Zhang J, Shen Y, Cai H, Liu YM, Qin G. Hepatitis B virus infection status and risk of type 2 diabetes mellitus: a meta-analysis. Hepatol Res. 2015;45(11):1100–9.

15

Inflammation and micronutrient biomarkers predict clinical HIV treatment failure and incident active TB in HIV-infected adults

Rupak Shivakoti[1,17]* ⬤, Nikhil Gupte[1], Srikanth Tripathy[2,18], Selvamuthu Poongulali[3], Cecilia Kanyama[4], Sima Berendes[5,19], Sandra W. Cardoso[6], Breno R. Santos[7], Alberto La Rosa[8], Noluthando Mwelase[9], Sandy Pillay[10], Wadzanai Samaneka[11], Cynthia Riviere[12], Patcharaphan Sugandhavesa[13], Robert C. Bollinger[1,15], Ashwin Balagopal[1], Richard D. Semba[14], Parul Christian[15,20], Thomas B. Campbell[16], Amita Gupta[1] and for the NWCS 319 and PEARLS Study Team

Abstract

Background: Various individual biomarkers of inflammation and micronutrient status, often correlated with each other, are associated with adverse treatment outcomes in human immunodeficiency virus (HIV)-infected adults. The objective of this study was to conduct exploratory factor analysis (EFA) on multiple inflammation and micronutrient biomarkers to identify biomarker groupings (factors) and determine their association with HIV clinical treatment failure (CTF) and incident active tuberculosis (TB).

Methods: Within a multicountry randomized trial of antiretroviral therapy (ART) efficacy (PEARLS) among HIV-infected adults, we nested a case-control study ($n = 290$; 124 cases, 166 controls) to identify underlying factors, based on EFA of 23 baseline (pre-ART) biomarkers of inflammation and micronutrient status. The EFA biomarker groupings results were used in Cox proportional hazards models to study the association with CTF (primary analysis where cases were incident World Health Organization stage 3, 4 or death by 96 weeks of ART) or incident active TB (secondary analysis).

Results: In the primary analysis, based on eigenvalues> 1 in the EFA, three factors were extracted: (1) carotenoids), (2) other nutrients, and (3) inflammation. In multivariable-adjusted models, there was an increased hazard of CTF (adjusted hazard ratio (aHR) 1.47, 95% confidence interval (CI)1.17–1.84) per unit increase of inflammation factor score. In the secondary incident active TB case-control analysis, higher scores of the high carotenoids and low interleukin-18 factor was protective against incident active TB (aHR 0.48, 95% CI 0.26–0.87).

Conclusion: Factors identified through EFA were associated with adverse outcomes in HIV-infected individuals. Strategies focused on reducing adverse HIV outcomes through therapeutic interventions that target the underlying factor (e.g., inflammation) rather than focusing on an individual observed biomarker might be more effective and warrant further investigation.

Keywords: HIV, Inflammation, Antiretroviral therapy, Tuberculosis, IL-18, Exploratory factor analysis

* Correspondence: rs3895@cumc.columbia.edu
[1]Department of Medicine, Johns Hopkins University School of Medicine, Baltimore, MD, USA
[17]Present Address: Department of Epidemiology, Columbia University Mailman School of Public Health, 722 West 168th St, Room 705, New York, NY 10032, USA
Full list of author information is available at the end of the article

Background

Single biomarkers have been assessed in antiretroviral therapy (ART)-naïve HIV-infected adults in multiple studies, and results show that specific biomarkers of inflammation or micronutrient concentrations are associated with adverse outcomes [1–4]. Various markers of inflammation, including C-reactive protein (CRP), soluble CD14 (sCD14), and various cytokines (e.g., interleukin-6 and 18 (IL-6 and IL-18)), are associated with increased mortality and morbidity [1–6]. Morbidity includes increased clinical treatment failure (CTF), risk of incident active TB, and even longer-term outcomes such as cardiovascular disease. Similarly, studies have shown that levels of various micronutrients such as vitamin D, selenium, and iron can also affect various HIV outcomes [7–11].

However, many of the inflammation markers are correlated with each other, such as in cases where they might be activated by the same stimuli or signaling pathway [12]. The nutritional biomarkers might also correlate with each other, for example, if different micronutrients are part of the same or similar foods [13]. Furthermore, there is evidence that inflammation and micronutrient status can directly affect each other. For example, studies show that circulating levels of selenium and zinc are reduced during the acute phase response [14, 15]. As a result, studies on the association of these biomarkers with outcomes might benefit from considering the relationship between these biomarkers.

Data reduction methods, such as exploratory factor analysis (EFA), have been useful in dealing with multicollinearity [16]. EFA is a statistical method for data reduction, in which numerous observed variables (e.g., circulating biomarkers) that co-vary with each other are assumed to reflect a smaller number of underlying unobserved variables ("factors") [17]. An important point to note for these analyses is that each individual will receive a score for each factor (i.e., an individual whose pattern poorly matches the factor gets a lower score), and the association of a specific factor with an outcome is compared between individuals with high and low scores of that factor, rather than between different factors.

Various studies have shown that factor analysis can identify biologically meaningful "biomarker superfamilies" which can be utilized to stratify individuals in high- and low-risk subgroups [12, 18–20] based on their factor score and potentially identify therapeutics that target the underlying factor rather than the individual observed variables. An example of the public health potential for EFA is evident in the field of nutrition and obesity where dietary patterns (e.g., high fat/low fiber pattern) are identified based on EFA and are part of the intervention (e.g., to consume less of that pattern) [21, 22].

The goal of this study was to conduct EFA on multiple observed biomarkers of inflammation and micronutrient status in HIV-infected adults initiating ART, in order to identify biomarker groupings that are hypothesized to represent underlying biological processes (factors) and to determine whether these factors were associated with adverse HIV outcomes including CTF (CTF as primary outcome) and incident active tuberculosis (TB) (TB as secondary outcome). To address this research question, we conducted nested case-control studies within a multicountry randomized clinical trial of ART efficacy (PEARLS) [23].

Methods
Study design and population

PEARLS was conducted from 2005 to 2010 (NCT00084136) [23] in 1571 ART-naïve HIV-infected adults from diverse settings to compare the efficacy of three different ART regimens: (1) efavirenz plus twice-daily lamivudine-zidovudine; (2) atazanavir plus didanosine EC and emtricitabine, all given once daily; or (3) efavirenz plus emtricitabine-tenofovir DF once daily. The primary efficacy outcome was treatment failure. PEARLS trial participants who met the inclusion criteria (including age greater than 18 years old and CD4+ T cell count less than 300 cells/mm^3) were recruited from nine different countries: Brazil ($n = 231$), Haiti ($n = 100$), India ($n = 255$), Malawi ($n = 221$), Peru ($n = 134$), South Africa ($n = 210$), Thailand ($n = 100$), the USA ($n = 210$), and Zimbabwe ($n = 110$). Pregnant women and individuals with an acute illness or severe anemia were excluded from the study. Detailed inclusion and exclusion criteria for PEARLS are described elsewhere [23].

For this study, we nested a case-control analysis ($n = 290$; 124 cases, 166 controls) within PEARLS to assess the association of baseline (pre-ART initiation) biomarkers of inflammation and micronutrients with CTF. CTF was defined as an incident World Health Organization (WHO) stage 3 or 4 event (including incident active TB) or death within 96 weeks post-ART initiation [24]. While all the cases from the parent study with available biomarker values were selected, controls (who did not develop clinical failure by 96 weeks) were selected based on random subsampling of the parent cohort stratified by country (the same approach used for secondary case controls).

Three other secondary nested case-control analyses were performed: severe outcome case control ($N = 254$; 81 cases and 173 controls), virologic failure case control ($N = 260$; 90 cases and 170 controls), and incident active TB case control ($N = 220$; 47 cases and 173 controls) analyses. The outcomes analyzed for these case controls were (1) severe outcomes defined as death, serious bacterial infections or sepsis, and opportunistic infections (including TB), (2) virologic failure defined as HIV-1 RNA levels ≥ 1000 copies/mL for two successive visits at ≥ 16 weeks after ART initiation, and (3) incident active TB defined as pulmonary or extrapulmonary TB that developed during the follow-up period (96 weeks post-ART initiation). We use the term "incident active TB" to define anyone who presented with signs or symptoms of TB disease and resulted in having confirmed or probable TB disease after entry into the study; the term does not distinguish between recently acquired TB through transmission, reactivation of TB, and subclinical/unmasked TB. Using standardized AIDS Clinical Trials Group (ACTG) definitions, incident active TB was defined as one of the following: confirmed pulmonary TB, probable pulmonary TB, confirmed extrapulmonary TB, probable extrapulmonary TB, and TB immune reconstitution inflammatory syndrome (TB-IRIS). While the diagnostic information is described in detail elsewhere [6], cases were considered confirmed if TB was isolated by culture, and they were considered probable based on signs and symptoms, acid-fast bacilli stain, x-rays, and TB treatment initiation. The definitions were standardized across the various sites, and the data for each diagnosis were reviewed by five physicians in the study team.

Data collection and laboratory analysis

Clinical history, including outcome assessment, was collected at baseline and at 2, 4, and 8 weeks post-ART initiation. After 8 weeks, clinical history was collected every 4 weeks through 24 weeks and every 8 weeks after that through 96 weeks. Plasma and serum samples were collected at baseline and other relevant time points and stored at $-80\,°C$.

The exposure variables (23 markers of inflammation and micronutrient status) were measured from plasma and serum samples collected at baseline (pre-ART initiation). Inflammation markers assessed in this study were interferon-γ (IFN-γ), IL-6, IFN-γ inducible protein (IP)-10, IL-18, tumor necrosis factor-α (TNF-α), CRP, sCD14, and EndoCAb immunoglobulin M (IgM). Luminex multiplex enzyme-linked immunosorbent assays (ELISAs) (R&D Systems, Minneapolis, MN, USA) were used to measure plasma levels of IFN-γ, IL-6, and TNF-α, while IP-10 was measured by MSD multiplex ELISAs (Meso Scale Discovery, Rockville, MD, USA). Single-plex ELISAs were used to measure plasma CRP, sCD14 (both R&D Systems), IL-18 (eBiosciences), and EndoCAb IgM (Cell Sciences, Canton, MA, USA). Further details on the inflammation markers are described elsewhere [6, 25].

The micronutrient markers assessed in this study were markers of vitamin A (retinol), vitamin B_6, vitamin B_{12}, vitamin D, vitamin E (α-tocopherol and γ-tocopherol), iron (ferritin and soluble transferrin receptor), selenium, and various carotenoids (α-carotene, β-carotene, β-cryptoxanthin, lutein, lycopene, and zeaxanthin). Details of assessment are described elsewhere [26]. Briefly,

serum ferritin (ALPCO, Salem, NH, USA) and soluble transferrin receptor (R&D Systems) were measured using an ELISA, while radioimmunoassay (DiaSorin, Saluggia, Italy) was used to measure total (D_2 and D_3) serum 25-hydoxyvitamin. High-performance liquid chromatography (HPLC) was used to measure serum vitamin B_6, retinol (vitamin A), and the carotenoids, as previously described [26]. Abbott AxSYM (Abbott Laboratories, Lake Bluff, IL, USA), an automated immunochemical analyzer, was used to measure serum vitamin B_{12}, while serum selenium was assessed with a Perkins-Elmer AAnalyst 600 graphite furnace atomic absorption spectrometer.

Potential confounders measured at baseline and included in multivariable models were body mass index (BMI), CD4+ T cell count, plasma HIV RNA, hemoglobin, and albumin. Plasma HIV-1 RNA was measured using the Roche Amplicor Monitor Assay (v1.5; Roche Molecular Systems, Branchburg, NJ, USA). Serum hemoglobin, albumin, and CD4+ T cell count were measured in the individual site laboratories that met the quality assurance standards of the NIH ACTG Network laboratory [23].

Statistical analyses

Twenty-three immune and micronutrient biomarkers were used to perform EFA, and the principal factor method was used, which is the default factor analysis method utilized by STATA software. In the principal factor method, the factor loadings are calculated using squared multiple correlations. While we also considered the proportion of variance explained, the final numbers of factors were extracted based on scree plots and eigenvalues (number of observed variables which the factor represents) greater than 1, as commonly done in EFA studies [27]. For simpler interpretation, factors were treated as orthogonal (where it is assumed that the factors themselves are not correlated to each other) and were rotated through the varimax method, which improves interpretability of orthogonal factors by rotating the axes so that each observed variable will load strongly on one of the factors [12]. Factor loadings above 0.3 were considered significant [28]; loadings are regression coefficients that describe the relationship between an unmeasured variable (i.e., an underlying factor which is not directly measured) and an observed/measured biomarker (a similar idea to correlation but not the same). The common characteristics among the high loading biomarkers for each factor were used for interpreting and naming the factors.

Based on the EFA, factor scores were generated for each participant, with higher scores indicating a higher standing in the scale (i.e., a better match to that factor). The factor scores of the individuals were used in univariable and multivariable Cox proportional hazard models to determine the association of each factor with outcome

(CTF, severe outcomes, or TB). Sex, age, country, BMI, baseline TB status, CD4 count, viral load, treatment arm (ART regimen), anemia, and hypoalbuminemia were adjusted for in multivariable models. Baseline TB status is a binary variable referring to prior (i.e., the patient had TB disease and TB treatment prior to study initiation) or prevalent TB (i.e., under TB treatment at baseline). Race was not used in multivariable models due to co-linearity with country. STATA version 13 was used for data analysis.

Note that although the source population for the severe outcomes and TB case controls was the same PEARLS study as for the CTF case control, the specific study population for each case control is different (due to the different case definitions). As a result, although factors are extracted independent of the outcome, the different case controls themselves could have different factor profiles since each case control has a different sample population.

Results

Study population characteristics
The baseline characteristics of the cases and controls in the CTF case-control population differed significantly by the following baseline characteristics: country ($p = 0.001$), BMI ($p = 0.001$), prior TB diagnosis ($p = 0.01$), CD4 T cell count, hypoalbuminemia, and anemia ($p < 0.001$ for all) (Table 1).

EFA and association with clinical treatment failure
From the CTF case-control EFA analysis, three underlying factors (Additional file 1: Table S1) were extracted based on correlations among the observed biomarkers (eigenvalues > 1). In an EFA, the names of the factors are given by the researchers after carefully examining what is common between the observed variables/biomarkers that have high loadings (correlation equivalent) on each factor.

Factor 1 (carotenoids) had high factor loadings (> 0.30) of carotenoids including α-carotene, β-carotene, β-cryptoxanthin, lutein, and zeaxanthin. Factor 2 (other nutrients) had high loadings of selenium, vitamin B_6, vitamin E (α-tocopherol), lycopene, α-carotene, and β-cryptoxanthin (the last three are carotenoids as well). Factor 3 (inflammation) had high loadings of C-reactive protein (CRP), soluble CD14 (sCD14), interleukin 18 (IL-18), and ferritin (an indicator of iron stores but also an acute phase protein) (Additional file 1: Table S1). As is common in factor analysis, some biomarkers (e.g., vitamin D) did not have high loadings in any of the three extracted factors.

Higher scores of the carotenoids and other nutrients factors were associated with reduced hazards of CTF in univariable models, but not in multivariable models that

Table 1 Characteristics of population by CTF cases and control status

Characteristic	All n = 290	CTF n = 124 (43%)	Controls n = 166 (57%)	p value[a]
Gender				
Male	160 (55)	71 (44)	89 (56)	0.55
Female	130 (45)	53 (41)	77 (59)	
Age (years)	35.0 (29.0–42.0)	35.5 (29.5–42.0)	35.0 (29.0–42.0)	0.81
Country				
Brazil	44 (15)	16 (36)	28 (64)	0.001
Haiti	34 (12)	11 (32)	23 (68)	
India	23 (8)	18 (78)	5 (22)	
Malawi	38 (13)	22 (58)	16 (42)	
Peru	19 (7)	4 (21)	15 (79)	
South Africa	38 (13)	20 (53)	18 (47)	
Thailand	23 (8)	6 (26)	17 (74)	
USA	44 (15)	17 (39)	27 (61)	
Zimbabwe	27 (9)	10 (37)	17 (63)	
Body mass index (kg/m²)				
< 18.5	29 (10)	18 (62)	11 (38)	0.001
18–25	192 (66)	89 (46)	103 (54)	
≥ 25	69 (24)	17 (25)	52 (75)	
Prior TB diagnosis				
Yes	59 (20)	34 (58)	25 (42)	0.01
No	231 (80)	90 (39)	141 (61)	
Treatment arm				
A	100 (35)	58 (56)	45 (44)	0.72
B	108 (37)	54 (42)	39 (58)	
C	82 (28)	67 (29)	27 (71)	
CD4 count (cells/mm³)				
< 100	103 (36)	50 (69)	22 (31)	< 0.001
100–200	93 (32)	45 (49)	46 (51)	
> 200	94 (34)	43 (41)	63 (59)	
Log viral load (copies/mL)				
< 4	21 (7)	6 (29)	15 (71)	0.18
4–5	98 (34)	38 (39)	60 (61)	
> 5	171 (59)	80 (47)	91 (53)	
Hypoalbuminemia				
Yes (≤ 3.5 g/dL)	77 (19)	51 (41)	26 (16)	< 0.001
No (> 3.5 g/dL)	215 (81)	73 (59)	140 (84)	
Anemia				
Yes	168 (58)	87 (54)	81 (46)	< 0.001
No	121 (42)	36 (50)	85 (50)	

Data are presented as number (%) of the CTF case control. Anemia is defined based on hemoglobin cutoffs for males (< 13.0 g/dL) and non-pregnant females (< 12.0 g/dL). [a]Fisher's exact test was used to calculate the p values for categorical variables, and the rank sum test for continuous variables adjusted for sex, age, country, BMI, baseline TB status, CD4 count, viral load, treatment arm, anemia, and hypoalbuminemia (Table 2). In contrast, higher scores of inflammation factor were associated with increased hazards of CTF in both univariable (hazard ratio (HR) 1.53; 95% confidence interval (CI) 1.32–1.77) and multivariable (adjusted HR (aHR) 1.47; 95% CI 1.17–1.84) analyses (Table 2).

As CTF is a composite diagnosis that includes multiple outcomes with a range in severity, we also assessed whether similar patterns were observed when we limited our analysis to more severe outcomes. In the severe outcome case-control population, cases and controls differed significantly by the following baseline characteristics: country (p = 0.01), BMI (p = 0.003), prior TB (p = 0.02), CD4 count, hypoalbuminemia, and anemia (all $p < 0.001$) (data not shown). For this severe outcome analysis, three factors were extracted based on the EFA (eigenvalues > 1). The factors extracted in this analysis had a remarkably similar profile to our prior analysis where CTF was the outcome (Additional file 2: Table S2). Factor 1 (carotenoids) and factor 2 (other nutrients) had high loadings of the same markers, while factor 3 (inflammation) had an additional marker with high loading (IP-10) (Additional file 2: Table S2). Similar to our analysis with CTF, higher scores of the carotenoids and other nutrients factor were associated with reduced hazards of severe outcomes in univariable but not multivariable models (Table 3). In contrast, higher scores of the inflammation factor had increased hazards of severe outcomes only in multivariable models (aHR 1.60; 95% CI 1.24–2.06) (Table 3).

In addition to severe outcomes, we also conducted a virologic failure case-control analysis. The factor profiles were very similar to those of the CTF and severe outcomes analysis, where three factors were extracted and had the same high loading markers (Additional file 3: Table S3). As with the CTF analysis, higher scores of the inflammation factor (but not the other two factors) were associated with increased hazards of virologic failure in both univariable (HR 1.32; 95% CI 1.11–1.56) and multivariable models (aHR 1.36; 95% CI 1.05–1.75) (Additional file 4: Table S4).

Table 2 Association of each factor with clinical treatment failure

	Univariable analysis HR (95% CI)	Multivariable analysis HR (95% CI)
Factor 1 (Carotenoids)	0.71 (0.56–0.90)	0.77 (0.57–1.05)
Factor 2 (Other nutrients)	0.79 (0.63–0.87)	0.83 (0.57–1.32)
Factor 3 (Inflammation)	1.53 (1.32–1.77)	1.47 (1.17–1.84)

The association of each factor with CTF was determined in univariable and multivariable Cox regression models. Sex, age, country, treatment arm, body mass index (BMI), baseline TB status, CD4 count, viral load, anemia, and hypoalbuminemia were adjusted for in the multivariable models. N = 290 (124 cases, 166 controls)

Table 3 Association of each factor with severe outcomes

	Univariable analysis HR (95% CI)	Multivariable analysis HR (95% CI)
Factor 1 (Carotenoids)	0.71 (0.52–0.95)	0.86 (0.58–1.26)
Factor 2 (Other nutrients)	0.75 (0.57–0.98)	0.78 (0.49–1.26)
Factor 3 (Inflammation)	0.97 (0.61–1.53)	1.60 (1.24–2.06)

The association of each factor with severe outcomes was determined in univariable and multivariable Cox regression models. Sex, age, country, treatment arm, body mass index (BMI), baseline TB status, CD4 count, viral load, anemia, and hypoalbuminemia were adjusted for in the multivariable models. Severe outcomes were defined as death, serious bacterial infections/sepsis, and opportunistic infections. N = 254 (81 cases, 173 controls)

EFA and association with incident active TB

In the incident active TB case-control population, cases and controls differed significantly by the following baseline characteristics: BMI (p = 0.001), prior TB (p = 0.02), CD4 count (p = 0.02), country, hypoalbuminemia, and anemia (all $p < 0.001$) (data not shown). The EFA analysis of base­line biomarkers in the incident active TB case-control ana­lysis also yielded three factors (eigenvalues > 1). However, the profiles of the factors and their association with incident active TB had some important differences from the CTF analyses (Additional file 5: Table S5). In this analysis, factor 1 (high carotenoids and low IL-18) had high loadings of α-carotene, β-carotene, β-cryptoxanthin, lutein, and zeaxanthin, as well as high negative loadings of IL-18, ferritin, and γ-tocopherol. Factor 2 (other nutrients) had high loadings of selenium, vitamin A (retinol), vitamin B₆, vitamin E (α-tocopherol), lycopene, α-carotene, and β-cryptoxanthin. Factor 3 (inflammation) had high loadings of IFN-γ, TNF-α, IL-6 and IP-10 (Additional file 5: Table S5).

Interestingly, higher scores of factor 1 (high carotenoids and low IL-18) were associated with reduced hazards of TB incidence in both univariable (HR 0.56; 95% CI 0.37–0.82) and multivariable analyses (aHR 0.48; 95% CI 0.26–0.87) (Table 4). Higher scores of factor 2 (other nutrients) were associated with reduced hazards of TB incidence in univariable but not in multivariable models. Unlike the results with CTF, factor 3 (inflammation) was not associated with increased hazards of incident active TB in both univariable (HR 1.15; 95% CI 0.83–1.54) and multivariable models (aHR 0.91; 95% CI 0.57–1.45) (Table 4).

Table 4 Association of each factor with incident active TB

	Univariable analysis HR (95% CI)	Multivariable analysis HR (95% CI)
Factor 1 (High carotenoids and low IL-18)	0.56 (0.38–0.82)	0.48 (0.26–0.87)
Factor 2 (Other nutrients)	0.65 (0.45–0.95)	0.98 (0.48–2.05)
Factor 3 (Inflammation)	1.15 (0.83–1.54)	0.91 (0.57–1.45)

The association of each factor with incident active TB was determined in univariable and multivariable Cox regression models. Baseline variables including sex, age, country, treatment arm, body mass index (BMI), CD4 count, viral load, baseline TB status, anemia, and hypoalbuminemia were adjusted for in the multivariable models. N = 220 (47 cases, 173 controls)

Sensitivity analyses

Although incident active TB meets the definition for both CTF and severe outcomes, the inclusion of TB as an element of these outcomes (CTF and severe outcomes) could potentially affect the derivation of the factors and association of the factor with the outcomes. As a result, we have conducted sensitivity analyses that remove incident active TB from the CTF ($N = 242$) and severe outcome ($N = 208$) analyses. The factor profiles were similar, and the results are consistent with the original analysis for the both the CTF (aHR 1.50; 95% CI 1.15–1.98 for factor 3) and severe outcomes (aHR 1.95; 95% CI 1.35–2.82 for factor 3) analysis (data not shown).

Our case-control analysis of incident active TB included individuals with prevalent TB at baseline (pre-ART initiation). In a sensitivity analysis removing those with prevalent TB at baseline, the profile of factors remained similar, and our results were consistent (aHR 0.46; 95% CI 0.23–0.91 for factor 1) (data not shown).

Discussion

In our study of HIV-infected individuals initiating ART, underlying factors were extracted from multiple biomarkers of baseline nutritional and immunological status, and the association of these factors with adverse HIV outcomes (CTF and incident active TB) was assessed. Higher scores of the inflammation factor were associated with increased hazards of CTF. Interestingly, higher scores of the high carotenoids and low IL-18 factor were associated with reduced hazards of incident active TB. Our results, utilizing analytical approaches that account for correlations (e.g., EFA) between multiple biomarkers, support findings from other studies on the association of inflammation and micronutrients with HIV outcomes, while suggesting that it may be valuable to focus on potential interventions that address the underlying factor rather than any one particular biomarker.

In the CTF analysis, when we assessed the relationship of each factor with outcome, only the inflammation factor was associated with increased hazards of CTF. There is increasing evidence of inflammation being associated with adverse HIV outcomes, and the high loading markers including IL-18, CRP, and sCD14 have all been individually associated with adverse HIV outcomes in studies including those from this cohort [1–6]. Although using factors, based on measurement of multiple biomarkers, to risk stratify individuals is not practical in a clinical setting when compared to single markers that are also predictive, our results can inform interventions that seek to reduce inflammation. The utility of such an approach can be seen in assessment of food insecurity, where responses from multiple questions are reduced to a single variable (although not through EFA) of food insecurity, which has shown to be associated with various

adverse health outcomes in HIV [29–31] and is a target for intervention [32]. While confirming the important role of these specific cytokines, our results also suggest that a more effective approach to reduce adverse HIV outcomes might be to focus on interventions that reduce the underlying inflammation (factor) represented by various correlated markers rather than focusing on only one of the markers which might represent a more specific type of inflammation (e.g., sCD14 for monocyte activation).

Notably the extracted factors in the incident active TB analyses were distinct from those in the CTF analyses. Factor 1 comprised high carotenoids and low IL-18, and the inflammation factor had high loadings of IFN-γ, TNF-α, IL-6, and IP-10. A major reason for the profiles of the factors being different between the CTF and TB case-control analyses is that the outcomes are different (TB accounts for 31% of the cases in CTF; 100% in TB case control). The relationship between carotenoids and IL-18 is intriguing, and some studies have shown that IL-18 levels can be affected by β-carotene metabolism [33, 34].

In our association studies, only the high carotenoids and low IL-18 factors were associated with reduced hazards of incident active TB. Given the findings that over-activation of inflammation (e.g., type I IFNs) results in increased incidence of TB [35], it is biologically plausible that inflammasome activation and increase in IL-18 could also result in higher incident TB [36]. The potential protective relationship of carotenoids with incident TB warrants further investigations, but potential mechanisms include an effect on immunity (e.g., inflammation, macrophage function, mucosal immunity) and oxidative stress [37–40]. Plasma carotenoids are considered a biomarker of fruit and vegetable intake [41, 42], and prior studies have observed that higher intakes of fruits and vegetables are protective against risk of TB [43, 44]. A new study from HIV-uninfected individuals [45] also suggests that low carotenoid levels might be associated with increased risk of TB.

The inflammation factor was not associated with development of incident active TB. A closer look at the high loading biomarkers (IFN-γ, TNF-α, IL-6, IP-10) suggests that while they are also pro-inflammatory, they have a different profile from the ones that load highly in the CTF inflammation factor (sCD14, CRP, IL-18, ferritin). The high loading biomarkers in the incident active TB inflammation factor are the classical Th1 cytokines important in anti-TB immunity [35], and they have not been consistently associated with adverse outcomes in HIV.

In our prior analyses on the association of an individual marker with an outcome (CTF or TB) using this same dataset [6, 7, 46], specific markers that were independently associated (e.g., vitamin D) with the outcome do not have significant loadings on any of the dominant factors. However, it is important to note that it is possible for a specific marker to still be independently associated with an outcome despite not being a part of one of the extracted factors. Factors are chosen based on correlations between the observed variables and are independent of the outcome; thus, the individual marker might or might not strongly load into any of the extracted factors. Future studies should test whether interventions that target the individual marker (e.g., vitamin D) and/or the underlying factor (e.g., inflammation) may improve clinical outcomes. Examples of potential therapeutics that may affect the underlying factor include diet (e.g., high-carotenoid foods or supplements for TB) and probiotics (to reduce microbial translocation and immune activation), along with medications to reduce inflammation (e.g., statins and aspirin) and treat co-morbidities (e.g., cytomegalovirus and helminth infections). Future studies will need to address how these interventions will affect the factors and ultimately HIV and TB outcomes.

The strengths of our study include the assessment of exposure prior to the outcome, the assessment of multiple outcomes, and addressing potential collinearity between multiple correlated biomarkers by using EFA. A limitation of this study is the CTF definition for the primary outcome, which is a composite definition based on multiple outcomes ranging from death to less severe outcomes. While this is based on a WHO definition that is widely used, we conducted a secondary analysis with more severe outcomes as well as virologic failure and observed a similar pattern. In this study, we are also unable to distinguish between TB recently acquired through transmission, TB reactivation, and subclinical/unmasked TB. The parent study was not designed to distinguish between TB reactivation and TB recently acquired through transmission. About 30% of the incident active TB cases developed within 3 months of ART initiation, which suggests that they might be subclinical or unmasked TB. However, we found a similar strength of associations but were underpowered to reach statistical significance at the $p < 0.05$ level when focusing our analyses only on new TB cases occurring after 3 months post-ART initiation. Another limitation of our study is that we did not assess food insecurity. Given the literature on the association of food insecurity with adverse HIV outcomes [29–31] along with its link to nutrition and immunity [47], a better understanding of the relationship between the extracted factors and food insecurity may have provided further insight into potential interventions.

Conclusion

In conclusion, our results suggest that groupings of nutritional and immunological biomarkers underlying specific factors are associated with adverse events and that an approach focusing on interventions targeting the underlying factor rather than any single observed variable warrants investigation. In addition, our results focus on a group of inflammatory biomarkers that further confirm the central role of inflammation in adverse HIV outcomes, while also suggesting that carotenoids potentially protect against TB.

Abbreviations

ACTG: AIDS Clinical Trials Group; aHR: Adjusted hazard ratio; ART: Antiretroviral therapy; BMI: Body mass index; CI: Confidence interval; CRP: C-reactive protein; CTF: Clinical treatment failure; EFA: Exploratory factor analysis; ELISA: Enzyme-linked immunosorbent assay; HIV: Human immunodeficiency virus; sCD14: Soluble CD14; TB: Tuberculosis

Acknowledgements

The authors thank the PEARLS study participants for volunteering their time and effort; we also thank the other PEARLS study team members.

Funding

This work was supported by the National Institute of Allergy and Infectious Diseases (grant numbers UM1 AI068634, UM1 AI068636, UM1 AI106701, UM1 AI069465, and R01 AI080417). RS was supported by the National Institute of Child Health and Human Development (grant number K99 HD089753) of the National Institutes of Health. The content is solely the responsibility of the authors and does not necessarily represent the official views of the National Institutes of Health. The parent trial A5175 was also supported in part by Boehringer Ingelheim, Bristol-Myers Squibb, Gilead Sciences, and GlaxoSmithKline. The funders had no role in study design, data collection or analysis, publication decision, or manuscript preparation.

Authors' contributions

RS designed the research question, conducted the data analysis, and wrote the primary version of the manuscript. NG conducted the data analysis and contributed to the interpretation. AB, PC and RCB contributed to data interpretation and manuscript review. SB, ALR, SWC, NM, CK, SP, WS, CR, PS, BRS, SP, and ST contributed to data collection and manuscript review. RDS contributed to study design, laboratory testing, and review of the manuscript. TBC contributed to study design, data collection, oversight of study implementation, and manuscript review. AG obtained funding and contributed to study design and manuscript writing and review. All authors meet the criteria for authorship as recommended by the International Committee of Medical Journal Editors (ICMJE) and were fully responsible for all aspects of manuscript development. All authors read and approved the final manuscript.

Competing interests

Thomas B. Campbell is an advisory board member for Gilead Sciences and Theratechnologies, Inc. Amita Gupta and Rupak Shivakoti have received grant funding from Gilead Foundation. All other authors declare that they have no competing interests.

Author details

[1]Department of Medicine, Johns Hopkins University School of Medicine, Baltimore, MD, USA. [2]National AIDS Research Institute, Pune, India. [3]YR Gaitonde Center for AIDS Research and Education, Chennai, India. [4]UNC Lilongwe, Lilongwe, Malawi. [5]Malawi College of Medicine-Johns Hopkins University Research Project, Blantyre, Malawi. [6]STD/AIDS Clinical Research Laboratory, Instituto de Pesquisa Clinica Evandro Chagas, Fundacao Oswaldo Cruz, Rio de Janeiro, Brazil. [7]Hospital Nossa Senhora de Conceiçã, Porto Alegre, Brazil. [8]Asociacion Civil Impacta Salud y Educacion, Lima, Peru. [9]Department of Medicine, University of Witwatersrand, Johannesburg, South Africa. [10]Durban International Clinical Research Site, Durban University of Technology, Durban, South Africa. [11]University of Zimbabwe Clinical

Research Centre, Harare, Zimbabwe. [12]Les Centres GHESKIO, Port-Au-Prince, Haiti. [13]Research Institute for Health Sciences, Chiang Mai, Thailand. [14]Department of Ophthalmology, Johns Hopkins University School of Medicine, Baltimore, MD, USA. [15]Department of International Health, Johns Hopkins Bloomberg School of Public Health, Baltimore, MD, USA. [16]Department of Medicine, Division of Infectious Diseases, University of Colorado School of Medicine, Aurora, CO, USA. [17]Present Address: Department of Epidemiology, Columbia University Mailman School of Public Health, 722 West 168th St, Room 705, New York, NY 10032, USA. [18]Present Address: National Institute of Research in Tuberculosis, Chennai, India. [19]Present Address: Liverpool School of Tropical Medicine, Liverpool, UK. [20]Present Address: Bill and Melinda Gates Foundation, Seattle, USA.

References

1. Boulware DR, Hullsiek KH, Puronen CE, Rupert A, Baker JV, French MA, Bohjanen PR, Novak RM, Neaton JD, Sereti I. Higher levels of CRP, D-dimer, IL-6, and hyaluronic acid before initiation of antiretroviral therapy (ART) are associated with increased risk of AIDS or death. J Infect Dis. 2011;203(11): 1637–46.

2. Deeks SG. Immune dysfunction, inflammation, and accelerated aging in patients on antiretroviral therapy. Top HIV Med. 2009;17(4):118–23.

3. Deeks SG, Tracy R, Douek DC. Systemic effects of inflammation on health during chronic HIV infection. Immunity. 2013;39(4):633–45.

4. Ledwaba L, Tavel JA, Khabo P, Maja P, Qin J, Sangweni P, Liu X, Follmann D, Metcalf JA, Orsega S, et al. Pre-ART levels of inflammation and coagulation markers are strong predictors of death in a South African cohort with advanced HIV disease. PLoS One. 2012;7(3):e24243.

5. Balagopal A, Gupte N, Shivakoti R, Cox AL, Yang WT, Berendes S, Mwelase N, Kanyama C, Pillay S, Samaneka W, et al. Continued elevation of interleukin-18 and interferon-gamma after initiation of antiretroviral therapy and clinical failure in a diverse multicountry human immunodeficiency virus cohort. Open Forum Infect Dis. 2016;3(3):ofw118.

6. Tenforde MW, Gupte N, Dowdy DW, Asmuth DM, Balagopal A, Pollard RB, Sugandhavesa P, Lama JR, Pillay S, Cardoso SW, et al. C-reactive protein (CRP), interferon gamma-inducible protein 10 (IP-10), and lipopolysaccharide (LPS) are associated with risk of tuberculosis after initiation of antiretroviral therapy in resource-limited settings. PLoS One. 2015;10(2):e0117424.

7. Havers F, Smeaton L, Gupte N, Detrick B, Bollinger RC, Hakim J, Kumarasamy N, Andrade A, Christian P, Lama JR, et al. 25-Hydroxyvitamin D insufficiency and deficiency is associated with HIV disease progression and virological failure post-antiretroviral therapy initiation in diverse multinational settings. J Infect Dis. 2014;210(2):244–53.

8. Shivakoti R, Gupte N, Yang WT, Mwelase N, Kanyama C, Tang AM, Pillay S, Samaneka W, Riviere C, Berendes S, et al. Pre-antiretroviral therapy serum selenium concentrations predict WHO stages 3, 4 or death but not virologic failure post-antiretroviral therapy. Nutrients. 2014;6(11):5061–74.

9. Baum MK, Campa A, Lai S, Sales Martinez S, Tsalaile L, Burns P, Farahani M, Li Y, van Widenfelt E, Page JB, et al. Effect of micronutrient supplementation on disease progression in asymptomatic, antiretroviral-naive, HIV-infected adults in Botswana: a randomized clinical trial. JAMA. 2013;310(20):2154–63.

10. Drain PK, Kupka R, Mugusi F, Fawzi WW. Micronutrients in HIV-positive persons receiving highly active antiretroviral therapy. Am J Clin Nutr. 2007; 85(2):333–45.

11. Isanaka S, Mugusi F, Hawkins C, Spiegelman D, Okuma J, Aboud S, Guerino C, Fawzi WW. Effect of high-dose vs standard-dose multivitamin supplementation at the initiation of HAART on HIV disease progression and mortality in Tanzania: a randomized controlled trial. JAMA. 2012;308(15):1535–44.

12. Wada NI, Bream JH, Martinez-Maza O, Macatangay B, Galvin SR, Margolick JB, Jacobson LP. Inflammatory biomarkers and mortality risk among HIV-suppressed men: a multisite prospective cohort study. Clin Infect Dis. 2016;63(7):984–90.

13. Bodnar LM, Wisner KL, Luther JF, Powers RW, Evans RW, Gallaher MJ, Newby PK. An exploratory factor analysis of nutritional biomarkers associated with major depression in pregnancy. Public Health Nutr. 2012;15(6):1078–86.

14. Rayman MP. Selenium and human health. Lancet. 2012;379(9822):1256–68.

15. Craig GM, Evans SJ, Brayshaw BJ. An inverse relationship between serum zinc and C-reactive protein levels in acutely ill elderly hospital patients. Postgrad Med J. 1990;66(782):1025–8.

16. Knafl GJ, Grey M. Factor analysis model evaluation through likelihood cross-validation. Stat Methods Med Res. 2007;16(2):77–102.

17. Fabrigar LR, Wegener DT, MacCallum RC, Strahan EJ. Evaluating the use of exploratory factor analysis in psychological research. Psychol Methods. 1999; 4(3):272–99.

18. Manhenke C, Orn S, von Haehling S, Wollert KC, Ueland T, Aukrust P, Voors AA, Squire I, Zannad F, Anker SD, et al. Clustering of 37 circulating biomarkers by exploratory factor analysis in patients following complicated acute myocardial infarction. Int J Cardiol. 2013;166(3):729–35.

19. Braunwald E. Biomarkers in heart failure. N Engl J Med. 2008;358(20):2148–59.

20. Chan D, Ng LL. Biomarkers in acute myocardial infarction. BMC Med. 2010;8:34.

21. Newby PK, Muller D, Hallfrisch J, Andres R, Tucker KL. Food patterns measured by factor analysis and anthropometric changes in adults. Am J Clin Nutr. 2004;80(2):504–13.

22. Ambrosini GL. Conference on 'Childhood Nutrition and Obesity: Current Status and Future Challenges' Symposium 3: effects of early nutrition on later health childhood dietary patterns and later obesity: a review of the evidence. Proc Nutr Soc. 2014;73(1):137–46.

23. Campbell TB, Smeaton LM, Kumarasamy N, Flanigan T, Klingman KL, Firnhaber C, Grinsztejn B, Hosseinipour MC, Kumwenda J, Lalloo U, et al. Efficacy and safety of three antiretroviral regimens for initial treatment of HIV-1: a randomized clinical trial in diverse multinational settings. PLoS Med. 2012;9(8):e1001290.

24. WHO. The use of antiretroviral drugs for treating and preventing HIV infection. 2013. https://www.ncbi.nlm.nih.gov/pubmed/24716260.

25. Balagopal A, Asmuth DM, Yang WT, Campbell TB, Gupte N, Smeaton L, Kanyama C, Grinsztejn B, Santos B, Supparatpinyo K, et al. Pre-cART elevation of CRP and CD4+ T-cell immune activation associated with HIV clinical progression in a multinational case-cohort study. J Acquir Immune Defic Syndr. 2015;70(2):163–71.

26. Shivakoti R, Christian P, Yang WT, Gupte N, Mwelase N, Kanyama C, Pillay S, Samaneka W, Santos B, Poongulali S, et al. Prevalence and risk factors of micronutrient deficiencies pre- and post-antiretroviral therapy (ART) among a diverse multicountry cohort of HIV-infected adults. Clin Nutr. 2016;35(1):183–9.

27. Flood A, Rastogi T, Wirfalt E, Mitrou PN, Reedy J, Subar AF, Kipnis V, Mouw T, Hollenbeck AR, Leitzmann M, et al. Dietary patterns as identified by factor analysis and colorectal cancer among middle-aged Americans. Am J Clin Nutr. 2008;88(1):176–84.

28. Mraity HA, England A, Cassidy S, Eachus P, Dominguez A, Hogg P. Development and validation of a visual grading scale for assessing image quality of AP pelvis radiographic images. Br J Radiol. 2016;89(1061):20150430.

29. Spinelli MA, Frongillo EA, Sheira LA, Palar K, Tien PC, Wilson T, Merenstein D, Cohen M, Adedimeji A, Wentz E, et al. Food insecurity is associated with poor HIV outcomes among women in the United States. AIDS Behav. 2017; 21(12):3473–7.

30. Anema A, Chan K, Chen Y, Weiser S, Montaner JS, Hogg RS. Relationship between food insecurity and mortality among HIV-positive injection drug users receiving antiretroviral therapy in British Columbia, Canada. PLoS One. 2013;8(5):e61277.

31. Aibibula W, Cox J, Hamelin AM, McLinden T, Klein MB, Brassard P. Association between food insecurity and HIV viral suppression: a systematic review and meta-analysis. AIDS Behav. 2017;21(3):754–65.

32. Weiser SD, Bukusi EA, Steinfeld RL, Frongillo EA, Weke E, Dworkin SL, Pusateri K, Shiboski S, Scow K, Butler LM, et al. Shamba Maisha: randomized controlled trial of an agricultural and finance intervention to improve HIV health outcomes. AIDS. 2015;29(14):1889–94.

33. He M, Cornelis MC, Kraft P, van Dam RM, Sun Q, Laurie CC, Mirel DB, Chasman DI, Ridker PM, Hunter DJ, et al. Genome-wide association study identifies variants at the IL18-BCO2 locus associated with interleukin-18 levels. Arterioscler Thromb Vasc Biol. 2010;30(4):885–90.

34. Wu L, Guo X, Wang W, Medeiros DM, Clarke SL, Lucas EA, Smith BJ, Lin D. Molecular aspects of beta, beta-carotene-9', 10'-oxygenase 2 in carotenoid metabolism and diseases. Exp Biol Med (Maywood). 2016;241(17):1879–87.

35. O'Garra A, Redford PS, McNab FW, Bloom CI, Wilkinson RJ, Berry MP. The immune response in tuberculosis. Annu Rev Immunol. 2013;31:475–527.

36. Sutinen EM, Pirttila T, Anderson G, Salminen A, Ojala JO. Pro-inflammatory interleukin-18 increases Alzheimer's disease-associated amyloid-beta production in human neuron-like cells. J Neuroinflammation. 2012;9:199.

37. Chew BP, Park JS. Carotenoid action on the immune response. J Nutr. 2004; 134(1):257S–61S.

38. Bai SK, Lee SJ, Na HJ, Ha KS, Han JA, Lee H, Kwon YG, Chung CK, Kim YM. beta-Carotene inhibits inflammatory gene expression in lipopolysaccharide-stimulated macrophages by suppressing redox-based NF-kappaB activation. Exp Mol Med. 2005;37(4):323–34.

39. Mehendale SM, Shepherd ME, Brookmeyer RS, Semba RD, Divekar AD, Gangakhedkar RR, Joshi S, Risbud AR, Paranjape RS, Gadkari DA, et al. Low carotenoid concentration and the risk of HIV seroconversion in Pune, India. J Acquir Immune Defic Syndr. 2001;26(4):352–9.

40. Imamura T, Bando N, Yamanishi R. Beta-carotene modulates the immunological function of RAW264, a murine macrophage cell line, by enhancing the level of intracellular glutathione. Biosci Biotechnol Biochem. 2006;70(9):2112–20.

41. Burrows TL, Hutchesson MJ, Rollo ME, Boggess MM, Guest M, Collins CE. Fruit and vegetable intake assessed by food frequency questionnaire and plasma carotenoids: a validation study in adults. Nutrients. 2015;7(5):3240–51.

42. Campbell DR, Gross MD, Martini MC, Grandits GA, Slavin JL, Potter JD. Plasma carotenoids as biomarkers of vegetable and fruit intake. Cancer Epidemiol Biomark Prev. 1994;3(6):493–500.

43. Franke MF, del Castillo H, Pereda Y, Lecca L, Cardenas L, Fuertes J, Murray MB, Bayona J, Becerra MC. Modifiable factors associated with tuberculosis disease in children: a case-control study. Pediatr Infect Dis J. 2014;33(1):109–11.

44. Hemila H, Kaprio J, Pietinen P, Albanes D, Heinonen OP. Vitamin C and other compounds in vitamin C rich food in relation to risk of tuberculosis in male smokers. Am J Epidemiol. 1999;150(6):632–41.

45. Aibana O, Franke MF, Huang CC, Galea JT, Calderon R, Zhang Z, Becerra MC, Smith ER, Ronnenberg AG, Contreras C, et al. Impact of vitamin a and carotenoids on the risk of tuberculosis progression. Clin Infect Dis. 2017;65(6):900–9.

46. Tenforde MW, Yadav A, Dowdy DW, Gupte N, Shivakoti R, Yang WT, Mwelase N, Kanyama C, Pillay S, Samaneka W, et al. Vitamin A and D deficiencies associated with incident tuberculosis in HIV-infected patients initiating antiretroviral therapy in multinational case-cohort study. J Acquir Immune Defic Syndr. 2017;75(3):e71–9.

47. Vaidya A, Bhosale R, Sambarey P, Suryavanshi N, Young S, Mave V, Kanade S, Kulkarni V, Deshpande P, Balasubramanian U, et al. Household food insecurity is associated with low interferon-gamma levels in pregnant Indian women. Int J Tuberc Lung Dis. 2017;21(7):797–803.

The impact of demographic changes, exogenous boosting and new vaccination policies on varicella and herpes zoster

Alessia Melegaro[1,2]* (ID), Valentina Marziano[3], Emanuele Del Fava[2], Piero Poletti[3], Marcello Tirani[4], Caterina Rizzo[5] and Stefano Merler[3]

Abstract

Background: The present study aims to evaluate the cost-effectiveness of the newly introduced varicella and herpes zoster (HZ) vaccination programmes in Italy. The appropriateness of the introduction of the varicella vaccine is highly debated because of concerns about the consequences on HZ epidemiology and the expected increase in the number of severe cases in case of suboptimal coverage levels.

Methods: We performed a cost-utility analysis based on a stochastic individual-based model that considers realistic demographic processes and two different underlying mechanisms of exogenous boosting (temporary and progressive immunity). Routine varicella vaccination is given with a two-dose schedule (15 months, 5–6 years). The HZ vaccine is offered to the elderly (65 years), either alone or in combination with an initial catch-up campaign (66–75 years). The main outcome measures are averted cases and deaths, costs per quality-adjusted life years gained, incremental cost-effectiveness ratios, and net monetary benefits associated with the different vaccination policies.

Results: Demographic processes have contributed to shaping varicella and HZ epidemiology over the years, decreasing varicella circulation and increasing the incidence of HZ. The recent introduction of varicella vaccination in Italy is expected to produce an enduring reduction in varicella incidence and, indirectly, a further increase of HZ incidence in the first decades, followed by a significant reduction in the long term. However, the concurrent introduction of routine HZ vaccination at 65 years of age is expected to mitigate this increase and, in the longer run, to reduce HZ burden to its minimum. From an economic perspective, all the considered policies are cost-effective, with the exception of varicella vaccination alone when considering a time horizon of 50 years. These results are robust to parameter uncertainties, to the two different hypotheses on the mechanism driving exogenous boosting, and to different demographic projection scenarios.

Conclusions: The recent introduction of a combined varicella and HZ vaccination programme in Italy will produce significant reductions in the burden of both diseases and is found to be a cost-effective policy. This programme will counterbalance the increasing trend of zoster incidence purely due to demographic processes.

Keywords: Varicella, Chickenpox, Herpes zoster, Shingles, Vaccination, Italy, Cost-effectiveness, Modelling, Individual-based models, Demography, Immunisation

* Correspondence: alessia.melegaro@unibocconi.it
[1]Department of Social and Political Sciences, Bocconi University, Milano, Italy
[2]Carlo F. Dondena Centre for Research on Social Dynamics and Public Policy, Bocconi University, Milano, Italy
Full list of author information is available at the end of the article

Background

Varicella zoster virus (VZV) is a DNA virus belonging to the *Herpesviridae* family that affects only humans. Infection by VZV can result in two distinct diseases: varicella or chickenpox, which is a highly communicable and widespread childhood disease, and herpes zoster (HZ) or shingles, caused by the reactivation of VZV, which remains latent in the dorsal root ganglia after primary varicella infection. Although it is usually a mild disease with a relatively low percentage of complications, especially when occurring in immunocompetent children, varicella is highly contagious and may lead to more severe consequences and disabling symptoms in adults. Reactivation of the virus, usually occurring in the elderly or immuno-compromised patients, leads to HZ infection. This is characterised by a vesicular eruption along the course of the nerve and is commonly associated with pain. Complications of HZ occur in up to 20% of the cases among those aged 50 or older, with post-herpetic neuralgia (PHN) being the most common, persistent, and intractable chronic sequela [1, 2].

A live attenuated vaccine against varicella was developed in 1974 and introduced in some countries starting from 1995 [3]. In Italy, eight regions (Apulia, Basilicata, Calabria, Sardinia, Sicily, Tuscany, Veneto, and Friuli-Venezia Giulia) have gradually introduced childhood varicella vaccine into their immunisation programmes starting in 2003, in children aged 13–15 months and 5–6 years [4]. Since 2017, a two-dose schedule has been introduced nationally for all newborns as one of the ten vaccines (hexavalent, plus measles, mumps, rubella, and varicella) that have become compulsory for school attendance [5]. Nonetheless, in many developed countries, the introduction of varicella vaccination into the national schedule still represents an ongoing open discussion. Indeed, VZV mass immunisation would reduce varicella circulation, but it may potentially increase the incidence of more severe varicella cases among adults [6] and reduce the partial protection against HZ provided by VZV re-exposure (called "exogenous boosting"), thus increasing HZ incidence [7]. Results from HZ surveillance programmes in countries that have introduced VZV mass immunisation do not provide univocal evidence. Some countries detected an increase in HZ incidence following mass immunisation, while others did not observe any effect on it [8, 9]. Conversely, an increase in HZ incidence has been reported in the past decades across various countries before the introduction of varicella vaccination programmes [10]. This pattern appears consistent with results from modelling work that showed that past demographic changes and, in particular, the ageing of the population may have generated the remarkable growth of HZ incidence observed in Spain between 1997 and 2004, before the introduction of the varicella vaccination programme [11].

A live attenuated vaccine against HZ was licenced in 2006 [12, 13], and so far has been recommended in some countries, either in combination with the varicella vaccination (e.g. in the USA and recently in Italy) or alone (e.g. in France and the UK), making the evaluation of post-vaccination trends even more complex.

Previous transmission models of VZV infection suggested an increase in HZ incidence as a consequence of the reduction of exogenous boosting associated with varicella vaccination. However, the magnitude of this increase depends on modelling assumptions on the mechanism of VZV reactivation [14–19], whose biology has not yet been elucidated [20–25]. The cost-effectiveness analysis here is performed under two different assumptions regarding the mechanism of VZV reactivation. The first assumption, which has been widely adopted in past modelling approaches, hypothesises temporary complete immunity to HZ following re-exposure to VZV [16]. The second assumption relies instead on the explicit modelling of the development of a progressive partial immunity to HZ following each re-exposure to VZV, which better reflects the biological mechanisms driving the exogenous boosting [7]. So far, models including the latter mechanism have provided a better fit to the age-specific profile of HZ incidence in several countries [26], Italy included [18].

Also, the cost-effectiveness of varicella vaccination programmes was shown to be highly dependent on the assumptions about the boosting mechanism [27, 28]. Varicella vaccination appeared cost-effective when the model excluded the effect of boosting on the epidemiology of HZ [27, 29]. Conversely, when the latter effect was included, the cost-effectiveness of the programme became questionable, due to detrimental effects of varicella vaccination on HZ in the short and the medium term [30, 31].

The aim of this work is to provide a thorough evaluation of the expected effectiveness and cost-effectiveness of the recently introduced Italian varicella and HZ vaccination programme. For this purpose, a stochastic individual-based model (IBM) will be used, developed considering the observed demographic processes (such as the decline of fertility). Alternative immunisation strategies will be considered, and the sensitivity of our results to the two different assumptions about the exogenous boosting will be assessed.

Methods

In this study, we use a stochastic IBM for VZV transmission and reactivation in Italy, informed with historical demographic data and available demographic projections [32, 33] and calibrated on the age-specific varicella serological profile and age-specific HZ incidence.

The proposed modelling approach is similar to that adopted to investigate historical epidemiological trends of measles across different countries and varicella in Spain [11, 34, 35].

The model is used to assess the economic impact of different varicella and HZ vaccination strategies on the future epidemiology of the two diseases through a cost-effectiveness analysis. Details of the demographic and epidemiological data used to parameterise the model are provided in Additional file 1: Figures S1 and S4.

We consider two epidemiological models, which differ in the assumption made to model the mechanism driving exogenous boosting and VZV reactivation [7], denoted respectively as *progressive immunity* (PI) and *temporary immunity* (TI) [16, 18]. The structures of the corresponding models are shown in Additional file 1: Figures S2 and S3. In both models, maternal antibodies confer protection against varicella infection to newborn babies for 6 months on average, after which children become susceptible to natural VZV (i.e. wild-type) infection. Susceptible individuals are exposed to a time- and age-dependent force of infection. After recovery, varicella-infected individuals acquire lifelong immunity against varicella. The generation time of varicella infection is assumed to be 3 weeks on average. In model PI, after recovery from varicella, individuals become susceptible to HZ. The rate of VZV reactivation decreases with the number of re-exposures to VZV, while it increases with both the time elapsed since the last re-exposure and the individual's age [18]. In model TI, individuals who recover from varicella acquire temporary full protection against HZ, and the VZV reactivation rate only depends on the individual's age [16]. In both models, HZ-susceptible individuals may either develop HZ, acquiring, after recovery, lifelong immunity to HZ disease, or they can be boosted through VZV re-exposure. In model PI, each boosting event progressively reduces the risk of VZV reactivation into HZ, whereas in model TI, it provides a temporary complete protection against HZ development. In both models, we assume that only a fraction of contacts with VZV-infected individuals results in an effective boosting event [36]. Epidemiological parameters of both models' structures are provided in the Additional file 1: Table S1 and S2.

Varicella vaccine is administered in our models starting from the year 2017. Vaccinated individuals either develop lifelong protection against varicella or they undergo vaccine failure. In the latter case, they remain susceptible to VZV and may experience a milder varicella infection, called "breakthrough varicella". Although individuals infected with breakthrough varicella can transmit the virus, they are assumed to be half as contagious as natural varicella cases [37].

Under model PI, individuals who have recovered from breakthrough varicella become susceptible to HZ, whereas under model TI, they become temporarily immune against HZ. In both models, varicella vaccinated individuals can develop HZ, either after recovery from

varicella breakthrough or directly from the vaccine strain, or can experience boosting. The VZV reactivation rate for varicella vaccinated individuals is lower than for those who experienced natural varicella [38]. Individuals successfully vaccinated against HZ acquire lifelong immunity to VZV reactivation, whereas those experiencing HZ vaccine failure remain susceptible to HZ.

Five different vaccination scenarios are considered and compared in an incremental cost-effectiveness analysis. The case of no intervention is also explored to assess the expected evolution of varicella and HZ epidemiology as driven by the changing demography only, had vaccination not been introduced. Following the new Italian National Immunisation Plan (NIP) 2017–2019 [39], we implement a routine varicella vaccination programme with a two-dose schedule (first dose at 15 months of age, second dose at 5–6 years of age) and an HZ vaccination programme with the live attenuated vaccine, targeted at individuals who are 65 years old. The two policies are evaluated either as single strategies or in combination. In addition, we also evaluate the effects of a catch-up campaign with the HZ vaccine targeting 66- to 75-year-old individuals. The resulting five programmes are the following: (1) routine varicella vaccination (V_R), (2) routine HZ vaccination (HZ_R), (3) routine HZ vaccination with HZ catch-up campaign (HZ_{R+CU}), (4) routine varicella and HZ vaccinations $(V_R HZ_R)$, and (5) routine varicella and HZ vaccinations with HZ catch-up campaign $(V_R HZ_{R+CU})$. Base case coverage levels for varicella and HZ vaccination are assumed to be equal to 80% and 60%, respectively. The vaccine efficacy per dose is set to 80% for the varicella vaccine, which implies an efficacy of 96% after two doses [40], while it is set to 50% for one dose of HZ vaccine [13]. The efficacy of varicella vaccine only refers to the protection against VZV infection. This means that a larger efficacy for the varicella vaccine generates in our model a larger proportion of individuals not developing varicella.

Finally, demographic changes are simulated in the period 2015–2100 as informed by temporal variations of the crude birth and age-specific mortality rates provided by the United Nations in the 2015 World Population Prospects [38].

The calibration of the models was carried out using Monte Carlo Markov chain (MCMC) methods applied to the binomial likelihood of the VZV seroprevalence profile in 1996–1997 [41] and to the Poisson likelihood of the age-specific HZ incidence in 2004 (Additional file 1: Figure S4) [2]. We calculated 95% prediction intervals (PIs) for the model-based estimates. More details are provided in Additional file 1 where the robustness of our results is assessed (Figures S5 and S6). Modelling and data analyses were conducted in C and R.

Cost-effectiveness analysis

Cost-effectiveness analysis is applied to the outcomes of the epidemiological model, and quality-adjusted life years (QALYs) gained are used to evaluate the impact of different policies in terms of reduction of disease burden. Varicella cases are differentiated between natural infection and breakthrough cases, as the latter are expected to incur lower QALY losses and generate lower costs (Additional file 1: Figure S11). For HZ, we distinguish between cases that develop post-herpetic neuralgia (PHN) and those that do not, as costs and benefits for the two conditions are expected to differ (Additional file 1: Figure S12). We consider both the direct costs of disease (general practitioner (GP) visits, treatment, and hospitalisation) and the costs of the vaccination programmes. We report on the effects of the different policies on varicella and HZ, in terms of both burden of illness (averted cases and deaths, by disease) and economic and quality of life impact (QALY gained ΔE, and net costs ΔC).

Cost-effectiveness outcomes are produced under the taxpayer perspective and evaluated at three different time horizons (TH = 25, 50, 85 years), assuming discount rates of either 3% or 0% per year for both future health benefits and costs. The 3% discount rate puts less weight on the cases predicted in the long term, while the 0% discount rate weighs cases at a greater distance in time as much as those closer to the origin.

We perform an incremental cost-effectiveness analysis to determine, for each model and time horizon, which policies are deemed cost-effective, using both the incremental cost-effectiveness ratio (ICER, computed as $\Delta C/\Delta E$) and the net monetary benefit (NMB, computed as $t\Delta E - \Delta C$), where the threshold t represents the opportunity cost of an additional QALY gained. We consider two possible cost-effectiveness (CE) thresholds t, one demand-based of 40,000 EUR [42], and one supply-based of 15,000 EUR [43]. The former threshold represents the dominating approach in all health care systems, including those in Italy [42], and it depends on how individuals value health compared to other types of consumptions. The latter, based on the estimated marginal productivity of the health care system, represents a direct measure of the health consequence of changes in the allocation of the available resources [43]. A sensitivity analysis is conducted to assess how cost-effectiveness analysis results change when assuming different values of the CE threshold t.

The base case analysis considers 1000 model realisations of varicella and HZ cases by age and over time, generated under the strategies under investigation. These are combined with the base case values of the economic and quality of life parameters (Tables 1 and 2). The robustness of model results to uncertainty in model parameters is assessed through a probabilistic sensitivity analysis (PSA) [44], where, using an empirical Bayesian approach, the prior distributions for the model parameters are either grounded on the respective base case values or are set by assuming little or no information about the parameters of interest (e.g. when any estimate of the variability of the parameter is not available) [45]. For evaluating the effects of the uncertainty around both epidemiological estimates and economic model parameters, we compute the NMB associated with 1000 different parameter sets, sample from their posterior distribution, and derive 95% credible intervals (CIs) from their posterior distribution. The uncertainty around the choice of the optimal strategy (i.e. generating the highest NMB), under both discount rates of 0% and 3%, is represented with (1) box plots of the posterior distribution of the NMB and (2) net benefit charts showing how the median NMB changes for a variety of values of the CE threshold [46]. Finally, six additional scenarios under the PSA are evaluated to assess the sensitivity of our results to (1) two different coverage levels of varicella vaccination (70%, 95%), (2) two extreme assumptions on the role of exogenous boosting (assuming either low or high reduction of the HZ risk due to VZV re-exposure), and (3) two different demographic scenarios on the total fertility rate in the future (a lower and a higher crude birth rate).

Results

Under the no vaccination scenario, both model structures predict a stable overall incidence of varicella over time (Fig. 1a), as well as an increase in HZ rate, which will stabilise only after some decades (Fig. 1d–f and Fig. 2). This growth can be ascribed to two factors, i.e. the population ageing that acts equally in both models, and the delayed effect, stronger for model PI, of the decline in the fertility rate which occurred during the last century on the individual risk of HZ development. Indeed, the decline of fertility in the past reduced both varicella circulation and the frequency of VZV re-exposure. In particular, during the period 2017–2100, model TI forecasts a peak in the total HZ incidence of about 15.1% (95% PI 8.1–22.3%) with respect to 2017 and a stable incidence level in the long term that is 2.6% (95% PI −5.2 to 10.9%) higher than in 2017. On the other hand, model PI forecasts a peak in HZ incidence with respect to 2017 that amounts to 61.4% (95% PI 44.9–77.1%) and a stable incidence level in the long term that is 48.3% (95% PI 33.4–62.8%) higher than in 2017 (Fig. 2).

The recently introduced combined varicella and zoster vaccination strategy (V_RHZ_R), at baseline coverage levels of 80% and 60%, respectively, is expected to produce a sudden and enduring reduction in varicella incidence as well as a significant increase in the average age at

Table 1 Epidemiological and quality of life (QALY) parameters of the economic model. We report the base case values and the standard deviations, taken either from the literature or from administrative data, the shapes of the prior distribution, the 95% CI from the posterior distribution of the parameters, and the source of the base case values

Parameter	Base case values	Standard deviations	Prior Distribution	95% CI Posterior distribution	Source
Epidemiological parameters					
Proportion of HZ cases developing PHN[c]	0.049 (by age)	0.0023 (by age)	Beta	–	[2]
Hosp. rate for natural varicella (NV) per model TI/PI (per 1000 cases)	2.35/2.36 (by age)	0.61/0.62 (by age)	Beta	–	Estimate[a]
Breakthrough varicella (BV) vs. NV hosp. rate	0.25	0.05	Beta	[0.16–0.35]	[58, 59]
Hosp. rate for HZ per model TI/PI (per 1000 cases)	13.60/13.12 (by age)	4.49/4.63 (by age)	Beta	–	Estimate[a]
Hosp. rate for PHN per model TI/PI (per 1000 cases)	41.55/40.77 (by age)	9.53/10.39 (by age)	Beta	–	Estimate[a]
Case fatality rate for NV (per 1000 hospitalised)	4.01 (by age)	2.98 (by age)	Beta	–	Estimate[b]
BV vs. NV case fatality rate	0.005	0.0022	Beta	[0.002–0.01]	[59, 60]
HZ-PHN case fatality rate (per 1000 hospitalised)	12.70 (by age)	5.43 (by age)	Beta	–	Estimate[b]
No. GP consultations per NV case					
< 14 years	2	0.2	Gamma	[1.63–2.43]	[59]
≥ 15 years	1	0.2	Gamma	[0.64–1.43]	[59]
No. GP consultations per BV case	0.5	0.05	Gamma	[0.41–0.60]	[59]
Quality of life measures					
Overall weighted health state index (EQ-5D$_{index}$)	0.84 (by age)	0.21 (by age)	Beta		[61]
Weighted health state index varicella					
< 14 years	0.81	0.031	Beta	[0.76–0.86]	[31]
≥ 15 years	0.73	0.025	Beta	[0.68–0.78]	[62]
Prob. severe NV cases	0.65	0.0063	Beta	[0.64–0.66]	[63]
Prob. severe BV cases	0.25	0.011	Beta	[0.23–0.27]	[63]
Reduction in QALY loss Mild vs. severe varicella cases	0.25	0.10	Beta	[0.08–0.47]	[48]
QALY loss HZ					
20 years	0.022	0.0018	Beta	[0.019–0.026]	[48]
40 years	0.031	0.0030	Beta	[0.026–0.037]	[48]
60 years	0.064	0.0082	Beta	[0.049–0.081]	[48]
80 years	0.19	0.030	Beta	[0.14–0.25]	[48]

[a]Average number of hospitalisations by age due to varicella, HZ, and PHN (Hospital Discharge Register, 2001–2012) divided by the predicted pre-vaccination incidence generated by the epidemiological model. PHN incidence is derived by multiplying the estimated HZ incidence by the probability of HZ cases developing PHN [2]

[b]Average number of deaths by age due to varicella (Italian National Health Institute, 2001–2012) and HZ (European Union detailed mortality database, 2001–2012) divided by the respective estimates of the hospitalisation rates

[c]PHN cases lasting at least 3 months

varicella infection (Fig. 1b). Moreover, although in the short and the medium term the current programme might provide an increase in HZ incidence compared to the pre-vaccination level (though still lower than under the no vaccination scenario), in the long term it is expected to reduce the burden of HZ disease in Italy to its minimum, with small differences between the two models (Fig. 1d–f and Fig. 2, Additional file 1: Figures S9 and S10). In particular, we expect a reduction of 70.7% (95% PI 34.7–91.5%) in HZ incidence with respect

to the no vaccination scenario under model PI, and of 68.6% (95% PI 61.8–74.1%) under model TI (Fig. 1f), with an upwards shift in the average age at VZV reactivation into HZ. Indeed, for both models, while the age group that is mostly affected by HZ in 2017 is 55–64 years (accounting on average for 21.1% and 20.3% of the total cases in models PI and TI, respectively), in the long term the models forecast that most cases would occur in the age group 75–84 under model PI (40% on average) and in the age group 85–99 under model TI (26.8% on average).

Table 2 Cost of disease and vaccination parameters of the economic model. We report the base case values and the standard deviations, taken either from the literature or from administrative data, the shapes of the prior distribution, the 95% CI from the posterior distribution of the parameters, and the source of the base case values

Parameter	Base case values (EUR)	Standard deviation (EUR)	Prior Distribution	95% CI Posterior distribution	Source
Cost of disease parameters					
GP consultation cost for NV[a]					
< 14 years	29.07	2.05	Gamma	[25.14–33.27]	[64]
≥ 15 years	19.00	1.25	Gamma	[16.65–21.53]	[65]
GP treatment cost for NV[a]					
< 14 years	13.64	1.61	Gamma	[10.72–16.96]	[66]
≥ 15 years	26.10	2.00	Gamma	[22.35–30.14]	[65]
Hospitalisation cost for NV					
< 14 years	2683.25	1780.56	Gamma	[411.80–7128.02]	Hospital Discharge Register (HDR) Lombardy
≥ 15 years	2720.29	2573.64	Gamma	[348.73–9463.01]	HDR Lombardy
Outpatient cost for HZ (incl. Visit, treatment, and diagnostics)[a]	144.03	114.48	Gamma	[11.53–438.21]	[2]
Outpatient cost for PHN (incl. Visit, treatment, and diagnostics)[a]	523.72	520.05	Gamma	[13.95–1905.90]	[2]
Hospitalisation cost for HZ					
< 49 years	2073.50	2260.35	Gamma	[176.35–8238.92]	HDR Lombardy
≥50 years	2020.23	1332.60	Gamma	[307.63–5313.47]	HDR Lombardy
Hospitalisation cost for PHN					
< 49 years	1500.74	1714.41	Gamma	[78.93–6132.75]	HDR Lombardy
≥50 years	1927.25	1892.80	Gamma	[75.02–7058.80]	
Vaccination parameters					
Cost per dose of varicella vaccination	31.46		Fixed	–	Purchase price[b]
Cost per dose of HZ vaccination	87.00		Fixed	–	Invitation for bid
Admin. cost per dose of vaccination[a]	7.56		Fixed	–	[59]

[a]These costs are adjusted for the inflation at 2015, using the Italian Consumer Price Index
[b]Purchase price of the vaccine for varicella per dose, paid by Lombardy Regional Health System

Nonetheless, the overall reduction in HZ incidence obtained with the combined programme (V_RHZ_R) implies a much lower cumulative number of HZ cases and HZ-related deaths than those expected with no vaccination, under any time horizon (Additional file 1: Tables S3 and S4, with 3% and 0% discount rates, respectively).

The effect of the introduction of a varicella vaccination policy alone (V_R) on natural HZ incidence in the short and the medium term strongly depends on the model considered. In the first decades after introduction, no evident variation with respect to the no vaccination scenario is expected under model TI, whereas a 15% increase of HZ incidence is estimated under model PI (Fig. 2). In the long term, since varicella vaccination would reduce the replacement of the HZ-susceptible individuals generated by natural varicella, we would find that HZ incidence is less than half of that expected under no vaccination (Fig. 1f), with levels even lower than those in the pre-vaccination period (Fig. 2). Conversely, a

routine HZ vaccination programme would mitigate the increase of HZ incidence both in the absence (HZ_R) and in the presence of varicella vaccination (V_RHZ_R), in both the short and the medium term. However, the policy including only HZ vaccination would not affect the replacement of the HZ-susceptible individuals caused by varicella infection, and therefore result in the long term in a much higher level of HZ incidence than that achieved through policy V_R (Fig. 1f). Indeed, according to model PI, in the long term, V_R and HZ_R would respectively lead to a 60.6% (95% PI 12.6–88.2%) and an 18.1% (95% PI 15.9%–20.4%) reduction in HZ incidence with respect to no vaccination (although the undiscounted cumulative number of zoster cases remains slightly higher under policy V_R (Additional file 1: Table S4).

Under both models and time horizons (except for TH = 50 under the PI model) and assuming a discount rate of 3%, we found the combined policy with varicella vaccination and HZ vaccination with catch-up (V_RHZ_{R+CU}) to

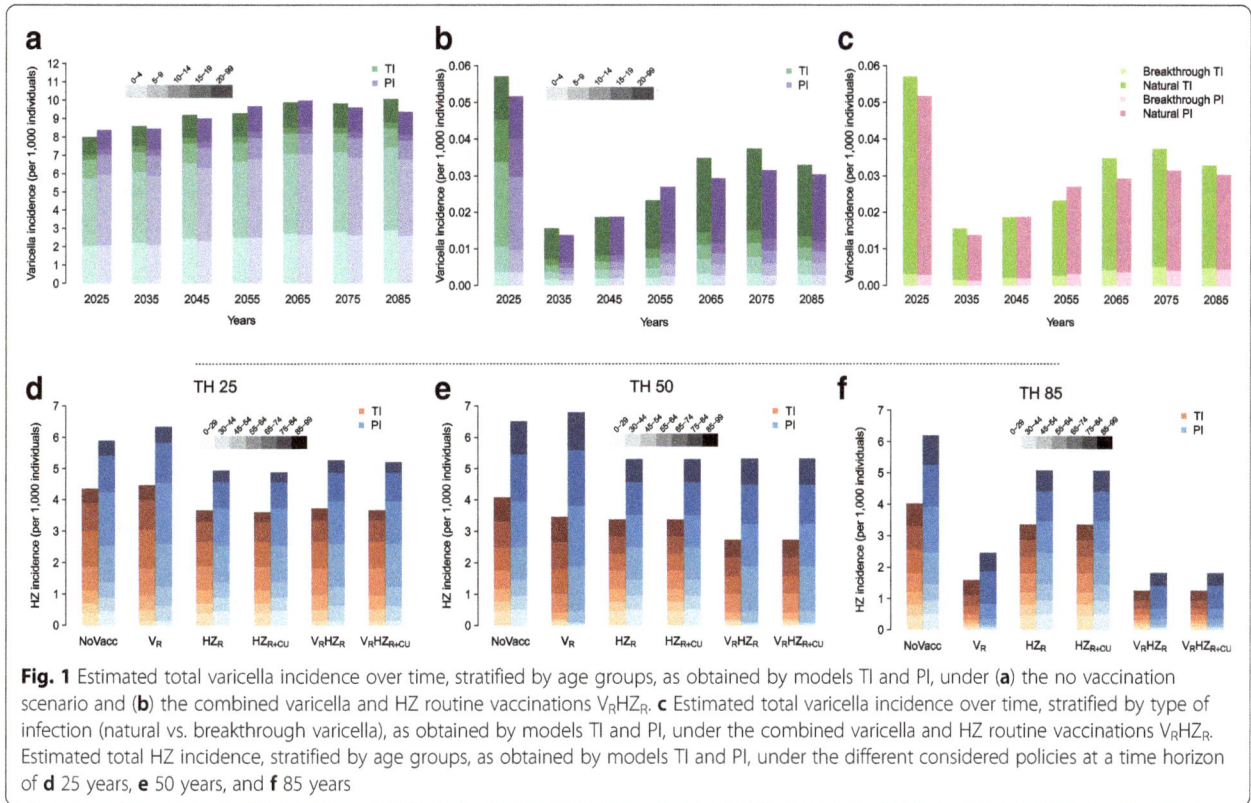

Fig. 1 Estimated total varicella incidence over time, stratified by age groups, as obtained by models TI and PI, under (**a**) the no vaccination scenario and (**b**) the combined varicella and HZ routine vaccinations $V_R HZ_R$. **c** Estimated total varicella incidence over time, stratified by type of infection (natural vs. breakthrough varicella), as obtained by models TI and PI, under the combined varicella and HZ routine vaccinations $V_R HZ_R$. Estimated total HZ incidence, stratified by age groups, as obtained by models TI and PI, under the different considered policies at a time horizon of **d** 25 years, **e** 50 years, and **f** 85 years

be the most cost-effective in terms of ICER and NMB, no matter what the chosen threshold (Table 3). However, for TH = 50 years and when considering model PI, the most cost-effective policy remains the one with the HZ vaccination and catch-up campaign ($HZ_{R + CU}$) (Table 3).

Varicella vaccination alone (V_R) was never found to perform better than the other strategies, even though it strongly dominated the no vaccination scenario under model TI, resulting in cost savings in the medium and in the long term (Table 3). Conversely, V_R performed worse under model PI, where it turned out to be always dominated and even generated QALY losses in the medium and in the long term as a consequence of the increase in cumulative HZ cases in the first decades following the introduction of vaccination (Additional file 1: Table S3). Similar conclusions can be drawn when considering a discount rate of 0% (Additional file 1: Table S4). Also with undiscounted values, we found the combined policy

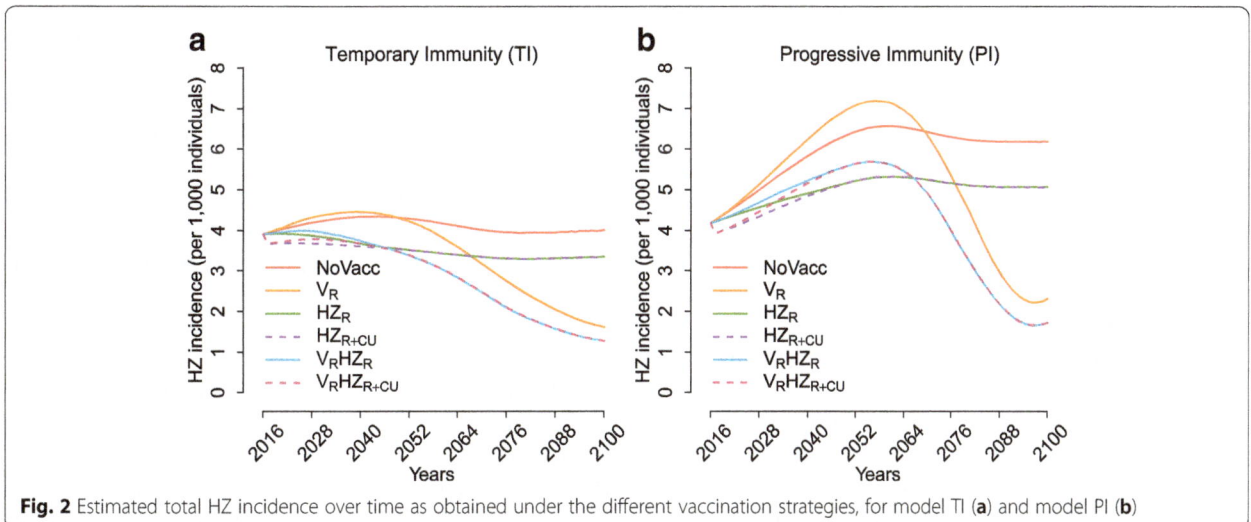

Fig. 2 Estimated total HZ incidence over time as obtained under the different vaccination strategies, for model TI (**a**) and model PI (**b**)

Table 3 Cost-utility analysis for the different vaccination policies, by model and by time horizon

Model TI						Model PI					
Policy	Total cost[a]	QALY loss[b]	ICER[c]	NMB$_k$[d]	NMB$_v$[e]	Policy	Total cost[a]	QALY loss[b]	ICER[c]	NMB$_k$[d]	NMB$_v$[e]
					Time horizon = 25 years						
No vacc.	1812	455	–	–	–	No vacc.	2023	538	–	–	–
V$_R$	1831	446	2219	110	324	V$_R$	2066	537	WD	−37	−28
HZ$_R$	2540	413	WD	−94	963	HZ$_R$	2722	481	WD	143	1548
V$_R$HZ$_R$	2555	402	WD	50	1371	V$_R$HZ$_R$	2757	477	WD	166	1667
HZ$_{R+CU}$	2823	380	WD	109	1975	HZ$_{R+CU}$	2995	444	WD	436	2782
V$_R$HZ$_{R+CU}$	2836	369	12,989	265	2414	V$_R$HZ$_{R+CU}$	3028	439	10,175	476	2944
					Time horizon = 50 years						
No vacc.	2668	691	–	–	–	No vacc.	3145	885	–	–	–
V$_R$	2643	680	Cost-saving	190	466	V$_R$	3240	924	SD	−679	−1654
V$_R$HZ$_R$	3563	576	WD	820	3679	HZ$_R$	3989	745	6031	1255	4754
HZ$_R$	3601	593	SD	531	2970	V$_R$HZ$_R$	4047	767	SD	878	3844
V$_R$HZ$_{R+CU}$	3841	543	8722	1052	4760	HZ$_{R+CU}$	4258	707	6984	1563	6022
HZ$_{R+CU}$	3880	560	SD	749	4017	V$_R$HZ$_{R+CU}$	4313	727	SD	1204	5156
					Time horizon = 85 years						
No vacc.	3092	798	–	–	–	No vacc.	3724	1059	–	–	–
V$_R$	2962	759	Cost-saving	717	1695	V$_R$	3704	1072	1517	−174	−497
V$_R$HZ$_R$	3984	634	8170	1570	5674	V$_R$HZ$_R$	4572	874	4375	1934	6571
HZ$_R$	4119	676	SD	805	3859	HZ$_R$	4627	878	SD	1824	6367
V$_R$HZ$_{R+CU}$	4264	600	8266	1799	6752	V$_R$HZ$_{R+CU}$	4842	834	6829	2257	7881
HZ$_{R+CU}$	4402	643	SD	1020	4904	HZ$_{R+CU}$	4898	839	SD	2128	7632

All outcomes are reported with a 3% discount rate for both benefits and costs
[a]Accounting for cost of disease and cost of policy, in million EUR
[b]In thousands
[c]SD strong dominance (a policy is dominated when the alternative is less costly and more effective), WD weak dominance (a policy is dominated when its ICER is larger than that of a policy with higher effectiveness). The ICER is measured in EUR/QALY gained
[d]Based on the marginal productivity of the national health system (t = 15,000 EUR) and calculated with respect to no vaccination, in million EUR
[e]Based on the consumers' willingness to pay (t = 40,000 EUR) and calculated with respect to no vaccination, in million EUR

V$_R$HZ$_{R+CU}$ to be the most cost-effective for all models and time horizons, except for TH = 50 under model TI, where the policy HZ$_{R+CU}$ was the most cost-effective (Additional file 1: Table S5).

Under the PSA, we found that, for a CE threshold of 15,000 EUR, V$_R$ consistently underperforms compared to the other strategies, irrespective of the model used and the assumed discount rate. Its worst performance, with the NMB decreasing as the CE threshold increases, is expected under model PI with discount rate equal to 3%, because of the higher (negative) impact of varicella vaccination on HZ epidemiology (Fig. 3h). On the contrary, under model TI, V$_R$ always generates a strictly positive NMB, but it is always dominated by the other strategies, except for CE thresholds lower than 8000 EUR (Fig. 3g).

Under both models, the combination of the two vaccinations, V$_R$HZ$_R$ and V$_R$HZ$_{R+CU}$, maximises the NMBs when considering undiscounted outcomes (Fig. 3a and b), with the latter strategy being the most

cost-effective above a CE threshold of 8000 EUR (Fig. 3e and f). However, when assuming a 3% discount rate, we find that, under model PI, the reductions in HZ incidence in the long term are not enough to counterbalance the short-term increase in HZ infections induced by varicella vaccination. Hence, the resulting NMB distribution of the combined programmes is quite similar to those generated by HZ$_R$ and HZ$_{R+CU}$ (Fig. 3d and h). In particular, increasing the CE threshold, the strategy V$_R$HZ$_{R+CU}$ converges to a probability of about 60% of being the most cost-effective, while the strategy HZ$_{R+CU}$ converges to about 40% (Additional file 1: Figure S14D). This result shows that the introduction of an HZ catch-up programme for those aged 66–75 is always beneficial, as it usually produces an increase in the estimated NMB.

Interestingly, we found that the input parameters for the epidemiological model, rather than those for the economic model, represented the most influential source

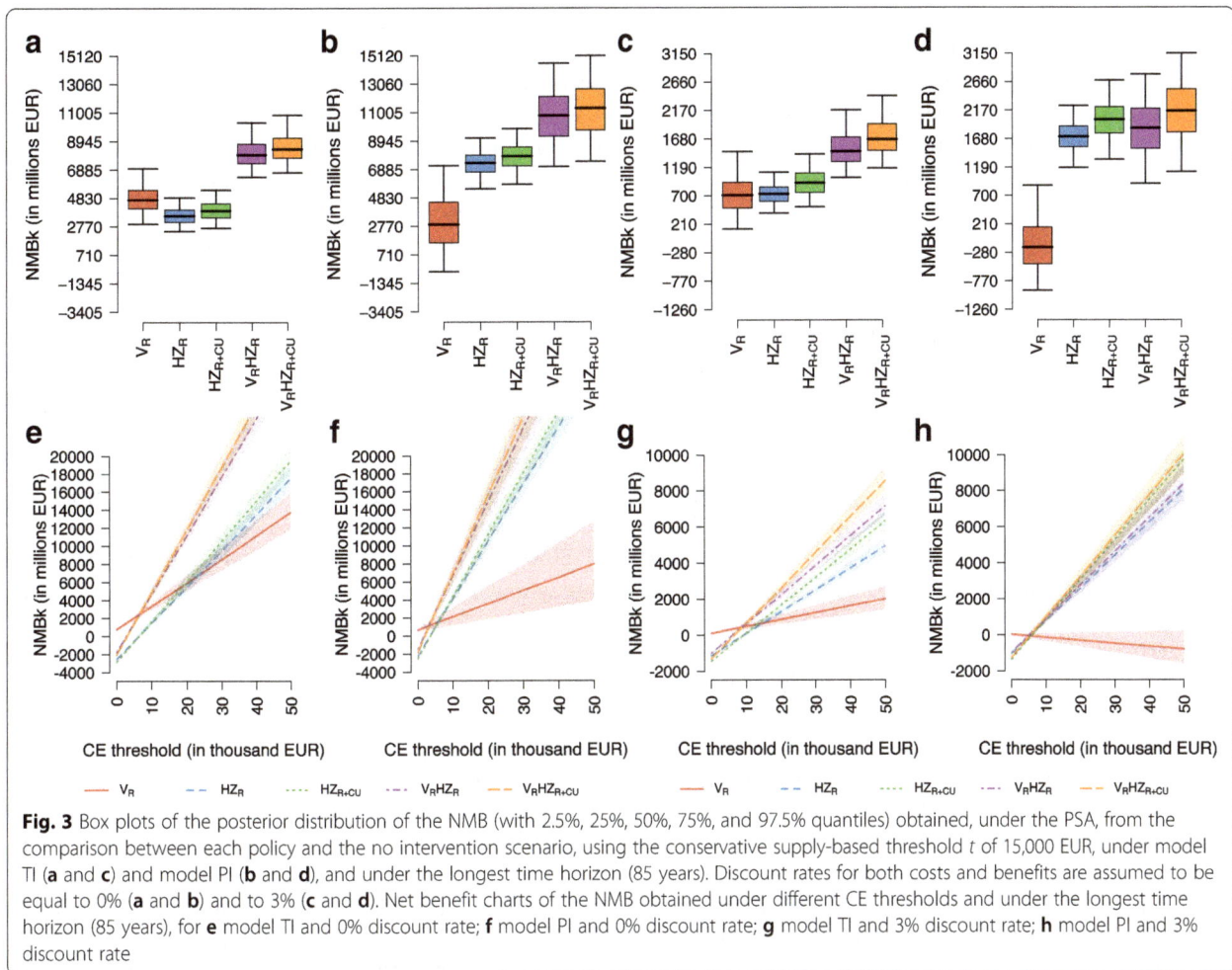

Fig. 3 Box plots of the posterior distribution of the NMB (with 2.5%, 25%, 50%, 75%, and 97.5% quantiles) obtained, under the PSA, from the comparison between each policy and the no intervention scenario, using the conservative supply-based threshold t of 15,000 EUR, under model TI (**a** and **c**) and model PI (**b** and **d**), and under the longest time horizon (85 years). Discount rates for both costs and benefits are assumed to be equal to 0% (**a** and **b**) and to 3% (**c** and **d**). Net benefit charts of the NMB obtained under different CE thresholds and under the longest time horizon (85 years), for **e** model TI and 0% discount rate; **f** model PI and 0% discount rate; **g** model TI and 3% discount rate; **h** model PI and 3% discount rate

of uncertainty on the posterior distribution of the NMB (Additional file 1: Figure S26 and Table S6).

Remarkably, the obtained results are quite robust to variations in the varicella vaccination coverage levels, although upwards or downwards variations in the coverage generate, respectively, a decrease or an increase in the estimated NMBs (Additional file 1: Figures S15 and S16). When we assume a weaker boosting effect, i.e. a low reduction of the HZ risk due to VZV re-exposure, the distribution of the NMBs for the single HZ policies shifts downwards, and the combined policies $V_R HZ_{R+CU}$ and $V_R HZ_R$ outperform the single ones (Additional file 1: Figure S17). Conversely, by considering a stronger role of boosting, both combined policies ($V_R HZ_R$ and $V_R HZ_{R+CU}$) underperform compared to those solely based on HZ vaccination (HZ_R and HZ_{R+CU}), while V_R never proves cost-effective, even in the long term (Additional file 1: Figure S18). Considering the uncertainty in future demographic changes, scenarios assuming a higher future birth rate result in a higher varicella and a lower HZ incidence. However, under a high birth rate scenario, the population would also increase, leading to a higher number of HZ

cases, despite the drop in the incidence. Nevertheless, in the long term, the results of the cost-effectiveness analysis are robust to the uncertainty in the demography, with the combined strategies generating the highest NMBs under both the low and the high birth rate scenarios (Additional file 1: Figures S23 and S24).

Discussion

Principal findings

The results of this study suggest that the recent introduction of the combined varicella and HZ vaccination programmes in Italy is expected to produce a significant reduction of the disease burden caused by VZV infection and reactivation in the long term. The new policy appears to be economically acceptable from a public health payer perspective under different model assumptions on the mechanism of exogenous boosting. In the base case analysis, under the progressive immunity (PI) model, we found that the combined programme would annually prevent, with respect to no vaccination, an average of 435,000 undiscounted cases of varicella, more than 77,000 cases of HZ, and 81 HZ-related deaths per year at a cost of 4375 EUR per QALY gained. Instead, under the temporary immunity (TI) model, we would predict a reduction of almost 437,000 varicella cases, 59,000 HZ cases, and 45 HZ-related deaths per year at a cost of 8170 EUR per QALY gained. From our modelling results, the projected impact would be further improved by adding an HZ catch-up campaign targeting persons 66–75 years old to the implemented national programme. The inclusion of this targeted immunisation activity could prevent on average 3542 additional cases of HZ and 6 deaths per year under model PI, or 3079 HZ cases and 5 deaths under model TI, always maximising the estimated NMB of the strategy. The NMBs are mostly sensitive to the uncertainty on epidemiological parameters, and the ICER values strongly depend on parameters related to HZ and PHN, such as the outpatient and inpatient costs and the corresponding QALY loss (Additional file 1: Figure S25). Overall results appeared robust to changes in model parameters and to different assumptions on exogenous boosting. However, when considering a post-vaccination time horizon of 25 years, varicella vaccination produced an increase in HZ incidence, the magnitude of which depended on whether we assumed a *progressive* or a *temporary* immunity model.

Individual strategies were also evaluated, and model results showed that, whereas HZ vaccination is expected to cost-effectively reduce the burden of HZ disease, varicella vaccination would negatively impact the overall burden of VZV in the short and the medium term. Hence, the introduction of this strategy on its own would not be considered cost-effective from the health care payer perspective.

Strengths and limitations
The obtained results are relevant as they thoroughly evaluate the impact of these newly introduced vaccination programmes, taking into consideration all potential direct and indirect, both positive and negative, effects of the vaccines in Italy, exploring the current uncertainty on the mechanism, either temporary or progressive, underlying exogenous boosting. This latter aspect differentiates this study from previous work, where the cost-effectiveness was evaluated either considering no exogenous boosting or assuming a TI mechanism. In the former case, findings showed that varicella vaccination was always cost-effective (under the health payer perspective) or even cost-saving (under the societal perspective) [27, 29], while in the latter case, it was generally not cost-effective [30, 31] (except for France [47]), except when considering the long term [29, 48]. Moreover, the model also improves on the previous analyses in the way demographic processes are accommodated. Indeed, the model explicitly considers realistic changes in the Italian population age structure over time to take into account temporal trends in VZV epidemiology that are not directly

ascribable to the immunisation programme, but rather to the ageing of the population and to the reduction in the expected number of susceptible children. A similar approach was also recently considered for modelling varicella and HZ epidemiology in Germany [49]. In their study, the authors evaluated the effect of population ageing and migration flows on the epidemiology of the two diseases, along with vaccination policies, but they did not assess the cost-effectiveness and economic acceptability of the programmes.

Our work is based on the underlying assumption of long-lasting protection induced by the HZ vaccine, which might appear to contrast with recent evidence of declining effectiveness (from 60 to 70% in the first years to 30 to 40% in the eighth year) [50]. Although we acknowledge that this can be considered a limitation of our work, we believe that our assumption of a constant vaccine efficacy of 50% can be seen as an average level of protection throughout the observation period. To address the issue of waning vaccine-induced immunity, a second dose of vaccine has been suggested [51]. We took into consideration this possibility by doubling the price of the considered live attenuated HZ vaccine to mimic a two-dose HZ vaccination policy. We found that HZ vaccination would still be cost-effective in the long run, even under the lower threshold of the ICER. Clearly, more work is needed in this direction, also in the light of the fact that some countries are currently considering replacing the live attenuated HZ vaccine with a new recombinant one [52, 53]. This new vaccine has recently been licenced by the US Food and Drug Administration and recommended for healthy adults aged 50 and above to prevent shingles and related complications [54]. Although its reported high efficacy is expected to enhance the cost-effectiveness of the HZ vaccination, both alone and in combination with the varicella vaccine [55], the two-dose schedule and the high price might counterbalance the positive effects.

Finally, our model assumed that the varicella vaccination was first administered to all newborn babies in Italy beginning in 2017, despite the vaccination having gradually been available in some regions since 2003. Considering that the coverage in these regions has reached moderate or high levels in recent years [56, 57], our results might underestimate the impact of varicella vaccination on VZV circulation in Italy and consequently overestimate varicella and HZ incidence, mostly in the short term [4].

Implications for policy makers
Our findings are especially relevant when considering the very recent changes in the Italian National Immunisation Plan (NIP) 2017–2019. The NIP 2017–2019 has introduced recommendations for six new additional vaccinations, which will be administered free of charge: four vaccinations targeted to infants and children (i.e. vaccines

against rotavirus, varicella, group B meningococcal disease, and human papillomavirus for boys), and two to the elderly (i.e. vaccines against pneumococcal disease and herpes zoster). These recommendations have sparked a lively and heated debate on the appropriateness of the new childhood programmes and on the fact that varicella is one of the ten vaccines (hexavalent, plus measles, mumps, rubella, and varicella) that have been introduced as compulsory for school attendance (only starting from those born in 2017). So far, Italy has shown high regional heterogeneity regarding immunisation schedules and outcomes; thus, a new structured national plan will promise a better harmonisation in the vaccine offer and uptake. At the same time, the NIP requirements for school entry should ensure the achievement and maintenance of the high vaccination coverage rates that are necessary for the desired herd immunity effects.

Conclusions

Our study has shown that the newly introduced combined varicella and HZ vaccination strategy in Italy is expected to be effective and cost-effective in reducing the burden of disease and the loss of quality of life. Moreover, the programme is expected to counterbalance the increasing trend in HZ incidence that is estimated in the absence of any vaccination programme and is thus purely due to demographic change. In particular, under the more realistic assumption of PI for the exogenous boosting, this decline would amount to around 435,000 undiscounted cases of varicella and more than 77,000 cases of HZ (and 81 HZ-related deaths) per year at a cost of 4375 EUR per QALY gained. We also found that an additional catch-up campaign for HZ vaccination targeting people aged 66–75 would further increase the benefits of the combined programme, leading to an additional reduction of 3542 cases of HZ and 6 HZ-related deaths per year, at a cost of 6829 EUR per QALY gained.

Our work shows the importance of using models with non-stationary populations, in particular accounting for changing demography, when assessing the impact of vaccination policies on the epidemiology of those infectious diseases that are highly dependent on people mixing. This can surely provide a more thorough understanding of the expected outcomes and therefore help policy makers to design effective preventive strategies.

Abbreviations

CE: Cost-effectiveness; CI: Credible interval; GP: General practitioner; HZ: Herpes zoster; IBM: Individual-based model; ICER: Incremental cost-effectiveness ratio; MCMC: Monte Carlo Markov chain; NIP: National Immunisation Plan; NMB: Net monetary benefit; PHN: Post-herpetic neuralgia; PI: Progressive immunity; PSA: Probabilistic sensitivity analysis; QALY: Quality-adjusted life year; TH: Time horizon; TI: Temporary immunity; VZV: Varicella zoster virus

Acknowledgements
We are grateful to Dr. Maria Gramegna and Alessandra Piatti from Regione Lombardia for providing us with the Hospital Discharge Register data on varicella and HZ for the Lombardy region. We also thank Prof. Giovanni Fattore and Carlo Federici from Bocconi University for the helpful discussions and for providing feedback on our work. We thank the reviewers for their very useful comments and suggestions.

Funding
The research leading to these results has received funding from the European Research Council (ERC) under the European Union's Seventh Framework Programme (FP7/2007–2013) and ERC Grant agreement number 283955 (DECIDE). The funder had no role in the design of the study, collection, analysis, or interpretation of data, or in writing the manuscript.

Authors' contributions
AM, MT, and PP conceived the project. MT collected all data on economic parameters. VM, PP, and SM designed the computer model and carried out the computer simulations and analysis. EDF and AM designed the economic model. EDF performed the cost-effectiveness analysis. CR provided epidemiological expertise. AM, VM, and EDF drafted the manuscript. All authors commented on the drafts and contributed to the final version. AM is the guarantor of the study. All authors read and approved the final manuscript.

Competing interests
PP has received personal fees from Merck & Co. Inc. for consultancy activity outside of the submitted work. All other authors declare that they have no competing interests.

Author details
[1]Department of Social and Political Sciences, Bocconi University, Milano, Italy. [2]Carlo F. Dondena Centre for Research on Social Dynamics and Public Policy, Bocconi University, Milano, Italy. [3]Center for Information and Communication Technology, Bruno Kessler Foundation, Trento, Italy. [4]Department of Hygiene and Preventive Medicine, ATS, Bergamo, Italy. [5]Department of Infectious Disease, Istituto Superiore di Sanità, Roma, Italy.

References
1. Gauthier A, Breuer J, Carrington D, Martin M, Rémy V. Epidemiology and cost of herpes zoster and post-herpetic neuralgia in the United Kingdom. Epidemiol Infect. 2008;137:38–47.
2. Gialloreti LE, Merito M, Pezzotti P, Naldi L, Gatti A, Beillat M, et al. Epidemiology and economic burden of herpes zoster and post-herpetic neuralgia in Italy: a retrospective, population-based study. BMC Infect Dis. 2010;10:230–11.
3. Goldman GS, King PG. Review of the United States universal varicella vaccination program: herpes zoster incidence rates, cost-effectiveness, and vaccine efficacy based primarily on the Antelope Valley Varicella Active Surveillance Project data. Vaccine. 2013;31:1680–94.
4. Bechini A, Boccalini S, Baldo V, Castiglia P, Gallo T, Giuffrida S, et al. Impact of universal vaccination against varicella in Italy. Hum Vaccin Immunother. 2015;11:63–71.

5. Signorelli C, Guerra R, Siliquini R, Ricciardi W. Italy's response to vaccine hesitancy: an innovative and cost effective National Immunization Plan based on scientific evidence. Vaccine. 2017;35:4057–9.

6. Brisson M, Edmunds WJ, Gay NJ. Varicella vaccination: impact of vaccine efficacy on the epidemiology of VZV. J Med Virol. 2003;70:S31–7.

7. Hope-Simpson RE. The nature of herpes zoster: a long-term study and a new hypothesis. Proc R Soc Med. 1965;58:9–20.

8. Jumaan AO, Yu O, Jackson LA, Bohlke K, Galil K, Seward JF. Incidence of herpes zoster, before and after varicella-vaccination-associated decreases in the incidence of varicella, 1992–2002. J Infect Dis. 2005;191:2002–7.

9. Reynolds MA, Chaves SS, Harpaz R, Lopez AS, Seward JF. The impact of the varicella vaccination program on herpes zoster epidemiology in the United States: a review. J Infect Dis. 2008;197:S224–7.

10. Kawai K, Gebremeskel BG, Acosta CJ. Systematic review of incidence and complications of herpes zoster: towards a global perspective. BMJ Open. 2014;4:e004833.

11. Marziano V, Poletti P, Guzzetta G, Ajelli M, Manfredi P, Merler S. The impact of demographic changes on the epidemiology of herpes zoster: Spain as a case study. Proc R Soc B. 2015;282:20142509.

12. Mitka M. FDA approves shingles vaccine: herpes zoster vaccine targets older adults. J Am Med Assoc. 2006;296:157–8.

13. Oxman MN, Levin MJ, Johnson GR, Schmader KE, Straus SE, Gelb LD, et al. A vaccine to prevent herpes zoster and postherpetic neuralgia in older adults. N Engl J Med. 2009;352:2271–84.

14. Karhunen M, Leino T, Salo H, Davidkin I, Kilpi T, Auranen K. Modelling the impact of varicella vaccination on varicella and zoster. Epidemiol Infect. 2010;138:469–81.

15. Poletti P, Melegaro A, Ajelli M, Del Fava E, Guzzetta G, Faustini L, et al. Perspectives on the impact of varicella immunization on herpes zoster. A model-based evaluation from three European countries. PLoS One. 2013;8:e60732.

16. Brisson M, Melkonyan G, Drolet M, De Serres G, Thibeault R, De Wals P. Modeling the impact of one- and two-dose varicella vaccination on the epidemiology of varicella and zoster. Vaccine. 2010;28:3385–97.

17. van Hoek AJ, Melegaro A, Zagheni E, Edmunds WJ, Gay NJ. Modelling the impact of a combined varicella and zoster vaccination programme on the epidemiology of varicella zoster virus in England. Vaccine. 2011;29:2411–20.

18. Guzzetta G, Poletti P, Del Fava E, Ajelli M, Scalia Tomba G, Merler S, et al. Hope-Simpson's progressive immunity hypothesis as a possible explanation for herpes zoster incidence data. Am J Epidemiol. 2013;177:1134–42.

19. Guzzetta G, Poletti P, Merler S, Manfredi P. The epidemiology of herpes zoster after varicella immunization under different biological hypotheses: perspectives from mathematical modeling. Am J Epidemiol. 2016;183:765–73.

20. Terada K, Kawano S, Yoshihiro K, Morita T. Proliferative response to varicella-zoster virus is inversely related to development of high levels of varicella-zoster virus specific IgG antibodies. Scand J Infect Dis. 2009;25:775–8.

21. Vossen MTM, Gent M-R, Weel JFL, de Jong MD, van Lier RAW, Kuijpers TW. Development of virus-specific CD4+ T cells on reexposure to varicella-zoster virus. J Infect Dis. 2004;190:72–82.

22. Ogunjimi B, Smits E, Hens N, Hens A, Lenders K, Ieven M, et al. Exploring the impact of exposure to primary varicella in children on varicella-zoster virus immunity of parents. Viral Immunol. 2011;24:151–7.

23. Thomas SL, Wheeler JG, Hall AJ. Contacts with varicella or with children and protection against herpes zoster in adults: a case-control study. Lancet. 2002;360:678–82.

24. Brisson M, Gay NJ, Edmunds WJ, Andrews N. Exposure to varicella boosts immunity to herpes-zoster: implications for mass vaccination against chickenpox. Vaccine. 2002;20:2500–7.

25. Gaillat J, Gajdos V, Launay O, Malvy D, Demoures B, Lewden L, et al. Does monastic life predispose to the risk of Saint Anthony's fire (herpes zoster)? Clin Infect Dis. 2011;53:405–10.

26. Marangi L, Mirinaviciute G, Flem E, Scalia Tomba G, Guzzetta G, Freiesleben de Blasio B et al. The natural history of varicella zoster virus infection in Norway: Further insights on exogenous boosting and progressive immunity to herpes zoster. PLoS ONE. 2017; 12: e0176845–17

27. Damm O, Ultsch B, Horn J, Mikolajczyk RT, Greiner W, Wichmann O. Systematic review of models assessing the economic value of routine varicella and herpes zoster vaccination in high-income countries. BMC Public Health. 2015;15:222.

28. van Lier A, Lugnér A, Opstelten W, Jochemsen P, Wallinga J, Schellevis F, et al. Distribution of health effects and cost-effectiveness of varicella vaccination are shaped by the impact on herpes zoster. EBioMedicine. 2015;2:1494–9.

29. Bilcke J, van Hoek AJ, Beutels P. Childhood varicella-zoster virus vaccination in Belgium: cost-effective only in the long run or without exogenous boosting? Hum Vaccin Immunother. 2014;9:812–22.

30. Brisson M, Edmunds WJ. The cost-effectiveness of varicella vaccination in Canada. Vaccine. 2002;20:1113–25.

31. Brisson M, Edmunds WJ. Varicella vaccination in England and Wales: cost-utility analysis. Arch Dis Child. 2003;88:862–9.

32. Human Mortality Database University of California, Berkeley (USA), and Max Planck Institute for Demographic Research (Germany) http://www.mortality.org. Accessed 3 May 2018.

33. Database of the Italian Institute of Statistics. Italian National Institute of Statistics (ISTAT), Rome, Italy. http://demo.istat.it/. Accessed 3 May 2018.

34. Merler S, Ajelli M. Deciphering the relative weights of demographic transition and vaccination in the decrease of measles incidence in Italy. Proc R Soc B. 2014;281:20132676.

35. Trentini F, Poletti P, Merler S, Melegaro A. Measles immunity gaps and the progress towards elimination: a multi-country modelling analysis. Lancet Infect Dis. 2017;17:1089–97.

36. Johnson RW. Zoster-associated pain: what is known, who is at risk and how can it be managed? Herpes. 2007;14((Suppl 2)):30–4.

37. Seward JF, Zhang JX, Maupin TJ, Mascola L, Jumaan AO. Contagiousness of varicella in vaccinated cases: a household contact study. J Am Med Assoc. 2004;292:704–8.

38. Civen R, Chaves SS, Jumaan AO, Wu H, Mascola L, Gargiullo PM, et al. The incidence and clinical characteristics of herpes zoster among children and adolescents after implementation of varicella vaccination. Pediatr Infect Dis J. 2009;28:954–9.

39. Ministero della Salute. Piano Nazionale Prevenzione Vaccinale. Rome: Gazzetta Ufficiale; 2017.

40. Vázquez M, LaRussa PS, Gershon AA, Steinberg SP, Freudigman K, Shapiro ED. The effectiveness of the varicella vaccine in clinical practice. N Engl J Med. 2001;344:955–60.

41. Gabutti G, Penna C, Rossi M, Salmaso S, Rota MC, Bella A, et al. The seroepidemiology of varicella in Italy. Epidemiol Infect. 2001;126:433–40.

42. Fattore G. Proposta di linee guida per la valutazione economica degli interventi sanitari in Italia. Pharmacoeconomics Ital Res Articles. 2009;11:83–93.

43. Woods B, Revill P, Sculpher M, Claxton K. Country-level cost-effectiveness thresholds: initial estimates and the need for further research. Value Health. 2016;19:929–35.

44. Baio G, Dawid AP. Probabilistic sensitivity analysis in health economics. Stat Methods Med Res. 2011;24:615–34.

45. Briggs AH. A Bayesian approach to stochastic cost-effectiveness analysis. Health Econ. 1999;8:257–61.

46. Stinnett AA, Mullahy J. Net health benefits: a new framework for the analysis of uncertainty in cost-effectiveness analysis. Med Dec Making. 1998;18:202–12.

47. Littlewood KJ, Ouwens MJNM, Sauboin C, Tehard B, Alain S, Denis F. Cost-effectiveness of routine varicella vaccination using the measles, mumps, rubella and varicella vaccine in France: an economic analysis based on a dynamic transmission model for varicella and herpes zoster. Clin Ther. 2015;37:830–7.

48. van Hoek AJ, Melegaro A, Gay NJ, Bilcke J, Edmunds WJ. The cost-effectiveness of varicella and combined varicella and herpes zoster vaccination programmes in the United Kingdom. Vaccine. 2012; 30:1225–34.

49. Horn J, Damm O, Greiner W, Hengel H, Kretzschmar ME, Siedler A, et al. Influence of demographic changes on the impact of vaccination against varicella and herpes zoster in Germany – a mathematical modelling study. BMC Med. 2018;16:1–9.

50. Morrison VA, Johnson GR, Schmader KE, Levin MJ, Zhang JH, Looney DJ, et al. Long-term persistence of zoster vaccine efficacy. Clin Infect Dis. 2015;60:900–9.

51. Tseng H-F, Harpaz R, Luo Y, Hales CM, Sy LS, Tartof SY, et al. Declining effectiveness of herpes zoster vaccine in adults aged ≥ 60 years. J Infect Dis. 2016;213:1872–5.

52. Lal H, Cunningham AL, Godeaux O, Chlibek R, Díez-Domingo J, Hwang S-J, et al. Efficacy of an adjuvanted herpes zoster subunit vaccine in older adults. N Engl J Med. 2015;372:2087–96.

53. Cunningham AL, Lal H, Kovac M, Chlibek R, Hwang S-J, Díez-Domingo J, et al. Efficacy of the herpes zoster subunit vaccine in adults 70 years of age or older. N Engl J Med. 2016;375:1019–32.

54. Span P. No excuses, people: get thenew shingles vaccine. New York City: The New York Times; 2017. https://nyti.ms/2ho3vmE. Accessed 3 May 2018

The impact of demographic changes, exogenous boosting and new vaccination policies on varicella...

207

55. Marchetti S, Guzzetta G, Flem E, Mirinaviciute G, Scalia Tomba G, Manfredi P. Modeling the impact of combined vaccination programs against varicella and herpes zoster in Norway. Vaccine 2018; 36: 1116–125.

56. Trucchi C, Gabutti G, Rota MC, Bella A. Burden of varicella in Italy, 2001–2010: analysis of data from multiple sources and assessment of universal vaccination impact in three pilot regions. J Med Microbiol. 2015;64:1387–94.

57. Signorelli C, Odone A, Cella P, Iannazzo S, D'Ancona F, Guerra R. Infant immunization coverage in Italy (2000-2015). Ann Ist Super Sanità. 2017; 53:231-7.

58. Vázquez M, Shapiro ED. Varicella vaccine and infection with varicella-zoster virus. N Engl J Med. 2005;352:439–40.

59. Thiry N, Beutels P, Van Damme P, Van Doorslaer E. Economic evaluations of varicella vaccination programmes. PharmacoEconomics. 2003;21:13–38.

60. Coudeville L, Brunot A, Szucs TD, Dervaux B. The economic value of childhood varicella vaccination in France and Germany. Value Health. 2005; 8:209–22.

61. Kind P, Hardman G, Macran S. UK population norms for EQ-5D. Centre for Health Economics Discussion Paper Series. Report No. 172. York: University of York; 1999. p. 1–98.

62. Bala MV, Wood LL, Zarkin GA, Norton EC, Gafni A, O'Brien B. Valuing outcomes in health care: a comparison of willingness to pay and quality-adjusted life-years. J Clin Epidemiol. 1998;51:667–76.

63. Chaves SS, Zhang J, Civen R, Watson BM, Carbajal T, Perella D, et al. Varicella disease among vaccinated persons: clinical and epidemiological characteristics, 1997-2005. J Infect Dis. 2008;197(Suppl 2):S127–31.

64. Fornaro P, Gandini F, Marin M, Pedrazzi C, Piccoli P, Tognetti D, et al. Epidemiology and cost analysis of varicella in Italy: results of a sentinel study in the pediatric practice. Pediatr Infect Dis J. 1999;18:414–9.

65. Zotti CM, Maggiorotto G, Migliardi A. I costi della varicella. Ann Ig. 2002;14:29–33.

66. Giaquinto C, Sturkenboom M, Mannino S, Arpinelli F, Nicolosi A, Cantarutti L. Epidemiologia ed esiti della varicella in Italia: risultati di uno studio prospettico sui bambini (0–14 anni) seguiti dai pediatri di libera scelta (Studio Pedianet). Ann Ig. 2002;14:21–7.

Selective serotonin reuptake inhibitor use during early pregnancy and congenital malformations

Shan-Yan Gao[1], Qi-Jun Wu[1], Ce Sun[1], Tie-Ning Zhang[2], Zi-Qi Shen[3], Cai-Xia Liu[3], Ting-Ting Gong[3], Xin Xu[1], Chao Ji[1], Dong-Hui Huang[1], Qing Chang[1] and Yu-Hong Zhao[1*]

Abstract

Background: In 2005, the FDA cautioned that exposure to paroxetine, a selective serotonin reuptake inhibitor (SSRI), during the first trimester of pregnancy may increase the risk of cardiac malformations. Since then, the association between maternal use of SSRIs during pregnancy and congenital malformations in infants has been the subject of much discussion and controversy. The aim of this study is to systematically review the associations between SSRIs use during early pregnancy and the risk of congenital malformations, with particular attention to the potential confounding by indication.

Methods: The study protocol was registered with PROSPERO (CRD42018088358). Cohort studies on congenital malformations in infants born to mothers with first-trimester exposure to SSRIs were identified via PubMed, Embase, Web of Science, and the Cochrane Library databases through 17 January 2018. Random-effects models were used to calculate summary relative risks (RRs).

Results: Twenty-nine cohort studies including 9,085,954 births were identified. Overall, use of SSRIs was associated with an increased risk of overall major congenital anomalies (MCAs, RR 1.11, 95% CI 1.03 to 1.19) and congenital heart defects (CHD, RR 1.24, 95% CI 1.11 to 1.37). No significantly increased risk was observed when restricted to women with a psychiatric diagnosis (MCAs, RR 1.04, 95% CI 0.95 to 1.13; CHD, RR 1.06, 95% CI 0.90 to 1.26). Similar significant associations were observed using maternal citalopram exposure (MCAs, RR 1.20, 95% CI 1.09 to 1.31; CHD, RR 1.24, 95% CI 1.02 to 1.51), fluoxetine (MCAs, RR 1.17, 95% CI 1.07 to 1.28; CHD, 1.30, 95% CI 1.12 to 1.53), and paroxetine (MCAs, RR 1.18, 95% CI 1.05 to 1.32; CHD, RR 1.17, 95% CI 0.97 to 1.41) and analyses restricted to using women with a psychiatric diagnosis were not statistically significant. Sertraline was associated with septal defects (RR 2.69, 95% CI 1.76 to 4.10), atrial septal defects (RR 2.07, 95% CI 1.26 to 3.39), and respiratory system defects (RR 2.65, 95% CI 1.32 to 5.32).

Conclusions: The evidence suggests a generally small risk of congenital malformations and argues against a substantial teratogenic effect of SSRIs. Caution is advisable in making decisions about whether to continue or stop treatment with SSRIs during pregnancy.

Keywords: Antidepressant, Congenital malformations, Cohort studies, Pregnancy, Serotonin uptake inhibitors, Meta-analysis

* Correspondence: zhaoyh@sj-hospital.org
[1]Department of Clinical Epidemiology, Shengjing Hospital of China Medical University, No. 36, San Hao Street, Shenyang, Liaoning, China
Full list of author information is available at the end of the article

Background

Selective serotonin reuptake inhibitors (SSRIs) have become the first-line pharmaceuticals for the treatment of depression, anxiety, and other psychiatric disorders since they were introduced into the market [1]. About 63% to 85% of pregnant women with exposure to antidepressant are treated with SSRIs [2–4]. SSRIs are thought to be effective for treating psychiatric disorders by increasing the synaptic bioavailability of the neurotransmitter serotonin (5-HT), which readily crosses the placenta and can affect certain kinds of cells and tissues during embryogenesis, which may result in certain congenital malformations, especially cardiac malformations [5–8]. In December 2005, the US Food and Drug Administration (FDA) cautioned that the use of paroxetine, as individual SSRI during the first trimester of pregnancy may increase the risk of cardiac malformations [9]. Since then, the associations between the use of SSRIs during pregnancy and the risk of congenital malformations in offspring have been the subject of much discussion and controversy [10].

The number of published meta-analyses regarding the associations between maternal use of SSRIs and congenital malformations has more than tripled during the last 5 years (20 meta-analyses to date). However, some of these studies produced conflicting results due to varying study designs and exposure times. Most inconsistently reported were congenital heart defects (CHD) (Additional file 1: Table S1). Furthermore, none of these meta-analyses attempted to comprehensively investigate the associations between the use of SSRIs and individual SSRIs and the risks of specific congenital malformations. Some of the previous meta-analyses [11–23] examined the risks of certain congenital malformations [overall major congenital anomalies (MCAs) and cardiac malformations] with maternal use of SSRIs and/or individual SSRIs. Other meta-analyses [24–28] examined the risks of specific (cardiac) malformations with the use of only one or two specific SSRIs. Reefhuis and colleagues [29] examined the risks of 15 congenital malformations categories with the use of individual SSRIs during early pregnancy; however, recall bias derived from case-control studies might have been inherent in those data. A large number of cohort studies were published recently that explore the aforementioned associations from Europe and other regions, but the results are still inconsistent [30–47].

Depression and anxiety have been associated with adverse pregnancy outcomes and health behaviors [48–50]. Thus, some researchers have expressed concerns that the underlying depression or psychiatric illness might increase the risks of congenital malformations in infants [51–53]. To the best of our knowledge, no previous meta-analyses have assessed potential confounding by

indication (underlying psychiatric diagnosis) by comparing women using SSRIs vs. those with unmedicated psychiatric illness during the first trimester of pregnancy.

We performed a detailed systematic review and large-scale meta-analysis of current evidence from cohort studies to investigate whether there is any relationship between maternal use of SSRIs during early pregnancy and congenital malformations in infants. Particular attention is given to the potential for confounding by indication.

Methods

The report of this systemic review and meta-analysis followed the recommendations of the Preferred Reporting Items for Systematic Reviews and Meta-Analyses (PRISMA) group [54]. Before study selection, the protocol for this review was registered with PROSPERO (CRD42018088358).

Data sources and searches

PubMed, Embase, Web of Science, and The Cochrane Library were searched from database inception to 17 January 2018. The search strategy combined medical subject heading (MeSH) and Embase subject heading (EMTREE) terms with other unindexed or free-text terms. Details of the full search strategy are provided in Additional file 2. Reference lists of retrieved articles and previous systematic and narrative reviews were searched manually to retrieve all relevant documents. No language restrictions were imposed.

Study selection

Cohort studies or randomized controlled trials that reported original data were eligible for inclusion if they reported any congenital malformations in infants born to mothers with any exposure to SSRIs or individual SSRIs (citalopram, fluoxetine, paroxetine, sertraline, escitalopram, or fluvoxamine) during the first trimester, had a comparison group that included pregnant women who were not exposed to any antidepressants and/or teratogens (folic acid antagonists, angiotensin-converting enzyme inhibitors, anticonvulsants, coumarin derivatives, and retinoids), and, if a risk estimate was not reported, provided necessary distribution of exposure, non-exposure, cases, and non-cases, from which a risk estimate could be calculated.

The titles and abstracts of retrieved articles were evaluated by two independent reviewers (S-YG and CS). The full texts of potentially eligible studies that seemed to meet the inclusion criteria were then obtained and independently reviewed by the two reviewers. Any disagreements were identified and resolved by discussion or by consultation with a third reviewer (Q-JW). If data were duplicated in more than one study, we included the study with the largest number of cases.

Data extraction

A standardized, pre-designed spreadsheet was used for data extraction from the included studies. The study quality and synthesis of evidence were assessed. The following data were extracted into the spreadsheet: first author, publication year, geographic location, study period, data source, sample size (cases and cohorts), types of birth, definition of outcome, outcome with their risk estimates and 95% confidence intervals (CIs), and adjusted confounders. Congenital malformations were identified and defined according to the European Surveillance of Congenital Anomalies (EUROCAT) Guide 1.3 and ICD-10 and ICD-9 codes (Additional file 3: Table S1). The primary outcomes of interest were overall MCAs and specific CHD. The secondary outcomes of interest were other system-specific malformations (nervous system defects; eye defects; ear, face, and neck defects; respiratory system defects; orofacial cleft; digestive system defects; urogenital system defects; urinary system defects; genital system defects; musculoskeletal system defects; limb; and abdominal wall defects. Two reviewers (T-NZ and Z-QS) extracted data independently; any disagreements were resolved by discussion with a third reviewer (S-YG) where necessary.

For a study [36] that reported a different follow-up duration, the estimate of the follow-up duration during the first 6 years of life was extracted. For studies [31, 40, 44, 45, 47, 55–61] that did not report any adjusted risk estimate, we used the crude risk estimate. If a study lacked required data, they were requested by contacting the study authors by email.

Risk of bias assessment

We used the Newcastle-Ottawa scale [62] to assess the risk of bias of cohort studies, which included studies based on the selection of study participant groups (four stars), the comparability of study groups (two stars), and the ascertainment of outcome (three stars). Studies were considered to have low risk of bias if they achieved a full rating in at least two categories of selection, comparability, or outcome assessment [63].

Statistical analysis

For a study [64] that separately reported the risk estimates of SSRIs but did not report combined estimates, the effective count method proposed by Hamling et al. [65] was used to recalculate the effect estimate. Another study [56] reported results separately (but not combined) for CHD (bulbus cordis anomalies and anomalies of cardiac septal closure and other congenital anomalies of heart), nervous system malformations (spina bifida and other congenital anomalies of nervous system), digestive system defects (cleft palate and cleft lip, other congenital anomalies of

upper alimentary tract, and other congenital anomalies of digestive system), and musculoskeletal system defects (certain congenital musculoskeletal deformities, other congenital musculoskeletal anomalies, and other congenital anomalies of limbs); here, the results were pooled using a fixed-effect model to obtain an overall combined estimate before combining these estimates with the remaining studies (Additional file 3: Table S1). Similar analyses also were performed for limb defects (limb reduction and clubfoot) [31, 34]. If the selected study did not include a risk estimate, the unadjusted risk estimate and the 95% CI were calculated from the raw data for simplicity [31, 38, 44, 45, 57, 59, 61, 66]. Because the odds ratio is an excellent approximation of the risk ratio in the case of rare outcomes, the results were referred to as relative risks (RRs) [67]; therefore, all results were reported as RR for simplicity. Estimates were pooled using the DerSimonian and Laird random-effects model to calculate summarized RRs and 95% CI [68].

We used the I^2 statistic to assess heterogeneity in effect measures between the studies. I^2 values of 25, 50, and 75% were considered to represent low, moderate, and high heterogeneity, respectively [69]. If ≥ 8 studies were available, potential sources of heterogeneity were explored by conducting subgroup analyses according to the following parameters: study quality (high risk vs. low risk), geographic location (Europe vs. Northern America or other regions), and adjustment for potential confounders (adjusted vs. unadjusted) including maternal age, socioeconomic status, smoking, alcohol drinking, body mass index (BMI) during pregnancy, pregnancy complications, and parity. Heterogeneity between subgroups was evaluated by meta-regression analysis. The potential for publication bias was examined through Begg's and Egger's tests [70, 71]. To determine the influence of an individual study in each main analysis of the estimated RR, we conducted a sensitivity analysis that recalculated the pooled effect by omitting one study at a time. Analyses were performed with Stata version 11.0 (StataCorp, College Station, TX). A two-tailed P value less than 0.05 was considered as statistically significant.

Results

Search results

We identified 10,919 potentially eligible articles in PubMed, Embase, Web of Science, and The Cochrane Library. Two additional studies were identified in a manual search of the reference lists. The titles and abstracts were screened, and 79 articles qualified for full-text review (Fig. 1). The authors of two studies failed to respond to requests for additional data. Finally, 29 cohort studies (published between 1996 and 2017) providing 649 data points that contributed to the quantitative

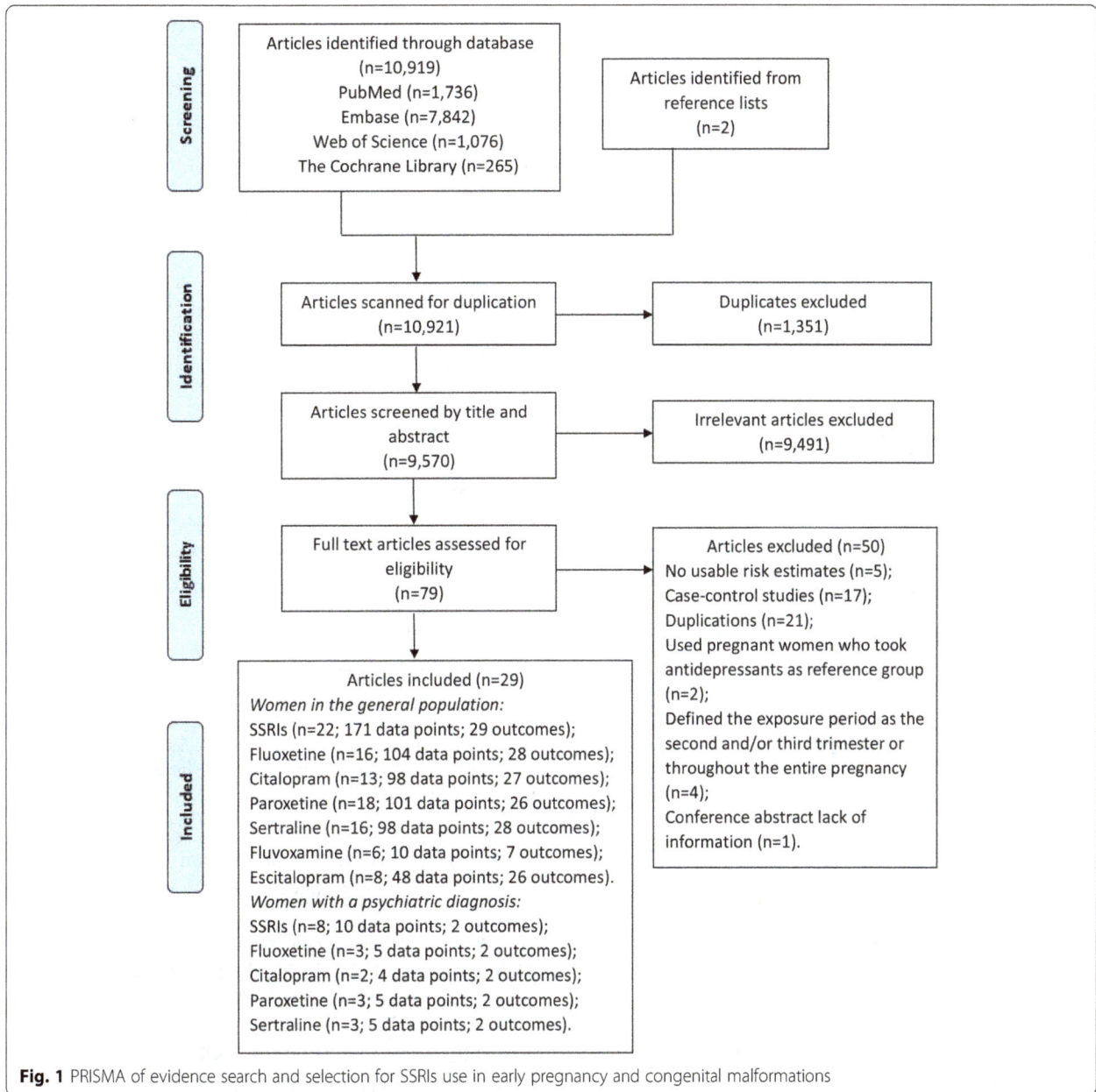

Fig. 1 PRISMA of evidence search and selection for SSRIs use in early pregnancy and congenital malformations

synthesis met all inclusion and exclusion criteria, which included a total of 9,085,954 individuals for analysis. These included 25 studies focused on women in the general population, 8 studies focused on women with a psychiatric disorder, and 6 studies focused on both; 7,926,215 untreated pregnant women without psychiatric disorders, 1,916,076 SSRI-untreated women with psychiatric disorders, and 59,894 SSRI-treated women with psychiatric disorders; 7,590,399 individuals from Europe (15 studies), 1,206,094 from North America (10 studies), and 289,461 from Japan and Israel (4 studies). The key characteristics of the included studies are presented in Additional file 3: Table S2.

Bias assessment

Analysis of the included studies using Newcastle-Ottawa criteria indicated that 23 studies were low risk and 6 were high risk for bias. All studies achieved a total score of 4 to 9 (median = 8) (Additional file 3: Table S3).

Exposure to SSRIs
Risk of major congenital anomalies

Nine studies [34, 37–40, 43, 60, 61, 72] for the comparison of women receiving SSRIs versus women in the general population were included for this analysis. The pooled RR was 1.11 (95% CI 1.03 to 1.19, I^2 = 38.4%, P = 0.11, Figs. 2 and 3, Additional file 3: Table S4), with no

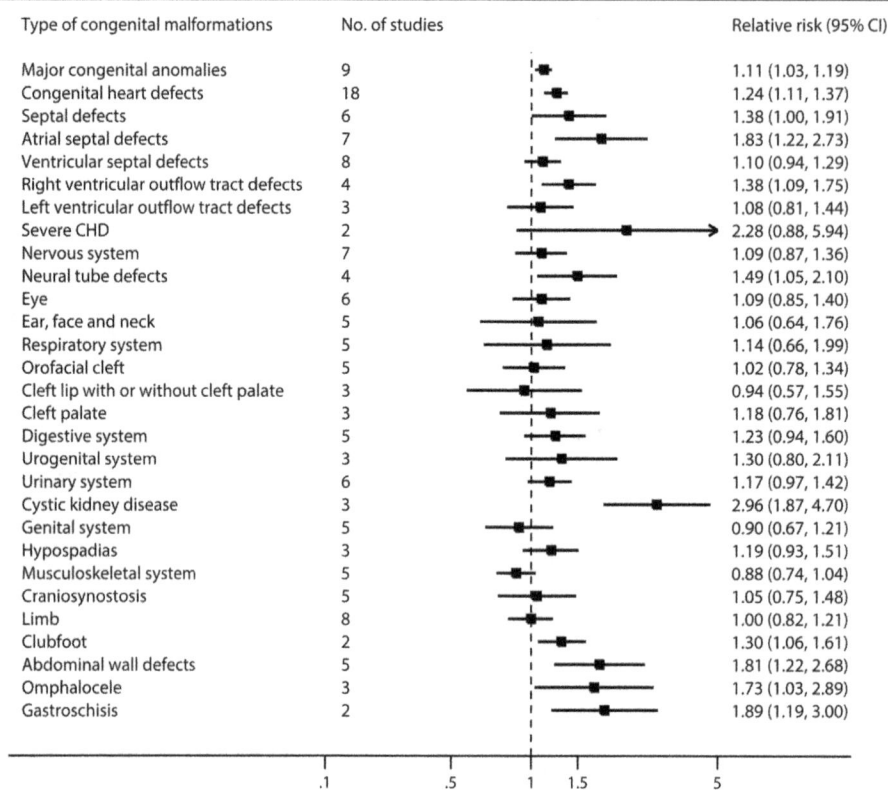

Type of congenital malformations	No. of studies	Relative risk (95% CI)
Major congenital anomalies	9	1.11 (1.03, 1.19)
Congenital heart defects	18	1.24 (1.11, 1.37)
Septal defects	6	1.38 (1.00, 1.91)
Atrial septal defects	7	1.83 (1.22, 2.73)
Ventricular septal defects	8	1.10 (0.94, 1.29)
Right ventricular outflow tract defects	4	1.38 (1.09, 1.75)
Left ventricular outflow tract defects	3	1.08 (0.81, 1.44)
Severe CHD	2	2.28 (0.88, 5.94)
Nervous system	7	1.09 (0.87, 1.36)
Neural tube defects	4	1.49 (1.05, 2.10)
Eye	6	1.09 (0.85, 1.40)
Ear, face and neck	5	1.06 (0.64, 1.76)
Respiratory system	5	1.14 (0.66, 1.99)
Orofacial cleft	5	1.02 (0.78, 1.34)
Cleft lip with or without cleft palate	3	0.94 (0.57, 1.55)
Cleft palate	3	1.18 (0.76, 1.81)
Digestive system	5	1.23 (0.94, 1.60)
Urogenital system	3	1.30 (0.80, 2.11)
Urinary system	6	1.17 (0.97, 1.42)
Cystic kidney disease	3	2.96 (1.87, 4.70)
Genital system	5	0.90 (0.67, 1.21)
Hypospadias	3	1.19 (0.93, 1.51)
Musculoskeletal system	5	0.88 (0.74, 1.04)
Craniosynostosis	5	1.05 (0.75, 1.48)
Limb	8	1.00 (0.82, 1.21)
Clubfoot	2	1.30 (1.06, 1.61)
Abdominal wall defects	5	1.81 (1.22, 2.68)
Omphalocele	3	1.73 (1.03, 2.89)
Gastroschisis	2	1.89 (1.19, 3.00)

Fig. 2 Risk of congenital malformations in infants, according to maternal exposure to SSRIs. Relative risks and 95% confidence intervals are presented to show the risk of congenital malformations among infants born to women with exposure to SSRIs during the first trimester, as compared with the risk among infants born to women in the general population without such exposure. SSRIs, selective serotonin reuptake inhibitors

evidence of publication bias (Begg's $P = 0.92$, Eggers's $P = 0.83$). No significantly increased risk was observed when restricted to women with a psychiatric diagnosis (RR 1.04, 95% CI 0.95 to 1.13, $I^2 = 2.5\%$, $P = 0.38$, Fig. 3) [2, 33, 37, 72].

Risk of specific congenital heart defects
Eighteen studies [31, 32, 34–40, 42–44, 46, 55, 56, 58, 61, 72] in the general population were included for this analysis. The pooled RR was 1.24 (95% CI 1.11 to 1.37, $I^2 = 59.0\%$, $P = 0.001$, Figs. 2 and 4, Additional file 3: Table S4), with no evidence of publication bias (Begg's $P = 0.23$, Eggers's $P = 0.45$). No significantly increased risk was observed when restricted to women with a psychiatric diagnosis (RR 1.06, 95% CI 0.90 to 1.26, $I^2 = 33.9\%$, $P = 0.18$, Fig. 4) [31, 37, 41, 55, 64, 72].

Maternal use of SSRIs during the first trimester was associated with an increased risk in septal defects [36, 37, 40, 42, 43, 72] (RR 1.38, 95% CI 1.00 to 1.91, $I^2 = 67.4\%$, $P = 0.009$), atrial septal defects (ASD) [31, 35, 37, 39, 40, 61, 72] (RR 1.83, 95% CI 1.22 to 2.73, $I^2 = 72.0\%$, $P = 0.002$), and right ventricular outflow tract defects (RVOTD) [34, 39, 55, 72] (RR 1.38, 95% CI 1.09 to 1.75, $I^2 = 33.0\%$, $P = 0.21$) (Figs. 2 and 5; Additional file 3:

Table S4). No evidence of publication bias was detected in any of these studies (all $P > 0.05$).

Risk of other system-specific malformations
Maternal use of SSRIs during the first trimester was associated with an increased risk of neural tube defects [31, 37, 39, 46] (RR 1.49, 95% CI 1.05 to 2.10, $I^2 = 0$, $P = 0.43$), cystic kidney disease [34, 40, 46] (RR 2.96, 95% CI 1.87 to 4.70, $I^2 = 0$, $P = 0.81$), clubfoot [31, 34] (RR 1.30, 95% CI 1.06 to 1.61, $I^2 = 0$, $P = 0.65$), abdominal wall defects [30, 31, 37, 46, 72] (RR 1.81, 95% CI 1.22 to 2.68, $I^2 = 0$, $P = 0.86$), omphalocele [31, 34, 39] (RR 1.73, 95% CI 1.03 to 2.89, $I^2 = 0$, $P = 0.73$), and gastroschisis [31, 34] (RR 1.89, 95% CI 1.19 to 3.00, $I^2 = 0$, $P = 0.56$) (Fig. 2, Additional file 3: Table S4).

Exposure to individual SSRIs
Citalopram
Eight studies [34, 37, 39, 40, 43, 60, 61, 72] in the general population provided data for MCAs in infants. The pooled RR was 1.20 (95% CI 1.09 to 1.31, $I^2 = 13.4\%$, $P = 0.33$), with no evidence of publication bias (Begg's $P = 0.54$, Eggers's $P = 0.77$). No significantly increased risk was observed when restricted to

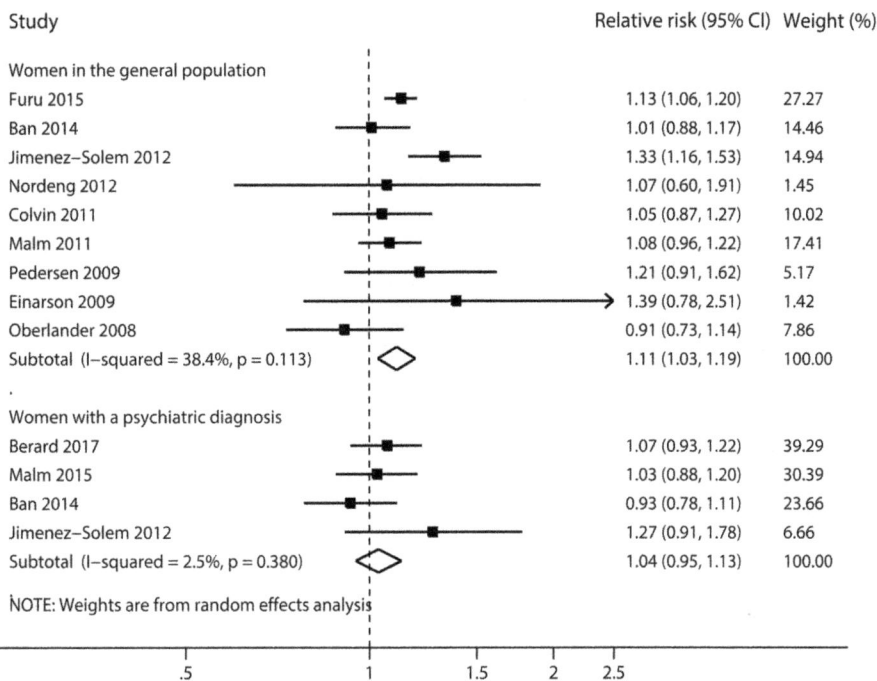

Fig. 3 Risk of major congenital anomalies in infants, according to maternal exposure to SSRIs. Relative risks and 95% confidence intervals are presented to show the risk of major congenital anomalies among infants born to women with exposure to SSRIs during the first trimester, as compared with the risk among infants born to women without such exposure. SSRIs, selective serotonin reuptake inhibitors

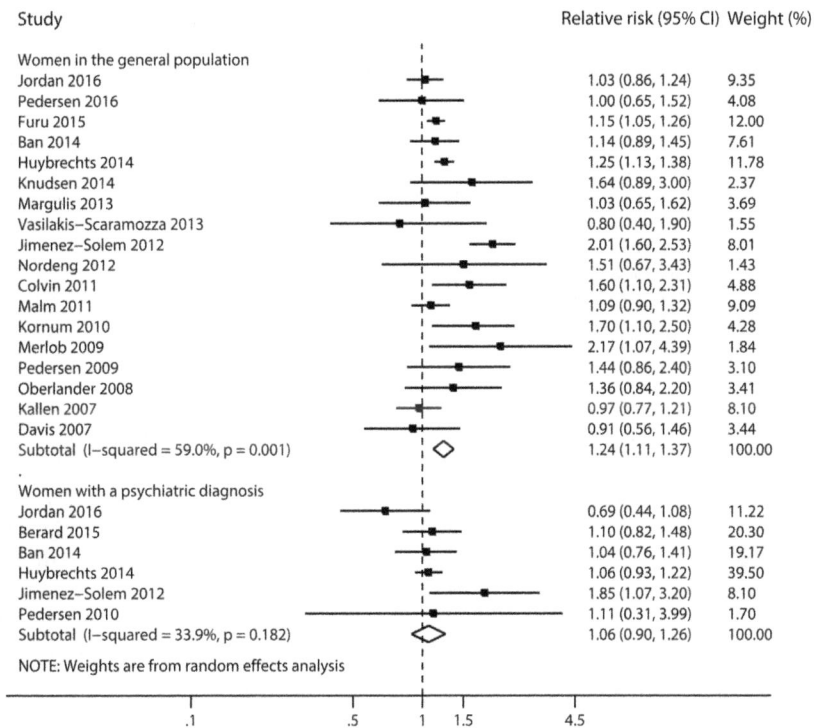

Fig. 4 Risk of congenital heart defects in infants, according to maternal exposure to SSRIs. Relative risks and 95% confidence intervals are presented to show the risk of congenital heart defects among infants born to women with exposure to SSRIs during the first trimester, as compared with the risk among infants born to women without such exposure. SSRIs, selective serotonin reuptake inhibitors

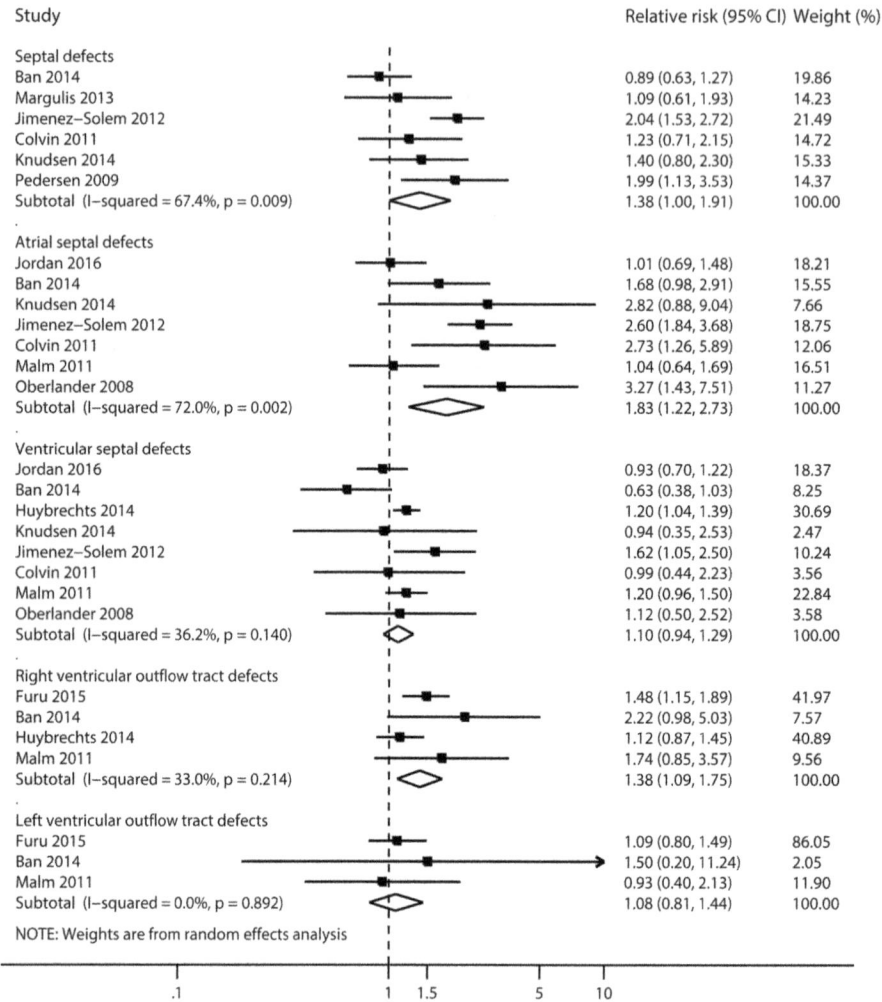

Fig. 5 Risk of septal defects in infants, according to maternal exposure to SSRIs. Relative risks and 95% confidence intervals are presented to show the risk of septal defects among infants born to women with exposure to SSRIs during the first trimester, as compared with the risk among infants born to women in the general population without such exposure. SSRIs, selective serotonin reuptake inhibitors

women with a psychiatric diagnosis (RR 1.17, 95% CI 0.84 to 1.62, I^2 = 66.0%, $P=0.09$) [2, 72] (Additional file 3: Table S5, Additional file 4).

Eleven studies [31, 34, 37, 39, 40, 42–44, 46, 61, 72] provided data for CHD in infants in the general population. The pooled RR was 1.24 (95% CI 1.02 to 1.51, I^2 = 52.5%, $P=0.02$), with no evidence of publication bias (Begg's $P=0.23$, Eggers's $P=0.32$). No significantly increased risk was observed when restricted to women with a psychiatric diagnosis (RR 1.08, 95% CI 0.75 to 1.56, I^2 = 0, $P=0.75$) [2, 72] (Additional file 3: Table S5, Additional file 5).

Citalopram use during the first trimester was associated with an increased risk of septal defects [37, 40, 42, 43] (RR 1.81, 95% CI 1.22 to 2.68, I^2 = 0, $P=0.55$), RVOTD [34, 39] (RR 1.59, 95% CI 1.08 to 2.35, I^2 = 0, $P=0.54$), eye defects [31, 37, 40, 72] (RR 2.00, 95% CI 1.13 to 3.54, I^2 = 0, $P=0.55$), urinary system defects [31, 37, 40, 72] (RR

1.72, 95% CI 1.27 to 2.33, I^2 = 0, $P=0.72$), and hypospadias [31, 34] (RR 1.87, 95% CI 1.23 to 2.83, I^2 = 0, $P=0.43$) (Additional file 3: Table S5).

Fluoxetine
Eleven studies [34, 37–40, 43, 45, 57, 60, 61, 72] in the general population provided data for MCAs in infants. The pooled RR was 1.17 (95% CI 1.07 to 1.28, I^2 = 0, $P=0.50$), with no evidence of publication bias (Begg's $P=0.28$, Eggers's $P=0.62$). No significantly increased risk was observed when restricted to women with a psychiatric diagnosis (RR 0.84, 95% CI 0.67 to 1.05, I^2 = 0, $P=0.83$) [2, 72] (Additional file 3: Table S6, Additional file 6).

Fourteen studies [31, 34, 37–40, 42–46, 55, 61, 72] provided data for CHD in infants in the general population. The pooled RR was 1.30 (95% CI 1.12 to 1.53, I^2 = 29.3%, $P=0.14$), with no evidence of publication bias (Begg's $P=0.23$, Eggers's $P=0.32$). No significantly increased risk was observed when restricted to women with a psychiatric diagnosis (RR 0.94, 95% CI 0.65 to 1.37, I^2 = 41.9%, P = 0.18) [2, 55, 72] (Additional file 3: Table S6, Additional file 7).

Fluoxetine use during the first trimester was associated with an increased risk of septal defects [37, 40, 42, 43] (RR 1.65, 95% CI 1.02 to 2.67, I^2 = 0, P = 0.99), RVOTD [34, 39, 55] (RR 1.63, 95% CI 1.11 to 2.41, I^2 = 18.0%, P = 0.30), neural tube defects [31, 37, 39] (RR 2.28, 95% CI 1.28 to 4.06, I^2 = 0, P = 0.76), and ear, face, and neck defects [31, 40] (RR 3.45, 95% CI 1.28 to 9.29, I^2 = 0, P = 0.41) (Additional file 3: Table S6).

Paroxetine

Eleven studies [34, 37–40, 43, 45, 47, 60, 61, 72] provided data for MCAs in infants in the general population. The pooled RR was 1.18 (95% CI 1.05 to 1.32, I^2 = 0, P = 0.64), with no evidence of publication bias (Begg's P = 0.09, Eggers's P = 0.14). No significantly increased risk was observed when restricted to women with a psychiatric diagnosis (RR 1.17, 95% CI 0.97 to 1.41, I^2 = 0, P = 0.34) [2, 72] (Additional file 3: Table S7, Additional file 8).

Sixteen studies [31, 34, 37–40, 42–45, 55, 56, 61, 66, 72] in the general population provided data for CHD in infants. The pooled RR was 1.35 (95% CI 1.19 to 1.53, I^2 = 0, P = 0.71), with no evidence of publication bias (Begg's P = 0.69, Eggers's P = 0.21). No significantly increased risk was observed when restricted to women with a psychiatric diagnosis (RR 1.27, 95% CI 0.89 to 1.80, I^2 = 72.3%, P = 0.03) [2, 55, 72] (Additional file 3: Table S7, Additional file 9).

Paroxetine use during the first trimester was associated with an increased risk of RVOTD [34, 39, 55] (RR 2.15, 95% CI 1.04 to 4.44, I^2 = 67.0%, P = 0.049), eye defects [31, 56, 72] (RR 2.26, 95% CI 1.26 to 4.04, I^2 = 0, P = 0.53), and cleft palate [31, 39] (RR 2.82, 95% CI 1.26 to 6.32, I^2 = 0, P = 0.83) (Additional file 3: Table S7).

Sertraline

Nine studies [34, 37–40, 43, 60, 61, 72] provided data for MCAs in infants. The pooled RR was 1.10 (95% CI 0.99 to 1.22, I^2 = 0, P = 0.69), with no evidence of publication bias (Begg's P = 0.92, Eggers's P = 0.85). No significantly increased risk was observed when restricted to women with a psychiatric diagnosis (RR 1.12, 95% CI 0.87 to 1.44, I^2 = 0, P = 0.79) [2, 72] (Additional file 3: Table S8, Additional file 10).

Thirteen studies [31, 34, 37–40, 42–44, 46, 55, 61, 72] provided data for CHD in infants. The pooled RR was 1.42 (95% CI 1.12 to 1.80, I^2 = 63.9%, P = 0.001), with no evidence of publication bias (Begg's P = 0.50, Eggers's P = 0.26). No significantly increased risk was

observed when restricted to women with a psychiatric diagnosis (RR 1.12, 95% CI 0.92 to 1.35, I^2 = 0, P = 0.80) [2, 55, 72] (Additional file 3: Table S8, Additional file 11).

Sertraline use during the first trimester was associated with an increased risk of septal defects [37, 40, 42, 43] (RR 2.69, 95% CI 1.76 to 4.10, I^2 = 16.8%, P = 0.31), ASD [31, 37, 39, 40] (RR 2.07, 95% CI 1.26 to 3.39, I^2 = 0, P = 0.54), respiratory system defects [37, 39, 40, 72] (RR 2.65, 95% CI 1.32 to 5.32, I^2 = 0, P = 0.45), limb defects [31, 34, 37, 72] (RR 1.42, 95% CI 1.03 to 1.95, I^2 = 0, P = 0.54), and clubfoot [31, 34] (RR 1.72, 95% CI 1.11 to 2.65, I^2 = 0, P = 0.77) (Additional file 3: Table S8).

Escitalopram/fluvoxamine

Maternal use of escitalopram during the first trimester was associated with an increased risk of clubfoot [31] (RR 2.18, 95% CI 1.16 to 4.08), abdominal wall defects [31] (RR 3.52, 95% CI 1.56 to 7.93), and gastroschisis [31] (RR 3.95, 95% CI 1.46 to 10.68) (Additional file 3: Table S9). There was no statistically significant association between first-trimester exposure to fluvoxamine and MCAs [34, 39, 60, 61] (RR 0.77, 95% CI 0.49 to 1.21, I^2 = 0, P = 0.79, Additional file 3: Table S10).

Subgroup and sensitivity analyses

The results of subgroup and meta-regression analyses are presented in Additional file 3: Table S11-S15. Subgroup analyses indicated that the low risk of bias studies and European studies were generally consistent with the main results; however, they were not all statistically significant. No statistically significant source of heterogeneity was identified in meta-regression analyses. The sensitivity analysis omitted one study at a time, which showed the results appeared to be robust to the influence of individual studies. By contrast, the pooled RR of MCAs was 1.06 with SSRIs (95% CI 0.85 to 1.32, I^2 = 0, P = 0.67) after excluding the study by Huybrechts et al. [55].

Discussion

This comprehensive systemic review and meta-analysis of cohort studies including more than nine million births found generally small increased risks in 18 of 29 congenital malformations categories in infants born to mothers with exposure to SSRIs and individual SSRIs during early pregnancy, especially for MCAs and CHD. We found the RRs for the association between use of SSRIs and outcomes were lower in the restricted cohorts. Though the 95% CIs of the comparisons made between studies in general population and studies in mothers with a psychiatric diagnosis contained an overlap, we still cannot exclude the possibility of confounding by indication.

SSRIs and congenital malformations

We identified a small but significant association between maternal use of SSRIs during the first trimester and MCAs in infants. This observed increase was consistent with the results of previous meta-analyses [15, 19] However, the association was attenuated after controlling for psychiatric diagnosis. Although the effects of SSRIs could never be completely separated from a psychiatric illness itself, such estimates are likely to be influenced by potential confounding by indication. Jimenez-Solem and colleagues [37] first differentiated between the consequences of SSRI use and the underlying disease, and found an increased risk of MCAs among infants born to women who took SSRIs during the first trimester, whereas the correlation was not significant for women who paused their use of SSRIs during the first trimester in a nationwide cohort study. Ban and colleagues [72] compared risks between pregnant women with medicated and unmedicated depression based on a population-based cohort study. Although results for MCAs were not statistically significant, the point estimate slightly decreased in comparison with pregnant women treated with SSRIs.

There was an association between first-trimester exposure to SSRIs and the risk of CHD. Some biological evidence possibly supports the observed increase [8, 73], but the results were inconsistent in three meta-analyses [14, 15, 19]. This difference is probably due to variations in sample size, study design, and time of exposure. The meta-analysis by Wang and colleagues [14] included four population-based cohort studies enrolling 1,996,519 participants and found no significant associations between the use of SSRIs and heart defects (Additional file 1: Table S1). In recent years, fourfold population-based cohort studies including nearly eight million participants have been conducted to examine the aforementioned relationship, and the results were consistent with our primary results (our unreported data). Myles and colleagues [15] synthesized evidence from nine cohort studies combined with case-control studies; however, high heterogeneity might have been inherent in those data. Nikfar and colleagues [19] assessed the risk of cardiovascular malformations with the use of SSRIs during pregnancy, but not during the first trimester. Similarly, the association was markedly attenuated after controlling for psychiatric diagnosis.

Individual SSRIs and congenital malformations
Citalopram

The observed increase in MCAs and CHD with maternal use of citalopram during the first trimester was inconsistent with all previous meta-analyses [11, 12, 14, 15]. A recent meta-analysis by Kang and colleagues [11], including five cohort studies and one case-control study, reported no significant associations between exposure to citalopram and the risk of CHD during pregnancy. However, over twofold cohort studies were eligible for inclusion in our analysis. Data for 2.3 million births from a previous cohort study [34] were re-analyzed by an aggregate meta-analysis by Selmer and colleagues [12]; this cohort study was included in our meta-analysis. Results between the meta-analysis and the included study were similar regarding the association of citalopram use and CHD. Our findings regarding the effect of citalopram use on neural tube defects and hypospadias were inconsistent with the study by Reefhuis and colleagues [29], which used Bayesian analysis to combine summarized results from published literature with data from the US National Birth Defects Prevention Study.

Fluoxetine

The main results of this meta-analysis of fluoxetine use during early pregnancy were consistent with our previous study [26] and a recent meta-analysis by Selmer and colleagues [12]. Our data on fluoxetine-associated ventricular septal defects (VSD) and RVOTD were consistent with the study of Reefhuis and colleagues [29]. Our data also showed significant associations between fluoxetine use and the risk of system-specific malformations (neural tube defects and ear, face, and neck defects). However, these results require corroboration due to the limited number of individual studies.

Paroxetine

Our data show a significant association between the use of paroxetine and the risks of MCAs and CHD. The results were consistent with a recent meta-analysis by Berard and colleagues [27], but were inconsistent with a previous meta-analysis by Bar-Oz and colleagues [22]. Bar-Oz and colleagues conducted the analysis in 2007, and thus only included three cohort and case-control studies. Two meta-analyses assessed the risk of system-specific malformations from exposure to paroxetine and yielded inconsistent results due to the varying study design. One meta-analysis of cohort and cases studies [27] identified an increased risk of septal defects and ASD with paroxetine use; the other meta-analysis of case-control studies [29] identified an increased risk of ASD, gastroschisis, and omphalocele with paroxetine use (but not cleft palate or hypospadias).

Sertraline

Although the findings of this meta-analysis were consistent with our previous study [25], our data regarding the association of sertraline use with septal defects were inconsistent with the results of Reefhuis and colleagues [29]. Our data also showed significant associations between sertraline use and the risk of system-specific malformations (respiratory system defect, limb defect, and clubfoot). These results require corroboration due to the limited number of individual studies.

Escitalopram

The main results of this meta-analysis were consistent with previous meta-analyses [12, 29] regarding the risks of CHD and septal defects from exposure to escitalopram during early pregnancy. One of our included studies [31] reported statistically significant associations between escitalopram use and the risk of system-specific malformations (limb defect, clubfoot, abdominal wall defects, and gastroschisis) in three population-based cohorts that included 519,117 fetuses and infants.

Potential mechanism

Potential biological mechanisms of SSRI use and the increased risk of congenital malformations is based on studies of drug metabolite levels in cord blood in human [74]. In vitro, a growing body of evidence has suggested that the neurotransmitter serotonin (5-HT) plays a crucial role as a signaling molecule in cardiogenesis [8, 75]. Consequently, disruption of the 5-HT signaling caused by the use of SSRIs may result in several different types of CHD [73, 76].

Strengths and limitations of the study

Our study has several strengths. First, this meta-analysis of current evidence from cohort studies includes the largest sample size (more than nine million births) analyzed to date and combines the results with the most comprehensive data related to associations between the use of SSRIs and all individual SSRIs during early pregnancy and the risks of 29 categories of congenital malformations. Second, this meta-analysis pays particular attention to the potential confounding by indication. Third, for ethical reasons, there are no randomized controlled trials; therefore, the quality of evidence from cohort studies could provide clinicians and pregnant women with a reference in clinical practice.

There are limitations in our meta-analysis related to evidence synthesis and quality. First, the definition of outcomes varied among studies, particularly the definition of CHD, which could contribute to the high heterogeneity in our study. CHD has a specific definition and coding in the EUROCAT guide, but not in the ICD codes; however, most of the individual studies defining outcomes were based on ICD codes such as ICD-10 and ICD-9 (Additional file 3: Table S1-S2). We also failed to find any specific coding in either the ICD codes or EUROCAT subgroups related to MCAs, septal defects, RVOTD, and left ventricular outflow tract defects. Furthermore, the definitions of outcomes might depend on the authors of individual studies. For example, Ban and colleagues [72] defined septal defects as ASD, VSD, and atrioventricular septal defects, whereas Pedersen and colleagues [43] defined the defects as ASD and VSD. Additionally, the follow-up duration may also be a potential source of heterogeneity. On the one hand, some types of CHD (e.g., VSDs) may be self-healing [77]. On the other hand, due to the serious malformations are usually symptomatic with early detection, whereas milder malformations are sometimes identified at later age [36].

Second, the majority of individual studies only included live births. Stillbirth, spontaneous abortion, or induced abortion caused by severe malformations [78, 79] were not always recorded or observable and would have been missed, which could introduce selection bias and underestimate the strength of the associations between the use of SSRIs during early pregnancy and congenital malformations in infants [80]. The restriction of results according to different data sources also could also result in potential bias. The pooled effects of this study were dominated by record-linkage studies. However, data collected from prescription registries, dispensation registries, or drug reimbursement registries that rely on dispensed prescription information to determine maternal use of SSRIs would lead to misclassification of exposure [81, 82]. The dispensing of SSRIs may not always precisely reflect the specific time of exposure or verify that SSRIs were actually taken as prescribed. Selection bias presents a potential limitation in teratology information service studies, as women recruited during early pregnancy who feel the need for counseling about the teratogenic potential of SSRIs may be at higher risk than those who have no concerns [83].

Third, the event rate of congenital malformations in infants is very low, and individual studies may not have consistently adjusted for potential confounders. Therefore, we included adjusted or unadjusted risk estimates in our meta-analysis. Unadjusted risk estimates should be interpreted with caution, but the main results were still robust after removing crude risk estimates in the sensitivity analysis. Due to the lack of information on other potential confounders such as folic acid supplementation and familial-related factors, we could not fully rule out the possibility of residual confounding. For example, the study by Furu and colleagues [34] reported results from sibling design in addition to the full cohort. The results of sibling-controlled analyses showed attenuated risk compared with the full cohort. Thus, the small observed increased risk could be explained by familial-related factors or other lifestyle-related factors not adjusted for. In addition, we lacked information about the restricted cohorts regarding severity of disease. Eliminating the potential teratogenicity of SSRIs from a potential effect of the underlying psychiatric diagnoses remains a challenge.

Fourth, as we could not obtain an estimate for the incidence of MCAs and CHD events in the general population or in women with a psychiatric diagnosis, we could not provide an absolute risk increase of MCAs and CHD associated with exposure to SSRIs in the general population and in women with a psychiatric diagnosis. However, we obtained some examples from the published studies to give a suggestion of the increased absolute risk. Ban and colleagues [72] reported that children born to women with diagnosed depression unmedicated in early pregnancy had higher absolute risks of overall MCAs than children of mothers with no depression (absolute risk increase: 15 per 10000 births). Futhermore, Alwans et al. and Huybrechts et al. [55, 84] found a small increase in the absolute risk of CHD with exposure to SSRIs. Although the absolute risk of MCAs and CHD were highly likely to remain small, it is still of concern to pregnant women.

Fifth, it should be recognized that the implicated system-specific malformations and controlled psychiatric diagnosis studies are rare. The small number of included studies limited the statistical power of the study, which limited our ability to perform subgroup analyses to further investigate these issues and interpret the results. There was insufficient evidence to estimate fetal outcomes for the dosage of SSRIs use during pregnancy. Thus, we were unable to conduct a dose-response analysis.

Finally, since the study focused on non-exposure, i.e., pregnant women who were not exposed to any antidepressants and/or teratogens, rather than pregnant women who were exposed to other individual SSRIs, we could not determine if any of the individual SSRIs was preferable over others.

Conclusions
The results of this meta-analysis highlight the complexity of this topic and the need to better understand the potential effect of the underlying psychiatric diagnosis. Continued evaluation of the association between maternal use of SSRIs and congenital malformations is warranted, and there is a pressing need for new studies on the effects of individual SSRIs (and their dosage) on system-specific malformations, specifically in women with underlying psychiatric diagnosis. The accumulated evidence suggests a generally small risk of congenital malformations and argues against a substantial teratogenic effect of SSRIs. Caution is advisable in making decisions about whether to continue or stopping treatment with SSRIs during pregnancy. Stopping treatment in mothers with major depression could be more harmful for the infant than continuing use of SSRIs. This information could be helpful for pregnant women and their healthcare providers to make more informed decisions about treatment.

Additional files

Additional file 1: Table S1. Characteristics of prior meta-analyses of selective serotonin reuptake inhibitors (SSRIs) use in pregnancy and congenital malformations. (DOC 816 kb)

Additional file 2: Appendix 1. Search strategy. (DOCX 26 kb)

Additional file 3: Table S1. EUBOCAT Guide 1.3, ICD-10, and ICD-9 codes used to identify and define congenital malformations. **Table S2.** Characteristics of cohort studies of selective serotonin reuptake inhibitors (SSRIs) use in first-trimester and congenital malformations. **Table S3.** Risk of bias of included reports from cohort studies as assessed with the Newcastle-Ottawa scale. Table S4. Exposure to selective serotonin reuptake inhibitors (SSRIs) during the first trimester of pregnancy and risk of congenital malformations in infants: results of meta-analyses. **Table S5.** Exposure to citalopram during the first trimester of pregnancy and risk of congenital malformations in infants: results of meta-analyses. **Table S6.** Exposure to fluoxetine during the first trimester of pregnancy and risk of congenital malformations in infants: results of meta-analyses. **Table S7.** Exposure to paroxetine during the first trimester of pregnancy and risk of congenital malformations in infants: results of meta-analyses. **Table S8.** Exposure to sertraline during the first trimester of pregnancy and risk of congenital malformations in infants: results of meta-analyses. **Table S9.** Exposure to escitalopram during the first trimester of pregnancy and risk of congenital malformations in infants: results of meta-analyses. **Table S10.** Exposure to fluvoxamine during the first trimester of pregnancy and risk of congenital malformations in infants: results of meta-analyses. **Table S11.** Subgroup analysis of selective serotonin reuptake inhibitors (SSRIs) and risk of congenital malformations in infants: results of meta-analyses. **Table S12.** Subgroup analysis of citalopram and risk of congenital malformations in infants: results of meta-analyses. **Table S13.** Subgroup analysis of fluoxetine and risk of congenital malformations in infants: results of meta-analyses. **Table S14.** Subgroup analysis of paroxetine and risk of congenital malformations in infants: results of meta-analyses. **Table S15.** Subgroup analysis of sertraline and risk of congenital malformations in infants: results of meta-analyses. (DOC 1162 kb)

Additional file 4: Figure S1. Risk of major congenital anomalies in infants, according to maternal exposure to citalopram. (TIF 1083 kb)

Additional file 5: Figure S2. Risk of congenital heart defects in infants, according to maternal exposure to citalopram. (TIF 1123 kb)

Additional file 6: Figure S3. Risk of major congenital anomalies in infants, according to maternal exposure to fluoxetine. (TIF 1141 kb)

Additional file 7: Figure S4. Risk of congenital heart defects in infants, according to maternal exposure to fluoxetine. (TIF 1177 kb)

Additional file 8: Figure S5. Risk of major congenital anomalies in infants, according to maternal exposure to paroxetine. (TIF 1135 kb)

Additional file 9: Figure S6. Risk of congenital heart defects in infants, according to maternal exposure to paroxetine. (TIF 1244 kb)

Additional file 10: Figure S7. Risk of major congenital anomalies in infants, according to maternal exposure to sertraline. (TIF 1112 kb)

Additional file 11: Figure S8. Risk of congenital heart defects in infants, according to maternal exposure to sertraline. (TIF 1185 kb)

Abbreviations
ASD: Atrial septal defect; CHD: Congenital heart defect; CIs: Confidence intervals; EUROCAT: European Surveillance of Congenital Anomalies; MCAs: Major congenital anomalies; RR: Relative risk; RVOTD: Right ventricular outflow tract defect; SSRIs: Selective serotonin reuptake inhibitors; VSD: Ventricular septal defect

Acknowledgements
We would like to thank BioMed Proofreading for English proofreading.

Funding
This study was funded by National Key R&D Program of China (no. 2017YFC0907400 to Y-HZ); the Science and Technology Project of Liaoning Province (no. 2013225079 to Y-HZ); the Natural Science Foundation of China

(no. 81602918 to Qi-Jun Wu), the Doctoral Start-up Foundation of Liaoning Province (no. 201501007 to Qi-Jun Wu), the Younger research fund of Shengjing Hospital (grant 2014sj09 to Qi-Jun Wu), and the Outstanding Youth Foundation of China Medical University (no. YQ20170002 to Qi-Jun Wu). The funders had no role in the study design, data collection, data analysis and interpretation, or the content of the final manuscript.

Authors' contributions

YG, Q-JW, and Y-HZ designed the study and formulated the clinical question. S-YG and CS performed the literature search and, with Q-JW, reviewed the search results for study inclusion. T-NZ, Z-QS, and S-YG designed the data extraction form and extracted the data. All authors collected, managed, and analyzed the data. S-YG drafted the manuscript. All authors prepared, reviewed, revised, and approved the manuscript. Y-HZ had full access to all data in the study and is responsible for data integrity and the accuracy of data analysis. All authors read and approved the final manuscript.

Competing interests

The authors declare that they have no competing interests.

Author details

[1]Department of Clinical Epidemiology, Shengjing Hospital of China Medical University, No. 36, San Hao Street, Shenyang, Liaoning, China. [2]Department of Pediatrics, Shengjing Hospital of China Medical University, Shenyang, China. [3]Department of Obstetrics and Gynecology, Shengjing Hospital of China Medical University, Shenyang, China.

References

1. Ornoy A, Koren G. Selective serotonin reuptake inhibitors in human pregnancy: on the way to resolving the controversy. Semin Fetal Neonatal Med. 2014;19(3):188–94.
2. Berard A, Zhao J, Sheehy O. Antidepressant use during pregnancy and the risk of major congenital malformations in a cohort of depressed pregnant women: an updated analysis of the Quebec Pregnancy Cohort. BMJ Open. 2017;7:e0133721.
3. Jimenez-Solem E, Andersen JT, Petersen M, Broedbaek K, Andersen NL, Torp-Pedersen C, et al. Prevalence of antidepressant use during pregnancy in Denmark, a nation-wide cohort study. PLoS One. 2013;8(4):e63034.
4. Taouk LH, Matteson KA, Stark LM, Schulkin J. Prenatal depression screening and antidepressant prescription: obstetrician-gynecologists' practices, opinions, and interpretation of evidence. Arch Womens Ment Health. 2018; 21(1):85–91.
5. Liu Y, Zhou X, Zhu D, Chen J, Qin B, Zhang Y, et al. Is pindolol augmentation effective in depressed patients resistant to selective serotonin reuptake inhibitors? A systematic review and meta-analysis. Hum Psychopharmacol. 2015;30(3):132–42.
6. Hendrick V, Stowe ZN, Altshuler LL, Hwang S, Lee E, Haynes D. Placental passage of antidepressant medications. Am J Psychiatry. 2003;160(5):993–6.
7. Laine K, Heikkinen T, Ekblad U, Kero P. Effects of exposure to selective serotonin reuptake inhibitors during pregnancy on serotonergic symptoms in newborns and cord blood monoamine and prolactin concentrations. Arch Gen Psychiatry. 2003;60(7):720–6.
8. Sadler TW. Selective serotonin reuptake inhibitors (SSRIs) and heart defects: potential mechanisms for the observed associations. Reprod Toxicol. 2011; 32(4):484–9.
9. U.S Food and Drug Administration (FDA). Public Health Advisory: Paroxetine. 2005. https://wayback.archive-it.org/7993/20170112033310/http://www.fda. gov/Drugs/DrugSafety/PostmarketDrugSafetyInformationforPatients andProviders/ucm051731.htm. Accessed 27 Aug 2018.; 2018.
10. Nembhard WN, Tang X, Hu Z, MacLeod S, Stowe Z, Webber D. Maternal and infant genetic variants, maternal periconceptional use of selective serotonin reuptake inhibitors, and risk of congenital heart defects in offspring: population based study. BMJ. 2017;356:j832.
11. Kang HH, Ahn KH, Hong SC, Kwon BY, Lee EH, Lee JS, et al. Association of citalopram with congenital anomalies: a meta-analysis. Obstet Gynecol Sci. 2017;60(2):145–53.
12. Selmer R, Haglund B, Furu K, Andersen M, Nørgaard M, Zoëga H, et al. Individual-based versus aggregate meta-analysis in multi-database studies of pregnancy outcomes: the Nordic example of selective serotonin reuptake inhibitors and venlafaxine in pregnancy. Pharmacoepidem DR S. 2016; 25(10):1160–9.
13. Kowalik E, Ward K, Ye Y. SSRI use in pregnancy and congenital heart defects: a metaanalysis of population-based cohort studies. Pharmacotherapy. 2016;36(12):e302.
14. Wang S, Yang L, Wang L, Gao L, Xu B, Xiong Y. Selective Serotonin Reuptake Inhibitors (SSRIs) and the Risk of Congenital Heart Defects: A Meta-Analysis of Prospective Cohort Studies. J Am Heart Assoc. 2015;4(5):e001681.
15. Myles N, Newall H, Ward H, Large M. Systematic meta-analysis of individual selective serotonin reuptake inhibitor medications and congenital malformations. Aust NZ J Psychiat. 2013;47(11):1002–12.
16. Painuly N, Painuly R, Heun R, Sharan P. Risk of cardiovascular malformations after exposure to paroxetine in pregnancy: meta-analysis. Psychiatrist. 2013; 37(6):198–203.
17. Riggin L, Frankel Z, Moretti M, Pupco A, Koren G. The fetal safety of fluoxetine: a systematic review and meta-analysis. Journal of obstetrics and gynaecology Canada. JOGC. 2013;35(4):362–9.
18. Yan Y, Cheng Y, Crowe B, Chhabra-Khanna R, Camporeale A, Marangell L. First trimester fluoxetine use and major malformations: a meta-analysis of epidemiological studies. Pharmacoepidem DR S. 2013;22:168–9.
19. Nikfar S, Rahimi R, Hendoiee N, Abdollahi M. Increasing the risk of spontaneous abortion and major malformations in newborns following use of serotonin reuptake inhibitors during pregnancy: a systematic review and updated meta-analysis. Daru. 2012;20:75.
20. Wurst KE, Poole C, Ephross SA, Olshan AF. First trimester paroxetine use and the prevalence of congenital, specifically cardiac, defects: a meta-analysis of epidemiological studies. Birth Defects Res Part A Clin Mol Teratol. 2010;88(3): 159–70.
21. O'Brien L, Einarson TR, Sarkar M, Einarson A, Koren G. Does paroxetine cause cardiac malformations? J Obstet Gynaecol Can. 2008;30(8):696–701.
22. Bar-Oz B, Einarson T, Einarson A, Boskovic R, O'Brien L, Malm H, et al. Paroxetine and congenital malformations: meta-analysis and consideration of potential confounding factors. Clin Ther. 2007;29(5):918–26.
23. Addis A, Koren G. Safety of fluoxetine during the first trimester of pregnancy: a meta-analytical review of epidemiological studies. Psychol Med. 2000;30(1):89–94.
24. Zhang TN, Gao SY, Shen ZQ, Li D, Liu CX, Lv HC, et al. Use of selective serotonin-reuptake inhibitors in the first trimester and risk of cardiovascular-related malformations: a meta-analysis of cohort studies. Sci Rep. 2017;7: 43085.
25. Shen ZQ, Gao SY, Li SX, Zhang TN, Liu CX, Lv HC, et al. Sertraline use in the first trimester and risk of congenital anomalies: a systemic review and meta-analysis of cohort studies. Brit J Clin Pharmaco. 2017;83(4):909–22.
26. Gao SY, Wu QJ, Zhang TN, Shen ZQ, Liu CX, Xu X, et al. Fluoxetine and congenital malformations: a systematic review and meta-analysis of cohort studies. Brit J Clin Pharmaco. 2017;83(10):2134–47.
27. Bérard A, Iessa N, Chaabane S, Muanda FT, Boukhris T, Zhao JP. The risk of major cardiac malformations associated with paroxetine use during the first trimester of pregnancy: a systematic review and meta-analysis. Brit J Clin Pharmaco. 2016;81(4):589–604.
28. Grigoriadis S, VonderPorten EH, Mamisashvili L, Roerecke M, Rehm J, Dennis CL, et al. Antidepressant exposure during pregnancy and congenital malformations: is there an association? A systematic review and meta-analysis of the best evidence. J Clin Psychiat. 2013;74(4):e293–308.
29. Reefhuis J, Devine O, Friedman JM, Louik C, Honein MA. Specific SSRIs and birth defects: bayesian analysis to interpret new data in the context of previous reports. BMJ-Brit Med J. 2015;351:h3190.
30. Nishigori H, Obara T, Nishigori T, Mizuno S, Metoki H, Hoshiai T, et al. Selective serotonin reuptake inhibitors and risk of major congenital anomalies for pregnancies in Japan: a nationwide birth cohort study of the Japan Environment and Children's Study. Congenit Anom. 2017;57(3):72–8.
31. Jordan S, Morris JK, Davies GI, Tucker D, Thayer DS, Luteijn JM, et al. Selective Serotonin Reuptake Inhibitor (SSRI) antidepressants in pregnancy and congenital anomalies: Analysis of linked databases in Wales, Norway and Funen, Denmark. Plos One. 2016;11(12):e0165122.

32. Petersen I, Evans SJ, Gilbert R, Marston L, Nazareth I. Selective serotonin reuptake inhibitors and congenital heart anomalies: comparative cohort studies of women treated before and during pregnancy and their children. J Clin Psychiat. 2016;77(1):e36–42.

33. Malm H, Sourander A, Gissler M, Gyllenberg D, Hinkka-Yli-Salomäki S, McKeague IW, et al. Pregnancy complications following prenatal exposure to SSRIs or maternal psychiatric disorders: results from population-based national register data. AM J Psychiat. 2015;172(12):1224–32.

34. Furu K, Kieler H, Haglund B, Engeland A, Selmer R, Stephansson O, et al. Selective serotonin reuptake inhibitors and venlafaxine in early pregnancy and risk of birth defects: population based cohort study and sibling design. BMJ. 2015;350:h1798.

35. Knudsen TM, Hansen AV, Garne E, Andersen AMN. Increased risk of severe congenital heart defects in offspring exposed to selective serotonin-reuptake inhibitors in early pregnancy - an epidemiological study using validated EUROCAT data. BMC Pregnancy Childbirth. 2014;14(1):333.

36. Margulis AV, Abou-Ali A, Strazzeri MM, Ding Y, Kuyateh F, Frimpong EY, et al. Use of selective serotonin reuptake inhibitors in pregnancy and cardiac malformations: a propensity-score matched cohort in CPRD. Pharmacoepidem DR S. 2013;22(9):942–51.

37. Jimenez-Solem E, Andersen JT, Petersen M, Broedbaek K, Jensen JK, Afzal S, et al. Exposure to selective serotonin reuptake inhibitors and the risk of congenital malformations: A nationwide cohort study. BMJ Open. 2012;2(3):e001148.

38. Nordeng H, Van Gelder MMHJ, Spigset O, Koren G, Einarson A, Eberhard-Gran M. Pregnancy outcome after exposure to antidepressants and the role of maternal depression: results from the Norwegian mother and child cohort study. J Clin Psychopharm. 2012;32(2):186–94.

39. Malm H, Artama M, Gissler M, Ritvanen A. Selective serotonin reuptake inhibitors and risk for major congenital anomalies. Obstet Gynecol. 2011;118(1):111–20.

40. Colvin L, Slack-Smith L, Stanley FJ, Bower C. Dispensing patterns and pregnancy outcomes for women dispensed selective serotonin reuptake inhibitors in pregnancy. Birth Defects Res Part A Clin Mol Teratol. 2011;91(4):268.

41. Petersen I, Gilbert R, Evans S, Marston L, Nazareth I. SSRI and risk of congenital cardiac abnormalities. Pharmacoepidem DR S. 2010;19:S211.

42. Kornum JB, Nielsen RB, Pedersen L, Mortensen PB, Norgaard M. Use of selective serotonin-reuptake inhibitors during early pregnancy and risk of congenital malformations: updated analysis. Clin Epidemiol. 2010;2:29–36.

43. Pedersen LH, Henriksen TB, Vestergaard M, Olsen J, Bech BH. Selective serotonin reuptake inhibitors in pregnancy and congenital malformations: population based cohort study. BMJ. 2009;339:b3569.

44. Merlob P, Birk E, Sirota L, Linder N, Berant M, Stahl B, et al. Are selective serotonin reuptake inhibitors cardiac teratogens? Echocardiographic screening of newborns with persistent heart murmur. Birth Defects Res Part A Clin Mol Teratol. 2009;85(10):837–41.

45. Diav-Citrin O, Shechtman S, Weinbaum D, Wajnberg R, Avgil M, Di Gianantonio E, et al. Paroxetine and fluoxetine in pregnancy: a prospective, multicentre, controlled, observational study. Brit J Clin Pharmaco. 2008;66(5):695–705.

46. Kallen BA, Otterblad OP. Maternal use of selective serotonin re-uptake inhibitors in early pregnancy and infant congenital malformations. Birth Defects Res A Clin Mol Teratol. 2007;79(4):301–8.

47. Vial T, Cournot MP, Bernard N, Carlier P, Jonville-Bero AP, Jean-Pastor MJ, et al. Paroxetine and congenital malformations: a prospective comparative study. Drug Saf. 2006;29(10):970.

48. Grote NK, Bridge JA, Gavin AR, Melville JL, Iyengar S, Katon WJ. A meta-analysis of depression during pregnancy and the risk of preterm birth, low birth weight, and intrauterine growth restriction. Arch Gen Psychiatry. 2010;67(10):1012–24.

49. Szegda K, Markenson G, Bertone-Johnson ER, Chasan-Taber L. Depression during pregnancy: a risk factor for adverse neonatal outcomes? A critical review of the literature. J Matern Fetal Neonatal Med. 2014;27(9):960–7.

50. Ogunyemi D, Jovanovski A, Liu J, Friedman P, Sugiyama N, Creps J, et al. The contribution of untreated and treated anxiety and depression to prenatal, intrapartum, and neonatal outcomes. AJP Rep. 2018;8(3):e146–57.

51. Pedersen LH. The risks associated with prenatal antidepressant exposure: time for a precision medicine approach. Expert Opin Drug Saf. 2017;16(8):915–21.

52. Susser LC, Sansone SA, Hermann AD. Selective serotonin reuptake inhibitors for depression in pregnancy. Am J Obstet Gynecol. 2016;215(6):722–30.

53. Koren G, Nordeng H. Antidepressant use during pregnancy: the benefit-risk ratio. Am J Obstet Gynecol. 2012;207(3):157–63.

54. Moher D, Liberati A, Tetzlaff J, Altman DG. Preferred reporting items for systematic reviews and meta-analyses: the PRISMA statement. BMJ. 2009;339:b2535.

55. Huybrechts KF, Palmsten K, Avorn J, Cohen LS, Holmes LB, Franklin JM, et al. Antidepressant use in pregnancy and the risk of cardiac defects. N Engl J Med. 2014;370(25):2397–407.

56. Davis RL, Rubanowice D, McPhillips H, Raebel MA, Andrade SE, Smith D, et al. Risks of congenital malformations and perinatal events among infants exposed to antidepressant medications during pregnancy. Pharmacoepidemiol Drug Saf. 2007;16(10):1086–94.

57. Chambers CD, Johnson KA, Dick LM, Felix RJ, Jones KL. Birth outcomes in pregnant women taking fluoxetine. N Engl J Med. 1996;335(14):1010–5.

58. Vasilakis-Scaramozza C, Aschengrau A, Cabral H, Jick SS. Antidepressant use during early pregnancy and the risk of congenital anomalies. Pharmacotherapy. 2013;33(7):693–700.

59. Klieger-Grossmann C, Weitzner B, Panchaud A, Pistelli A, Einarson T, Koren G, et al. Pregnancy outcomes following use of escitalopram: a prospective comparative cohort study. J Clin Pharmacol. 2012;52(5):766–70.

60. Einarson A, Choi J, Einarson TR, Koren G. Incidence of major malformations in infants following antidepressant exposure in pregnancy: results of a large prospective cohort study. Can J Psychiatr. 2009;54(4):242–6.

61. Oberlander TF, Warburton W, Misri S, Riggs W, Aghajanian J, Hertzman C. Major congenital malformations following prenatal exposure to serotonin reuptake inhibitors and benzodiazepines using population-based health data. Birth Defects Res Part B Dev Reprod Toxicol. 2008;83(1):68–76.

62. Wells GA, Shea BJ, O'Connell D, Peterson J, Welch V, Losos M, et al. The Newcastle–Ottawa scale (NOS) for assessing the quality of non-randomized studies in meta-analysis. Appl Eng Agric. 2014;18(6):727–34.

63. Odutayo A, Wong CX, Hsiao AJ, Hopewell S, Altman DG, Emdin CA. Atrial fibrillation and risks of cardiovascular disease, renal disease, and death: systematic review and meta-analysis. BMJ. 2016;354:i4482.

64. Bérard A, Zhao JP, Sheehy O. Sertraline use during pregnancy and the risk of major malformations. Am J Obstet Gynecol. 2015;212(6):791–5.

65. Hamling J, Lee P, Weitkunat R, Ambuhl M. Facilitating meta-analyses by deriving relative effect and precision estimates for alternative comparisons from a set of estimates presented by exposure level or disease category. Stat Med. 2008;27(7):954–70.

66. Einarson A, Pistelli A, DeSantis M, Malm H, Paulus WD, Panchaud A, et al. Evaluation of the risk of congenital cardiovascular defects associated with use of paroxetine during pregnancy. AM J Psychiat. 2008;165(6):749–52.

67. Rothman KJ. Development DD. Modern Epidemiology. 3rd ed; 2014.

68. Dersimonian R, Laird N. Meta-analysis in clinical trials. Control Clin Trials. 1986;7(3):177.

69. Higgins JP, Thompson SG, Deeks JJ, Altman DG. Measuring inconsistency in meta-analyses. BMJ. 2003;327(7414):557–60.

70. Begg CB, Mazumdar M. Operating characteristics of a rank correlation test for publication bias. Biometrics. 1994;50(4):1088–101.

71. Egger M, Davey SG, Schneider M, Minder C. Bias in meta-analysis detected by a simple, graphical test. BMJ. 1997;315(7109):629–34.

72. Ban L, Gibson JE, West J, Fiaschi L, Sokal R, Smeeth L, et al. Maternal depression, antidepressant prescriptions, and congenital anomaly risk in offspring: a population-based cohort study. Bjog-Int J Obstet GY. 2014;121(12):1471–81.

73. Sari Y, Zhou FC. Serotonin and its transporter on proliferation of fetal heart cells. Int J Dev Neurosci. 2003;21(8):417–24.

74. Sit DK, Perel JM, Helsel JC, Wisner KL. Changes in antidepressant metabolism and dosing across pregnancy and early postpartum. J Clin Psychiatry. 2008;69(4):652–8.

75. Yavarone MS, Shuey DL, Tamir H, Sadler TW, Lauder JM. Serotonin and cardiac morphogenesis in the mouse embryo. Teratology. 1993;47(6):573–84.

76. Choi DS, Kellermann O, Richard S, Colas JF, Bolanos-Jimenez F, Tournois C, et al. Mouse 5-HT2B receptor-mediated serotonin trophic functions. Ann N Y Acad Sci. 1998;861:67–73.

77. Gentile S. Early pregnancy exposure to selective serotonin reuptake inhibitors, risks of major structural malformations, and hypothesized teratogenic mechanisms. Expert Opin Drug Metab Toxicol. 2015;11(10):1585–97.

78. Carmi R, Gohar J, Meizner I, Katz M. Spontaneous abortion--high risk factor for neural tube defects in subsequent pregnancy. Am J Med Genet. 1994;51(2):93–7.

79. Bukowski R, Carpenter M, Conway D, Coustan D, Dudley DJ, Goldenberg RL, et al. Causes of death among stillbirths. Jama-J Am Med Assoc. 2011; 306(22):2459–68.
80. Ehrenstein V, Sorensen HT, Bakketeig LS, Pedersen L. Medical databases in studies of drug teratogenicity: methodological issues. Clin Epidemiol. 2010;2:37–43.
81. Tuccori M, Montagnani S, Testi A, Ruggiero E, Mantarro S, Scollo C, et al. Use of selective serotonin reuptake inhibitors during pregnancy and risk of major and cardiovascular malformations: an update. Postgrad Med. 2010; 122(4):49–65.
82. Alwan S, Friedman JM. Safety of selective serotonin reuptake inhibitors in pregnancy. CNS Drugs. 2009;23(6):493–509.
83. Alwan S, Friedman JM, Chambers C. Safety of selective serotonin reuptake inhibitors in pregnancy: a review of current evidence. CNS Drugs. 2016; 30(6):499–515.
84. Alwan S, Reefhuis J, Rasmussen SA, Olney RS, Friedman JM. Use of selective serotonin-reuptake inhibitors in pregnancy and the risk of birth defects. N Engl J Med. 2007;356(26):2684–92.

Permissions

All chapters in this book were first published in MEDICINE, by BioMed Central; hereby published with permission under the Creative Commons Attribution License or equivalent. Every chapter published in this book has been scrutinized by our experts. Their significance has been extensively debated. The topics covered herein carry significant findings which will fuel the growth of the discipline. They may even be implemented as practical applications or may be referred to as a beginning point for another development.

The contributors of this book come from diverse backgrounds, making this book a truly international effort. This book will bring forth new frontiers with its revolutionizing research information and detailed analysis of the nascent developments around the world.

We would like to thank all the contributing authors for lending their expertise to make the book truly unique. They have played a crucial role in the development of this book. Without their invaluable contributions this book wouldn't have been possible. They have made vital efforts to compile up to date information on the varied aspects of this subject to make this book a valuable addition to the collection of many professionals and students.

This book was conceptualized with the vision of imparting up-to-date information and advanced data in this field. To ensure the same, a matchless editorial board was set up. Every individual on the board went through rigorous rounds of assessment to prove their worth. After which they invested a large part of their time researching and compiling the most relevant data for our readers.

The editorial board has been involved in producing this book since its inception. They have spent rigorous hours researching and exploring the diverse topics which have resulted in the successful publishing of this book. They have passed on their knowledge of decades through this book. To expedite this challenging task, the publisher supported the team at every step. A small team of assistant editors was also appointed to further simplify the editing procedure and attain best results for the readers.

Apart from the editorial board, the designing team has also invested a significant amount of their time in understanding the subject and creating the most relevant covers. They scrutinized every image to scout for the most suitable representation of the subject and create an appropriate cover for the book.

The publishing team has been an ardent support to the editorial, designing and production team. Their endless efforts to recruit the best for this project, has resulted in the accomplishment of this book. They are a veteran in the field of academics and their pool of knowledge is as vast as their experience in printing. Their expertise and guidance has proved useful at every step. Their uncompromising quality standards have made this book an exceptional effort. Their encouragement from time to time has been an inspiration for everyone.

The publisher and the editorial board hope that this book will prove to be a valuable piece of knowledge for researchers, students, practitioners and scholars across the globe.

List of Contributors

Trisha Greenhalgh, Joe Wherton, Chrysanthi Papoutsi, Gemma Hughes, Christine A'Court and Sara Shaw
Department of Primary Care Health Sciences, University of Oxford, Oxford OX2 6GG, UK

Jenni Lynch
School of Health and Social Work, University of Hertfordshire, Hatfield, UK

Sue Hinder
RAFT Research consultancy, Clitheroe, UK

Rob Procter
Department of Computer Science, University of Warwick, Coventry, UK

Rajeev K. Tyagi, Patrick J. Gleeson, Ludovic Arnold, Eric Prieur, Jean-Louis Pérignon and Pierre Druilhe
The Vac4All Initiative, 26 Rue Lecourbe, 75015 Paris, France

Rajeev K. Tyagi, Patrick J. Gleeson, Ludovic Arnold, Eric Prieur, Jean-Louis Pérignon and Pierre Druilhe
Biomedical Parasitology Unit, Institut Pasteur, Paris, France

Rachida Tahar
Faculté de Pharmacie, Université Paris Descartes, COMUE Sorbonne Paris Cité, Paris, France
Institut de Recherche pour le Développement, UMR MERIT 216, Paris, France

Laurent Decosterd
Division of Clinical Pharmacology, Centre Hospitalier Universitaire Vaudois, Lausanne, Switzerland

Piero Olliaro
Centre for Tropical Medicine and Global Health, Nuffield Department of Medicine, University of Oxford, Oxford, UK

Rajeev K. Tyagi
Amity Institute of Microbial Technology, Amity University, Noida, Uttar Pradesh, India

Patrick J. Gleeson
Centre de Recherche sur l'Inflammation, INSERM U1149, Faculté de Médecine, Université Diderot-Site Bichat, 16 rue Henri Huchard, 75018 Paris, France

Jean-Louis Pérignon
Present Address: Laboratoire de Biochimie, Hôpital Necker-Enfants Malades, Paris, France

Tadashi Kato
Aratama Kokorono Clinic, Nagoya, Japan

Toshi A. Furukawa
Department of Health Promotion of Human Behavior, Kyoto University Graduate School of Medicine / School of Public Health, Yoshida Konoe-cho, Sakyo-ku, Kyoto 606-8501, Japan

Akio Mantani
Mantani Mental Clinic, Hiroshima, Japan

Masaki Kondo
Department of Psychiatry and Cognitive-Behavioral Medicine, Nagoya City University Graduate School of Medical Sciences, Nagoya, Japan

Yasumasa Okamoto
Department of Neuropsychiatry, Hiroshima University Graduate School of Biomedical & Health Sciences, Hiroshima, Japan

Hirokazu Fujita
Center to Promote Creativity in Medical Education, Kochi Medical School, Kochi University, Nankoku, Japan

Naohiro Yonemoto
Department of Biostatistics, Kyoto University Graduate School of Medicine / School of Public Health, Kyoto, Japan

Shiro Tanaka
Department of Clinical Biostatistics, Kyoto University Graduate School of Medicine / School of Public Health, Kyoto, Japan

Gwenan M. Knight, Jonathan A. Otter and Alison H. Holmes
National Institute of Health Research Health Protection Research Unit in Healthcare Associated Infections and Antimicrobial Resistance, Imperial College London, Commonwealth Building, Hammersmith Campus, Imperial College London, Du Cane Road, London W12 0NN, UK

Gwenan M. Knight and Eimear T. Brannigan
Infectious Diseases and Immunity, Commonwealth Building, Hammersmith Campus, Imperial College London, Du Cane Road, London W12 0NN, UK

Eleonora Dyakova, Siddharth Mookerjee, Frances Davies, Eimear T. Brannigan, Jonathan A. Otter and Alison H. Holmes
Imperial College Healthcare NHS Trust, London, UK

Elizabeth Cecil, Alex Bottle, Richard Ma and Sonia Saxena
Department of Primary Care and Public Health, Imperial College London Charing Cross Campus, London W6 8RP, UK

Dougal S. Hargreaves
Institute of Child Health, University College London, London, England

Ingrid Wolfe
Department of Primary Care and Public Health Sciences, King's College London, London, England

Arch G. Mainous III
Department of Health Services Research, Management and Policy, University of Florida, Gainesville, FL, USA

Jean T. Coulibaly, Gordana Panic, Jana Kovač, Beatrice Barda and Jennifer Keiser
Department of Medical Parasitology and Infection Biology, Swiss Tropical and Public Health Institute, Basel, Switzerland

Jean T. Coulibaly, Gordana Panic, Jana Kovač, Beatrice Barda, Jan Hattendorf and Jennifer Keiser
University of Basel, Basel, Switzerland

Jean T. Coulibaly
Unité de Formation et de Recherche Biosciences, Université Félix Houphouët-Boigny, Abidjan, Côte d'Ivoire

Richard B. Yapi
Centre Suisse de Recherches Scientifiques, Abidjan, Côte d'Ivoire

Yves K. N'Gbesso
Departement d'Agboville, Centre de Santé Urbain d'Azaguié, Azaguié, Côte d'Ivoire

Jan Hattendorf
Department of Epidemiology and Public Health, Swiss Tropical and Public Health Institute, Basel, Switzerland

Amytis Heim, Philippe Ravaud, Gabriel Baron and Isabelle Boutron
INSERM, U1153 Epidemiology and Biostatistics Sorbonne Paris Cité Research Center (CRESS), Methods of Therapeutic Evaluation of Chronic Diseases Team (METHODS), Paris, France

Amytis Heim, Philippe Ravaud, Gabriel Baron and Isabelle Boutron
Paris Descartes University, Sorbonne Paris Cité, Paris, France

Philippe Ravaud, Gabriel Baron and Isabelle Boutron
Centre d'Epidémiologie Clinique, Hôpital Hôtel-Dieu, Assistance Publique des Hôpitaux de Paris, Paris, France

Horace C. W. Choi, Mark Jit, Gabriel M. Leung and Joseph T. Wu
WHO Collaborating Centre for Infectious Disease Epidemiology and Control, School of Public Health, Li Ka Shing Faculty of Medicine, The University of Hong Kong, 1/F North Wing, Patrick Manson Building, 7 Sassoon Road, Pok Fu Lam, Hong Kong

Horace C. W. Choi, Leung and Kwok-Leung Tsui
Department of Systems Engineering and Engineering Management, City University of Hong Kong, Kowloon Tong, Hong Kong

Horace C. W. Choi
Department of Clinical Oncology, Li Ka Shing Faculty of Medicine, The University of Hong Kong, Pok Fu Lam, Hong Kong

Mark Jit
Modelling and Economics Unit, Public Health England, London, UK
Department of Infectious Disease Epidemiology, London School of Hygiene and Tropical Medicine, London, UK

Florence Y. Lai, Mintu Nath, Stephen E. Hamby, John R. Thompson, Christopher P. Nelson and Nilesh J. Samani
Department of Cardiovascular Sciences, University of Leicester, Leicester, UK

Florence Y. Lai, Mintu Nath, Stephen E. Hamby, Christopher P. Nelson and Nilesh J. Samani
NIHR Leicester Biomedical Research Centre, Glenfield Hospital, Leicester, UK

John R. Thompson
Department of Health Sciences, University of Leicester, Leicester, UK

Pauline Heus, Johanna A. A. G. Damen, Rob J. P. M. Scholten, Johannes B. Reitsma, Karel G. M. Moons and Lotty Hooft
Cochrane Netherlands, University Medical Center Utrecht, Utrecht University, Utrecht, The Netherlands

Pauline Heus , Johanna A. A. G. Damen, Romin Pajouheshnia, Rob J. P. M. Scholten,Johannes B. Reitsma, Karel G. M. Moons and Lotty Hooft
Julius Center for Health Sciences and Primary Care, University Medical Center Utrecht, Utrecht University, Utrecht, The Netherlands

Gary S. Collins and Douglas G. Altman
Centre for Statistics in Medicine, NDORMS, Botnar Research Centre, University of Oxford, Oxford, UK

Maria Panagioti, David Reeves, Mark Hann, Kelly Howells, Lisa Riste and Peter Bower
NIHR School for Primary Care Research, Centre for Primary Care, Manchester Academic Health Science Centre, University of Manchester, Williamson Building, Oxford Road, Manchester M13 9PL, UK

Rachel Meacock and Beth Parkinson
Manchester Centre for Health Economics, Division of Population Health, Health Services Research & Primary Care, Manchester Academic Health Science Centre, University of Manchester, Manchester M13 9PL, UK

Karina Lovell and Amy Blakemore
School of Nursing, Midwifery & Social Work, University of Manchester, Manchester M13 9PL, UK.

Peter Coventry and Lisa Riste
Mental Health and Addiction Research Group, Department of Health Sciences and Hull York Medical School, University of York, York YO10 5DD, UK.

Thomas Blakeman
NIHR Collaboration for Leadership in Applied Health Research and Care – Greater Manchester and Manchester Academic Health Science Centre, University of Manchester, Manchester M13 9PL, UK

Mark Sidaway
Salford Royal NHS Foundation Trust, Stott Lane, Salford M6 8HD, UK

Kirsten E Wiens, Lauren P Woyczynski, Jorge R Ledesma, Jennifer M Ross, Molly H Biehl, Sarah E Ray, Natalia V Bhattacharjee, Nathaniel J Henry, Robert C Reiner Jr, Hmwe H Kyu, Christopher J L Murray and Simon I Hay
Institute for Health Metrics and Evaluation, University of Washington, 2301 5th Ave, Suite 600, Seattle, WA 98121, USA

Jennifer M Ross
Departments of Global Health and Medicine, University of Washington, Seattle, WA, USA

Roberto Zenteno-Cuevas
Public Health Institute, University of Veracruz, Veracruz, Mexico

Amador Goodridge and Jennifer M Ross
Tuberculosis Biomarker Research Unit, Instituto de Investigaciones Científicas y Servicios de Alta Tecnología (INDICASAT-AIP), City of Knowledge, Panama, Panama

Irfan Ullah
Gomal Centre of Biochemistry and Biotechnology, Gomal University, Dera Ismail Khan, Khyber Pakhtunkhwa, Pakistan
Programmatic Management of Drug-Resistant TB Unit, BSL-II TB Culture Laboratory, Mufti Mehmood Memorial Teaching Hospital, Dera Ismail Khan, Khyber Pakhtunkhwa, Pakistan

Barun Mathema
Department of Epidemiology, Mailman School of Public Health, Columbia University, New York, NY, USA

Joel Fleury Djoba Siawaya
Unité de Recherche et de Diagnostics Spécialisés, Laboratoire National de Santé Publique, Libreville, Gabon

Centre Hospitalier Universitaire Mère-Enfant Fondation Jeanne EBORI, Libreville, Gabon

A. Colver, H. McConachie, A. Le Couteur, K. D. Mann, M. S. Pearce, L. Vale and H. Merrick
Institute of Health & Society, Sir James Spence Institute, Royal Victoria Infirmary, Newcastle University, Queen Victoria Road, Newcastle upon Tyne NE1 4LP, UK

A. Colver, G. Dovey-Pearce and A. Colver
Northumbria Healthcare NHS Foundation Trust, North Tyneside General Hospital, Rake Lane, North Shields NE29 8NH, UK

A. Le Couteur and J. R. Parr
Northumberland, Tyne and Wear NHS Foundation Trust, St. Nicholas Hospital, Jubilee Road, Newcastle upon Tyne NE3 3XT, UK

J. E. McDonagh
Centre for Musculoskeletal Research and Manchester Academic Health Science Centre, University of Manchester, Stopford Building, Oxford Rd, Manchester M13 9PT, UK
NIHR Manchester Biomedical Research Centre, Manchester University NHS Foundation Trust, Manchester Royal Infirmary, Oxford Rd, Manchester M13 9WL, UK

J. R. Parr
Institute of Neuroscience, Sir James Spence Institute, Newcastle University, Queen
Victoria Road, Newcastle upon Tyne NE1 4LP, UK
Great North Children's Hospital, Newcastle Upon Tyne Hospitals NHS Foundation Trust, Royal Victoria Infirmary, Queen Victoria Road, Newcastle upon Tyne NE1 4LP, UK

Jiahui Si, Canqing Yu, Chenxi Qin, Jun Lv and Liming Li
Department of Epidemiology and Biostatistics, School of Public Health, Peking University Health Science Center, 38 Xueyuan Road, Beijing 100191, China

Yu Guo, Zheng Bian and Liming Li
Chinese Academy of Medical Sciences, Beijing, China

Ling Yang, Yiping Chen and Zhengming Chen
Clinical Trial Service Unit & Epidemiological Studies Unit (CTSU), Nuffield Department of Population Health, University of Oxford, Oxford, UK

Li Yin
Hunan Center for Disease Control & Prevention, Changsha, Hunan, China

Hui Li
Liuzhou Traditional Chinese Medical Hospital, Liuzhou, Guangxi, China

Jian Lan
Liuzhou Center for Disease Control & Prevention, Liuzhou, Guangxi, China

Junshi Chen
China National Center for Food Safety Risk Assessment, Beijing, China

Jun Lv
Peking University Institute of Environmental Medicine, Beijing, China

Rupak Shivakoti and Nikhil Gupte
Department of Medicine, Johns Hopkins University School of Medicine, Baltimore, MD, USA

Rupak Shivakoti
Department of Epidemiology, Columbia University Mailman School of Public Health, 722 West 168th St, Room 705, New York, NY 10032, USA

Srikanth Tripathy
National AIDS Research Institute, Pune, India

Srikanth Tripathy
National Institute of Research in Tuberculosis, Chennai, India

Wadzanai Samaneka
University of Zimbabwe Clinical Research Centre, Harare, Zimbabwe

Cynthia Riviere
Les Centres GHESKIO, Port-Au-Prince, Haiti

Patcharaphan Sugandhavesa
Research Institute for Health Sciences, Chiang Mai, Thailand

Parul Christian
Department of International Health, Johns Hopkins Bloomberg School of Public Health, Baltimore, MD, USA
Bill and Melinda Gates Foundation, Seattle, USA

Thomas B. Campbell
Department of Medicine, Division of Infectious Diseases, University of Colorado School of Medicine, Aurora, CO, USA

Alessia Melegaro and Alessia Melegaro
Department of Social and Political Sciences, Bocconi University, Milano, Italy

Alessia Melegaro and Emanuele Del Fava
Carlo F. Dondena Centre for Research on Social Dynamics and Public Policy, Bocconi University, Milano, Italy

Valentina Marziano, Piero Poletti and Stefano Merler
Center for Information and Communication Technology, Bruno Kessler Foundation, Trento, Italy

Marcello Tirani
Department of Hygiene and Preventive Medicine, ATS, Bergamo, Italy

Caterina Rizzo
Department of Infectious Disease, Istituto Superiore di Sanità, Roma, Italy

Shan-Yan Gao, Qi-Jun Wu, Ce Sun, Xin Xu, Chao Ji, Dong-Hui Huang, Qing Chang and Yu-Hong Zhao
Department of Clinical Epidemiology, Shengjing Hospital of China Medical University, No. 36, San Hao Street, Shenyang, Liaoning, China

Tie-Ning Zhang
Department of Pediatrics, Shengjing Hospital of China Medical University, Shenyang, China

Zi-Qi Shen, Cai-Xia Liu and Ting-Ting Gong
Department of Obstetrics and Gynecology, Shengjing Hospital of China Medical University, Shenyang, China

Index

www.ingramcontent.com/pod-product-compliance
Lightning Source LLC
Chambersburg PA
CBHW061245190326
41458CB00011B/3584